ENDOTOXIN

ADVANCES IN EXPERIMENTAL MEDICINE AND BIOLOGY

Recent Volumes in this Series

Volume 249
MINERAL ABSORPTION IN THE MONOGASTRIC GI TRACT:
Chemical, Nutritional, and Physiological Aspects
Edited by Frederick R. Dintzis and Joseph A. Laszlo

Volume 250
PROGRESS IN POLYAMINE RESEARCH:
Novel Biochemical, Pharmacological, and Clinical Aspects
Edited by Vincenzo Zappia and Anthony E. Pegg

Volume 251
IMMUNOBIOLOGY OF PROTEINS AND PEPTIDES V: Vaccines—Mechanisms, Design, and Applications
Edited by M. Zouhair Atassi

Volume 252
DRUGS, SYSTEMIC DISEASES, AND THE KIDNEY
Edited by Alberto Amerio, Pasquale Coratelli, Vito M. Campese, and Shaul G. Massry

Volume 253A
PURINE AND PYRIMIDINE METABOLISM IN MAN VI, Part A:
Clinical and Molecular Biology
Edited by Kiyonobu Mikanagi, Kusuki Nishioka, and William N. Kelley

Volume 253B
PURINE AND PYRIMIDINE METABOLISM IN MAN VI, Part B:
Basic Research and Experimental Biology
Edited by Kiyonobu Mikanagi, Kusuki Nishioka, and William N. Kelley

Volume 254
MECHANISMS OF LYMPHOCYTE ACTIVATION AND IMMUNE REGULATION II
Edited by Sudhir Gupta and William E. Paul

Volume 255
CALCIUM PROTEIN SIGNALING
Edited by H. Hidaka

Volume 256
ENDOTOXIN
Edited by Herman Friedman, T. W. Klein, Masayasu Nakano, and Alois Nowotny

---

A Continuation Order Plan is available for this series. A continuation order will bring delivery of each new volume immediately upon publication. Volumes are billed only upon actual shipment. For further information please contact the publisher.

ENDOTOXIN

Edited by

Herman Friedman
and T. W. Klein
The University of South Florida
Tampa, Florida

Masayasu Nakano
Jichi Medical School
Tochigi-Ken, Japan

and

Alois Nowotny
University of Pennsylvania
Philadelphia, Pennsylvania

SPRINGER SCIENCE+BUSINESS MEDIA, LLC

Library of Congress Cataloging in Publication Data

International Symposium on Endotoxins (1988: Jichi Medical School)
Endotoxin.

(Advances in experimental medicine and biology; v. 256)
"Proceedings of the International Symposium on Endotoxins, a satellite symposium of the Fourth International Conference on Immunopharmacology, held May 11-13, 1988, at Jichi Medical School, Tochigi-Ken, Japan"—T.p. verso.
Includes bibliographies and index.
1. Endotoxins—Physiological effect—Congresses. I. Friedman, Herman, 1931–
II. International Conference on Immunopharmacology (4th: 1988: Osaka, Japan) III. Title. IV. Series. [DNLM: 1. Endotoxins—congresses. WD1 AD559 v.256 QW 630 I623e 1988]
QP632.E4I56 1988 615.9′5299 89-15966

DOI 10.1007/978-1-4757-5140-6

Proceedings of the International Symposium on Endotoxins, a Satellite Symposium of the Fourth International Conference on Immunopharmacology, held May 11-13, 1988, at Jichi Medical School, Tochigi-Ken, Japan

Originally published by Plenum Press, New York in 1990
MyCopy version of the original edition 1990

This volume is dedicated to
L. JOE BERRY

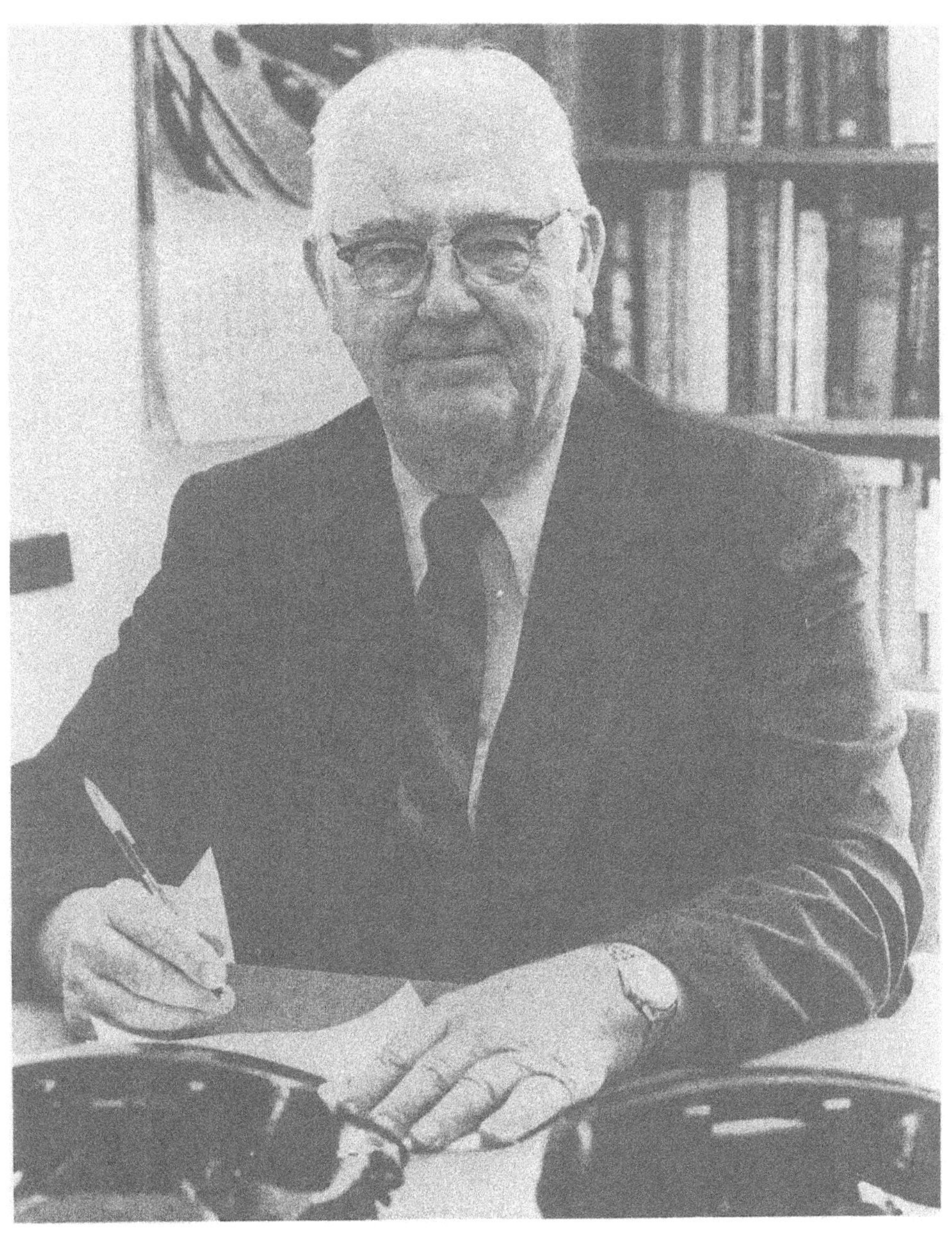

L. JOE BERRY
1910-1987

IN MEMORIAM - L. JOE BERRY

It rarely happens that one finds scientific excellence combined with true human greatness. L. Joe Berry had both and much more.

He was born in Birmingham, Alabama in 1910, and received his Ph.D. in biology at the University of Texas in Austin. In the early years of his distinquished scientific career, he worked on plant physiology, studying the effect of various physical factors on root development and growth. A few years later he published his first paper on the role of phagocytosis in natural defenses against pathogenic microorganisms. The scope of his work broadened, and for several years he and his associates studied the effect of extrinsic factors such as high altitudes or extreme cold temperature exposures on the susceptibility to infectious microorganisms. His interest grew rapidly with new developments in the biochemical events and resistance to infectious diseases. The host metabolisms during and after infections became the center of his research interest and this led inevitably to the studies of Gram negative endotoxins and their effects on it. The findings of L. Joe Berry, his students and his associates in this field laid the foundation of our present-day understanding of the major metabolic events occurring during endotoxemia. They studied the activities of several enzymes with particular emphasis on tryptophane pyrrolase and phosphoenlopyruvate carboxykinase. The pursuit of this unique avenue did not prevent him from extending his research and from contributing significantly to our knowledge in various corollary fields such as regulation of the reticuloendothelial system's functions, the isolation and use of ribosomal vaccines and other potentially useful bacterial cell components as immunogens.

His academic career is studded with awards, distinctions and with some of the highest honors for his accomplishments. He started as a teaching assistant at the University of Texas in Austin and became instructor in the same institution. He married a charming Texan girl, Virginia Goolsby in 1934. She was his lifelong companion, the most reliable and most dedicated co-worker in his office, a patron of the students, the most gracious hostess to friends and colleagues who enjoyed their hospitality. Tia, as she was affectionately called by everyone who knew her, and their son James, daughter-in-law and grandchildren, were the strongest supporters of Joe in every aspect of their rich and successful life. In 1940, they moved to Bryn Mawr College near Philadelphia, where he became Professor of Biology in 1952 and later chairman of the same department. He was elected Secretary of the Faculty and in 1969, acting Provost of this famous college. Later on, Tia and Joe returned to the University of Texas in Austin where he received his Ph.D. 31 years earlier. He was Chairman of the Department of Microbiology until the age of 65, and continued his research in the same department until his untimely death.

L. Joe Berry was also very active in professional associations. He was one of the most dynamic leaders in the American Society for Microbiology. He served as editor of the Journal of Bacteriology and of Infection and Immunity. He was the President of the ASM Eastern Pennsylvania branch and, later on, the President of the Texas branch of the ASM. He was the founder and the first Chairman of the Board of Education and Training of the ASM. There is a long list of various key roles he played in the ASM as well as in other societies. He was the President of the Reticuloendothelial Society, and served with great distinction on various NIH study sections and committees. In 1983, he became the Chairman of the Life Sciences Panel of the National Research Council. He was advisor of the Office of Naval Research, Chairman of the Research Review Committee of the Veterans Administration, and of the Research Advisory Board of the Alfred I. DuPont Institute. In 1968, he became Elected Associate Member of the Royal Society of Medicine, London, and he received the notification about this most prestigious distinction with humble modesty which was so characteristic of him.

We have not listed all the honors and awards he received - they were numerous - but neither these nor his heavy commitments in professional societies ever distracted him from being a passionately dedicated teacher. His former students say that in his busy schedule, he always found time for them, and he even spent time with the parents and friends of the students. The young people around him were always the first ones to get his attention, his generous help, fatherly advice and support. He had the same attitude towards colleagues. He was patient, accommodating and magnanimous to all of us. He had no enemies and he was the enemy of none. He never took himself too seriously. He remained a modest and unassuming scientist who simply loved people. He did not follow anybody's footsteps in his research; he cut his own path. He found a segment in endotoxinology which was remote from the main stream of interest at that time, but it fascinated him. He pursued this with the tenacity bestowed only on the greatest scientists. Neither fashionable new directions, nor more lucrative avenues regrarding grants made him vaccilate for a moment, although he was always fully aware of them. He was a towering Texan, a tower of strength, wisdom and genuine altruism.

His last endeavor was the initiation of the necessary steps to organize the International Endotoxin Society. He appointed two committees: one in charge of the nominations for the first election of officers, and the other to write the constitution of the society. He worked with these two committees and contacted leaders of endotoxin research in Europe, Asia and America, inviting them to join us in these organizational efforts. When everything showed unmistakable signs of success, on the morning of February 26, 1987, in Washington, D.C., Joe did not wake up. We have continued his efforts in the same vein, following his philosophy. The Society exists today, and in 1988 we dedicated the Endotoxin Symposium held at Jichi Medical School in Japan, to his memory.

In him we lost a dearly loved mentor, a superb scientist, and above all, an honest and true friend. But we did not lose him as a paragon of virtue. His rich life remains a shining example to be followed by us and by many future generations of scientists. With deep affection and gratitude and with even deeper sadness we dedicate this book to his everlasting memory.

Alois Nowotny
President of the IES

PREFACE

This volume is based on the proceedings of the International Symposium on Bacterial Endotoxins held in Japan, May 11-14, 1988 and sponsored by the International Endotoxin Society and the International Society for Immunopharmacology.

Speakers and participants of this symposium provided new information concerning fundamental and clinical aspects of endotoxin research conducted over the last half decade or so. Advances have been made in understanding the structure and nature of endotoxin molecules and their effects on a wide variety of both cellular and subcellular aspects of immunity, metabolism and physiology, both in vivo and in vitro.

Endotoxins are constituents of gram negative bacteria. Since their original discovery in the nineteenth century, many laboratories studied their chemical composition, their physico- and immunochemical properties, as well as their pharmacological and physiological effects on the host. Much is now known about the chemical structure of the endotoxins. There is also a growing body of information concerning the multiple effects of endotoxins on the host including immune mechanisms. Some effects have been found to be beneficial to the host and endotoxins are being used more frequently to induce important mediators of immunity as well as increasing resistance against infections by many microorganisms as well as inhibiting growth of tumors in experimental animal models and in man. The editors and the organizing committee believe this publication will provide a permanent collection of up to date research and review articles concerning the exploding information on endotoxin biology and chemistry presented by world renown chemists, microbiologists, immunologists, pharmacologists, pathologists and physiologists at this conference. In addition, the editors of this volume are convinced that the subject of endotoxins provides an important focal point for continued investigations of the dynamics of the host/parasite relationship. It is hoped that publication of this volume will provide a stimulus for further intensified study concerning both detrimental and beneficial effects of endotoxins on the host.

The leader of the organizing committee was Dr. M. Nakano of Jichi Medical School, Tochigi, Japan. Other members of the committee were Dr. Herman Friedman, University of South Florida College of Medicine, Tampa, Florida; Dr. John Hadden, University of South Florida, College of Medicine, Tampa, Florida; Dr. Nobuhiko Kasai, Showa University School of Pharmaceutical Sciences, Tokyo, Japan; Dr. Tadashi Kawai, Jichi Medical School, Tochigi, Japan, and Dr. Alois Nowotny, University of Pennsylvania, Center for Oral Health Research, Philadelphia, Pennsylvania, USA. It is anticipated that publication of this volume based on the conference will provide a stimulus for new perspectives in this rapidly growing field. The editors take this opportunity to express their most profound gratitude to Mrs. Sally Baker, Ms. Judith Flynn, Mrs. Ilona Friedman, and Mrs. Angie Pruitt for outstanding editorial assistance in the preparation of this volume.

H. Friedman
T. W. Klein
M. Nakano
A. Nowotny

March 1989

CONTENTS

SECTION I. SYNTHESIS, STRUCTURE AND FUNCTION

Chemical Synthesis of Endotoxin.................................. 3

S. Kusumoto, N. Kusunose, M. Imoto, T. Kamikawa, and T. Shiba

Structural Requirements of Lipid A for Endotoxicity and Other cal Activities - An Overview 13

S. Kotani and H. Takada

Natural Variants of Lipid A.. 45

H. Mayer, J. H. Krauss, A. Yokota, and J. Weckesser

Immunochemistry of Lipid A.. 71

N. Kasai, S. Arata, J. Mashimo, T. Hirayama, and M. Ueno

Bacterial Lipopolysaccharides: Relationship of Structure and Conformation to Endotoxic Activity, Serological Specificity and Biological Function... 81

E. Th. Rietschel, L. Brade, U. Schade, U. Seydel, U. Zähringer, K. Brandenburg, I. Helander, O. Holst, S. Kondo, H.M. Kuhn, B. Lindner, E. Röhrscheidt, R. Russa, H. Labischinski, Naumann, D. Naumann, and H. Brade

Structure-Activity Relationship of Chemically Synthesized Nonreducing Parts of Lipid A Analogs.. 101

J. Y. Homma, M. Matsuura and Y. Kumazawa

The Chemical Structure of the Lipopolysaccharide of A Rc-Type Mutant of Proteus Mirabilis Lacking 4-Amino-4-Deoxy-L Anauinose and its Susceptibility Towards Polymyxin B................................ 121

J. Radziejewska-Lubrecht, U. R. Bhat, H. Brade, W. Kaca, and H. Mayer

The Structure of O-Specific Polysaccharide of Proteus Vulgaris 019 Lipopolysaccharide.. 127

E. V. Vinogradov, W. Kaca, Y. A. Knirel, A. Rozalski, K. Kotelko, and N. K. Kochetkov

Endotoxins of Pseudomonas Fluorescens.............................. 131

G. M. Zdorovenko, S. N. Veremeychenko, I. Ya. Zakharova, and Yu.A. Knirel

Cloning and Expression of rfe Gene.................................. 137

M. Ohta, N, Kido, K. Jann, Y. Arakawa, T. Komatsu, H. Ito, and N. Kato

Cloning and Analysis of rfb Gene Synthesizing the Mannan O Side Chain of Escherichia coli O9 Lipopolysaccharide........................... 141

N. Kido, M. Ohta, H. Ito, K-I. Iida, Y. Arakawa, T. Komatsu, K. Jann, and N. Kato

SECTION II. ACTIVE SITES, CONTAMINANTS, QUALITATIVE AND QUANTITATIVE ASSAYS

The Activation of C3H/HeJ Cells by Certain Types of Lipopolysaccharides... 149

B. M. Sultzer and R. Castagna

Lipoamino Acids which are Similar to Bacterial Endotoxin in Both Structure and Biological Activity Related to Physiological Function.. 159

Y. Kawai, K. Akagawa, and I. Yano

Chemistry and Biology of a Novel Lipid Contaminant of Some Endotoxin Preparations with Selective Cytotoxicity to Transformed Cells........ 163

T. Keler, C. A. D. Smith, and A. Nowotny

Porin as a Component of Yersinia Pseudotuberculosis Endotoxin........ 185

Yu. S. Ovodov, T. F. Solovjeva, V. A. Khomenko, O. D. Novikova, G. M. Frolova, I. M. Yermak, and G. A. Neberezhnykh

Lipopolysaccharides of Non-Cholera Vibrios Possessing Common Antigen Factor to O1 Vibrio cholerae.. 189

K. Hisatsune, Y. Haishima, T. Iguchi, and S. Kondo

Immunocytochemical Localization of Bacterial Lipopolysaccharide with Colloidal-Gold Probes in Different Target Cells..................... 199

A. M. Municio, S. Abarca, J. L. Carrascosa, R. Garcia, I. Diaz-Laviada, M. J. Ainaga, M. T. Portoles, R. Pagani, C. Risco and M. A. Bosch

Development of a New Quantitative Method for Detection of Endotoxin by Fluorescence Labeling of 3-Hydroxy Fatty Acid......................... 203

K.I. Tanamoto

A New Endotoxin-Specific Assay...................................... 215

T. Obayashi

A New Perchloric Acid Treatment of Human Plasma for Detection of Endotoxin by an Endotoxin-Specific Chromogenic Test.................. 225

K. Inada, M. Yoshida, T. Takahashi, S. Tamura, S. Tanaka, S. Endo, T. Yoshida, H. Suda, and T. Komuro

SECTION III. MOLECULAR INTERACTIONS

Fluorescent Detection of Lipopolysaccharide Interactions with Model Membranes.. 233

D. M. Jacobs, H. Yeh, and R. M. Price

Interaction of Mg^{2+} and Ca^{2+} in In Vitro Hexagonal Assembly of R-Form Lipopolysaccharides.. 247

N. Kato, M. Ohta, N. Kido, H. Ito, and S. Naito

Biological Activities of Anti-LPS Factor and LPS Binding Peptide from Horseshoe Crab Amoebocytes... 257

M. Niwa, H. Hua, S. Iwanaga, T. Morita, T. Miyata, T. Nakamura, J. Aketagawa, T. Muta, F. Tokunaga, and K. Ohashi

Primary Structures and Functions of Anti-Lipopolysaccharide Factor and Tachyplesin Peptide Found in Horseshoe Crab Hemocytes................ 273

T. Muta, T. Nakamura, H. Furunaka, F. Tokunaga, T. Miyata, M. Niwa, and S. Iwanaga

Investigation of Endotoxin Binding Cationic Proteins from Granulocytes; Agglutination of Erythrocytes Sensitized with RE-LPS........... 287

M. Hirata, M. Yoshida, K. Inada, and T. Kirikae

Interaction of Bacterial Endotoxin (LPS) with Fluid Phase and Macrophage Membrane Associated C1Q, the FC-Recognizing Component of the Complement System.. 301

M. Loos, B. Euteneuer, and F. Clas

Further Characterization of Monoclonal Antibodies to Lipopolysaccharide of Salmonella Minnesota Strain R595 319

B. J. Appelmelk, J. Cohen, A. Silva, A. M. J.J. Verweij-van Vught, H. Brade, J. J. Maaskant, W. F. Schouten, O. Mol, A. Honing, L. G. Thijs, and D. M. MacLaren

Specificity and Function of Monoclonal Antibodies Reactive with Discrete Structural Elements of Bacterial Lipopolysaccharide............ 331

M. Pollack, K. Olishi, J. Chia, M. Evans, G. Guelde, and N. Koles

Mechanisms of Neutralization of Endotoxin by Monoclonal Antibodies to O and R Determinants of Lipopolysaccharide 341

T. Sagawa, Y. Hitsumoto, M. Kanoh, S. Utsumi, and S. Kimura

SECTION IV. CELLULAR INTERACTIONS

Possible Refractory Site on LPS-Induced Interleukin 1 Production in C3H/HeJ Peritoneal Macrophages.................................... 347

M. Nakano, Y. Terada, H. Matsumura, and H. Shinomiya

The Role of 13-Hydroxylinoleic Acid in the Activation of Macrophages by Lipopolysaccharide.. 361

U. F. Schade, I. Burmeister, R. Engel, H. Lode, and I. Kozka

Modulation of Interleukin 1 Production by Endotoxin, Pertussis Toxin, and Indomethacin.. 369

T. W. Klein, C. A. Newton, F. R. Vogel, H. Friedman, M. Lucas, A. Rodloff, and H. Hahn

Immunopharmacologic Aspects of Lipopolysaccharide Endotoxin Action with Special Reference to Cyclic Nucleotides........................ 375

J. W. Hadden

Mechanisms of Endotoxin Stimulation of Monocytes in Whole Blood...... 389

B. Osterud, J. O. Olsen, and L. Wilsgard

Comparative Study of Lipopolysaccharide- Lipid IVa-, and Lipid X-Induced Tumor Necrosis Factor Production in Murine Macrophage-Like Cell Lines.. 399

T. P. Birkland, R. D. Cornwell, D. T. Golenbock, and R. A. Proctor

Lipopolysaccharide-Induced Priming of the Murine Macrophage-Like Cell Line J774A.1 for Enhanced Production of Reactive Oxygen Intermediates is Blocked by Antiserum to Murine Interferon B..................... 403

T. P. Birkland and R. A. Proctor

Lipopolysaccharide-Containing Cytoplasmic Membranes as Immunostimulators of the Peritoneal Macrophages............................. 407

E. Ivanova, J. Gumpert, and A. Popov

Effects of Lipopolysaccharide or Recombinant Human-Interleukin-1β on Chemiluminescence by Peritoneal Macrophages from Normal and MRL-lpr-/lpr Mice... 413

C. Damais, L. Friteau, D. Lando, and B. Dugas

LPS-Mediated Triggering of T Lymphocytes in Immune Response Against Gram-Negative Bacteria.. 417

E. Jirillo, C. De Simone, V. Covelli, H. Kiyono, J. R. McGhee, and S. Antonaci

Involvement of I-A-Restricted B-B Cell Interaction in the Polyclonal B Cell Differentiation Induced by Lipopolysaccharide.................. 427

Y. Takahama, S. Ono, K. Ishihara, M. Muramatsu, and T. Hamaoka

Identification and Characterization of Lipopolysaccharide Receptor Molecules on Mammalian Lymphoid Cells................................ 445

M.-G. Lei, L. Flebbe, D. Roeder, and D. C. Morrison

Regulatory Mechanism of Expression of LPS Binding Site (S) and Signaling Events by LPS in Macrophages................................ 467

K. S. Akagawa, K. Kamoshita, T. Tomita, T. Yasuda, and T. Tokunaga

Endotoxin and Kupffer Cells in Liver Disease......................... 481

K. Tanikawa and M. Sata

SECTION V. HOST RESPONSES

Metabolic Fate of Endotoxin in Rat.................................. 499

M. Freudenberg and C. Galanos

Bacterial Endotoxin as a Probe to Investigate Viral Induced Immune Deficiencies.. 511

M. Bendinelli, D. Matteucci, P. G. Conaldi, and E. Soldaini

Immunoadjuvanticity of Endotoxins and Nontoxic Derivatives for Normal and Leukemic Immunocytes... 525

H. Friedman, T. Klein, S. Specter, C. Newton, and A. Nowotny

Various Aspects of Synergism between Endotoxin and MDP.............. 537

M. Parant and L. Chedid

The Mediation of Endotoxin-Induced Beneficial Effects by Cytokines.. 549

R. Urbaschek and B. Urbaschek

The Mechanism of Adjuvant Action of Bacterial Lipopolysaccharide in Subcutaneous Immunization.. 557

Y. Inoue and T. Yokochi

Lipid A, the Immunostimulatory Principle of Lipopolysaccharides?..... 561

H. Loppnow, I. Durrbaum, H. Brade, C. A. Dinarello, S. Kusumoto, E. Th. Rietschel, and H.-D. Flad

A Study of the Cellular and Molecular Mediators of the Adjuvant Action of a Nontoxic Monophosphoryl Lipid A................................ 567

A. G. Johnson and M. A. Tomai

Anti-LPS Region Antibody Responses and Cellular Immune Responsiveness in Typhoid Patients.. 581

C. M. Mastroianni, A. Misefari, E. Jirillo, C. DeSimone, V. Vullo, and S. Delia

Lipopolysaccharide, but not Lethal Infection, Releases Tumor Necrosis Factor in Mice.. 585

R. D. Cornwell, D. T. Golenbock, and R. A. Proctor

Biological Properties of Lipopolysaccharides Isolated from Bordetella.. 589

M. Watanabe, H. Takimoto, Y. Kumazawa, and K. Amano

Alterations of Responses to Bacterial Endotoxin by Bacteroides fragilis in Vivo and in Vitro.. 593

A. C. Rodloff, S. Ehlers, D. K. Blanchard, and H. Hahn

Mechanisms of the Lethal Action of Endotoxin and Endotoxin Hypersensitivity.. 603

C. Galanos, M. A. Freudenberg, and M. Matsuura

Septic Shock in the Elderly.. 621

A. Shibusawa and H. Ogata

Endotoxin-Induced Cytokines in Human Septicemia.................... 635

I. de Vries, S. J. H. van Deventer, J. Debets, H. R. Buller, J. W. ten Cate, W. Pauw, L. W. Statius van Eps, and A. Sturk

Lipid A Precursors Protect against Endotoxin Challenge.............. 641

R. A. Proctor

New Therapeutic Method against Septic Shock - Removal of Endotoxin Using Extracorporeal Circulation.................................... 653

M. Kodama, K. Hanasawa and T. Tani

Immunotherapy with Bacterial Endotoxins.............................. 665

J. A. Rudbach, J. L. Cantrell, J. T. Ulrich, and M. S. Mitchell

Stimulation of Nonspecific Resistance by Radio-Detoxified Endotoxin.. 677

L. Bertók

Monoclonal Antibody to Lipid A Prevents the Development of Haemodynamic Disorders in Endotoxemia.............................. 681

A. A. Shnyra, G. F. Kalantarov, T. N. Vlasik, I. N. Trakht, A. Ju. Mayatnikov, A. L. Tabachnik, D. V. Borovikov, and V. L. Golubykh

Endotoxin Size in Hemodialysis Solutions: Modifications in Presence of Concentrated Salt Solutions and Bacterial Products................ 685

V. Goury, A. C. Steinmetz, F. Vincent, A. Moufti, and J. C. Darbord

Protective Effect of Salmonella Typhimurium Re-LPS Antiserum......... 691

Yu Ching and Y. Shihao

Index.. 703

SECTION I.

SYNTHESIS, STRUCTURE AND FUNCTION

CHEMICAL SYNTHESIS OF ENDOTOXIN

S. Kusumoto, N. Kusunose, M. Imoto, T. Kamikawa, and T. Shiba

Department of Chemistry, Faculty of Science, Osaka University
Toyonaka, Osaka 560, Japan

INTRODUCTION

Total synthesis of lipid A's of Escherichia coli and many other bacterial species achieved in our laboratory (6, 7, 8) contributed not only to confirm their proposed chemical structures but also to establish unequivocally that these phosphorylated polyacyl glucosamine disaccharide with definite structures are responsible for most of the endotoxic activities of bacterial lipopolysaccharide (LPS) (4, 5). Furthermore, precise study on the biological activities could be carried out in relation to the acylation or phosphorylation patterns of the molecules with these pure synthetic preparations of lipid A's in hand (12, 13). Immunogenicity and antigenicity of lipid A could be analyzed as well (1, 2). As the results, evidences were obtained which indicated that the toxic and other biological activities of endotoxin could be separated by adequate modification of the structure such as distribution of the acyl groups. One might thus be able to utilize some of the beneficial biological activities by further research in this line.

In the meantime new knowledge has been accumulated on the significance of the inner core region on the biological activities of lipopolysaccharide (15). We then focused on the elucidation of the biological function of the inner core, particularly of 3-deoxy-D-manno-2-octulosonic acid (KDO) moieties, and started a new synthetic approach to LPS of E. coli Re mutant. It is the most simple natural LPS, whose structure was recently proposed as **1** by us and other groups (3 16), being comprised of only two moles of KDO and lipid A. This synthesis is important for the confirmation of the proposed structure **1** and simultaneously it provides a way to prepare many analogous compounds valuable for the purpose to evaluate on the molecular level the effect of each KDO moieties for various biological activities. In this paper we describe a new synthesis of KDO and its coupling to a lipid A part structure leading to the formation of a tetrasaccharide **2** corresponding to 1-dephospho derivative of Re LPS. Since direct comparison proved this synthetic compound to be identical with the natural specimen, the structure **1** of natural Re LPS was synthetically confirmed. Preparation of several related partial structures (**3**, **4**, and **5**) is also described.

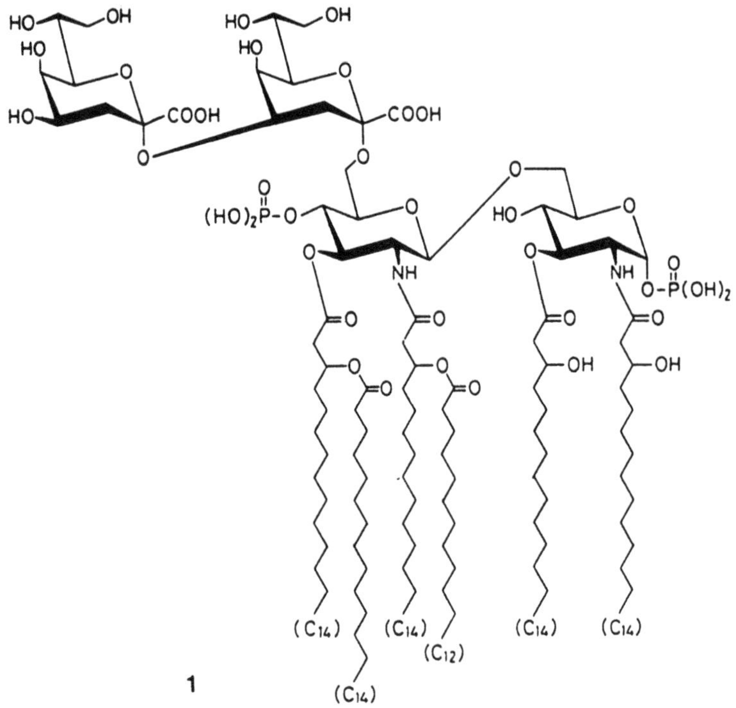

Fig 1. Chemical structure of Escherichia coli Re LPS.

MATERIAL AND METHODS

General

Reaction conditions employed for chemical conversions were same as described previously (8) unless otherwise noted. After each step, the product was purified by silica-gel column chromatography. The purities and the chemical structures were confirmed by means of TLC, ^{1}H NMR, and elemental analysis.

Benzyl (3-deoxy-2-fluoro-4,5:7,8-di-O-isopropylidene-α-D-manno-2-octulopyranosyl)onate (**12**)

The protected pyranosidic fluoride of KDO (**12**) was prepared from D-mannose as previously communicated in a preliminary form (9, 10). The synthetic scheme is shown in Fig 3.

Allyl 3-O-((R)-benzyloxytetradecanoyl)-2-((R)-benzyloxytetradecanoylamino)-2-deoxy-6-O-(2-deoxy-2-(R)-3-dodecanoyloxytetradecanoylamino)-3-O-((R)-3-tetradecanoyloxytetradecanoyl)-β-D-glucopyranosyl-α-D-glucopyranoside 4'-(Diphenyl phosphate) (**15a**), the Corresponding Intermediate (**15b**) of Precursor Ia, and Allyl 2-Deoxy-2-((R)-3-dodecanoyloxytetradecanoylamino)-3-O-((R)-3-tetradecanoyloxytetradecanoyl)-α-D-glucopyranoside 4'-(Diphenyl phosphate) (**13**)

The protected disaccharide intermediate (**15a**) with all acyl substituents of E. coli-type and 4'-phosphate was prepared according to the method described in our previous total synthesis of E. coli lipid A (8). The outline

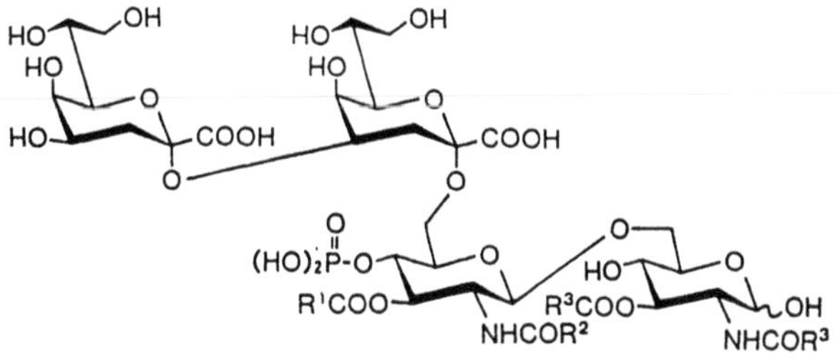

2 , 3 , 5 : R^1CO = (R)-3-tetradecanoyloxytetradecanoyl
R^2CO = (R)-3-dodecanoyloxytetradecanoyl
R^3CO = (R)-3-hydroxytetradecanoyl

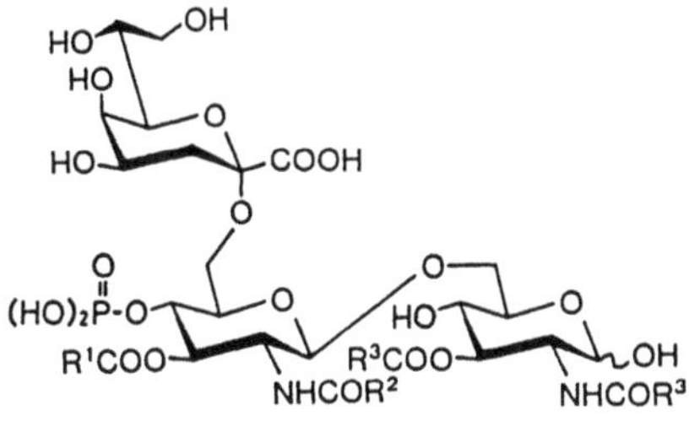

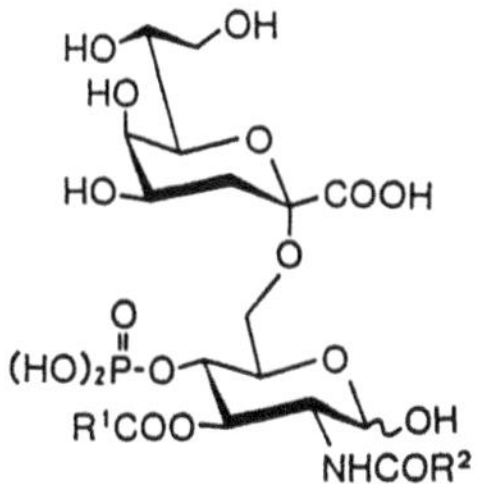

4 : R^1CO = R^2CO = R^3CO = (R)-3-hydroxytetradecanoyl

Fig 2. Part structures of Re LPS synthesized.

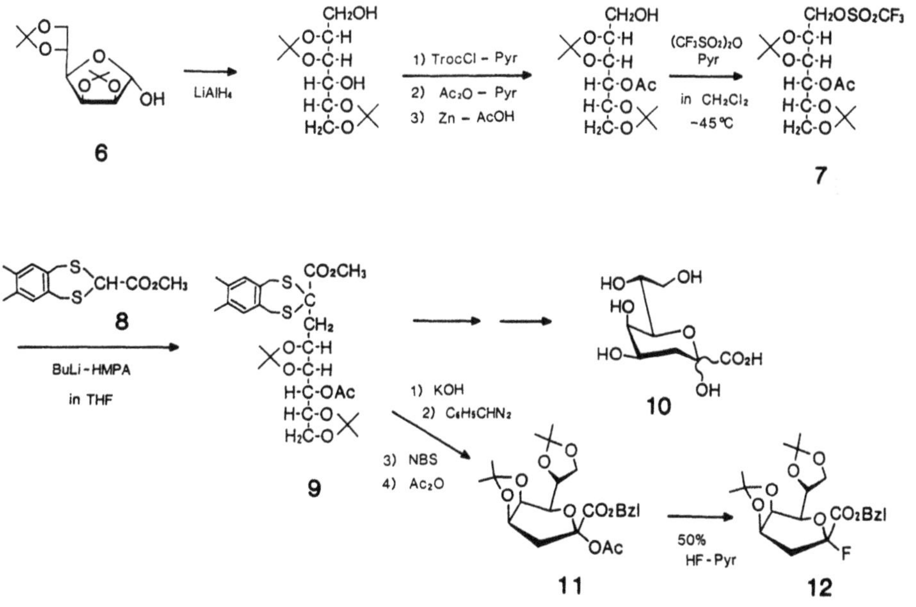

Fig 3. Synthetic scheme of a novel pyranosidic glycosyl donor **12** of KDO.

of the synthetic scheme is shown in Fig 5. The tetraacyl disaccharide 4'-phosphate intermediate (**15b**) corresponding to biosynthetic precursor of lipid A, Precursor Ia, was synthesized in a way similar to that shown in Fig 5. The 2-N,3-O-diacylated glucosamine 4-phosphate intermediate (**13**) corresponding to the non-reducing glucosamine part of **15a** was also prepared similarly.

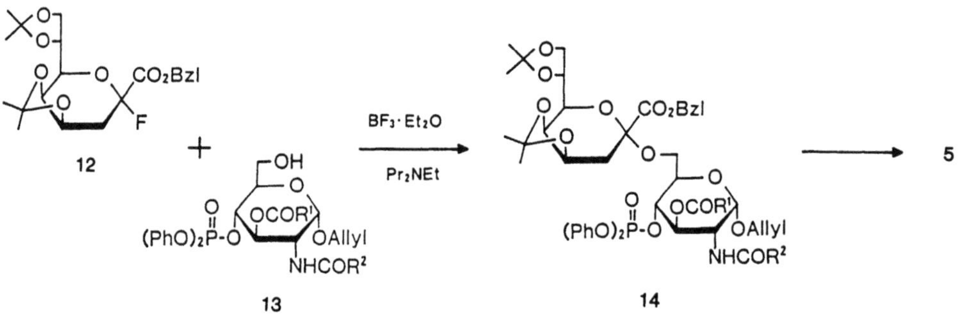

Fig 4. Synthetic scheme of a disaccharide part structure **5** containing KDO. (Explanation on page 8.)

Condensation of KDO Fluoride with 13, 15a, or 15b

A solution of the protected KDO fluoride (**12**) and the corresponding reaction partner (**13**, **15a**, or **15b**) in anhydrous dichloromethane was treated with boron trifluoride etherate in the presence of ethyldiisopropylamine at $0^{\circ}C$ under argon atmosphere as described (11).

Removal of the Protecting Groups

The conditions used for deprotection were same as previously reported (8, 11). The allyl glycosides were removed in two steps, i.e., isomerization into 1-propenyl group with an iridium complex followed by cleavage with iodine in aqueous THF. The isopropylidene groups on KDO were cleaved off by treating with trifluoroacetic acid containing 5% of water in dichloromethane at $0^{\circ}C$ (11). The persistent benzyl and phenyl groups were hydrogenolyzed with palladium black and platinum oxide as catalyst, respectively, at room temperature under atmosphere of hydrogen (5-8 kg/cm^2).

Purification of the Synthetic 1-Dephospho Re LPS (2)

The deprotection product was purified by means of centrifugal partition chromatography (CPC) with model CPC-B92 apparatus of Sanki Engineering Ltd, Kyoto, with a solvent system of chloroform-methanol-isopropanol-water-triethylamine (20:20:2.5:20:0.1) in descending mode (at 1300 rpm and flow rate of 3 ml/min). The product was obtained as colorless solid by precipitation with cold hydrochloric acid from an aqueous triethylamine solution $[\alpha]_D^{13}$ + 8.9° (c 0.49, chloroform-methanol 5:1). This product (**2**) was identified on TLC with the corresponding natural 1-dephospho derivative of natural Re LPS obtained as described below.

For further identification the product (**2**) was converted with ethereal dizomethane into the corresponding tetramethyl ester $[\alpha]_D^{13}$ + 15.2° (c 0.50, chloroform-methanol 9:1). The 500 MHz ^{1} NMR spectra of this methyl ester and its peracetate were identical with those of the corresponding derivatives obtained from natural Re LPS below.

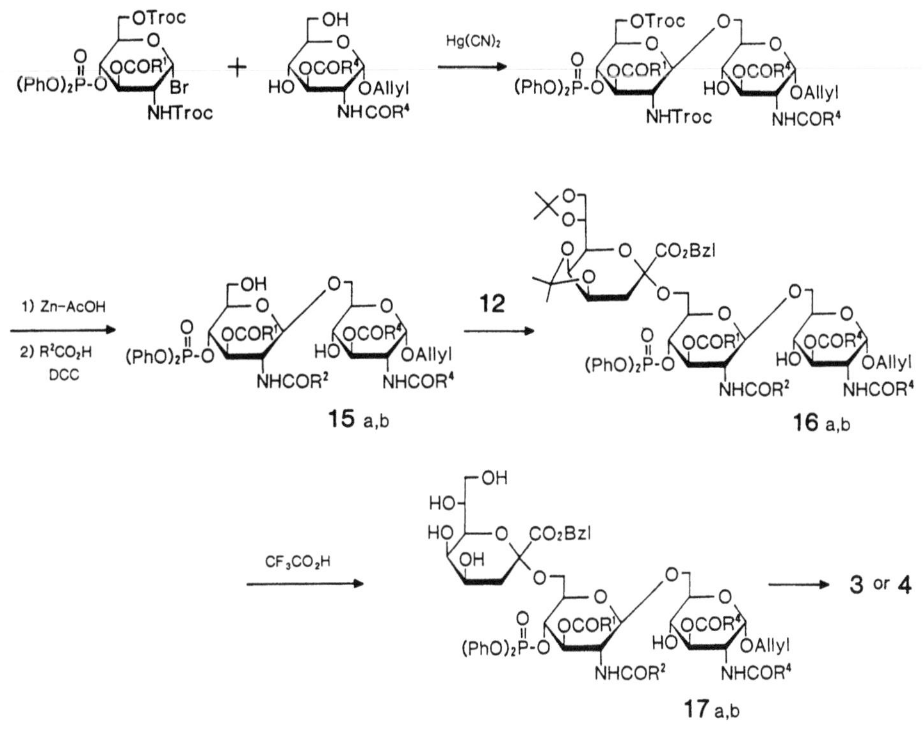

Hg(CN)$_2$

1) Zn–AcOH
2) R^2CO_2H
DCC

15 a,b

12

16 a,b

CF_3CO_2H

17 a,b

→ **3** or **4**

a : R^1CO = (R)-3-tetradecanoyloxytetradecanoyl
R^2CO = (R)-3-dodecanoyloxytetradecanoyl
R^4CO = (R)-3-benzyloxytetradecanoyl

b : R^1CO = R^2CO = R^4CO = (R)-3-benzyloxytetradecanoyl

Fig 5. Synthetic scheme of trisaccharide part structures 3 and 4.

Isolation of the 1-Dephospho Derivative of Natural E. coli Re LPS

LPS isolated from E. coli Re mutant strain F 515 cells was treated, after acid precipitation, with 2% acetic acid at 90°C for 10 min. The crude 1-dephospho derivative obtained by removal of the solvent in vacuo was treated with ethereal solution of diazomethane. The product was purified by preparative TLC on silica gel (chloroform-methanol 5:1) and lyophilized from dioxane $[\alpha]_D^{13}$ + 14.8° (c 0.48, chloroform-methanol 9:1).

RESULTS AND DISCUSSION

For the construction of the structure **2**, we employed a synthetic route to introduce two KDO moieties stepwise to a disaccharide intermediate of lipid A which already contains protected 4'-phosphate and all acyl groups at the correct positions. The required intermediate (**15a**) with free hydroxyl group at 6'-position could be obtained according to our previous work (8) via the route shown in Fig 5.

Paulsen et al., already reported syntheses of several KDO-containing oligosaccharides including the tetrasaccharide backbone of Re LPSs, α-KDO (2-4)-α -KDO-(2-6)-β -D-GlcN-(1-6)-D-GlcN. In their studies the α -glycosyl bromide of pyranosidic peracetylated KDO methyl ester was successfully employed. For the present synthesis, however, we need a different glycosyl donor of KDO containing such protective groups which can be removed later without affecting the acyl functions present in the lipid A part.

A novel glycosyl donor, flouoride of 4,5:7,8-di-O-isopropylidene derivative of KDO (**12**), which fill the above requirement was then prepared starting from readily available 2,3:5,6-di-O-isopropylidene-D-mannose (**6**) as illustrated in Fig 3. Thus, after lithium aluminum hydride reduction of **6** and protection of the 4-hydroxyl group by acetylation, the C-1 position was activated by trifluoromethanesulfonylation. The resultant triflate (**7**) was then coupled with methyl glyoxylate dithioacetal (**8**) in dry THF to give a product **9** which has the KDO skeleton with the required stereochemistry. Removal of all protecting groups of **9** afforded free KDO **10** which gave crystalline ammonium salt identical with an authentic specimen.

For the preparation of the glycosyl fluoride (**12**), **9** was hydrolyzed with potassium hydroxide and the product reesterified with phenyl diazomethane. After oxidative cleavage of the dithioacetal group with N-bromosuccinimide, the resultant pyranose form derivative was acetylated and then converted with hydrogen fluoride in pyridine into a crystalline fluoride **12**.

The α-ketosidic configuration and the boat conformation of the fluoride **12** was determined by single crystal X-ray analysis. From comparison of ^{1}H NMR data, it could be concluded that all 4,5:7,8-di-O-isopropylidene derivative of KDO exist in similar boat conformations. Furthermore, examination of the differences between chemical shift values of H-3eq and H-3ax proved to be useful as criteria of the anomeric configurations of these diisopropylidene derivatives, the α-anomers having larger Δ 3eq-3ax values (0.60-1.09 ppm) than the corresponding β-anomers (0.26-0.28 ppm) (10). It should be noted that in case of usual chair form derivatives of KDO, the reverse relation is observed, i.e., Δ 3eq-3ax values are larger in β-anomers than in α-anomers.

Coupling reaction by use of the KDO fluoride obtained above was examined with the monosaccharide derivative (**13**) which corresponds to the non-reducing half of E. coli lipid A. Reaction was affected with boron trifluoride as described in the Material and Methods section to give the desired disaccharide **14** in a satisfactory yield. Its anomeric α-configuration was assured by using the above NMR criteria. The corresponding β-anomer was formed only in trace amount in this reaction and could not be isolated. This result showed that the fluoride **12** is a useful glycosyl donor for our synthetic purpose. It is stable enough to be stored at room temperature and gives almost exclusively the desired α-linked KDO saccharide.

The fluoride was then coupled with the disaccharide acceptor of E. coli and precursor-type (**15a, b**) to give the corresponding trisaccharides (16a, b) respectively.

Prior to the condensation of the second mole of KDO to complete the desired tetrasaccharide structure, complete deprotection of the KDO-containing trisaccharides (**16a, b**) was next examined. On treatment of their dichloromethane solution with trifluoroacetic acid containing a small amount of water at $0^{o}C$, both isopropylidene groups of KDO moiety could be selectively removed. The ketosidic linkage of KDO was stable under these conditions and was not cleaved at all. Successive removal of allyl, benzyl and phenyl protecting groups afforded the free trisaccharide (**3** and **4**). Deprotection of the disaccharide **14** was performed in a similar way to give the free disaccharide **5** which represents the middle half of Re LPS molecule.

Compound **17a** was used as the substrate for the introduction of the second KDO molecule after selective monoacetonide formation at 7,8-position. Condensation of the KDO fluoride with the monoacetonide proceeded smoothly as above and a single tetrasaccharide product **19** was obtained. The desired α (2-4) structure of this product could be reasonably estimated on the basis of the much higher reactivity of the equatorial 4-hydroxyl group than that of the axial one on 5-position.

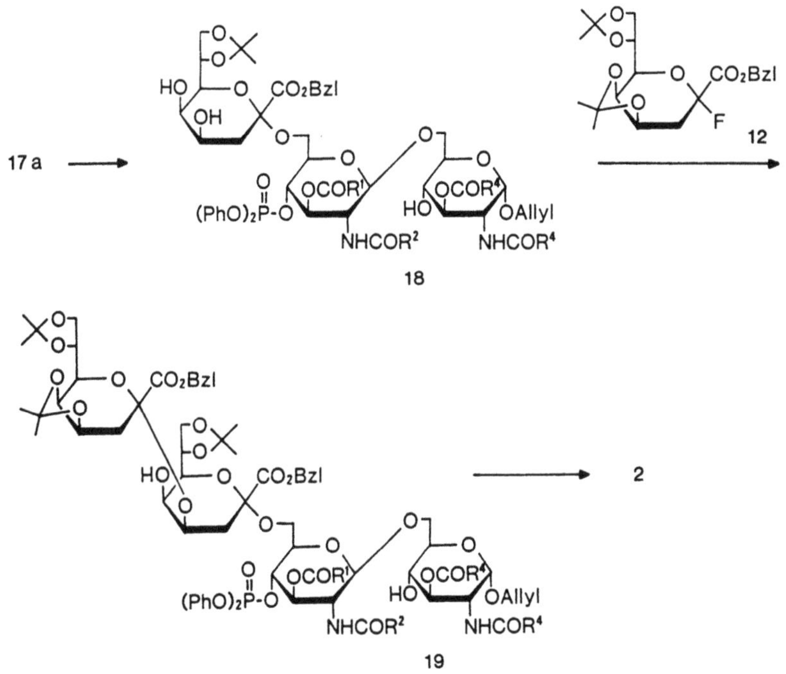

Fig 6. Synthetic scheme of 1-dephospho derivative **2** of Escherichia coli Re LPS.

Stepwise deprotection of **19** in a same manner as described for the trisaccharide above gave the synthetic 1-dephospho Re LPS **2**, which was identified on TLC with the main component of the 1-dephosphorylated product of natural LPS. For more strict identification, the natural derivative was isolated by preparative TLC after conversion into methyl ester. Synthetic and natural methyl esters and their peracetates gave identical ^{1}H NMR spectra respectively.

The chemical structure of Re LPS **1** proposed previously was thus synthetically confirmed by this work. Further, we are now able to obtain compounds with desired structures containing KDO and lipid A part by chemical means. Biological studies using such synthetic preparations are being undertaken and expected to give further informations concerning the biological significance of KDO moieties in LPS.

ACKNOWLEDGEMENT

We are greatly indebted to Drs. Chris Galanos and Otto Lüderitz of Max-Planck-Institut für Immunobiologie, Freiburg, FRG, for their generous gift of natural LPS of E. coli Re mutant.

REFERENCES

1. Arata, S., Mashimo, J., Kasai, N., Okuda, K., Aihara, Y., Kotani, S., Takada, H., Shimamoto, T., and Kusunose, N., 1988, Characterization of monoclonal lipid A antibodies with synthetic lipid a analogues. FEBS Microbiology Letters. 49: 479.

2. Brade, L., Brandenburg, K., Kuhn, H.-M., Kusumoto, S., Macher, T.I., Rietschel, E. Th., and Brade, H., 1987, The immunogenicity and antigenicity of lipid A are influenced by its physicochemical state and environment. Infect. Immun. 55: 2636.

3. Christian, R., Schulz, G., Waldstatten, P. and Unger, F. M., 1984, Zur Struktur der 3-Deoxyoktulosonsaure- (KDO-) Region des Lipopolysaccharids von Salmonella minnesota Re 595. Tetrahedron Lett. 25: 3433.

4. Galanos, C., Lehmann, V., Lüderitz, O., Rietschel, E. Th., Westphal, O., Brade, H., Brade, L., Freudenberg, M. A., Hansen-Hagge, T., Lüderitz, T., Mckenzie, G., Schade, U., Strittmatter, W., Tanamoto, K., Zähringer, U., Imoto, M., Yoshimura, H., Yamamoto, M., Shimamoto, T., Kusumoto, S., and Shiba, T., 1984, Endotoxic properties of chemically synthesized lipid A part structures - comparison of synthetic lipid A precursor and synthetic analogues with biosynthetic lipid A precursor and free lipid A. Eur. J. Biochem. 140: 221.

5. Galanos, C., Lüderitz, O., Rietschel, E. Th., Westphal, O., Brade, H., Brade, L., Freudenberg, M., Schade, U., Imoto, M., Yoshimura, H., Kusumoto, S., and Shiba, T., 1985, Synthetic and natural Escherichia coli free lipid A express identical endotoxic activities. Eur. J. Biochem. 148: 1.

6. Imoto, M., Yoshimura, H., Yamamoto, M., Shimamoto, T., Kusumoto, S., and Shiba, T., 1984, Chemical synthesis of phosphorylated tetraacyl disaccharide corresponding to a biosynthetic precursor of lipid A. Tetrahedron Lett. 25: 2667.

7. Imoto, M., Yoshimura, H., Sakaguchi, N., Kusumoto, S., and Shiba, T., 1985, Total synthesis of Escherichia coli lipid A. Tetrahedron Lett. 26: 1545.

8. Imoto, M., Yoshimura, H., Shimamoto, T., Sakaguchi, N., Kusumoto, S., and Shiba, T., 1987, Total synthesis of Escherichia coli Lipid A, the endotoxically active principle of cell-surface lipopolysaccharide. Bull. Chem. Soc. Jpn. 60: 2205.

9. Imoto, M., Kusumoto, S., and Shiba, T., 1987, A new synthesis of 3-deoxy--D-manno-2-octulosonic acid (KDO) from D-mannose. Tetrahedron Lett. 28: 6235.

10. Imoto, M., Kusunose, N., Matsuura, Y., Kusumoto, S., and Shiba, T., 1987, Preparation of novel pyranosyl fluoride of 3-deoxy-D-manno-2-octulosonic acid (KDO) feasible for synthesis of KDO α-glycosides. Tetrahedron Lett. 28: 6277.

11. Imoto, M., Kusunose, N., Kusumoto, S., and Shiba, T., 1988, Synthetic approach to bacterial lipopolysaccharide, preparation of trisaccharide part structure containing KDO and 1-dephospho lipid A. Tetrahedron Lett. 29: 2227.

12. Kanegasaki, S., Tanamoto, K., Yasuda, T., Homma, J. Y., Matsuura, M., Nakatsuka, M., Kumazawa, Y., Yamamoto, A., Shiba, T., Kusumoto, S., Imoto, M., Yoshimura, H., and Shimamoto, T., 1986, Structure-activity relationship of lipid A: comparison of biological activity of natural and synthetic lipid A's with different fatty acid compositions. J. Biochem. 99: 1203.

13. Kotani, S., Takada, H., Takahashi, I., Ogawa, T., Tsujimoto, M., Shimauchi, H., Ikeda, T., Okamura, H., Tamura, T., Harada, K., Tanaka, S., Shiba, T., Kusumoto, S., and Shimamoto, T., 1986, Immunobiological activities of synthetic lipid A analogs with low endotoxicity. Infect. Immun. 54: 673.

14. Paulsen, H. and Schüller, M., 1987, Synthese von KDO-haltigen Lipoid-A-Analoga. Liebigs Ann. Chem. 249.

15. Rietschel, E. Th., Brade, L., Schade, U., Seydel, U., Zähringer, U., Kusumoto, S., and Brade, H., 1988, Bacterial endotoxins: properties and structure of biologically active domains, "Surface Structures of Microorganisms and their Interaction with Mammalian Host," ed. U. Schwartz and M. Richmond, Verlag Chemie, Weinheim.

16. Zähringer, U., Lindner, B., Seydel, U., Rietschel, E. Th., Naoki, H., Unger, F. M., Imoto, M., Kusumoto, S., and Shiba, T., 1985, Structure of de-O-acylated lipopolysaccharide from Escherichia coli Re mutant strain F 515. Tetrahedron Lett. 26: 6321.

STRUCTURAL REQUIREMENTS OF LIPID A FOR ENDOTOXICITY AND OTHER BIOLOGICAL ACTIVITIES—AN OVERVIEW*

S. Kotani[1,2] and H. Takada[1]

[1]Department of Microbiology and Oral Microbiology, Osaka University Dental School, 1-8 Yamadaoka, Suita, Osaka 565
[2]Osaka College of Medical Technology, 1-30, Higashitenma 2-chome, Kita-ku, Osaka 530, Japan

INTRODUCTION

Lipopolysaccharide (LPS), a major constituent of outer membranes of gram-negative bacteria, exhibits a wide variety of bioactivities (Table 1) (61). In 1954 Westphal and Lüderitz proposed that the lipid moiety of LPS is responsible for most of endotoxicities, and designated it as lipid A (Fig 1) (60). However, this extremely important discovery was neither adequately nor unanimously accepted by endotoxin investigators at that time. One of the main reasons for this controversy is that the high hydrophobicity of the lipid A molecule made its manipulation as a test material for bioactivities difficult. Another reason is concerned with inherent microheterogeneity in fine structures even among preparations derived from the same bacterial

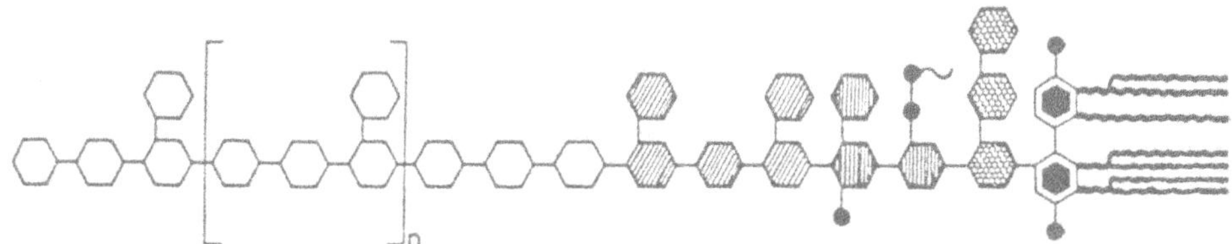

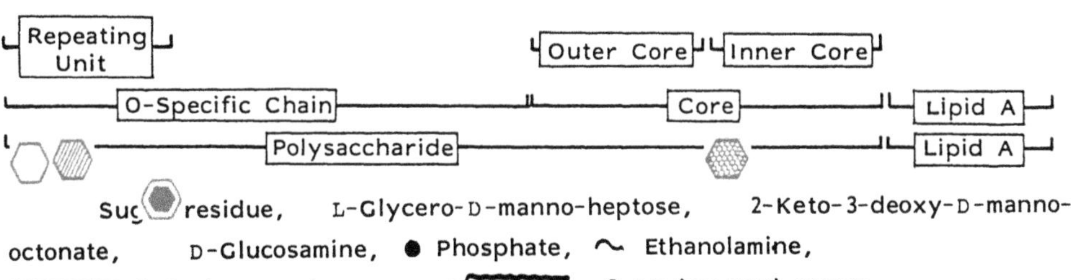

Fig 1. Schematic structure of **Salmonella** LPS. Taken from the review of Westphal et al. (61) with modifications.

*This overview is based on our recent review paper in CRC Critical Rev. Microbiol. (54).

Table 1. Bioactivities of LPS or lipid A[a]

Lethal toxicity	Adjuvant (immunomodulating) activity
Pyrogenicity	Increase of nonspecific resistance to infection
Preparative and provocative activity for local Shwartzman reaction	Induction of tumor necrosis
Induction of hypothermia in mice	Induction of tumor necrosis factor (TNF)
Induction of leukocytosis	Induction of interferon (IFN)
Induction of bone marrow necrosis	Induction of colony stimulating factor (CSF)
Depression of blood pressure	Induction of prostaglandin (PG) synthesis
Toxicity enhanced by BCG	Induction of tolerance to endotoxin
Toxicity enhanced by adrenalectomy	Induction of early refractory state to temperature change
Toxicity enhanced by galactosamine	
Enhanced dermal reactivity to epinephrine	Somnogenic effect[b]
Platelet aggregation	Analgesic effect[c]
Complement activation	Mitogenic activity for B lymphocytes
Hageman factor activation	Macrophage activation
Induction of plasminogen activator	Polymorphonuclear leukocyte activation
Limulus activity (activation of clotting enzyme cascade of amoebocyte lysate of horseshoe crab)	Endothelial cell activation
Embryonic bone resorption	Induction of mouse liver pyruvate kinase
Type C RNA virus release from mouse spleen cells	Inhibition of phosphoenolpyruvate carboxykinase

[a]Based on the review of Westphal et al. (61) with modifications and additions.
[b]Krueger et al. (34).
[c]Ogawa et al. (44).

strain, and with structural changes of a test lipid A specimen during preparation procedures. The former technical problem was nicely settled by Galanos who removed metal cations which lowered the solubility of lipid A, and then added triethylamine (TEA) to get a uniform TEA salt-form of lipid A which is highly soluble in water (8). Nevertheless, controversy due to microheterogeneity of bacterial lipid A preparations was not solved until lipid A could be synthesized successfully.

SYNTHETIC STUDY ON LIPID A

In the first half of the 1980s, investigators started synthetic studies on lipid A. Among them, Shiba, Kusumoto and their colleagues in Osaka University first succeeded in total synthesis of a lipid A whose whole structure corresponded to that proposed for lipid A isolated from **Escherichia coli** Re- mutant (17, 18). Bioactivities of this preparation have been extensively investigated by research groups in Japan and West Germany. As summarized in Table 2, the investigations lead us to the unanimous conclusion that the lipid A portion carries most, if not all, of the endotoxic and other bioactivities exhibited by bacterial LPS (12, 15, 31). Shiba's group has so far synthesized **Salmonella** and other enterobacterial types of lipid A's (33, unpublished data), biosynthetic precursors Ia(IVA) (16, 19) and Ib(IVB), the reducing moieties of lipid A's (37a), and a series of disaccharide lipid A analogs (32, unpublished).

Hasegawa and his colleagues, on the other hand, carried out a project which was focused on the preparation of nontoxic monosaccharide lipid A analogs with beneficial bioactivities which could be applicable in clinical medicine. They mainly synthesized compounds corresponding to the nonreducing moiety of lipid A's (7, 25, 26, 27, 28, 29, 45,). Bioactivities of these compounds were extensively studied by Homma's group (35, 36, 37, 39, 40).

There are other lines of synthetic studies on lipid A analogs; namely Charon's group reported the synthesis and immunobiological activities of glycolipids structurally related to lipid A (5, 6), and Achiwa's group recently synthesized 2-keto-3-deoxyoctonic acid (KDO)- and tetraacetyl-KDO-glucosamine-4-phosphate to compare their bioactivities with those of the corresponding compounds having no KDO (42, 50, 51).

Thus, a series of synthetic lipid A's and various disaccharide and monosaccharide analogs of them are now available for investigation of structure-bioactivity relationships of lipid A. These compounds also make it possible to elucidate the action mechanisms of lipid A under well-defined experimental conditions, that is, without ambiguity due to heterogeneity of preparations and contamination with bioactive materials other than the molecule in question.

STRUCTURE-BIOACTIVITY RELATIONSHIPS OF LIPID A

Fig 2 (upper half) illustrates the acylation patterns of test disaccharide preparations which correspond in structure to lipid A's of **Salmonella minnesota, E. coli, Chromobacterium,** biosynthetic precursors Ib and Ia, and their analogs. The lower half of the Fig 2 shows the acylation and phosphorylation patterns of test monosaccharide analogs which correspond to the reducing and non-reducing moiety of lipid A's. Compounds LA-16, 15, 22, 20 and 21-PP have 3-acyloxyacyl groups of more than one per disaccharide backbone, while LA-14, 18 and 24-PP have 3-hydroxyacyl groups but no double acyl groups. Compounds LA-17 and 23-PP have neither 3-hydroxy nor 3-acyloxyacyl groups.

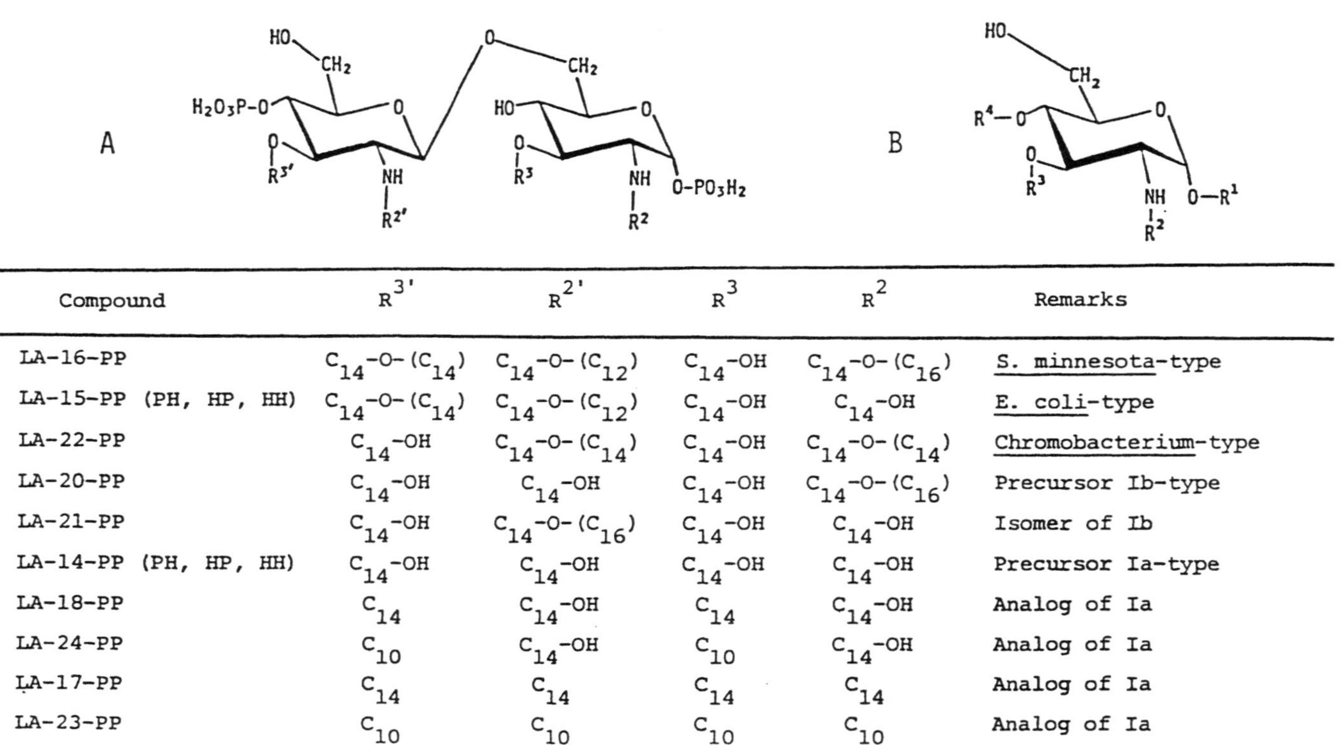

A

Compound	$R^{3'}$	$R^{2'}$	R^{3}	R^{2}	Remarks
LA-16-PP	C_{14}-O-(C_{14})	C_{14}-O-(C_{12})	C_{14}-OH	C_{14}-O-(C_{16})	_S. minnesota_-type
LA-15-PP (PH, HP, HH)	C_{14}-O-(C_{14})	C_{14}-O-(C_{12})	C_{14}-OH	C_{14}-OH	_E. coli_-type
LA-22-PP	C_{14}-OH	C_{14}-O-(C_{14})	C_{14}-OH	C_{14}-O-(C_{14})	_Chromobacterium_-type
LA-20-PP	C_{14}-OH	C_{14}-OH	C_{14}-OH	C_{14}-O-(C_{16})	Precursor Ib-type
LA-21-PP	C_{14}-OH	C_{14}-O-(C_{16})	C_{14}-OH	C_{14}-OH	Isomer of Ib
LA-14-PP (PH, HP, HH)	C_{14}-OH	C_{14}-OH	C_{14}-OH	C_{14}-OH	Precursor Ia-type
LA-18-PP	C_{14}	C_{14}-OH	C_{14}	C_{14}-OH	Analog of Ia
LA-24-PP	C_{10}	C_{14}-OH	C_{10}	C_{14}-OH	Analog of Ia
LA-17-PP	C_{14}	C_{14}	C_{14}	C_{14}	Analog of Ia
LA-23-PP	C_{10}	C_{10}	C_{10}	C_{10}	Analog of Ia

B

Compound	R^4	R^3	R^2	R^1	Remarks
401	H	C_{14}-OH	C_{14}-OH	P	Reducing moiety of LA-14-, 15-, and 21-PP (corresponds to lipid X)
408	H	C_{14}-OH	C_{14}-O-(C_{16})	P	Reducing moiety of LA-16- and 20-PP, and nearly equal to the reducing moiety of LA-22-PP (correspnds to lipid Y)
410	P	C_{14}-OH	C_{14}-OH	H	Nonreducing moiety of LA-14- and 20-PP
GLA-47	P	C_{14}-O-(C_{14})	C_{14}-O-(C_{14})	H	Analogous to the nonreducing moiety of LA-15- and 16-PP
GLA-27	P	C_{14}	C_{14}-O-(C_{14})	H	Analogous to the nonreducing moiety of LA-22-PP

Fig 2. Structures of synthetic lipid A's and their analogs that were most widely studied to demonstrate the structure-bioactivity relationships of lipid A. LA series compounds and compound 401, 408 and 410 were synthesized by Shiba's group (16, 17, 18, 19, 32, 33, 37a, 49, 55) and GLA series compounds were prepared by Hasegawa's group (26, 29). (A) lipid A's and disaccharide lipid A analogs; (B) monosaccharide lipid A analogs. Abbreviations: C_{10}, decanoyl; C_{12}, dodecanoyl; C_{14}, tetradecanoyl; C_{16}, hexadecanoyl; C_{14}-OH, (R)-3-hydroxytetradecanoyl; C_{14}-O-(C_{12}), (R)-3-dodecanoyloxytetradecanoyl; C_{14}-O-(C_{14}), (R)-3-tetradecanoyloxytetradecanoyl; C_{14}-O-(C_{16}), (R)-3-hexadecanoyloxytetradecanoyl; P, $PO(OH)_2$.

Table 2. Bioactivities of synthetic **E. coli**-type lipid A (LA-15-PP)

IN VIVO ACTIVITIES

Lethal toxicity; galactosamine-loaded mice (12, 15, 31), MDP-primed mice[a], tumor-bearing mice (59), chick embryos (31)

Tolerance induction against lethal toxicity of LPS (12)

Body weight decreasing effect (31)

Local Shwartzman reaction; preparatory (12, 15, 31) and provocative (15, 31) activity

Pyrogenicity (12, 15, 31)

Leukopenia induction (31)

Induction of tumor necrosis (12)

Induction of interferon (IFN) (33)

Adjuvant activity (adjuvanticity):
Guinea pigs; enhancement of antibody formation (31), induction of delayed-type hypersensitivity (31, 59)

Mice; enhancement of antibody formation (31, 33, 55)

Analgesic activity (44)

IN VITRO ACTIVITIES

Murine splenocyte stimulation:
Mitogenic effect (12, 15, 31)

Polyclonal B cell activating effect (31)

Macrophage stimulation:
Guinea pigs; enhancement of superoxide anion generation (31), enhancement of spreading (31), enhancement of glucosamine uptake (31), inhibition of thymidine uptake (31)

Mice; enhancement of prostaglandins (12, 33) and interleukin 1 (IL-1) generation (31)

Humans; enhancement of IL-1 generation (38)

Migration enhancement of human polymorphonuclear leukocytes (31)

Induction of IFN (15)

Complement activation (31)

Limulus activity (12, 15, 31)

Antigenicity: Immunogenicity (3, 4) and antigenic reactivity (3, 4, 15, 23)

[a]Takada, H., unpublished.

Endotoxic Activities

The extremely wide range of bioactivities of LPS's and lipid A's, many of which are interrelated with each other and some of which are held in common by other immunomodulators, makes the definition of endotoxic activities ambiguous. In this paper, we tentatively take the lethality, preparatory (and provocative) abilities for local Shwartzman reaction and pyrogenicity of test synthetic compounds as a typical potency of endotoxin, by the simple reason that enough data have already been available on these activities to discuss structure-endotoxicity relationships.

A. Lethal toxicity: Table 3 shows that among the test compounds, only compound LA-15-PP, a synthetic **E. coli**-type lipid A, exhibited strong lethal toxicity in chick embryos. Other compounds, including **S. minnesota**-type LA-16-PP, did not show any significant lethality. Although data are not available at present on LA-20-PP (precursor Ib-type), LA-21-PP (an isomer of Ib) and LA-22-PP (**Chromobacterium**-type lipid A), the structural requirement for the lethal toxicity in chick embryos seems to be very strict. Appropriate number (two, and if LA-20- and 21-PP will be proved highly lethal, one)

Table 3. Lethal toxicity of synthetic lipid A's and their analogs in chick embryos and galactosamine-loaded mice

Compound	LD50[a] (ng)	
	Chick embryos[b]	GalN-loaded mice[c]
LA-16-PP	- (10,000)[d]	5.0
LA-15-PP	74	7.9
LA-14-PP	- (10,000)	10.0
LA-18-PP	- (100,000)	≥ 126[e]
LA-17-PP	- (100,000)	≥ 100
401	- (20,000)	- (1,000)
408	- (10,000)	≥ 1,585
410	- (10,000)	- (1,000)
GLA-47	- (10,000)	- (1,000)
GLA-27	- (10,000)	≥ 1,259

[a]Median lethal dose calculated by Kärbar's method. Data were taken from Kotani et al. (31, 32, 33), Takada et al (52), and Takahashi et al. (55).
[b]Groups of chick embryos (11 days old) were injected intravenously with 0.1 ml of the test material and observed for death by intoxication for 48 hr.
[c]Groups of C57BL/6 mice were loaded by intraperitoneal injection of galactosamine (GalN; 16 mg/mouse). Then they were immediately challenged by intravenous injection of the test material and observed for death by intoxication for 24 hr.
[d]None of the test animals died at the highest test dose (in parenthesis).
[e]100% Death was not observed at the highest dose tested.

of 3-acyloxyacyl groups are required on β(1-6)-linked D-glucosamine disaccharide backbone for manifestation of full lethality. None of the monosaccharide lipid A analogs, including compounds having the double acyl groups were lethal at the higest test dose.

The lethality test in galactosamine-loaded mice which were made extremely susceptible to the lethal toxicity of LPS, lipid A and some bacterial products by the method of Galanos et al. (9), revealed structural requirements quite different from those in chick embryos (Table 3). Compounds LA-16 and 14-PP exhibited high toxicity comparable to LA-15-PP. Although data are not shown here, Rietschel's group reported that LA-20 and 21-PP showed high lethality comparable to LA-15-PP (49). Thus the presence of an adequate number of 3-acyloxyacyl groups on the disaccharide backbone structure are not prerequisite to the lethal toxicity in galactosamine-loaded mice. However, replacement (even partial) of 3-hydroxymyristic acids with non-hydroxylated myristic acids caused a marked decrease in the lethality, as shown by at least ten times less toxicity of LA-18 and 17-PP than LA-14-PP.

Table 4 shows that phosphate groups at the C-1 and C-4' positions may

Table 4. Endotoxic activities of 1- or 4'-monophosphoryl and dephospho analogs of LA-15-PP and LA-14-PP as compared with those of the parent compounds[a]

Compound	Lethal toxicity; LD_{50} (ng)		Shwartzman reaction (preparatory activity)	Pyrogenicity
	Chick embryos	GalN-loaded mice	min. effect. dose (μg)	min. effect. dose (μg)
LA-15-PP	74	7.9	1.25	0.01
LA-15-PH	±[b]	20.0	40	1.0
LA-15-HP	- (10,000)[c]	50.1	±[d]	±[e]
LA-15-HH	- (20,000)	- (1,000)	- (80)	- (31.6)
LA-14-PP	- (10,000)	10.0	- (80)	1.0
LA-14-PH	ND[f]	316	- (80)	3.0
LA-14-HP	ND	3,381	- (80)	3.0
LA-14-HH	ND	- (1,000)	- (80)	- (31.6)

[a]Assay methods were described in footnotes of Tables 3 and 5. Data were taken from Kotani et al. (30, 31) and Takada et al. (52).
[b]Two of ten and two of eleven embryos were killed by injection of 10,000 and 2,000 ng of LA-15-PH, respectively.
[c]None of the test animals exhibited a positive reaction at the highest test dose indicated in parentheses.
[d]One of three rabbits each exhibited a positive reaction by administration of 80, 40 and 20 μg/site of LA-15-HP.
[e]One of three rabbits exhibited positive reaction by injection of 1.0 μg/kg of LA-15-HP.
[f]Not determined.

play an important role in manifestation of the lethality in chick embryos, because either monophosphoryl or dephospho analogs of LA-15-PP were scarcely lethal. The lethality in galactosamine-loaded mice was also affected by the phosphorylation pattern: In both LA-15 and 14-series compounds, especially the latter, 1,4'-bisphosphoryl compounds were most active, followed by 4'-monophosphoryl and then by 1-monophosphoryl compounds. Dephospho compounds were hardly lethal.

Among the monosaccharide lipid A analogs tested, compound 408 and GLA-27 having one double acyl group per molecule, exhibited very low, but detectable lethality, whereas compounds having none or two 3-acyloxyacyl groups, compound 401 or 410 and compound GLA-47, respectively, did not show detectable lethality (Table 3).

Explanation for different structural requirements for lethal toxicity estimated by the above two assays await further studies. Lethal toxicity tests in normal mice may give information on this point, but limited availability of test synthetic compounds have so far not permitted us to do so, because larger doses are needed for the test.

B. Shwartzman reaction: Structural requirements of lipid A for the ability to prepare the rabbit skin for local Shwartzman reaction were similar to those in the lethal toxicity in chick embryos, although LA-16-PP which

Table 5. Ability of synthetic lipid A's and their analogs to prepare rabbit skin for the local Shwartzman reaction[a]

Compound	Minimum effective dose (μg)
LA-16-PP	80
LA-15-PP	1.25
LA-14-PP	- (80)[b]
LA-18-PP	- (80)
LA-17-PP	- (80)
401	- (80)
408	- (80)
410	- (80)
GLA-47	- (80)
GLA-27	- (80)

[a]Skin sites of more than two rabbits were prepared by intracutaneous injection of the test material. Twenty hours later, the rabbits received an intravenous injection of 100 μg (per animal) of **E. coli** 0127:B8 LPS (Difco) for provocation. The minimum dose to exhibit positive reaction in majority of the test rabbits was regarded as minimum effective dose. Data were taken from Kotani et al. (30, 31, 32, 33) and Takahashi et al. (55).

[b]No positive reaction was provoked at the site prepared with the highest test dose (80 μg/site).

showed only marginal lethal toxicity in chick embryos exhibited detectable preparatory activity (Table 5). The phosphorylation pattern also influenced the preparatory activity of the LA-15 series compounds, just as it did the lethal toxicity in chick embryos and galactosamine-loaded mice; the order of preparatory activity was PP → PH → HP → HH compounds (Table 4).

Preparatory and provocative activities of LA-20-PP and LA-21-PP, which have one 3-acyloxyacyl group in the amino group on the C-2 and C-2' position, respectively, have been studied by the Borstel/Freiburg group (49). Both compounds expressed similar definite preparative activity, although it was less than that of the reference LPS. Concerning the provocative activity, LA-21-PP was less active than LA-20-PP, which seems to be less active than LA-15-PP according to the finding of Galanos et al. (11) (Table 6). Thus structural requirements of lipid A analogs for provocation of a local Shwartzman reaction seem to be more strict than those for the preparative activity, although available data have so far been too limited to draw a general conclusion.

C. Pyrogenicity: Requirement of a suitable number of 3-acyloxyacyl groups on the disaccharide backbone for pyrogenicity is apparent as shown in Table 7. Compound LA-15-PP, which has two double acyl groups, was most pyrogenic in terms of minimum pyrogenic dose. The pyrogenicity of LA-20-PP and LA-21-PP, both of which have one double acyl group was not so different from

Table 6. Preparation and provocation of the local Shwartzman reaction by synthetic precursor Ib (IVB) (LA-20-PP), its isomer (LA-21-PP) and a reference LPS[a]

Pretreatment (day o, intradermal injection)		Degree of skin reaction after intravenous challenge (day 1, 50 μg) with		
Compound	Dose (μg)	LA-20-PP	LA-21-PP	LPS
LA-20-PP	100	4+	2+	3+
	50	3+	2+	2+
	25	2+	1+	2+
	12.5	1+	1+	1+
LA-21-PP	100	4+	2+	2+
	50	3+	2+	2+
	25	2+	1+	1+
	12.5	1+	0	1+
LPS[b]	50	5+	4+	5+
	25	4+	3+	4+

[a]Skin lesion provoked 4 hr after intravenous challenge was graded as follows: 5+, very strong; 4+, strong; 3+, medium; 2+, mild; 1+, slight; 0, no reaction. Quoted from Rietschel et al. (49).
[b]Lipopolysaccharide of **Salmonella abortus-equi.**

that of LA-15-PP, while LA-16-PP having three double acyl groups was significantly less pyrogenic than LA-15-PP. LA-14-PP having none was 100 times less pyrogenic than LA-15-PP. The presence of 3-acyloxyacyl groups in an appropriate number seems to be required for high pyrogenicity. Among other disaccharide bisphosphate compounds having no double acyl groups, some analogs exhibited weak pyrogenicity, but were never comparable in minimum pyrogenic dose to the compounds having double acyl groups.

All the acylated glucosamine phosphates tested showed only weak pyrogenicity, and their minimum pyrogenic dose was at least 1,000 times higher than that of LA-15-PP (Table 7).

Regarding the role of 1- or 4'-phosphate groups on the disaccharide backbone in pyrogenicity, the assay with LA-15 series compounds revealed that pyrogenicity decreased in the order of PP → PH → HP → HH compounds as in the

Table 7. Pyrogenicity of synthetic lipid A's and their analogs

Compound	Minimum pyrogenic dose (μg/kg)		
	Kotani's group[a]	Freiburg/Borstel group[b]	Homma's group[c]
LA-16-PP	0.1	0.4	0.1
LA-15-PP	0.01	0.004	0.001
LA-20-PP	ND[d]	0.01	ND
LA-21-PP	ND	0.05	ND
LA-14-PP	1.0	0.4	3.0
LA-18-PP	- (10.0)[e]	ND	1.0
LA-24-PP	1.0	ND	ND
LA-17-PP	10.0	ND	1.0
LA-23-PP	1.0	ND	ND
401	10.0	ND	ND
408	31.6	ND	ND
410	31.6	ND	ND
GLA-47	31.6	ND	- (30.0)
GLA-27	- (31.6)	ND	- (10.0)

[a]Taken from Kotani et al. (31, 32, 33) and Takahashi et al. (55).
[b]Taken from Galanos et al. (10, 12, 13) and Rietschel et al. (49).
[c]Taken from Kanegasaki et al. (21, 22), Homma et al. (15), and Matsuura et al. (39, 40).
[d]Not determined.
[e]No significant febrile response was detected at the highest test dose (in the parentheses).

other endotoxic activities. No difference was noted between LA-14-PH and -HP (Table 4), although Galanos's group (13) and Kanegasaki's group (22) reported that the pyrogenicity of the HP analog was stronger than that of PH analog.

Other in Vivo Bioactivities

A. Induction of interferon (IFN) and tumor necrosis factor (TNF): Table 8 summarizes the abilities of test compounds to induce IFN-α/β and TNF in appropriately primed mice. Potency of test lipid A analogs in this and

Table 8. Monokine induction in vivo by synthetic lipid A's and their analogs

Compound	Relative potency to induce		
	IFN-α/β[a]	TNF	
	(**P. acnes**-primed mice)	(BCG-primed mice)[b]	(**P. acnes**-primed mice)[c]
LA-16-PP	7	4	20
LA-15-PP	100	100	100
LA-14-PP	63	82	23
LA-18-PP	13	4	4
LA-17-PP	28	4	27
401	0.4	-[d]	ND[e]
408	0.2	0.1	ND
410	-	-	ND
GLA-47	-	-	(ND)[f]
GLA-27	ND	0.1	6

[a]ICR mice pretreated by intraperitoneal injection of heat-killed **P. acnes** 1 week before were intravenously injected with test compounds. Two hr later the levels of IFN-α/β induced in serum were determined with L929 cells and vesicular stomatitis virus system. Kotani et al. (31, 32, 33) and Takahashi et al. (55).

[b]ICR mice primed by percutaneous injection with **Mycobacterium bovis** BCG vaccine 2 weeks before were intravenously given with test compounds. Ninety min later, TNF activity in serum was assayed by the cytocidal effect on actinomycin D-treated L929 cells. Kotani et al. (31, 32, 33) and Takahashi et al. (55).

[c]ICR mice receiving the intraperitoneal injection of formalin-killed **P. acnes** 11 days before were intravenously injected with test compounds. TNF activity in serum 90 min after the injection was determined in terms of inhibition of [^{3}H] thymidine incorporation into L929 cells. Kanegasaki et al. (21, 22), Homma et al. (15), and Matsuura et al. (40).

[d]Not detected.

[e]Not determined.

[f]TNF was induced, but relative activity can not be obtained on the basis of Matsuura's report (39).

Table 9. Immunoadjuvant activity of synthetic lipid A's and their analogs to stimulate antibody production

Compound	Relative potency to stimulate antibody production against	
	SRBC[a]	BSA[b]
LA-16-PP	70	ND[c]
LA-15-PP	100	100
LA-14-PP	83	ND
LA-18-PP	ND	77
LA-17-PP	ND	83
401	2	ND
408	21	ND
GLA-47	65	ND
GLA-27	37	ND

[a]Activity to increase the number of anti-SRBC hemolytic PFC in the spleen of BALB/c mice by intraperitoneal injection with SRBC and test compound in PBS. Taken from Takahashi et al. (55).
[b]Activity to increase serum anti-BSA antibody level (determined by passive hemagglutination test) in BALB/c mice by subcutaneous injection with BSA and test compound incorporated in liposomes. Taken from Kotani et al. (32).
[c]Not determined.

the following assays is expressed as a relative value by assuming the potency of **E. coli**-type synthetic lipid A, LA-15-PP, to be 100, taking both minimum effective dose and extent of the effect into consideration. This treatment permits us to grasp the structural requirements of lipid A for these bioactivities, because assay results obtained under different experimental conditions could be roughly compared. Compound LA-15-PP exhibited strongest activities in both assays, and followed by LA-14-PP. The difference between these two compounds was not so marked as the difference in their endotoxicities. LA-16-PP as well as LA-17 or 18-PP was much less active than the above two compounds. Effect of phosphorylation pattern was examined on the TNF inducing ability of LA-15 series compounds in primed mice. LA-15-PP showed the strongest activity, followed by PH and then HP compounds (31).

All the test monosaccharide analogs of lipid A were practically inactive in induction of IFN-α/β and TNF in terms of relative potency (Table 8). Homma's group, however, reported weak, but definite TNF-inducing activity of GLA-27 in **P. acnes**-primed mice although higher doses are needed (39).

B. Immunoadjuvant activities: In terms of relative potency to that of LA-15-PP, all the test disaccharide lipid A analogs exhibited the ability to enhance the humoral immune response against sheep red blood cells (SRBC) and bovine serum albumin in BALB/c mice which was not so much different from LA-15-PP. Monosaccharide lipid A analogs, excepting compound 401, also exhibited definite adjuvant activity, and the activity of GLA-47 was close to that of the above disaccharide lipid A analogs (Table 9). Thus structural requirements of lipid A for adjuvanticity do not seem to be so strict as those for endotoxicities and IFN-α/β or TNF-inducing abilities.

The activity of LA-15 and LA-14 series compounds to induce delayed-type hypersensitivity to axobenzenarsonate-N-acetyl-(ABA)-L-tyrosine in guinea pigs was studied by Ukei et al. (59) (Table 10). Compound LA-15-PP showed the activity comparable to reference LPS and N-acetylmuramyl-L-alanyl-D-isoglutamine (MDP). The ability of LA-14-PP seemed to be less than that of LA-15-PP and to be comparable to that of LA-15-PH. Other test compounds gave marginally positive results.

C. Others: Galanos' group described the induction of tolerance to LPS by LA-15 and 14-PP. The activity of these two compounds was comparable to and somewhat less than that of reference bacterial lipid A, respectively (10, 12). They also found that LA-15-PP exhibited the antitumor activity comparable to that of bacterial **E. coli**-type lipid A in terms of necrosis and healing of Meth A fibrosarcoma carried by BALB/c mice (12). Ukei et al. (59) reported that both LA-14-PP and LA-15-HP were able to induce tumor necrosis in Meth A tumor established in BALB/c mice presensitized by **P. acnes.** LA-15-PH which is generally more bioactive than HP analogs, however, showed no activity, in this assay. LA-15-PP killed all the primed and tumor-bearing mice within one day.

Table 10. Adjuvant activity of LA-15 and 14 series compounds for induction of delayed-type hypersensitivity to ABA-Tyr in guinea pigs[a]

Compound	Induration, mm (mean ± SE)
LA-15-PP	15.0 ± 0.3
LA-15-PH	9.3 ± 1.1
LA-15-HP	4.3 ± 0.9
LA-14-PP	7.5 ± 1.7
LA-14-PH	5.0 ± 0.0
LA-14-HP	3.5 ± 0.2
LA-14-HH	2.8 ± 0.6
LPS (E. coli 055:B5)	15.0 ± 0.3
MDP	17.0 ± 0.5
Control (ABA-Tyr + FIA)	0.4 ± 0.3

[a]Groups of guinea pigs were immunized with ABA-Tyr (50 μg) in FIA with or without test compounds (50 μg). Two weeks later, skin tests were carried out by intradermal injection of ABA-BSA (50 μg/site) and the reaction was measured 48 hr later. Quoted from Ukei et al. (59).

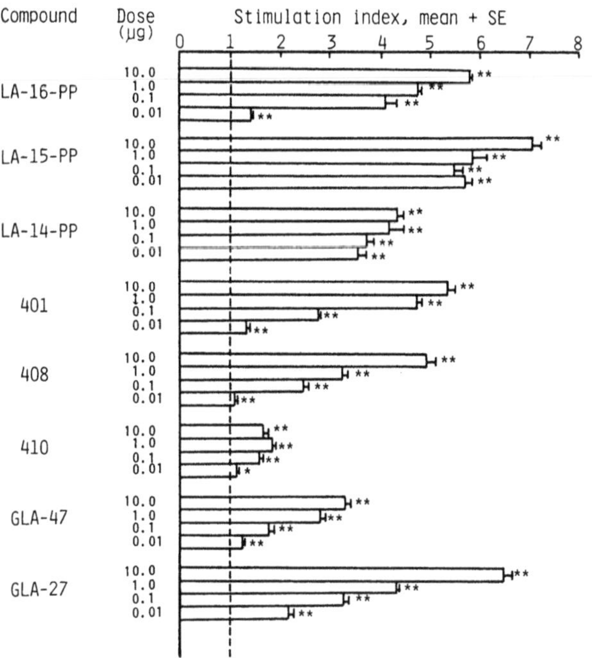

Fig 3. Mitogenic effect of synthetic lipid A's and their analogs on splenocytes of athymic nude (BALB/c nu/nu) mice. Splenocytes were cultured with test compounds for 24 hr, and then incubated with [^{3}H] thymidine for a further 24 hr. The increase in thymidine uptake was determined by the conventional method. *$P < 0.05$, **$P < 0.01$. Takahashi et al. (55).

In Vitro Bioactivities

Endotoxins are well known to modulate (mainly stimulate) various cells and enzyme cascades which are involved in defense mechanisms and homeostasis, under in vitro assay conditions. Among these activities, activation of lymphocytes, macrophages and complement cascade by synthetic lipid A's were extensively studied. Activation of the clotting enzyme cascade of amoebocyte lysates of horseshoe crab by synthetic lipid A's (**Limulus** test) has also been a target of study, because this test has been used for a long time as a possible substitute for the pyrogen test to estimate contaminating or coexistent LPS in a variety of materials. Difficulty encountered in studies on structural requirements of lipid A's for stimulatory effects on cultured lymphocytes and macrophages is that the same compounds frequently cause a different extent of stimulation from one assay to another even in seemingly the same assay conditions. This situation makes interpretation difficult. In the following description, therefore, we intended to compare the results obtained by the same assay performed with the same preparation of target cells as much as possible.

Analysis of immunodominant determinants on lipid A is also of interest. Disaccharide and monosaccharide lipid A analogs which are different in patterns of acylation and phosphorylation should be very useful as "analytical" reagents for this study. However, this topic will not be discussed here because of limited space (see Ref 1, 2, 3, 4, 23, 24).

A. Lymphocyte stimulation: Fig 3 summarizes the mitogenic activity of representative synthetic compounds on splenocytes of athymic nude mice,

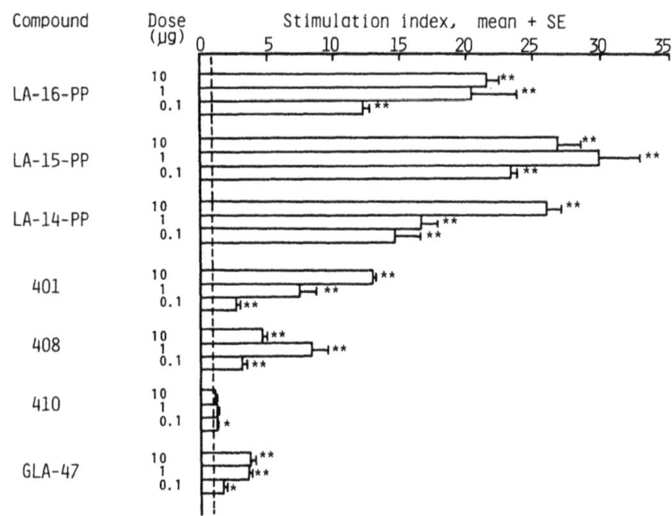

Fig 4. Polyclonal B cell activating effect of synthetic lipid A's and their analogs in BALB/c mice. *P < 0.05, **P < 0.01. Takahashi et al. (55).

essentially B cells. One can see that the effective dose and the extent of stimulation showed that LA-15-PP was the most mitogenic compound, followed by LA-14 and 16-PP. Incidentally, Rietschel's group observed that the mitogenic activity of LA-20-PP and LA-21-PP was comparable to that of LA-14 and 15-PP (49). The mitogenicity of LA-18-PP was somewhat weaker than that of LA-14-PP, which was comparable to that of LA-17-PP (32). Monophosphoryl compounds were generally less active than the respective parent bisphosphoryl compound. Differences in the activity between PH and HP compounds were at most slight, while dephospho compounds were scarcely active (31, 32, 33, 52).

Regarding monosaccharide lipid A analogs, all the test analogs, except compound 410, exhibited definite mitogenic activity. The mitogenicity of GLA-47 was minimal at a test dose of 10 μg (Fig 3). Thus, the structural requirements of lipid A for the mitogenic activity are generally not so strict as those for the bioactivities determined in vivo assays.

It may be noted that all the test synthetic lipid A and their analogs did not show any significant mitogenicity on splenocytes of LPS-nonresponsive C3H/HeJ mice, like bacterial lipid A and LPS (10, 13, 21, 22, 30, 32, 33, 49, 52, 55). This finding indicates that test synthetic compounds including monosaccharide lipid A analogs exert stimulatory effects on murine B cells by a mechanism common with bacterial products.

Polyclonal B cell activating (PBA) effects, determined in terms of increase in background plaque forming cell counts against SRBC or 2, 4, 6-trinitrophenylated SRBC (TNP-SRBC), possessed stricter structural requirements than those for the mitogenicity (Fig 4). LA-15-PP exhibited stronger activity than LA-14 and 16-PP. Remarkable differences were noted in the PBA activity between disaccharide and monosaccharide lipid A analogs. Both LA-18-PP and LA-17-PP (data not shown) also exhibited definite PBA effects, which were weaker than bacterial **E. coli** lipid A (32). Monophosphoryl compounds, both PH and HP compounds of LA-14 and LA-15 series, caused PBA, but to a lesser extent than the respective PP compound (31, 52).

B. Macrophage stimulation: The macrophage stimulating effects of

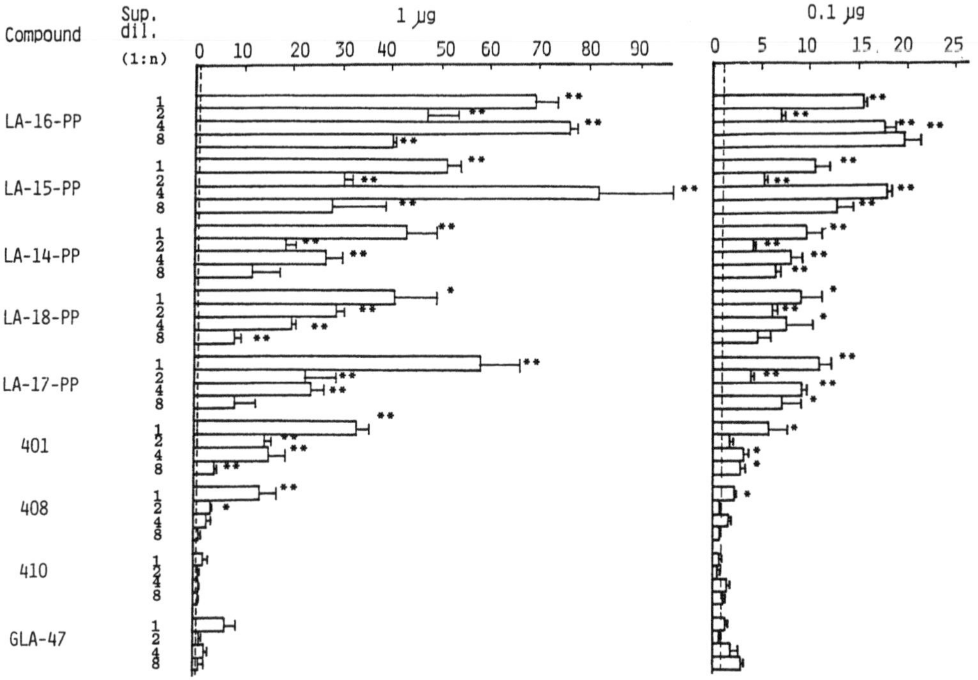

Fig 5. Enhanced IL-1 production by DBA/2 mice peritoneal macrophages stimulated by two different doses (0.1 and 1.0 μg) of synthetic lipid A's and their analogs. IL-1 activity was measured by mitogenic response of thymocytes from C3H/HeJ mice in the presence of a submitogenic dose of phytohemagglutinin (1 μg/ml). $*P < 0.05$, $**P < 0.01$. Takahashi et al. (56).

synthetic lipid A's and their analogs were extensively studied in terms of enhanced generation of IL-1 (32, 33, 38, 55, 56), prostaglandin E2 (10, 12, 13, 32, 33, 49, 55) and superoxide anion (31, 32, 33, 55), increased uptake of glucosamine (30, 31), increased spreading on tissue culture plate (30, 31, 55), and enhanced phagocytosis (52). Among these studies, that of Takahashi et al., (55, 56) was the most informative on structural requirements for macrophage stimulation by lipid A, because comparisons were made under essentially the same assay conditions. Fig 5 shows the structural dependency of enhancement of IL-1 generation by peritoneal macrophages from DBA/2 mice which were incubated with test synthetic lipid A's and their analogs. Compound LA-16-PP as well as LA-15-PP was a very powerful IL-1 inducer. The activity of disaccharide analogs having no 3-acyloxyacyl groups, such as LA-14, 18 and 17-PP, was less than that of compounds with double acyl groups. Among the monosaccharide lipid A analogs, compound 401 definitely enhanced the generation of IL-1, but the extent of enhancement was far less than that by disaccharide lipid A analogs. Other acyl glucosamine phosphates were scarcely active.

Although the effects of phosphorylation pattern on stimulation by LA-15 and 14 series compounds were not examined in Takahashi's study, Loppnow et al. (38) gave us informations on this point (Fig 6). They examined the activity of culture supernatant of human peripheral blood mononuclear cells incubated with test compounds for co-mitogenic activity in thymocyte assay and growth-promoting activity in the fibroblast assay. They found much stronger IL-1 inducing ability of LA-15-HP (compound 505) than LA-15-PP, LA-

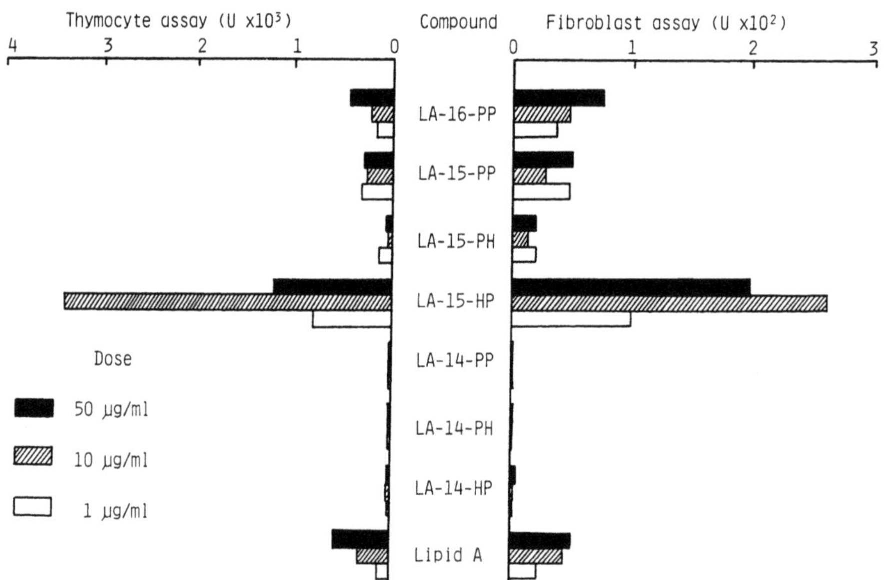

Fig 6. Induction of IL-1 in human peripheral blood mononuclear cell cultures by three different doses of synthetic lipid A's and their analogs. IL-1 activity was determined in terms of co-mitogenic activity in thymocyte assay and growth-promoting activity in fibroblast assay. Data are shown as units calculated by comparison with a standard. Quoted from Loppnow et al. (38).

16-PP (506 and 516, respectively), bacterial lipid A, and LPS. It may be added here, however, that LA-15-HP was less active than LA-15-PP, if the effective doses of both compounds were taken into consideration (Loppnow, personal communication). LA-15-PH was only slightly active, and LA-14 series compounds practically lacked the activity. Thus, the structural requirements of lipid A for enhanced IL-1 generation of macrophages seemed different from those for other bioactivities, although no cell-associated IL-1 activity was estimated in the above studies.

Structural requirements of lipid A for PGE_2 generation in resident peritoneal macrophages of ICR mice were essentially the same as those for other in vitro bioactivities, as shown in Fig 7. The activity of LA-15-PP was the strongest, judging from both the effective dose and the extent of enhanced PGE_2 generation, and this was followed by the activity of LA-14-PP and then by that of LA-16-PP. Significant differences were noted between the disaccharide and monosaccharide lipid A analogs. Although data were not shown, compounds LA-17-PP and LA-18-PP were comparably active to LA-14-PP (32, 33). Regarding precursor Ib-type LA-20-PP and its isomer, LA-21-PP, Rietschel's group found that these compounds stimulated PGE_2 release from murine resident peritoneal macrophages to a similar extent as LA-15-PP (49). Galanos, on the other hand, studied the role of phosphate groups, showing that all LA-14-PP, PH and HP compounds caused marked enhancement of PGE_2 production, and the stimulatory activity of LA-14-PP and -HP was higher than that of bacterial lipid A (10).

Structural requirements of lipid A for macrophage stimulation in terms of increase in superoxide anion release by guinea pig peritoneal macrophages (Fig 8) were similar to those for PGE_2 generation in murine macrophages.

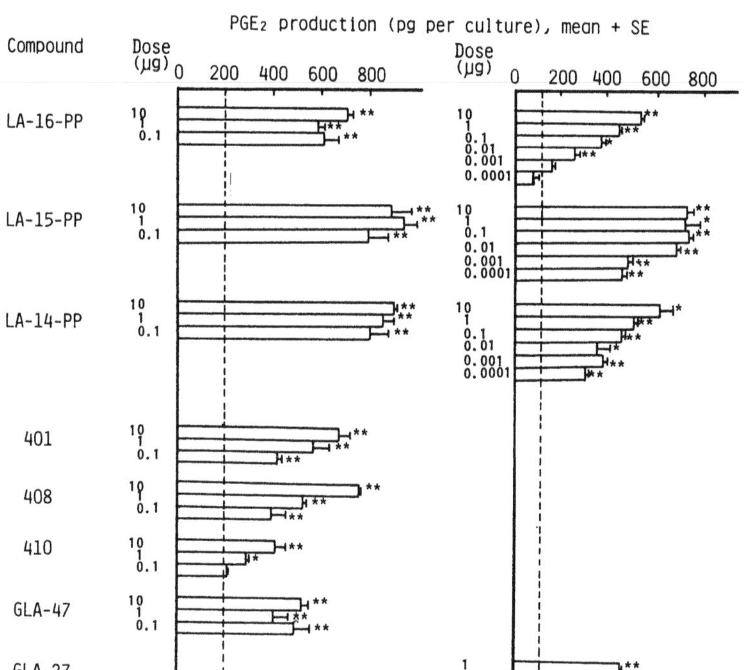

Fig 7. Enhanced PGE_2 production by murine resident peritoneal macrophages following stimulation with synthetic lipid A's and their analogs. Resident peritoneal macrophages of ICR mice were cultured with test compounds for 24 hr and PGE_2 generation determined by radioimmunoassay. $*P < 0.05$, $**P < 0.01$. Takahashi et al. (55).

However, differences among LA-16, 15, 18, and 17-PP and the respective PH compounds were not distinct unlike with those in PGE_2 generation (31, 32, 33).

The ability to enhance $[^{14}C]$ glucosamine uptake and spreading of guinea pig macrophages seemed to be more strictly dependent upon chemical structure than other macrophage stimulating activities (Fig 9). Monosaccharide analogs of lipid A, except compound GLA-27, were devoid of the activities. Considerable differences in activity were noted between PP compounds and the respective PH (or HP) compounds of the LA-15 series (31). No significant differences were found among the LA-14 series compounds (30).

C. Limulus activity: The **Limulus** test was carried out by both conventional gelation method, PreGel test, and colorimetric methods, namely toxicolor and endospecy tests. The difference between the latter two tests is the use of purified coagulation factor, factor C, in the endospecy test and the use of not extensively purified amoebocyte lysates contaminating factor G, which is sensitive to β(1-3)-**D**-glucan, in the toxicolor test (20, 43).

In the PreGel test (Table 11), all the test bisphosphoryl disaccharide compounds having 3-acyloxyacyl or 3-hydroxyacyl groups exhibited equally potent gelating activity, although LA-24-PP showed somewhat lower activity. Compounds LA-17-PP and LA-23-PP which have only nonhydroxylated acyl groups were ten and one hundred times less active than the above compounds, respec-

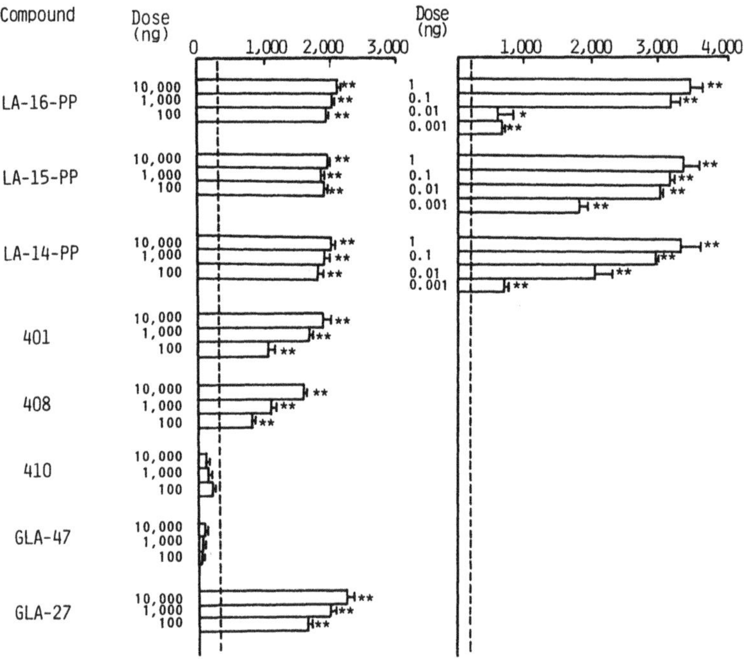

Fig 8. Production of O_2^- by guinea pig peritoneal macrophages stimulated with synthetic lipid A's and their analogs. Peritoneal macrophages induced by the injection of liquid paraffin were cultured with test compounds for 48 hr. The cultured cells then were stimulated by addition of wheat germ agglutinin and cytochalasin E. Superoxide anion (O_2^-) generation was determined in terms of reduction rate of cytochrome c added to the culture. $*P < 0.05$, $**P < 0.01$. Takahashi et al. (55).

tively. Acylated glucosamine phosphates were generally less active than disaccharide analogs of lipid A.

Both toxicolor and endospecy tests (Table 11) allowed clear distinction between the activity of disaccharide lipid A analogs having either 3-acyloxyacyl or 3-hydroxyacyl groups and those having only non-hydroxylated acyl groups. The compounds in the first groups, including bacterial products, were much more active than those in the second group. Among compounds in the first groups, those with one or two double acyl groups, LA-20 and 21-PP or LA-15 and 22-PP, respectively, were more reactive than those with three or none of the double acyl groups, LA-16 and 14-PP, respectively. Identical **Limulus** activity of LA-15-PP and LA-22-PP indicates that the site of the double acyl groups on the disaccharide bisphosphate backbone does not play a significant role in the activation of the horseshoe crab clotting enzyme cascade.

Monosaccharide lipid A analogs were much less reactive in both colorimetric tests than disaccharide analogs, irrespective of the fact that all of them have either 3-hydroxyacyl- or 3-acyloxyacyl group. The activity of monosaccharide lipid A analogs were thus comparable to those of disaccharide analogs having only non-hydroxylated acyl groups such as LA-17-PP and LA-23-PP.

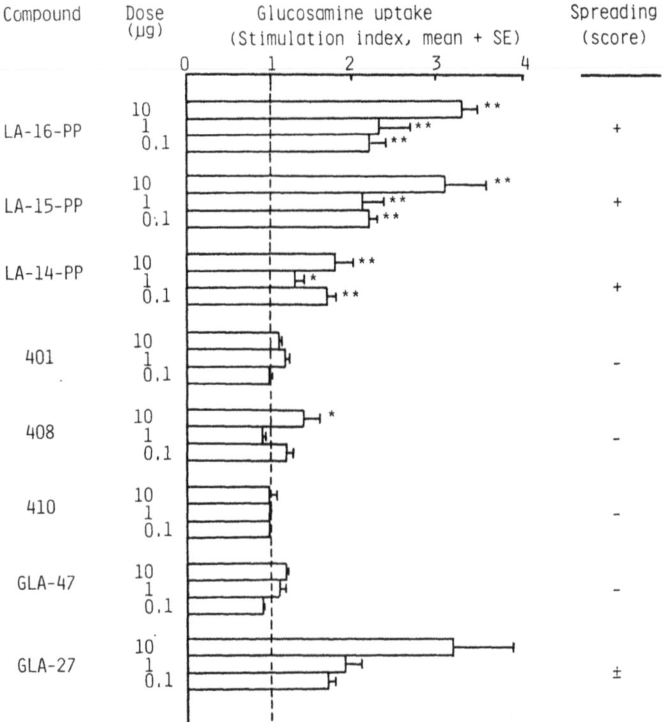

Fig 9. Stimulation of liquid paraffin-elicited guinea pig peritoneal macrophages by synthetic lipid A's and their analogs to increase [^{14}C] glucosamine uptake and spreading. Spreading was graded as follows: -, < 10%; ±, 10 to < 30%; +, ≥ 30%. *P < 0.05, **P < 0.01. Takahashi et al. (55).

The effects of phosphorylation pattern on the reactivity in PreGel and toxicolor tests are shown in Table 12. The reactivity in both tests decreased from strongly reactive PP compounds through PH derivative to HH compound, the last of which was hardly active.

As a whole the colorimetric tests were much more sensitive to changes in chemical structure and correlated better with pyrogenicity of the test compounds than the conventional gelation test, although the pyrogenicity is more dependent on chemical structure than even the colorimetric **Limulus** activity. This finding is noteworthy in view of the fact that the **Limulus** test has often been used as a substitute for the much more laborious pyrogenicity test in rabbits.

PROPOSED CLASSIFICATION OF BIOACTIVITIES OF LIPID A ON THE BASIS OF STRUCTURAL REQUIREMENTS

Different structural requirements of lipid A for various bioactivities tempt us to divide the bioactivities of lipid A's into several categories, as proposed in Table 13. Bioactivities in category I require an appropriate number (probably one or two) of 3-acyloxyacyl groups on the β(1-6)-linked **D**-glucosamine disaccharide bisphosphate backbone; namely LA-15, 20 and 21-PP are active, but other compounds are inactive or far less active (not enough data have so far been available on LA-22-PP). Most of the "typical" endotoxic activities belong to this category. This category may be further divided into two subcategories by degree of dependence on fine chemical

Table 11. Activation of the clotting enzyme cascade of **T. tridentatus** amoebocyte lysate by synthetic lipid A's and their analogs[a]

Compound	Equivalent of reference LPS[b] (mg/mg) by		
	PreGel Test	Toxicolor Test	Endospecy Test
LA-16-PP	10	1.50	1.41
LA-15-PP	10	5.52	5.18
LA-22-PP	10	5.50	5.10
LA-20-PP	10	4.28	4.33
LA-21-PP	10	8.90	8.00
LA-14-PP	10	1.98	1.56
LA-18-PP	10	0.24	0.25
LA-24-PP	1.0	0.56	0.56
LA-17-PP	1.0	0.00084	0.00071
LA-23-PP	0.1	0.000063	0.000040
401	0.1	0.00309	0.0032
408	1.0	0.00036	0.00030
410	0.1	0.00699	0.00571
GLA-47	1.0	0.00028	0.00016
GLA-27	1.0	0.000063	0.000040
(1-3) - β -D-glucan[c]	ND[d]	0.25	0.00

[a]Data were taken from Takada et al. (53).
[b]**E. coli** O111:B4 LPS (Difco).
[c]Prepared from **Alcaligenes faecalis** var. **myxogenes** IFO 13140 (Curdlan; Wako Pure Chemicals).
[d]Not determined.

structure. Subcategory I-1 type bioactivities show the greatest dependence on structure. Preparative activities for the Shwartzman reaction and the lethal toxicity in chick embryos (and probably in mice) belong to this subcategory. On the other hand, subcategory I-2 type bioactivities, such as pyrogenicity are exhibited by some monosaccharide lipid A analogs, although to a far less extent than that of the disaccharide bisphosphate compounds having an appropriate number of the double acyl groups.

Category II embraces most of the bioactivities other than endotoxicities listed in category I, and includes the lethality in galactosamine-loaded

Table 12. Activation of the clotting enzyme cascade of **T. tridentatus** amoebocyte lysate by LA-15 and 14 series compounds[a]

Compound	Equivalent of reference LPS[b] (mg/mg) by	
	PreGel Test	Toxicolor Test
LA-15-PP	10	5.52
LA-15-PH	10	0.83
LA-15-HP	1.0	0.044
LA-15-HH	0.001	0.00113
LA-14-PP	10	1.98
LA-14-PH	10	1.707
LA-14-HP	0.1	0.049
LA-14-HH	0.001	0.000062

[a]Data were taken from Takada et al. (53).
[b]**E. coli** O111:B4 LPS (Difco).

mice. This type of bioactivity is exhibited by LA-14-PP at a level similar to that of disaccharide bisphosphate compounds having 3-acyloxyacyl groups. This category may be further divided into two subcategories, II-1 and II-2, in consideration of bioactivities shown by monosaccharide lipid A analogs. The II-1 type bioactivities are scarcely exhibited by acylated glucosamine phosphate compounds, while the II-2 type bioactivities are exhibited by some monosaccharide lipid A analogs. Similar dependency on acylation pattern is noted among bioactivities belonging to category II as well as I; LA-15-PP shows the strongest activity in all the assays, and this was followed by LA-20 and 14-PP series compounds. Some monosaccharide lipid A analogs are active in limited assays on bioactivities of this category, but they showed generally weaker activity than the disaccharide analogs. Similar dependency on phosphorylation pattern is noted between bioactivities of categories I and II; generally, the strongest bioactivities of PP compounds were succeeded by PH compounds and then by HP compounds in the respective group of compounds. Dephospho derivatives were practically inactive.

The ability to activate human complement cascade and to stimulate macrophages to release IL-1 is different from other bioactivities listed in category I and II, with respect to dependency on chemical structure. Thus, these abilities are tentatively classified into category III. Although no description was made about the structural requirements of lipid A for complement activation in this article because of limited space, the activation of human complement cascade was caused by some monosaccharide analogs such as GLA-47 and GLA-27 (53). Their activity was very strong, and comparable to that of LA-15-PP. On the other hand, LA-14-PP, which exhibited distinct activities in other assays, scarcely caused complement avtivation, although compounds LA-14-PH and -HP resulted in distinct complement activation. Regarding enhanced IL-1 generation by macrophages, LA-16-PP was more active than LA-

Table 13. Classification of bioactivities of lipid A, proposed on the basis of structural requirements

CATEGORY I	
I-1	Lethal toxicity in chick embryos
	Shwartzman reaction
I-2	Pyrogenicity
CATEGORY II	
II-1	Lethal toxicity in galactosamine-loaded mice
	IFN-α/β inducing activity in **P. acnes**-primed mice
	TNF-inducing activity in **P. acnes**- or BCG-primed mice
	Immunoadjuvant activity (in vivo)
	Limulus activity (by colorimetric methods)
II-2	Murine splenocyte stimulating effects; mitogenicity, PBA activity (in vitro)
	Murine macrophage stimulating effects; enhancement of PGE_2 generation (in vitro)
	Guinea pig macrophage stimulating effects; enhancement of O_2^- generation and glucosamine incorporation (in vitro)
	Limulus activity (by gelation method)
CATEGORY III	
	Murine macrophage stimulating effects; enhancement of IL-1 generation (in vitro)
	Activation of complement cascade in human serum

15-PP, and LA-15-HP exhibited much higher activity than other disaccharide-type analogs, including LA-15-PP.

PROSPECT

Low Toxic Lipid A Analogs as a Possible Useful Immunostimulator

One of the purposes of the synthetic lipid A study is to create novel compounds which have good balance between endotoxicities and beneficial bioactivities such as immunoadjuvanticity, antitumor activity and the ability to induce useful cytokines. Systematic studies on structural requirements for various bioactivities by use of synthetic disaccharide and monosaccharide lipid A analogs have revealed that harmful endotoxic activities and some beneficial activities can be at least partly dissociated. Thus low toxic or "nontoxic" lipid A analogs which are applicable in clinical medicine may eventually be created. There are three approaches to this problem: 1) modi-

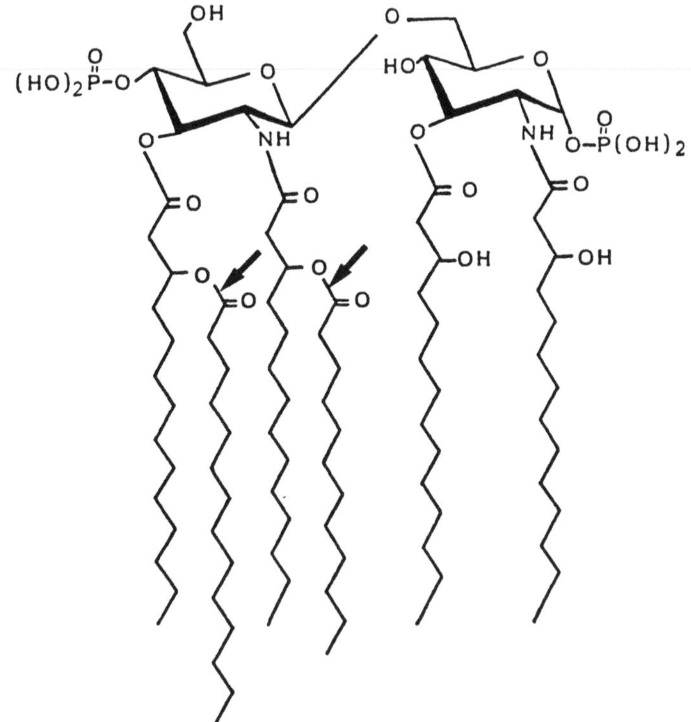

Fig 10. Proposed attacking sites (shown by arrows) on **S. typhimurium** lipid A of 3-acyloxyacyl hydrolase prepared from human peripheral blood neutrophiles. Quoted from Munford and Hall (41).

fication of acyl pattern on glucosamine disaccharide backbone; 2) modification of phosphorylation pattern of properly acylated disaccharide compounds; and 3) preparation of D-glucosamine phosphates adequately acylated. Although there is no space to discuss this subject, studies along these lines have already been started. But lipid A analogs so far synthesized do not necessarily satisfy our requirements.

It may be pertinent to add here monosphosphoryl lipid A (MPL) described by the late Dr. Edgar Ribi together with Takayama and Qureshi (47, 48, 57, 58). They prepared MPL from Re-LPS of **S. typhimurium** by hydrolysis in 0.1 N HCl in a methanol/water mixture (1:1, v/v) at 100 C. A partially purified preparation was composed of variously acylated 4'-monophosphoryl β(1-6)-linked D-glucosamine disaccharides. They investigated the ability of MPL to stimulate host resistance against microbial infections and tumor development with promising results. Although Ribi's MPL does not seem to be homogenous, one of the principal components responsible for the observed immunostimulatory activities may be an LA-15-PH type compound.

Degradation Products of Lipid A as Endogenous Immunostimulators

Studies on structure-bioactivity relationships of lipid A's have revealed that more typical endotoxic activities such as pyrogenicity, lethality and preparative activity to the Shwartzman reaction tended to be lost by a minor modification of the lipid A structure. Consequently, it is possible that lipid A's are degraded or modified in vivo to an appropriate structure and then may work as "endogenous immunomodulators" to regulate the defense and physiological mechanisms of the hosts.

Experimental evidence to support this speculation was recently given by Munford's group (14, 41, 46). They demonstrated that the granule fraction of human neutrophile leukocytes contained enzymes that were capable of partially deacylating the lipid A moiety of **S. typhimurium** LPS, as illustrated in Fig 10, to result in degradation products which were assumed to have a structure similar to LA-14-PP in lipid moiety. They speculated that during tissue invasion by gram-negative bacteria acyloxyacyl hydrolysis may be a defense mechanism that reduces the toxicity of LPS while preserving some of the potentially beneficial inflammatory and immune stimuli. Further studies along this line should help us to obtain a better understanding of the physiological roles of the interactions between host and endotoxins, which is a major cell surface component of gram-negative bacteria, many of which are indigenous to the host.

REFERENCES

1. Arata, S., Mashimo, J., Kasai, N., Okuda, K., Aihara, Y., Hasegawa, A., and Kiso, M., 1987, Analyses of antigenic reactivity of synthetic monosaccharide lipid A analogues with monoclonal antibodies. FEMS Microbiol. Lett. 44: 231.

2. Arata, S., Mashimo, J., Kasai, N., Okuda, K., Aihara, Y., Kotani, S., Takada, H., Shiba, T., Kusumoto, S., Shimamoto, T., Kusunose, N., 1988, Characterization of monoclonal lipid A antibodies with synthetic lipid A analogues. FEMS Microbiol. Lett. 49: 479.

3. Brade, L., Rietschel, E. T., Kusumoto, S., Shiba, T., and Brade, H., 1986, Immunogenicity and antigenicity of synthetic **Escherichia coli** lipid A. Infect. Immun. 51: 110.

4. Brade, L., Brandenburg, K., Kuhn, H.-M., Kusumoto, S., Macher, I., Rietschel, E. T., and Brade, H., 1987, The immunogenicity and antigenicity of lipid A are influenced by its physicochemical state and environment. Infect. Immun. 55: 2636.

5. Charon, D., Diolez, C., Mondange, M., Sarfati, S. R., Szabó, L., Szabó, P., and Trigalo, F., 1983, Synthetic studies on structural elements of the hydrophobic region present in bacterial endotoxins, in: "Bacterial Lipopolysaccharides: Structure, Synthesis, and Biological Activities", L. Anderson and F. M. Unger, ed., American Chemical Society, Washington DC, p. 301.

6. Charon, D., Chaby, R., Malinvaud, A., Mondange, M., and Szabó, L., 1985, Chemical synthesis and immunological activities of glycolipids structurally related to lipid A. Biochemistry 24: 2736.

7. Fujishima, Y., Kigawa, K., Ogawa, Y., Kiso, M., and Hasegawa, A., 1987, New synthetic immunomodulators combining a 4-O-phosphono-D-glucosamine derivative related to bacterial lipid A with 1-deoxy-N-acetylmuramoyl dipeptide analogs. Carbohyd. Res. 167: 317.

8. Galanos, C., and Lüderitz, O., 1975, Electrodialysis of lipopolysaccharides and their conversion to uniform salt forms. Eur. J. Biochem. 54: 603.

9. Galanos, C., Freudenberg, M. A., and Reutter, W., 1979, Galactosamine-induced sensitization to the lethal effects of endotoxin. Proc. Natl. Acad. Sci. U.S.A. 76: 5939.

10. Galanos, C., Lehmann, V., Lüderitz, O., Rietschel, E. T., Westphal, O.,

Brade, H., Brade, L., Freudenberg, M. A., Hansen-Hagge, T., Lüderitz, T., McKenzie, G., Schade, U., Strittmatter, W., Tanamoto, K., Zähringer, U., Imoto, M., Yoshimura, H., Yamamoto, M., Shimamoto, T., Kusumoto, S., and Shiba, T., 1984, Endotoxic properties of chemically synthesized lipid A part structures. Comparison of synthetic lipid A precursor and synthetic analogues with biosynthetic lipid A precursor and free lipid A. Eur. J. Biochem. 140: 1.

11. Galanos, C., Hansen-Hagge, T., Lehmann, V., and Lüderitz, O., 1985, Comparison of the capacity of two lipid A precursor molecules to express the local Shwartzman phenomenon. Infect. Immun. 48: 355.

12. Galanos, C., Lüderitz, O., Rietschel, E. T., Westphal, O., Brade, H., Brade, L., Freudenberg, M., Schade, U., Imoto, M., Yoshimura, H., Kusumoto, S., and Shiba, T., 1985, Synthetic and natural **Escherichia coli** free lipid A express identical endotoxic activities. Eur. J. Biochem. 148: 1.

13. Galanos, C., Lüderitz, O., Freudenberg, M., Brade, L., Schade, U., Rietschel, E. T., Kusumoto, S., and Shiba, T., 1986, Biological activity of synthetic hepta acyl lipid A representing a component of **Salmonella minnesota** R595 lipid A. Eur. J. Biochem. 160: 55.

14. Hall, C. L., and Munford, R. S., 1983, Enzymatic deacylation of the lipid A moiety of **Salmonella typhimurium** lipopolysaccharides by human neutrophils. Proc. Natl. Acad. Sci. U.S.A. 80: 6671.

15. Homma, J. Y., Matsuura, M., Kanegasaki, S., Kawakubo, Y., Kojima, Y., Shibukawa, N., Kumazawa, Y., Yamamoto, A., Tanamoto, K., Yasuda, T., Imoto, M., Yoshimura, H., Kusumoto, S., and Shiba, T., 1985, Structural requirements of lipid A responsible for the functions: a study with chemically synthesized lipid A and its analogues. J. Biochem. Tokyo 98: 395.

16. Imoto, M., Yoshimura, H., Yamamoto, M., Shimamoto, T., Kusumoto, S., and Shiba, T., 1984, Chemical synthesis of phosphorylated tetraacyl disaccharide corresponding to a biosynthetic precursor of lipid A. Tetrahedron Lett. 25: 2667.

17. Imoto, M., Yoshimura, H., Sakaguchi, N., Kusumoto, S., and Shiba, T., 1985, Total synthesis of **Escherichia coli** lipid A. Tetrahedron Lett. 26: 1545.

18. Imoto, M., Yoshimura, H., Shimamoto, T., Sakaguchi, N., Kusumoto, S., and Shiba, T., 1987, Total synthesis of **Escherichia coli** lipid A, the endotoxicity active principle of cell-surface lipopolysaccharide. Bull. Chem. Soc. Jpn. 60: 2205.

19. Imoto, M., Yoshimura, H., Yamamoto, M., Shimamoto, T., Kusumoto, S., and Shiba, T., 1987, Chemical synthesis of a biosynthetic precursor of lipid A with a phosphorylated tetraacetyl disaccharide structure. Bull. Chem. Soc. Jpn. 60: 2197.

20. Iwanga, S., Morita, T., Miyata, T., and Nakamura, T., 1985, Hemolymph coagulation system in **Limulus**, in: "Microbiology-1985", L. Schlessinger, ed., American Society for Microbiology, Washington DC, p. 29.

21. Kanegasaki, S., Kojima, Y., Matsuura, M., Homma, J. Y., Yamamoto, A., Kumazawa, Y., Tanamoto, K., Yasuda, T., Tsumita, T., Imoto, M., Yoshimura, H., Yamamoto, M., Shimamoto, T., Kusumoto, S., and Shiba, T., 1984, Biological activities of analogues of lipid A based chemically on

the revised structural model. Comparison of mediator-inducing, immunomodulating and endotoxic activities. Eur. J. Biochem. 143: 237.

22. Kanegasaki, S., Tanamoto, K., Yasuda, T., Homma, J. Y., Matsuura, M., Nakatsuka, M., Kumazawa, Y., Yamamoto, A., Shiba, T., Kusumoto, S., Imoto, M., Yoshimura, H., and Shimamoto, T., 1986, Structure-activity relationship of lipid A: Comparison of biological activities of natural and synthetic lipid A's with different fatty acid compositions. J. Biochem. Tokyo 99: 1203.

23. Kasai, N., Arata, S., Mashimo, J., Okuda, K., Aihara, Y., Kotani, S., Takada, H., Shiba, T., and Kusumoto, S., 1985, In vitro antigenic reactivity of synthetic lipid A analogues as determined by monoclonal and conventional antibodies. Biochem. Biophys. Res. Commun. 128: 607.

24. Kasai, N., Arata, S., Mashimo, J., Okuda, K., Aihara, Y., Kotani, S., Takada, H., Shiba, T., Kusumoto, S., Imoto, M., Yoshimura, H., and Shimamoto, T., 1986, Synthetic **Salmonella**-type lipid A antigen with high serological specificity. Infect. Immun. 51: 43.

25. Kiso, M., and Hasegawa, A., 1983, Synthetic studies on the lipid A component of bacterial lipopolysaccharide, in: "Bacterial Lipopolysaccharides: Structure, Synthesis, and Biological Activities", L. Anderson and F. M. Unger, ed., American Chemical Society, Washington DC, p. 277.

26. Kiso, M., Ishida, H., and Hasegawa, A., 1984, Synthesis of biologically active, novel monosaccharide analogs of lipid A. Agr. Biol. Chem. 48: 251.

27. Kiso, M., Ogawa, Y., Tanaka, S., Ishida, H., and Hasegawa, A., 1986, Synthesis of 1,5-anhydro-2-deoxy-4-O-phosphono-3-O-tetradecanoyl-2-[(3R)- and (3S)-3-tetradecanoyloxytetradecanamido]-D-glucitol (GLA-40) related to bacterial lipid A. J. Carbohyd. Chem. 5: 621.

28. Kiso, M., Tanaka, S., Tanahashi, M., Fujishima, Y., Ogawa, Y., and Hasegawa, A., 1986, Synthesis of 2-deoxy-4-O-phosphono-3-O-tetradecanoyl-2-[(3R)- and (3S)-3-tetradecanoyloxytetradecanamido]-D-glucose: A diastereoisomeric pair of 4-O-phosphono-D-glucosamine derivatives (GLA-27) related to bacterial lipid A. Carbohyd. Res. 148: 221.

29. Kiso, M., Tanaka, S., Fujita, M., Fujishima, Y., Ogawa, Y., Ishida, H., and Hasegawa, A., 1987, Synthesis of the optically active 4-O-phosphono-D-glucosamine derivatives related to the nonreducing-sugar subunit of bacterial lipid A. Carbohyd. Res. 162: 127.

30. Kotani, S., Takada, H., Tsujimoto, M., Ogawa, T., Harada, K., Mori, Y., Kawasaki, A., Tanaka, A., Nagao, S., Tanaka, S., Shiba, T., Kusumoto, S., Imoto, M., Yoshimura, H., Yamamoto, M., and Shimamoto, T., 1984, Immunobiologically active lipid A analogs synthesized according to a revised structural model of natural lipid A. Infect. Immun. 45: 293.

31. Kotani, S., Takada, H., Tsujimoto, M., Ogawa, T., Takahashi, I., Ikeda, T., Otsuka, K., Shimauchi, H., Kasai, N., Mashimo, J., Nagao, S., Tanaka, A., Tanaka, S., Harada, K., Nagaki, K., Kitamura, H., Shiba, T., Kusumoto, S., Imoto, M., and Yoshimura, H., 1985, Synthetic lipid A with endotoxic and related biological activities comparable to those of a natural lipid A from an **Escherichia coli** Re-mutant. Infect. Immun. 49: 225.

32. Kotani, S., Takada, H., Takahashi, I., Ogawa, T., Tsujimoto, M., Shimauchi, H., Ikeda, T., Okammura, H., Tamura, T., Harada, K., Tanaka,

S., Shiba, T., Kusumoto, S., and Shimamoto, T., 1986, Immunobiological activities of synthetic lipid A analogs with low endotoxicity. Infect. Immun. 54: 673.

33. Kotani, S., Takada, H., Takahashi, I., Tsujimoto, M., Ogawa, T., Ikeda, T., Harada, K., Okammura, H., Tamura, T., Tanaka, S., Shiba, T., Kusumoto, S., Imoto, M., Yoshimura, H., and Kasai, N., 1986, Low endotoxic activities of synthetic **Salmonella**-type lipid A with an additional acyloxyacyl group on the 2-amido group of β(1-6)glucosamine disaccharide 1,4'-bisphosphate. Infect. Immun. 52: 872.

34. Krueger, J. M., Kubillus, S., Shoham, S., and Davenne, D., 1986, Enhancement of slow-wave sleep by endotoxin and lipid A. Am. J. Physiol. 251: R591.

35. Kumazawa, Y., Matsuura, M., Homma, J. Y., Nakatsuru, Y., Kiso, M., and Hasegawa, A., 1985, B cell activation and adjuvant activities of chemically synthesized analogues of the nonreducing sugar moiety of lipid A. Eur. J. Immunol. 15: 199.

36. Kumazawa, Y., Matsuura, M., Maruyama, T., Homma, J. Y., Kiso, M., and Hasegawa, A., 1986, Structural requirements for inducing in vitro B lymphocyte activation by chemically synthesized derivatives related to the nonreducing **D**-glucosamine subunit of lipid A. Eur. J. Immunol. 16: 1099.

37. Kumazawa, Y., Nakatsuka, M., Takimoto, H., Furuya, T., Nagumo, T., Yamamoto, A., Homma, J. Y., Inada, K., Yoshida, M., Kiso, M., and Hasegawa, A., 1988, Importance of fatty acid substituents of chemically synthesized lipid A-subunit analogs in the expression of immunopharmacological activity. Infect. Immun. 56: 149.

37a. Kusumoto, S., Yamamoto, M., and Shiba, T., 1984, Chemical syntheses of lipid X and lipid Y, acyl glucosamine 1-phosphates isolated from **Escherichia coli** mutants. Tetrahedron Lett. 25: 3727.

38. Loppnow, E., Brade, L., Brade, H., Rietschel, E. T., Kusumoto, S., Shiba, T., and Flad, H. D., 1986, Induction of human interleukin 1 by bacterial and synthetic lipid A. Eur. J. Immunology. 16: 1263.

39. Matsuura, M., Kojima, Y., Homma, J. Y., Kubota, Y., Yamamoto, A., Kiso, M., and Hasegawa, A., 1984, Biological activities of chemically synthesized analogues of the nonreducing sugar moiety of lipid A. FEBS Lett. 167: 226.

40. Matsuura, M., Yamamoto, A., Kojima, Y., Homma, J. Y., Kiso, M., and Hasegawa, A., 1985, Biological activities of chemically synthesized partial structure analogues of lipid A. J. Biochem. Tokyo 98: 1229.

41. Munford, R. S., and Hall, C. L., 1986, Detoxification of bacterial lipopolysaccharides (endotoxins) by a human neutrophil enzyme. Science 234: 203.

42. Nakamoto, S., and Achiwa, K., 1987, Lipid A and related compounds. XVI. Synthesis of biologically active tetraacetyl-3-deoxy-D-manno-2-octulosonic acid (KDO)-(α2 →6)-**D**-glucosamine-4-phosphates, novel analogs of the nonreducing sugar moiety of lipid A. Chem. Pharm. Bull. 35: 4537.

43. Obayashi, T., Tamura, H., Tanaka, S., Ohki, M., Takahashi, S., Arai, M., Masuda, M., and Kawai, T., 1985, A new chromogenic endotoxin-specific

assay using recombined limulus coagulation enzymes and its clinical applications. Clinica Chim. Acta. 149: 55.

44. Ogawa, T., Kotani, S., Kusumoto, S., and Shiba, T., 1987, Analgesic action of endotoxic lipopolysaccharides, bacterial and synthetic lipid A's and their low toxic analogs in decreasing acetic acid-induced abdominal-writhing response in mice, in: "International Symposium on Pyrogen", Z. Haijun, ed., Chinese Pharmaceutical Association, p. 63.

45. Ogawa, Y., Fujishima, Y., Konishi, I., Kiso, M., and Hasegawa, A., 1987, The chemical modification of the C-1 substituent of a 4-O-phosphono-D-glucosamine derivative (GLA-27) related to bacterial lipid A. J. Carbohyd. Chem. 6: 399.

46. Pohlman, T. H., Munford, R. S., and Harlan, J. M., 1987, Deacylated lipopolysaccharide inhibits neutrophil adherence to endothelium induced by lipopolysaccharide in vitro. J. Exp. Med. 165: 1393.

47. Qureshi, N., Takayama, K., and Ribi, E., 1982, Purification and structural determination of nontoxic lipid A obtained from the lipopolysaccharide of **Salmonella typhimurium**. J. Biol. Chem. 257: 11808.

48. Ribi, E., Amano, K., Cantrell, J., Shwartzman, S., Parker, R., and Takayama, K., 1982, Preparation and antitumor activity of nontoxic lipid A. Cancer Immunol. Immunother. 12: 91.

49. Rietschel, E. T., Brade, L., Schade, U., Galanos, C., Freudenberg, M., Lüderitz, O., Kusumoto, S., and Shiba, T., 1987, Endotoxic properties of synthetic pentaacyl lipid A precursor Ib and a structural isomer. Eur. J. Biochem. 169: 27.

50. Shimizu, T., Akiyama, S., Masuzawa, T., Yanagihara, Y., Nakamoto, S., and Achiwa, K., 1987, Biological activities of chemically synthesized 2-keto-3-deoxyoctonicacid-($\alpha 2 \rightarrow 6$)-D-glucosamine analogs of lipid A. Infect. Immun. 55: 2287.

51. Shimizu, T., Akiyama, S., Masuzawa, T., Yanagihara, Y., Nakamoto, S., and Achiwa, K., 1987, Antitumor activity and lethal toxicity of chemically synthesized tetraacetyl-2-keto-3-deoxyoctonic acid-($\alpha 2 \rightarrow 6$)-D-glucosamine analogues of lipid A. Chem. Pharm. Bull. 35: 873.

52. Takada, H., Kotani, S., Tsujimoto, M., Ogawa, T., Takahashi, I., Harada, K., Katukawa, C., Tanaka, S., Shiba, T., Kusumoto, S., Imoto, M., Yoshimura, H., Yamamoto, M., and Shimamoto, T., 1985, Immunopharmacological activities of a synthetic counterpart of a biosynthetic lipid A precursor molecule and of its analogs. Infect. Immun. 48: 219.

53. Takada, H., Kotani, S., Tanaka, S., Ogawa, T., Takahashi, I., Tsujimoto, M., Komuro, T., Shiba, T., Kusumoto, S., Kusunose, N., Hasegawa, A., and Kiso, M., 1988, Structural requirements of lipid A species in activation of clotting enzymes from horseshoe crab, and the human complement cascade. Eur. J. Biochem. 175: 573.

54. Takada, H., and Kotani, S., 1989, Structural requirements of lipid A for endotoxicity and other biological activities. CRC Critic. Rev. Microbiol. (in press).

55. Takahashi, I., Kotani, S., Takada, H., Tsujimoto, M., Ogawa, T., Shiba, T., Kusumoto, S., Yamamoto, M., Hasegawa, A., Kiso, M., Nishijima, M.,

Amano, F., Akamatsu, Y., Harada, K., Tanaka, S., Okamura, H. and Tamura, T., 1987, Requirement of a properly acylated β(1-6)-**D**-glucosamine disaccharide bisphosphate structure for efficient manifestation of full endotoxic and associated bioactivities of lipid A. Infect. Immun. 55: 57.

56. Takahashi, I., Kotani, S., Takada, H., Shiba, T. and Kusumoto, S., 1988, Structural requirements of endotoxic lipopolysaccharides and bacterial cell walls in induction of interleukin-1. Blood Purification 6: 188.

57. Takayama, K., Qureshi, N., Raetz, C. R. H., Ribi, E., Peterson, J., Cantrell, J. L., Pearson, F. C., Wiggins, J., and Johnson, A. G., 1984, Influence of fine structure of lipid A on **Limulus** amoebocyte lysate clotting and toxic activities. Infect. Immun. 45: 350.

58. Takayama, K., Qureshi, N., Ribi, E., and Cantrell, J. L., 1984, Separation and characterization of toxic and nontoxic forms of lipid A. Rev. Infect. Dis. 6: 439.

59. Ukei, S., Iida, J., Shiba, T., Kusumoto, S., and Azuma, I., 1986, Adjuvant and antitumour activities of synthetic lipid A □ analogues. Vaccine 4: 21.

60. Westphal, O., and Lüderitz, O., 1954, Chemische Erforschung von Lipopolysacchariden gramnegativer Bakaterien. Angew. Chem. 66: 407.

61. Westphal, O., Lüderitz, O., Galanos, C., Mayer, H., and Rietschel, E. T., 1986, The story of bacterial endotoxin. Adv. Immunopharmacol. 3: 13.

NATURAL VARIANTS OF LIPID A

H. Mayer, J. H. Krauss, A. Yokota and J. Weckesser*

Max-Planck-Institut für Immunbiologie, D-7800 Freiburg i.Br.
and *Institut für Biologie II, Mikrobiologie, der Universität
D-7800 Freiburg i.Br., FRG

INTRODUCTION

Recent studies by several groups (46,58,61,63) have revealed that the now "classical" structure of enterobacterial lipid A, the 1,4'-bisphosphorylated β-1,6-linked glucosamine disaccharide with amide- and esterlinked 3-hydroxy fatty acids or 3-acyloxyacyl residues (25a,44), is not universally distributed amongst gram-negative bacteria. It is especially not frequently encountered in families being phylogenetically remote from Enterobacteriaceae, such as the phototrophic bacteria or the thiobacilli. (59,65).

Initially we called deviating lipid A structures "unusual" lipid A-types (28), but now we would like to refer to them rather as lipid A variants, because of studies during the past few years in which these deviating lipid A's have been recognized also in thiobacilli (70,71), in bradyrhizobia (31), in Nitrobacter (29) in Brucella (37) and in members of the Chromatiaceae and the Chlorobiaceae families (33), to name only a few examples. This indicates that lipid A is not that non-variable as assumed previously (14,43), but shows a remarkable variability in its backbone structure as well as in its substitution.

Furthermore, we will avoid the designation "lipid A-types" since it would implicate distinct and characteristic structures, but the more recent investigations have shown that transitional forms of lipid A variants are as well existing. In Rhodobacter sphaeroides, only part of the amide-linked 3-hydroxy fatty acid is replaced by 3-oxo-myristic acid (48), whereas in lipid A from Rhodobacter capsulatus 37b4 this replacement is almost complete (J. H. Krauss, Thesis, Univ. Freiburg, 1988). In species of the Chromatiaceae family we find glucosamine (GlcN) as the lipid A backbone sugar, but it is always accompanied by a small amount of 2,3-diamino-2,3-dideoxy-D-glucose (34).

In the following sections we want to compile our recent knowledge on the chemistry, the distribution and the biological properties of the lipid A variants investigated so far. Also discussed will be the potential significance of these structural pecularities as it relates to bacterial relatedness.

ANALYSIS AND DISTRIBUTION OF TAXONOMICALLY RELEVANT LIPID A CONSTITUENTS

It is of value to discuss structural characteristics of a few otherwise only rarely encountered sugar and fatty acid constituents identified in distinct lipid A variants. This list will have to be extended by other characteristic lipid A constituents when more detailed and broader investigations become available.

2,3-Diamino-2,3-dideoxy-D-glucose (DAG)

The diamino sugar, DAG, has so far only been encountered in nature as the backbone sugar of lipid A. Uronic acid derivatives of 2,3-diamino-2,3-dideoxy-hexoses are reported as part of the somatic antigens (O-chains) of different serotypes of Pseudomonas aeruginosa (21).

Since the first isolation and characterization of DAG in 1975 by Roppel et al. (46) and Keilich et al. (20), DAG has been detected in lipid A of about 25 bacterial species belonging to 12 different genera or families (see Table 1).

For a quick screening of LPS or lipid A isolates for the presence of DAG, hydrolysates (4 M HCl, 100°C, 18h) are usually subjected to high-voltage paper electrophoresis (3 kV, 10 V/cm, 1-2 h) using glucosamine (GlcN) and glucose (non-migrating in pyridine/acetic acid buffer of pH 5.3) as standards. DAG shows a considerably higher electrophoretic mobility than GlcN (M_{GlcN} = 1.16 at pH 5.3 and 1.49 at pH 2.8) and is thus easily detectable and separable from most other LPS components (30,59). Very characteristic is the orange-brown staining of DAG with ninhydrin when heated at 100°C (46).

GC-MS analyses of the alditol acetate derivative of DAG have been performed either on a packed OV17 column or on a DB-5 (30 m x 0.25 mm, i.d.) capillary column (ICT, Frankfurt a.M., F.R.G.), using a temperature program from 120°C to 300°C, with a ramp rate of 10°C/min. Both columns allow a separation of the alditol acetates of the three diaminohexoses available as standards with D-allo, D-gluco- and D-galacto-configuration (35) and which elute in this order (46).

The mass spectrum of the alditol acetate derivative of DAG obtained from lipid A of the pathogenic species <u>Brucella melitensis</u> (Fig 1.) ($NaBH_4$ reduced, 36, 37) was compared with that of (NaB_2H_4 reduced) authentic DAG, obtained by chemical synthesis (35). Both spectra differ only insignificantly since most fragments originate from the common primary fragment m/z 288.

The mass spectrum is, however, similar to that of another lipid A amino sugar, namely of the 4-amino-4-deoxy-L-arabinose. This component occurs frequently as a polar headgroup attached to the ester-linked phosphate group of the lipid A backbone (25,45) and shows also a yellow-brown staining with ninhydrin. 4-Amino-4-deoxy-L-arabinose is, in contrast to DAG an acidlabile sugar and when reduced with NaB_2H_4 and analyzed by GC-MS, affords a mass spectrum which is clearly discernible from that of DAG by showing fragments at m/z 289, 247 and 229, instead of those at m/e 288, 246 and 228, when reduced with $NaBH_4$ (Fig 2). 4-Amino-4-deoxy-L-arabinose has been detected in <u>Salmonella</u>, <u>Yersinia</u>, <u>Proteus</u>, <u>Providencia</u> and <u>morganella</u> (8, 23) and in strains of Rhodocyclus tenuis and Rhodocyclus purpureus (40, 56).

3-Oxo-myristic Acid (3-oxo-14:0)

The occurrence of 3-oxo-myristic acid was first reported from Vibrio

Table 1. Bacteria reported to contain diaminoglucose (DAG) in lipid A of their lipopolysaccharides: (a) phototrophic species and (b) non-phototrophic species.

	Genus	Species	DAG-content*
(a)	Rhodopseudomonas	R.viridis	+++
		R.sulfoviridis	+++
		R.palustris	+++
	Rhodopila	R.globiformis	+++
	Chromatium	C.vinosum	+
		C.tepidum	+
	Thiocapsa	T.roseopersicina	+
		T.pfennigii	+
	Thiocystis	T.violacea	+
	Ectothiorhodospira	E.vacuolata	+
	Chlorobium	C.vibrioforme	+
(b)	Pseudomonas	P.diminuta	+++
		P.vesicularis	+++
		P.carboxydovorans	++
	Thiobacillus	T.ferrooxidans	++
		T.thiooxidans	++
		T.novellus	+++
		T.sp.IFO14570	+++
	Bradyrhizobium	B.japonicum	++
		B.(R.)lupini	++
	Nitrobacter	N.hamburgensis	+++
		N.winogradskyi	+++
	Phenylobacterium	P.immobile	+++
	Brucella	B.melitensis	++
		B.abortus	++

*+++) lipid A contains exclusively DAG,
++) lipid A contains DAG, but may also contain GlcN,
+) lipid A contains only traces of DAG besides high amounts of GlcN.

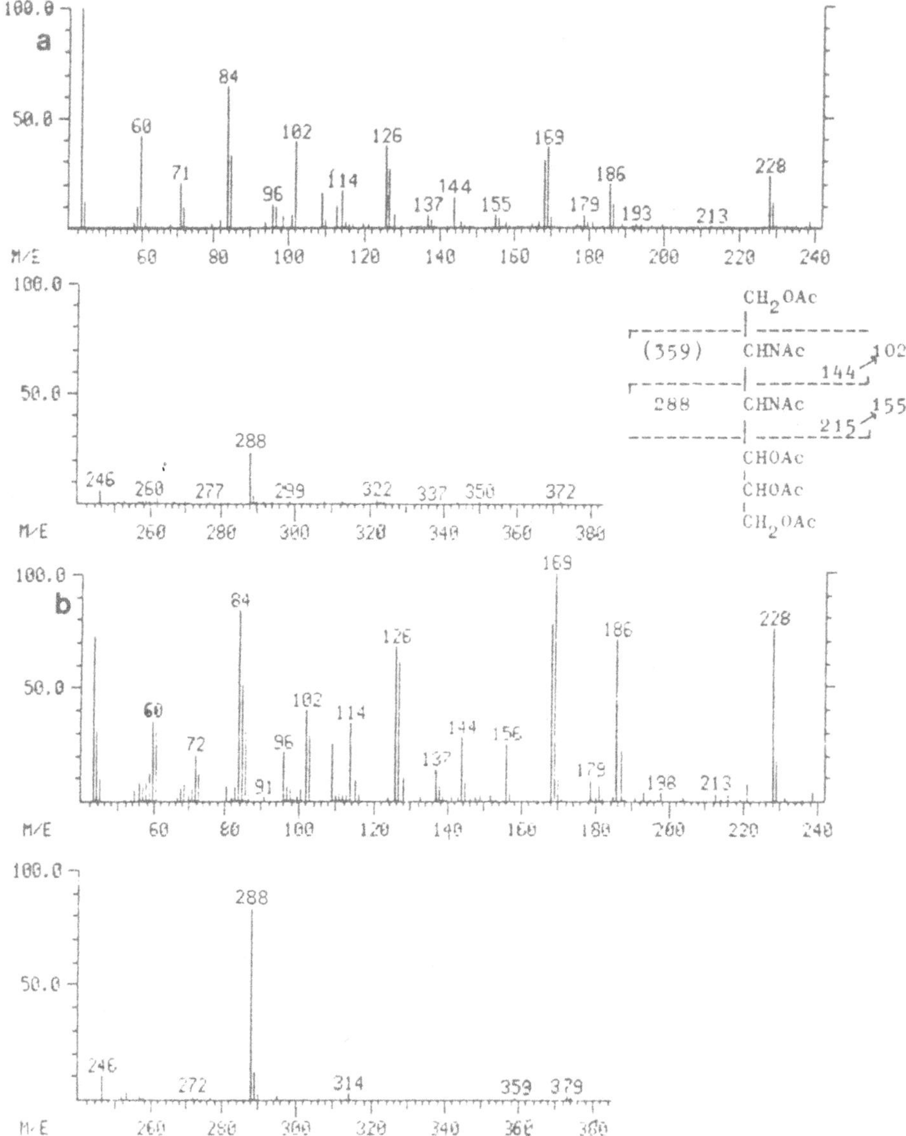

MS of alditol acetate of

(a) Brucella lipid A amino sugar, and

(b) authentic 2,3-diamino-D-glucose ($NaBD_4$-red.)

Fig 1. Mass spectra (as alditol acetate) of 2,3-diamino-2,3-dideoxy-D-glucose: (a) isolated from lipid A of Brucella melitensis (reduced with $NaBH_4$) (36, 37) (b) chemically synthesized standard reduced with NaB_2H_4 (35).

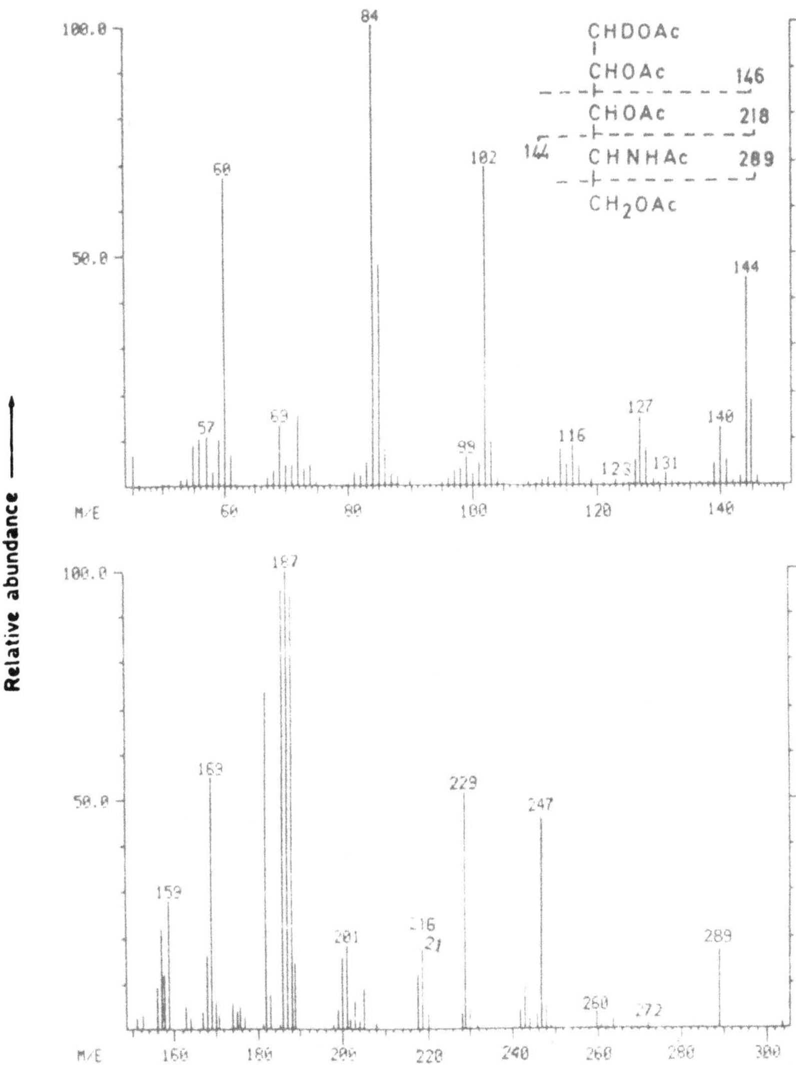

Fig 2. Mass spectrum of the alditol acetate of 4-amino-4-deoxy-L-arabinose (reduced with NaB_2H_4), isolated from a partial hydrolysate of LPS of Providencia rettgeri (3).

anguillarum (D. Shaw, St. John's, personal communication) and from Rhodobacter sphaeroides (53). It has now been observed that essentially all species and strains forming the α-3 branch of the phylogenetic tree of gram-negative bacteria, based on 16S rRNA sequence comparison (52,66), do contain this amide-linked fatty acid to a greater or lesser extent in their lipid A moieties (64 and J. H. Krauss, Thesis, Univ. Freiburg 1988).

This fatty acid (together with other fatty acids from lipid A) is liberated by water-free methanolysis and can be separated from the related 3-hydroxy-myristic acid on a SE-54 capillary column (25 m x 0.25 mm, i.d., operated isothermally at 180°C with He as carrier gas). Under these conditions 3-oxo-14:0 elutes at 9.24 min and 3-hydroxy-14:0 at 9.98 min.

The characteristic mass spectrum of this fatty acid (as methyl ester) was also studied (Fig 3). Fragments at m/e 116 (main fragment; originating from a cleavage between C-4 and C-5) and at m/e 183 (cleavage between C-2 and C-3 and formation of the fragment $C(=O)-(CH_2)_{10} \times CH_3^+$) in addition to the molecular ion [m/e 256], are characteristic of this fatty acid (48, 53).

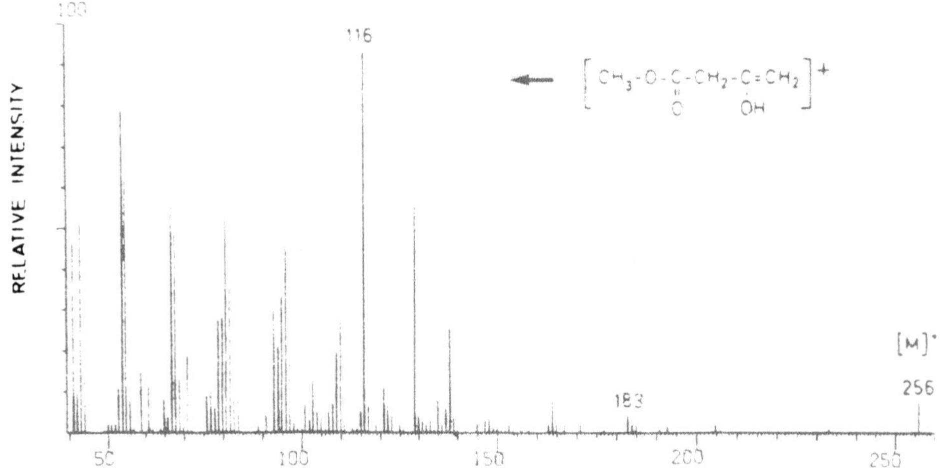

Fig 3. Mass spectrum of the 3-oxo-tetradecanoic acid methyl ester (3-oxo-14:0-methyl ester). Taken from Strittmatter et al. (53).

A survey of the species in which this fatty acid has been detected is given in Table 2.

Ester-linked Unsaturated Fatty Acids

Enterobacterial lipid A usually does not contain unsaturated fatty acids when bacteria are cultivated at temperatures between 35°-40°C. When cultivated, however, at significantly lower temperatures, e.g., at 12°C for Salmonella (68), or at 10°C for Yersinia enterocolitica (57), very significant amounts of mostly Δ^9-16:1 are incorporated in lipid A. These fatty acids are cis - Δ^9 unsaturated and as was shown for Salmonella replace the dodecanoic acid (12:0) linked to the 3-hydroxy group of the amide-linked hydroxy fatty acid at the non-reducing glucosaminyl-residue of the glucosamine disaccharide backbone (68,69). This incorporation of unsaturated fatty acids is ascribed to a process called "homeoviscous adaptation" which maintains the fluidity of the outer membrane (51). The ester-linked fatty acids described in Table 3, however, are not the Δ^9 unsaturated ones and they are

Table 2. Species containing amide-linked 3-oxo-myristic acid in lipid A of their lipopolysaccharides.

Genus	Species	Reference
Rhodobacter	R.sphaeroides	(53)
		(48)
	R.capsulatus	(39)
		Krauß, Thesis, 1988
	R.veldkampii	Krauß Thesis, 1988
Rhodopseudomona	R.blastica	(54)
Paracoccus	P.denitrificans	(64)
Thiobacillus	T.versutus	(71)
	T.sp. IFO14569	(71)

also present when cultivation was done at higher temperatures. These strains and species are mostly clustered in the α-2 and, especially, in the α-3 branch of purple bacteria (based on 16S rRNA homology studies), e.g., in members of the Rhodobacter genus.

Only a few of them have been completely characterized. The position of the double bond, usually not identifiable by mass spectrometric analysis of methyl esters, can be elegantly recognized by analysing the respective picolinyl esters by mass spectrometry at low ion energies (about 25-30 eV; 13). The mass spectrum of docosenoic acid picolinyl-ester (22:1) present in Rhodomicrobium vannielii (15) shows the typical Δ^{26} step between fragments at m/z 304 and 330, indicating a Δ^{14} double bond (Fig. 4).

Table 3. Species containing ester-linked unsaturated fatty acids or 3-hydroxylated fatty acids in their lipid A's upon growth under usual conditions (temperature and medium).

Species	Unsaturated fatty acid	16S rRNA group	Reference
Rhodobacter sphaeroides	Δ^{7}-14:1	α-3	(53)
Rhodobacter capsulatus	$\Delta^{?}$-12:1	α-3	Krauß, Thesis
Paracoccus dentrificans	$\Delta^{?}$-12:1	α-3	(64)
Thiobacillus versutus	$\Delta^{?}$14:1	α-3	(71)
Rhodomicrobium vannielii	Δ^{14}-22:1	α-2	(15)
Phenylobacterium immobile	cis-Δ^{5}-(3-OH)-12:1	α-2	(45)

Mannopyranosyl-groups in Lipid A

In a number of phosphate-free lipid A isolates, especially from phototrophic bacteria, e.g., in Rhodomicrobium vannielii, substantial amounts of D-mannose have been encountered (15). In all the species so far examined, mannose is in a terminal position and is β-pyranosidically linked. This was recognized by methylation analysis and by chromic acid oxidation, as well as by the lack of reactivity with concanavalin A, known to react with terminal-linked mannopyranosyl groups. More detailed analysis (15) has shown that mannose is located at C-4' of the non-reducing glucosamine of the backbone disaccharide. The substitution of the 4'-position is not complete, only 30% being mannosylated. The remaining hydroxyl groups seem to be also not free but very probably O-acetylated. This could be recognized by using the Ohno-methylation technique (38), which allows permanent labeling of the free hydroxyl groups by methylation at neutral pH without a removal of ester-linked fatty acids and phosphate groups. This technique yielded, as expected, 4-O-methyl-glucosamine (from GlcN I) and 6-O-methyl-glucosamine (from GlcN II), but no 4.6 di-O-methyl glucosamine from the reducing GlcN II. A list of

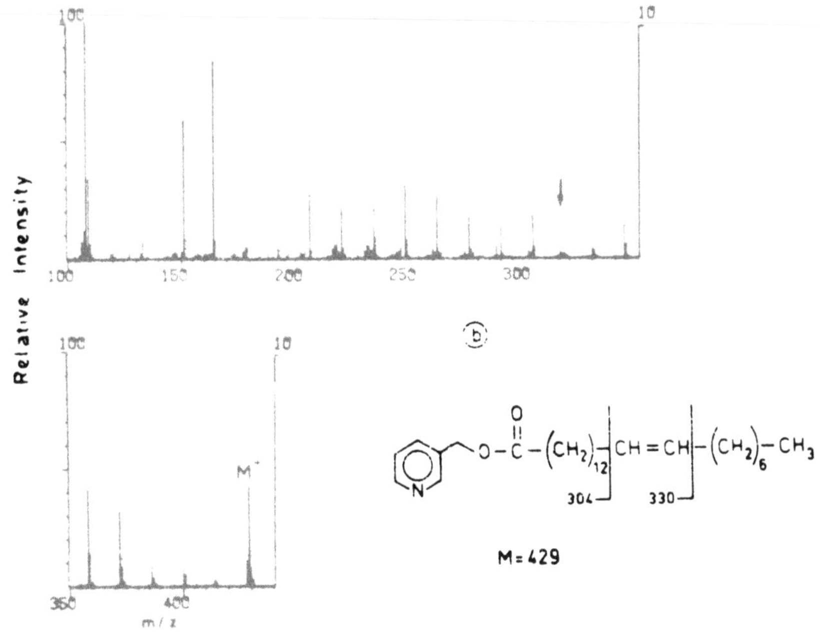

Fig 4. Mass spectrum of Δ^{14}-docosenoic acid picolinyl ester (Δ^{14}22:1 picolinyl ester). Taken from Holst et al. (15).

D-mannose-containing and phosphate-free lipid A's from photosynthetic bacteria, including Chromatiaceae, is given in Table 4.

If the finding that the attachment site of D-mannose at position 4 of the non-reducing glucosamine should be verified for other species, one could assume that the branching point in lipid A biosynthesis in these species would be where the tetra-acyl-glucosamine-disaccharide-1- (phosphate generated by the action of lipid A synthase; (41, 42), is not subjected to a following phosphorylation step as described for Enterobacteriaceae, but rather a partial mannosylation occurs. Mannose itself is not acylated, since it can be completely destroyed by periodate oxidation of lipid A.

LIPID A VARIANTS OF THE β-1-,6 GLUCOSAMINE-DISACCHARIDE TYPE

So far the lipid A variants encountered with glucosamine as backbone sugar share all the β-1,6 linked GlcN disaccharide as the sugar backbone. Four deviating lipid A structures have so far been investigated in more detail (Fig 5). The structures have previously been summarized and discussed (28, 77), with the exception of the lipid A of Rhodobacter capsulatus 37b4. We want to discuss them only briefly and focus the discussion on the recently identified structure present in R. capsulatus 37b4 (J. H. Krauss, Thesis, Univ. Freiburg, 1988).

Lipid A of Rhodocyclus tenuis is so far the only example where the otherwise unsubstituted OH-group of the backbone disaccharide at position C-4 is substituted by an additional sugar, namely by a D-glucosaminyl residue, carrying a free amino group (56). The low lethal toxicity of LPS which

Table 4. Lipid A's having additionally unacylated D-mannopyranosyl groups.

Genus	Species	Reference
Rhodomicrobium	R.vannielii	(15)
Rhodopseudomonas	R.acidophila	(54)
Chromatium	C.vinosum	(16)
	C.tepidum	(34)
Thiocapsa	T.roseopersicina	(17)
	T.pfennigii	(34)
Thiocystis	T.violacea	(34)

Species having additionally unacylated D-mannopyranose in their glucosamine-containing lipid A moiety of their LPSs.

amounts to about 1/100 of the Salmonella LPS lethality (11), is possibly due to this structural pecularity. In the passive hemolysis test, lipid A from R. tenuis showed extensive serological cross-reactivity with Salmonella lipid A (11).

Lipid A of Rhodomicrobium vannielii is phosphate-free and carries 30% β-linked D-mannopyranosyl residues attached to position C-4', i.e., at the position where usually the ester-linked phosphate group is attached (15). It has to be established whether the D-mannose-containing and phosphate-free lipid A's from Chromatiaceae have a similar lipid A structure or share only similar lipid A components.

Since this lipid A of R. vannielii is rather insoluble in water, serological cross-reactions could not be carried out. The toxicity of R. vannielii LPS amounts to about 1-10% of that of Salmonella.

Lipid A of Rhodobacter sphaeroides shows a much lower lethal toxicity amounting to 1/1000 - 1/10,000 of that of Salmonella LPS (53). The not so tight package of the lipid A fatty acids, caused by the kinks in the fatty acid chains of the 3-oxo-14:0 and of the unsaturated fatty acid (Δ^7 -14:1) (7, 48), might be the reason for this very low toxicity.

The lipid A structure of Rhodobacter capsulatus 37b4 has been elucidated (J. H. Krauss, Thesis, Univ. Freiburg, 1988). The chemical analysis of the backbone and its fatty acid substitution pattern were fully confirmed by laser-desorption-mass spectrometry (LD-MS) (50) of the dephosphorylated lipid A moiety (Fig 6). For analysis by LD-MS, LPS (about 30 mg) was treated with H_2F_2 (48%, 1 ml, 48 hr, 4°C) followed by subsequent acid hydrolysis to liberate dephosphorylated lipid A (0.1 N HCl, 1 h, 100°C) (50, and H.J.

Krauss, U. Seydel et al., in preparation). The LD-MS of the dephosphorylated lipid A, taken in the presence of Cs-salt, shows inter alia the quasi-molecular peak $(M + Cs)^+$ at m/z 1442 and ions at m/z 885 and 706 which represent the monosaccharidic partial lipid A structures, probably generated by the above discussed acidic treatment of the LPS molecule during the preparation of the dephosphorylated lipid A (44).

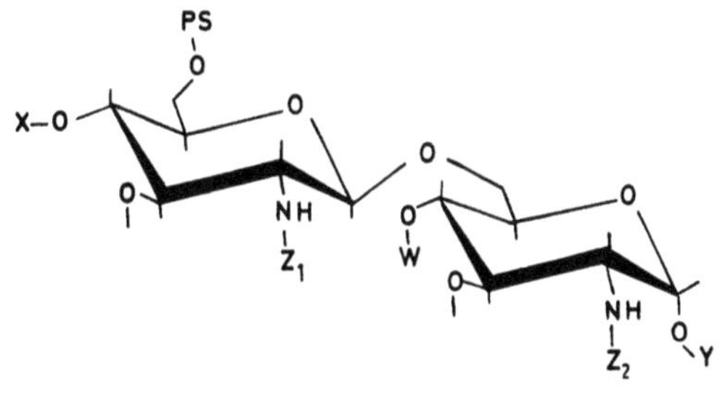

Species	W	X	Y	Z_1	Z_2
Rhodocyclus tenuis					
2761	GlcN	Ara4N-P	Araf-P	3-O(16:0)-10:0	3-OH-10:0
Rhodobacter capsulatus					
37b4	H	ETN-P	ETN-P(P)	3-oxo-14:0	3-oxo-14:0
Rhodobacter sphaeroides					
ATCC17023	H	P	P	3-O(Δ^7-14:1)14:0	3-oxo-14:0
Rhodomicrobium vannielii	H				
ATCC17100	H	Man/Ac	H	?	3-OH-16:0

Fig. 5. Structural make-up of lipid A from non- or low-toxic lipid A variants sharing the β-1.6-linked glucosaminyl-glucosamine backbone.

The low lethal toxicity (Table 5) must be due to the presence of the two amide-linked 3-oxo-14:0 molecules and the ester-linked unsaturated fatty acid (12:1), which do not allow a compact packing of the hydrophobic part of the lipid A moiety as in case of Salmonella (44). Since a complete serological cross reaction between lipid A of R. capsulatus and Salmonella lipid A was observed, this cross-reacting but almost non-toxic lipid A, is of considerable interest for pharmacological studies. Lipid A of R. sphaeroides which shows nearly identical biological properties as that from R. capsulatus is from a chemical point of view, an intermediate form between the Salmonella and the Rhodobacter capsulatus lipid A.

LIPID A VARIANTS OF THE DIAMINO-GLUCOSE-TYPE (LIPID A-DAG)

From the 25 species so far known to contain DAG in their lipid A moiety [Table 1], only a very few have been characterized thoroughly. This includes

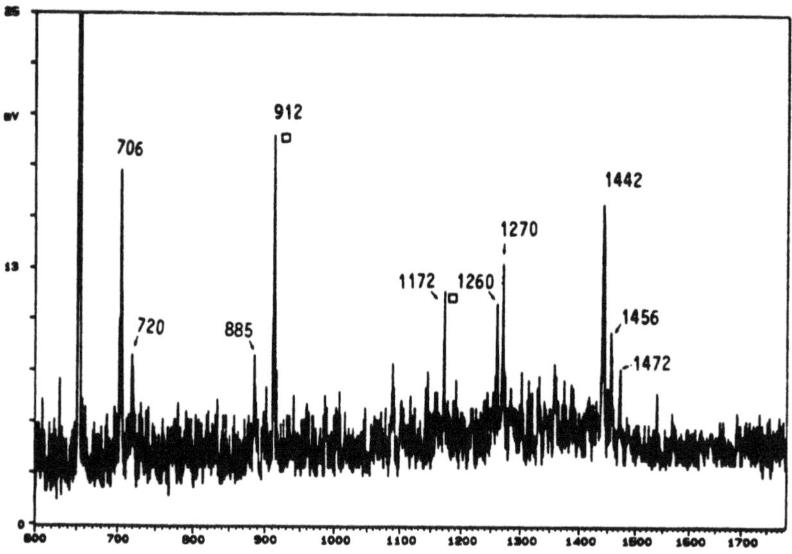

m/e 1442

$C_{72} O_{18} N_2 H_{128} Cs$

m/e 885

$C_{42} H_{75} O_{10} N Cs$

m/e 706

$C_{30} H_{55} O_9 N Cs$

Fig. 6. Laser-desorption mass spectrum (LD-MS) of the dephosphorylated lipid A from Rhodobacter capsulatus 37b4 (Krauss, Seydel, Mayer, Weckesser; in preparation) in the presence of Cs-salt.

lipid A-DA6 from Rhodopseudomonas viridis, from Phenylobacterium immobile and from Pseudomonas diminuta (18, 41, 61). It is remarkable that all three lipid A-DA6, isolates differ strongly in their chemical make-up, indicating that lipid A-DAG, like lipid A from the glucosamine type, represents a family of structurally related but characteristically different lipids.

Table 5. Biological properties of LPS's with different lipid A's.

Source of LPS	LIPID A charact. [HexN	FA-A	P]	Lethality* [x 10^{-2}µg/kg]	Pyrogenicity** [x 10^{-3}µg/kg]	TNF-Induction*** [Cr^{51} release]
Salmonella	GlcN	3-OH	+	1	1	+++
Rc. gelatinosus	GlcN	3-OH	+	1	1	+++
Rb. sphaeroides	GlcN	3-OH 3-Oxo	+	10^3 - 10^4	10^3	+
Rb. capsulatus	GlcN	3-Oxo	+	10^3 - 10^4	ND	+
Rp. viridis	DAG	3-OH	-	10^2 - 10^3	10^4	++/+++

µg/kg indicates µg LPS-TEN/kg animal. (TEN, triethylamine-salts of electrodialyzed LPS's).

* LD_{50} in mice (adrenalectomized or galactosamine-treated mice) (11, 53).
**MPD-3 values in the rabbit (11).
***With M.-L. Lohmann-Matthes: mouse macrophages, cytotoxicity versus L929 transformed fibroblasts as target cells (10 and unpublished results).

Two of the lipid moieties are monosaccharidic (Fig 7a and b) and the third one has been tentatively characterized as a phosphorylated disaccharide (Fig 7c) (18). Lipid A-DAG from Rhodopseudomonas viridis contains only 3-OH-14:0, but no ester-linked fatty acids at all. This fact was ascertained by analysis of water-phase LPS from six different strains of R. viridis (60).

The lipid A of Phenylobacterium immobile chloridazone-degrading soil bacterium (61), is also monosaccharidic. It contains a spectrum of amide- and ester-linked fatty acids, with a few of them, however, dominating (4). The main amide-linked fatty acid is 3-OH-12:0 and the main ester-linked fatty acids are 3-hydroxy-5c-dodecenoic (3-OH-12:1) and dodecanoic acid (12:0). Since the rare hydroxylated fatty acids were also present in the bound lipid fraction obtained from 17 different strains of Phenylobacterium immobile (4), one can assume that the same lipid ADA6 is present in all these strains. The tentative structure of P. immobile which includes only the main fatty acids is shown in Fig. 7b.

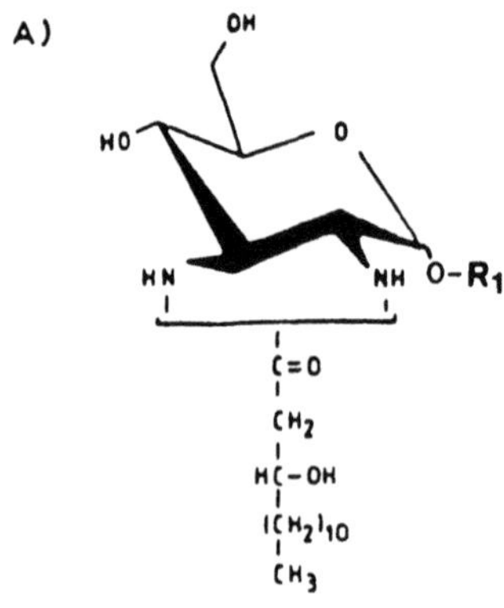

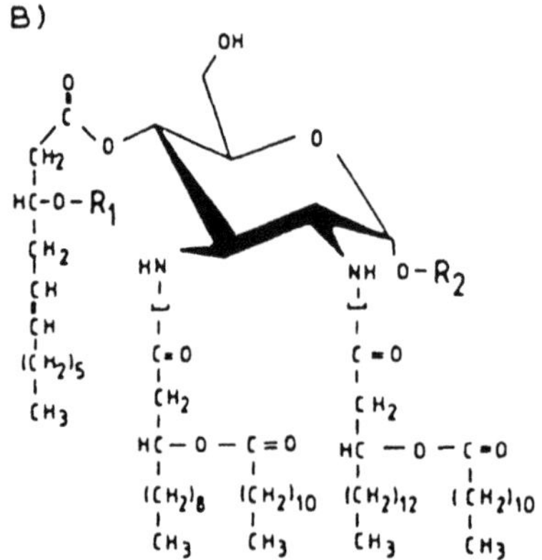

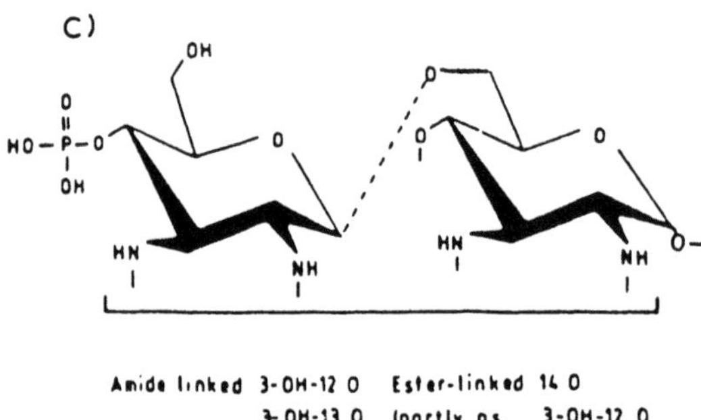

Fig. 7. Proposed structures (present knowledge) of different lipid A-DA6 isolates from (a) Rhodopseudomonas viridis, (b) Phenylobacterium immobile, (c) Pseudomonas diminuta. (Taken from (59)).

Pseudomonas diminuta lipid A-DA6 was investigated more thoroughly by Kasai et al., (19) and was identified by FAB-MS as a phosphorylated disaccharide of DAG with the phosphate being ester-linked. The structure shown in Fig 7c should only be taken as one of the possibilities of a structure fitting with the analytical results. In contrast to the findings with R. viridis LPS (and Rhodopseudomonas palustris Table 5) the lipid A-DA6 from P. diminuta was described as endotoxically highly active (18).

Further studies are urgently needed to clarify the detailed structures of at least some of the lipid A-DA6 types and to relate their structure to the biological properties observed with the respective LPSs. Also, the distribution of the lipid A-DA6 types amongst the species shown in Table 1 would be highly desirable.

"Mixed" Lipid Variants

From the existence of backbone disaccharides either with GlcN (Fig 5) or with DAG (from Pseudomonas diminuta) one can speculate whether also backbone disaccharides composed of one molecule of GlcN and one molecule of DAG, so-called "mixed" disaccharides, could exist in some lipid A variants.

That these mixed forms are even to be expected arises from biosynthetic studies carried out in vitro by C.H.R. Raetz (Madison) and F.M. Unger (Vienna/Edmonton), (personal communication). Lipid X (2,3-diacylglucosamine1-phosphate), a biosynthetic precursor of enterobacterial lipid A and its activated form (UDP-lipid X), as well as their diamino analogs, namely lipid X-DA6 and UDP-lipid X-DA6, were synthesized by Macher and Unger (26).

When lipid X and UDP-lipid X-DA6 or, inversely, lipid X-DAG and UDP-lipid X were incubated with lipid A synthase from E. coli, "mixed" tetra-acyl-disaccharide-1-phosphates were obtained with DAG either at the non-reducing or at the reducing end of the disaccharide (C.H.R. Raetz, personal communication). The rather low specificity of lipid A-synthase is also documented by the fact that 2,3-O,N-diacyl-kanosamine and 2,3-di-O-acyl-glucose also could be used as substrates (F.M. Unger, personal communication; 26).

With this knowledge one may assume that "mixed" lipid A backbones and possibly also transitional forms with nonstoichiometric ratios of the two amino sugars may well exist in lipid moieties of some bacterial species. Several observations made recently, speak for the existence of such "mixed" lipid A forms, although until today their existence has not yet definitely been proven. GlcN and DAG can be observed in lipid A isolates from Chromatiaceae (34), from some thiobacilli (70) and from Bradyrhizobium (Table 6), but the possibility still exists that two different lipid A species co-exist in these LPSs (59). So far, 3-amino-3-deoxy-D-glucose (kanosamine), has not been identified from bacterial LPSs, although the 2,3-diacyl derivative serves as substrate for lipid A synthase.

Biological Properties of Lipid A Variants

Only a few biological characteristics of LPS (or free lipid A) with lipid A variants have so far been investigated, namely lipid A antigenicity, lethal toxicity, pyrogenicity and induction of TNF synthesis and secretion (11 unpublished results with M. Freudenberg, Freiburg, and M.L. Lohmann-Matthes, Hannover (10). Some of the data are summarized in Table 5.

Using the passive hemolysis test and its inhibition (11), the serological cross-reactions of free lipid A from the strains shown in Table 5 were investigated. As a result of these studies one can summarize that all the glucosamine-containing lipid A's of Table 5 show complete serological cross-reaction with Salmonella lipid A, regardless of whether the lipid A antisera were obtained with lipid A from Salmonella or with lipid A variants (11, 53).

A clear serological differentiation was, however, observed with lipid ADA6 from Rhodopseudomonas viridis and R. palustris, which showed no serological cross-reactivity with Salmonella lipid A. They showed significant cross-reactivity, however, with each other (11), indicating at least partial sharing of epitopes.

High lethality, pyrogenicity and an effective stimulation of macrophages for TNF-production was observed with LPS of Rhodocyclus gelatinosus, being so far the only example of a highly toxic LPS occurring in phototrophic bacteria (11, 55). Lipid A of R. gelatinosus is similar in structure to Salmonella lipid A (28, 55), although the 3-OH-fatty acids are shorter (3-OH-10:0) than observed with Salmonella lipid A (3-OH-14:0)

All the other lipid A variants shown in Table 5 exhibit, in contrast, a very much reduced lethality and pyrogenicity and show only marginal activity in macrophage activation (Lohmann-Matthes, Hannover, personal communication). No significant difference was observed between LPS of Rhodobacter sphaeroides and Rhodobacter capsulatus, although the former has only a partial substitution of its amide-linked 3-hydroxy fatty acid by 3-oxo-14:0. As expected, the strongly deviating structure of R. viridis (and R. palustris, not shown), having the monosaccharidic lipid ADA6, has little toxicity and is very low in pyrogenicity. Lethality of lipid ADA6 is, however, not excluded necessarily as shown by Kasai with the disaccharidic lipid ADA6 from Pseudomonas diminuta showing about 1/10 of the toxicity of Salmonella lipid A.

Preliminary studies in collaboration with M.L. Lohmann-Matthes, Hannover, using either transformed fibroblast target cells (L929 cells) or TNF-sensitive tumor cells (Wehi 164; (10)) for the differentiation of excreted and membrane-associated TNF, showed the results given in Table 6. High activity of the toxic LPS-samples of Salmonella and Rhodocyclus gelatinosus, but only marginal activity in both tests by the Rhodobacter LPS were observed. The activity of Rhodopseudomonas viridis LPS in these tests is unexpected. The nontoxic LPS proved to be only slightly less active than the toxic LPS from R. gelatinosus.

No studies on the induction of IL-1 or interferon-γ in macrophages has been undertaken so far with lipid A variants.

The disaccharidic lipid ADA6, from Pseudomonas diminuta was active in the Limulus test and LPS and lipid A of this species were able to induce TNF-production in BCG-pretreated mice (18). Furthermore, studies with lipid X and lipid XDA6, obtained by chemical synthesis (26), were able to inhibit the ability of LPS to induce priming of human neutrophils in a concentration-dependent manner. At high concentrations of the inhibitors, however, lipid XDA6- but not lipid X- had the reverse effect in enhancing the priming activity. It is assumed that lipid X and lipid XDA6 (at low concentrations) compete with LPS for cellular binding sites. Furthermore, preliminary studies by Macher and Unger (26) show that lipid X and lipid XDA6 are promising candidates as immunomodulators with low toxicity. Surprisingly, the analogous derivatives with kanosamine (3-amino-3-deoxy-glucose) and glucose were essentially inactive in the test systems investigated so far.

Table 6. Characteristic constituents revealing uniformity or nonuniformity in the lipid moieties of some genera of gram-negative bacteria.

Genus	Species	Strains	GlcN	DAG	Others	P	3-OH-FA	3-Oxo-FA	DOC-PAGE	16S rRNA
Rhodocyclus	R.gelatinosus	12	●	–	-	●	10:0	-	R	β-1
	R.tenuis	8	●	–	$GlcNH_2$	●	10:0	-	SR-R	β-2
	R.purpureus	1	●	–	?	●	10:0	-	S	β-2
Rhodobacter	R.sphaeroides	3	●	–	-	●	10.0, 14:0	14:0	S-SR	α-3
	R.capsulatus	5	●	–	-	●	10:0, (14:0)	14:0	S-SR	α-3
	R.veldkampii	1	●	–	-	?	10:0, 14:0	14:0	SR	?
	R.sulfidophilus	1	●	–	-	?	10:0, 14:0	14:0	SR	?
Rhodomicrobium	R.vannielii	1	●	–	Man	-	16:0	-		α-2
Rhodopseudomonas	R.acidophila	1	●	–	Man	-	16:0	-	R	α-2
	R.viridis	8	–	●	-	-	14:0	-	S	α-2
	R.palustris	13	–	●	-	-	14:0, 16:0	-	S	α-2
Rhodopila	R.globiformis	1	–	●	-	-	14:0, 18:0, 19:0	-	S	α-1
Chromatium	C.vinosum	1	●	•	Man	-	14:0	-	S	γ-1
	C.tepidum	1	●	•	Man	-	14:0	-	S	γ-1
Thiocapsa	T.roseopersicina	1	●	•	Man	-	14:0	-	S	γ-1
	T.pfennigii	1	●	•	Man	-	14:0	-	S	γ-1
Thiocystis	T.violacea	1	●	•	Man	-	14:0	-	S	γ-1
Thiobacillus	T.versutus	2	●	–	-	●	10:0, 14:0	14:0	R	α-3
	T.sp. IFO14569	1	●	–	-	●	10:0, 14:0	14:0	R	α-3
	T.ferrooxydans	2	•	●	-	-	14:0	-	S	?
	T.thiooxydans	1	•	●	-	-	14:0	-	S	?
	T.novellus	1	–	●	-	-	14:0	-	S	?
	T.sp. IFO14570	1	–	●	-	-	12:0, 13:0, 18:0	-	S	?
Rhizobium	R.trifolii	Lit	●	–	-	●	14:0, 12:0	-	S	α-?
	R.leguminosarum	Lit	●	–	-		12:0, 14:0	-	S	α-2
Bradyrhizobium	B.japonicum	1	•	●	-	-	14:0, 12:0	-	S	α-2
	B.lupini	1	•	●	-	-	14:0, 12:0	-	S	α-2
Pseudomonas	P.aeruginosa	Lit	●	–	-	●	12:0, 14:0, 2-OH-14:0	-	S	γ-3
	P.syringae pv phaseolicola	1	●	–	-	●	12:0, 14:0, 2-OH-14:0		S	γ-3
	P.diminuta	3	–	●	-	-	14:0		R	α-2
	P.vesicularis	1	–	●	-	-	14:0		R	α-2
	"P.carboxydovorans"	1	•	●	-	-	14:0, 12:0, 18:0	-	(S)-R	α-2

Main 3-hydroxylated fatty acids are underlined; 16S rRNA-subdivision according to Woese et al., (2, 65, 66; and R, SR and S, indicating complete R-form, semirough and smooth form, are used as operational terms only (24, and Thesis J. H. Krauss, University, Freiburg, 1988). Data from 5, 6, 12, 31, 34, 47, 60, 63, 70 and 71.

Further studies are needed to evaluate, whether the low- and nontoxic lipid A variants can be used as potent inhibitors of the nonwanted toxic activities of enterobacterial LPS or lipid A. A good candidate would of course be the LPSs of Rhodobacter capsulatus and R. sphaeroides which show complete serological cross-reactions (sharing of the epitopes) with highly toxic enterobacterial lipid A but show only 1/1000-1/10,000 of the toxic effects.

Taxonomical and Phylogenetical Significance of Lipid A Composition and Structure

Table 6 lists characteristic constituents of lipid A from a number of species which belong to families or genera which have so far been studied in more detail (28). Especially those constituents are included which seem to have taxonomical significance, such as the backbone amino sugars, additional sugar constitutents directly attached to the lipid A backbone sugar(s), the phosphorus content, and the chemical nature of the hydroxy- or oxo-fatty acids. DOC-PAGE profiles, which allow to recognize the extent of O-chain heterogeneity and the S- or R-character of the LPS-species examined (22, 24) are likewise given. Available data on the 16S rRNA homology studies are also given in the table. They indicate the position of individual strains or species on the phylogenetical tree of bacteria (65, 66, 67).

Perusal of Table 6 indicates that, with the exception of the Chromatiaceae (with the genera Chromatium, Thiocapsa, and Thiocystis) and the well-studied Enterobacteriaceae (data not included), most other families and even genera do not show an uniform lipid A composition. Examples of this are the genera Rhodopseudomonas, Thiobacillus, Pseudomonas and the family Rhizobiaceae (31). It is evident, however, that a much better fitting of lipid A composition and classification is obtained, when the classification is based on the 16S rRNA homologies. Examples are the genera Rhodocyclus and Pseudomonas. This good correlation is especially obvious when more detailed data on the phylogenetic relatedness are available, as in case of the alpha-2 subgroup (Fig 8) (2). Although the cluster of strains (upper group of species in Fig 8) includes members of four different families (Pseudomonas, Rhodopseudomonas, Bradyrhizobium and Nitrobacter) all these strains were shown to have a similar and characteristic lipid A composition with 2,3-diamino-2,3-dideoxy-D-glucose as the (main) backbone sugar (31). The finding of a rather distant phylogenetic relationship (with SAB- values of about 0.47) (2) between rhizobia and bradyrhizobia, i.e., the fast- and the slow-growing Rhizobiaceae, is also indicated by very distinct differences in lipid A composition. It can be concluded that lipid A composition can be used as a criterion to prove or disprove phylogenetic relatedness of bacterial species. It may be stressed here that Enterobacteriaceae and Chromatiaceae, each of them showing uniform lipid A composition, also appear as two distinct phylogenetically coherent groups of species (52, 65).

Another group of species all having the rare amide-linked 3-oxo-myristic acid in their lipid A's, are the Rhodobacter species and the non-phototrophic Thiobacillus versutus (71) and Paracoccus denitrificans (64). All these strains are phylogenetically closely related and form the α-3 branch of the genealogical tree of purple bacteria (59, 66). So far, the only phototrophic species with 3-oxo-14:0 in lipid A and not included in the genus Rhodobacter is Rhodopseudomonas blastica (54). From its fatty acid profile (amide-linked 3-oxo-14:0 and ester-linked 3-OH-10:0) one may predict that R. blastica should also belong to the α-3 subgroup and not to the α-2 as do the other Rhodopseudomonas species.

Further studies on lipid A variants and on 16S rRNA homologies are

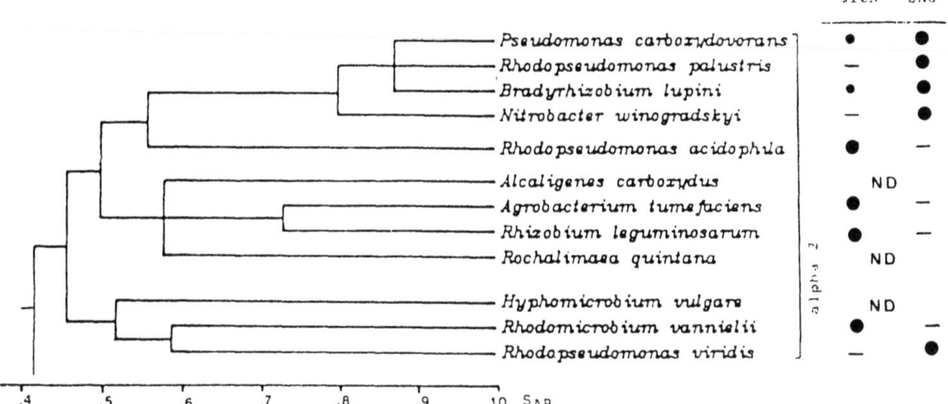

Fig. 8. Dendrogramm of the α-2 subgroup of purple bacteria, based on SAB values calculated by 16S rRNA homology studies. The nature of the lipid A backbone amino sugar is indicated. Modified according to Auling et al. (2, 31).

needed, especially in case of thiobacilli, to prove the general significance of lipid A composition and structure for recognizing distinct phylogenetical relationships of species.

DISCUSSION AND FINAL REMARKS

When the structures of all characterized lipid A variants are compared, a minimal partial structure, common to all of them, can be recognized. This common structural element (Fig 9) represents a 2-amino-hexose with D-gluco-configuration carrying an amide-linked 3-hydroxy- or 3-oxo-fatty acid with a chain length of at least 10 C-atoms and having an attachment site for KDO or a KDO-derivative (e.g., KDO-phosphate) (at position C-6). 2-Keto-octonate (KO) may replace KDO in case of Acinetobacter calcoaceticus (19).

With this information one may speculate whether lipid A is not primarily a highly elaborated and modifiable lipid anchor for KDO residue(s), known to be indispensible for the viability of the cell. KDO, in combination with divalent cations (Mg^{++} and Ca^{++}), plays an essential role in the organization and the interlinkage of the outer membrane components (45, 49). In addition, from the fact that LPS of the phototrophic Rhodocyclus gelatinosus is of very high toxicity, one must conclude that the endotoxic principle was invented assumingly early in evolution (62).

Water- and some soil-bacteria generally live at lower temperatures than endosymbionts or -parasites. Very often just these bacteria have a low content of ester-linked nonhydroxylated fatty acids in their LPSs and some of them are even unsaturated (60). The general lack or low content in acyl-oxy-acyl residues (68) may be due to the lower environmental temperature and the necessary fluidity of their outer membrane. The phosphate-containing lipid A's may also be modified by adapting to certain milieu changes (pH, poor or rich medium) (3a, 25) by a partial or a complete substitution of the backbone phosphates by cationic or neutral substituents, such as ethanolamine, 4-amino-4-deoxy-L-arabinose, D-glucosamine, or D-arabino-furanose (as in Rhodocyclus tenuis or in Yersinia pestis (8, 56).

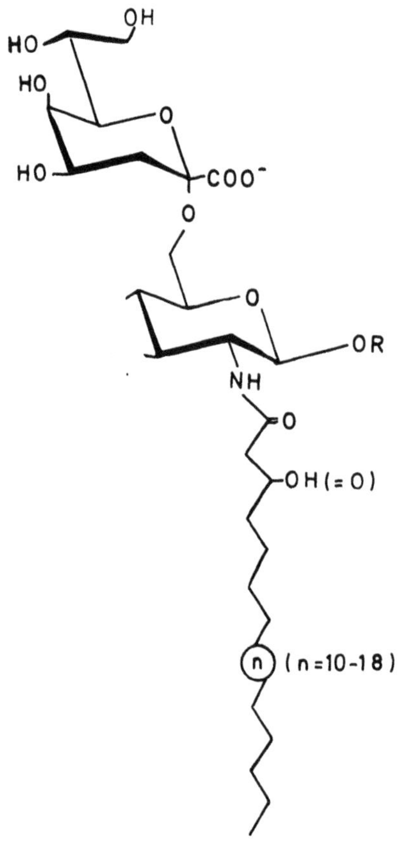

Fig. 9. The structural element common to all established lipid A variants: a 2-amino sugar with D-gluco-configuration, carrying an amide-linked 3-hydroxy- or 3-oxo-fatty acid and (at C_6) a ketosidically linked KDO or KDO-analogon.

Almost all lipid A variants have altered biological properties (low lethal toxicity and pyrogenicity), but, as proven for Rhodopseudomonas viridis lipid A and the synthetic lipid XDA6 (9, 26) are still able to elicit biological phenomena (activation of macrophages or production of TNF). They may serve as potent inhibitors of endotoxins in competing with them for cellular binding sites (9). Lipid A variants may represent a not yet explored reservoir of pharmacologically promising molecules. In addition, the possible value of non-toxic LPSs with various lipid A variants in increasing the resistance towards bacterial infections should be stressed here.

The currently established structures and constituents of lipid A variants indicate their significance in a number of cases as phenotypical markers for recognizing or confirming phylogenetical relationships of gram-negative bacteria. This was especially successful with the phototrophic bacteria, with thiobacilli and with Rhizobiaceae, where good correlations were found between 16S rRNA homologies and the lipid A composition.

REFERENCES

1. Ahamed, N. M., Mayer, H., Biebl, H. and Weckesser, J., 1982, Lipopolysaccharide with 2,3-diamino-2,3-dideoxyglucose containing lipid A in Rhodopseudomonas sulfovirids, FEMS Microbiol., 14:27-30.

2. Auling, G., Busse, J., Hahn, M., Hennecke, H., Kroppenstedt, R.-M., Probst, A. and Stackebrandt, E., Phylogenetic heterogeneity and chemotaxonomic properties of certain Gram-negative aerobic carboxydobacteria, Syst. Appl. Microbiol.1 10: 264-272.

3. Basu, S., Radziejewska-Lebrecht, J. and Mayer, H., 1986, Lipopolysaccharide of Providencia rettgeri, Chemical studies and taxonomical implication, Arch. Microbiol. 144: 213-218.

3a. Batley, M., Packer, N. H. and Redmond, J. W., 1985, Analytical studies of lipopolysaccharide and its derivatives from Salmonella minnesota R595, Biochem. Biophys. Acta. 821: 179-194.

4. Bellmann, W. and Lingens, F., 1985, Structural studies on the core oligosaccharide of Phenylobacterium immobile strain K_2 lipopolysaccharide. Chemical cynthesis of 3-hydroxy-5c-dodecenoic acid, Biol. Chem. Hoppe Seyler's 366: 567-575.

5. Carlson, R.W., 1982, The heterogeneity of Rhizobium lipopolysaccharides, J. Bacteriol. 158: 1012-1017.

6. Carlson, R. W., Shetters, R., Duh, J.-L., Turnbull, E., Hanley, B., Rolfe, B. G., Djordjevvie, M. A., 1987, The isolation and partial characterization of the lipopolysaccharides from several Rhizobium trifolii mutants affected in root hair infection, Plant Physiol. 84: 421-427.

7. Cotter, R. J., Honovich, J., Qureshi, N. and Takayama, K., 1987, Structural determination of lipid A from gram negative bacteria using laser desorption mass spectrometry, Biomed. Environ. Mass Spectrom. 14: 591-598.

8. Dalla Venezia, N., Minka, S., Bruneteau, M., Mayer, H. and Michel, G., 1985, Lipopolysaccharides from Yersinia pestis. Studies on lipid A of lipopolysaccharides I and II, Eur. J. Biochem., 151: 399-404.

9. Danner, R. L., Joiner, K. A. and Parrillo, J. E., 1987, Inhibiiton of endotoxin-induced priming of human neutrophils by lipid X and 3-aza-lipid X, J. Clin. Invest. 80: 605-612.

10. Decker, T., Lohmann-Matthes, M.-L. and Gifford, G. E., 1987, Cell associated tumor necrosis factor (TNF) as a filling mechanism of activated cytotoxic macrophages, J. Immunol. 138: 957-962.

11. Galanos, C., Roppel, J., Weckesser, J., Rietschel, E. Th. and Mayer, H., 1977, Biological activities of lipopolysaccharides and lipid A from Rhodospirillaceae, Infect. Immun., 16: 407-412.

12. Gross, M., Mayer, H., Widemann, C. and Rudolph, K., 1988, Comparative analysis of the lipopolysaccharides of a rough and a smooth strain of Pseudomonas syringae pv. phaseolicola, Arch. Microbiol., 149: 342-346.

13. Harvey, D. J., 1982, Picolinyl esters as derivatives for the structural determination of long chain branched and unsaturated fatty acids, Biomed. Mass Spectrom. 9: 33-38.

14. Hase, S. and Rietschel, E. Th., 1976, Isolation and analysis of the lipid A backbone. Lipid A structure of lipopolysaccharides from various bacterial groups, Eur. J. Biochem. 63: 101-107.

15. Holst, O., Borowiak, D., Weckesser, J. and Mayer, H., 1983, Structural studies on the phosphate-free lipid A of Rhodomicrobium vannielii ATCC 17100, Eur. J. Biochem. 137: 325-332.

16. Hurlbert, R. E., Weckesser, J., Mayer, H. and Fromme, F., 1976, Isolation and characterizatin of the lipopolysaccharide of Chromatium vinosum, Eur. J. Biochem., 68: 365-371.

17. Hurlbert, R. E., Weckesser, J., Tharanathan, R. N. and Mayer H., 1978, Isolation and characterization of the lipopolysaccharide of Thiocapsa roseopersicina, Eur. J. Biochem., 90: 241-246.

18. Kasai, N., Arata, S., Mashima, J. I., Akiyama, Y., Tanaka, C., Egawa, K. and Tanaka, S., 1987, Pseudomonas diminuta LPS with a new endotoxic lipid A structure, Biochem. Biophys. Res. Commun. 142: 972-978.

19. Kawahara, K., Brade, H., Rietschel, E. Th. and Zähringer, U., 1987, Studies on the chemical structure of the core-lipid A region of the lipopolysaccharide of Acinetobacter calcoaceticus NCTC 10305, Eur. J. Biochem. 163: 489-495.

20. Keilich, G., Roppel, J and Mayer, H., 1976, Characterization of a diaminohexose (2,3-diamino-2,3-dideoxy-D-glucose) from Rhodopseudomonas viridis lipopolysaccharides by circular dichroism, Carbohyd. Res. 5: 129-134.

21. Knirel, A. Y. and Kochetkov, N. K., 1987, 2,3-diamino-2,3-dideoxyuronic and 5,7-diamino-3,5,7,9-tetradeoxynonulosonic acids: new components of bacterial polysaccharides, FEMS Microbiol. Rev. 46: 381-385.

22. Komuro, T. and Galanos, C., 1986, Analysis of Salmonella lipopolysaccharides by sodium deoxycholate polyacrylamide gel electrophoresis, EOS-Rev. Immunol. 6: 147.

23. Kotelko, K., 1986, Proteus mirabilis: taxonomic positon, peculiarities of growth, components of the cell envelope, Curr. Top. Microbiol. Immunol. 129: 181.

24. Krauss, J. H., Weckesser, J. and Mayer, H., 1988, Electrophoretic analysis of lipopolysaccharides of purple nonsulfur bacteria, J. System. Bacteriol. 38:.

25. Lehmann, V., Redmond, J., Egan, A. and Minner, I., 1978, The acceptor for polar head groups of the lipid A component of Salmonella lipopolysaccharides, Eur. J. Biochem. 86: 487-496.

25a. Lüderitz, O., Galanos, C., Lehmann, V., Mayer, H., Rietschel, E. Th. and Weckesser, J., 1978, Chemical structure and biological activities of lipid A's from various bacterial families, Naturwissenschaften 65: 579-585.

26. Macher, I. and Unger, F.M., 1987, Monosaccharide derivatives related to the lipid A of enterobacteria, 4th European Carbohydrate Symposium, July 12-17, Darmstadt, FRG, B-34.

27. Mayer, H., 1984, Significance of lipopolysaccharide structure for questions of taxonomy and phylogenetical relatedness of gram-negative bacteria, in: "The cell membrane", E. Harber, ed., Plenum Press, New York, London pp. 71-83.

28. Mayer, H. and Weckesser, J., 1984, Unusual lipid A's: structures, taxonomical relevance and potential value for endotoxin research, in: "Handbook of endotoxin, Vol. 1, Chemistry of endotoxin, E. Th. Rietschel, ed., Elsevier Science Publishers, Amersterdam, pp. 221-247.

29. Mayer, H., Bock, E. and Weckesser, J., 1983, 2,3-diamino-2,3-dideoxyglucose containing lipid A in the Nitrobacter strain X_{14}, FEMS Microbiol. Lett. 17: 93-96.

30. Mayer, H., Tharanathan, R. N. and Weckesser, J., 1988, Analysis of lipopolysaccharides of Gram-negative bacteria, in: "Methods in Microbiology", G. Gottschalk, ed., Vol. 18, pp. 157-207, Academic Press, New York.

31. Mayer, H., Krauss, J. H., Puvanesarajah, Stacey, G. and Auling, G., 1988, Lipid A with diaminoglucose in lipopolysaccharides from slow-growing Rhizobiaceae and from Pseudomonas carboxydovorans, Arch. Microbiol. 151: 111-116.

32. Meissner, J., Borowiak, D., Fischer, U. and Weckesser, J., 1988, Lipopolysaccharide with lipid A_{DAG} in the phototropic Ectohiorhodospira vacuolata, Arch. Microbiol. 149: 245-248.

33. Meissner, J., Fischer, U. and Weckesser, J., 1987, The lipopolysaccharide of the green sulfur bacterium Chlorobium vibrioforme f. thiosulfatophilum, Arch. Microbiol. 149: 125-129.

34. Meissner, J., Pfennig, N., Krauss, J., Mayer, H. and Weckesser, J., 1988, Lipopolysaccharides of the Chromatiaceae species Thiocystis violacea, Thiocapsa pfennigii, and Chromatium tepidum, J. Bacteriol. 170: 3267-3272.

35. Meyer zu Reckendorf, W., 1964, Die Synthesen der 2,3-Diamino-2,3-didesoxy-D-allose, der 2,3-Diamino-2,3-didesoxy- α-D-glucose und der 2,6-Diamino-2,6-dideoxy- α-D-allose, Chem. Ber. 97: 1175-1285.

36. Moreno, E. and Mayer, H., 1988, Brucella Lipids, in: "Brucella", CNC (London). (in press)

37. Moreno, E., Borowiak, D. and Mayer, H., 1987, Brucella lipopolysaccharides and polysaccharides, Ann. Inst. Pasteur Microbiol. 138: 102-105.

38. Ohno, K., Nishiyama, H. and Nagase, H., 1979, A mild methylation of alcohols with diazomethane catalyzed by silica gel, Tetrahedron Lett. 45: 4405-4406.

39. Omar, A. S., Flammann, H. T., Borowiak, D. and Weckesser, J., 1983, Lipopolysaccharides of two strains of the phototrophic bacterium Rhodopseudomonas capsulata, Arch. Microbiol. 134: 212-216.

40. Radziejewska-Lebrecht, Feige, U., Mayer H. and Weckesser, J., 1981, Structure of the heptose region of lipopolysaccharides from Rhodospirillum tenue, J. Bacteriol. 145: 138-144.

41. Raetz, C. R. H., 1987, Biosynthesis and pharmacological properties of Escherichia coli lipid A, in: "Bacterial outer membranes as model systems", M. Inouye, ed., pp. 229-245, John Wiley and Sons, Inc.

42. Raetz, C. R. H., 1984, Escherichia coli mutants that allow elucidation of the precursors and biosynthesis of lipid A, in: "Handbook of Endotoxin", E. Th. Rietschel, ed., pp. 248-268, Elsevier Science Publishers, Amsterdam.

43. Rietschel, E. Th. and Lüderitz, O., 1980, Struktur von Lipopolysaccharid und Taxonomic gram-negativer Bakterien, Forum Mikrobiol. 3: 12-20.

44. Rietschel, E. Th., Wollenweber, H. W., Brade, H., Zahringer, U., Lindner, B., Seydel, U., Bradaczek, H., Barnickel, G., Labischinski, H. and Griesbrecht, P., 1984, Structure and conformation of the lipid A component of lipopolysaccharides, in: "Handbook of Endotoxin", Vol. 1, Chemistry of Endotoxin, E. Th. Rietschel, ed. pp. 187-200, Elsevier Science Publishers B. V., Amsterdam.

45. Rietschel, E. Th., Galanos, C., Lüderitz, O. and Westphal, O., 1982, The chemistry and biology of lipopolysaccharides and their lipid A component, in: "Immunopharmacology and the regulation of leukocyte function", D. R. Webb, ed., Marcel Dekker, Inc. New York, Basel, pp. 183-229.

46. Roppel, J., Mayer, H. and Weckesser, J., 1975, Identification of a 2,3--diamino-2,3-dideoxyhexose in the lipid A component of lipopolysaccharides of Rhodopseudomonas viridis and Rhodopseudomonas palustris, Carbohydr. Res. 40: 31-40.

47. Russa, R., Lüderitz, O. and Rietschel, E. Th., 1985, Structural analyses of lipid A from lipopolysaccharides of nodulating and nonnodulating Rhizobiium trifolii, Archiv. Microbiol. 141: 284-289.

48. Salimath, P. V., Weckesser, J., Strittmatter, W. and Mayer, H., 1983, Structural studies on the nontoxic lipid A from Rhodopseudomonas sphaeroides ATCC 17023, Eur. J. Biochem. 136: 195-200.

49. Schinler, M. and Osborn, M. J., 1979, Interaction of divalent cations polymyxin B with lipopolysaccharide, Biochem. 18: 4425-4430.

50. Seydel, U., Lindner, B., Zahringer, U., Rietschel, E. Th., Kusumoto, S. and Shiba, S., 1984, Laser desorption mass spectrometry of synthetic lipid A like compounds, Biomed. Mass Spectrom. 11: 132-141.

51. Siensky, M., 1974, Homeoviscous adaptation - a hoeostatic process that regulates the viscosity of membrane lipids in Escherichia coli, Proc. Nat. Acad. Sci. (Wash.) 71: 522-525.

52. Stackebrandt, E., 1986, Das hierarchische System der Eubakterien: Problem und Losungsansatze, Form Mikrobiologie 9: 255-260.

53. Strittmatter, W., Weckesser, J., Salimath, P. V. and Galanos, C., 1983, Nontoxic lipopolysaccharides from Rhodopseudomonas sphaeroides ATCC 17023, J. Bacteriol. 153-158.

54. Tegtmeyer, B., Weckesser, J., Mayer, H. and Imhoff, J. F., 1985, Chemical composition of the lipopolysaccharides of Rhodobacter sulfidophilus, Rhodopseudomonas acidophila and Rhodopseudomonas blastica, Arch. Microbiol. 143: 32-36.

55. Tharanathan, R. N., Salimath, P. V., Weckesser, J. and Mayer, H., 1985, The structure of lipid A from the lipopolysaccharide of Rhodopseudomonas gelatinosa 29/1, Arch. Microbiol. 141: 279-283.

56. Tharanathan, R. N., Weckesser, J. and Mayer, H., 1978, Structural studies on the D-arabinose-containing lipid A from Rhodospirillum tenue 2761, Eur. J. Biochem. 84: 385-394.

57. Wartenberg, K., Knapp, W., Ahamed, N. M., Widemann, C. and Mayer, H., 1983, Temperature-dependent changes in the sugar and fatty acid composition of lipopolysaccharides from Yersinia enterocolitica strains, Zbl. Bakt. Hyg., I., Abt. Orig. A253: 523-530.

58. Weckesser, J. and Mayer, H., 1987, Lipopolysaccharides of phototrophic bacteria, a contribution to phylogeny and endotoxin research, Forum Mikrobiologie, 108: 242-248.

59. Weckesser, J. and Mayer, H, 1987, Different lipid A types in lipopolysaccharides of phototrophic and related non-phototrophic bacteria, FEMS Microbiol. Rev.54: 143-154.

60. Weckesser, J., Drews, G., and Mayer, H., 1979, Lipopolysaccharides of photosynthetic prokaryotes, Ann. Rev. Microbiol. 33: 215-239.

61. Weisshaar, R. and Lingens, F., 1983, The lipopolysaccharide of a chloridazon-degrading bacterium, Eur. J. Biochem. 137: 155-161.

62. Westphal, O., Luderitz, O., Galanos, C., Mayer, H. and Rietschel, E. Th., 1985, The story of bacterial endotoxin, Adv. Immunopharmacol. 13-34.

63. Wilkinson, S. G. and Taylor, D. P., 1978, Occurrence of 2,3-diamino-2, 3-dideoxy-D-glucose in lipid A from lipopolysaccharide of Pseudomonas diminuta, J. Gen. Microbiol. 109: 367-370.

64. Wilkinson, B. J., Hindahl, M. S., Galbraith, L. and Wilkinson, S. G., 1986, Lipopolysaccharide of Paracoccus denitrificans ATCC 13543, FEMS Microbiol. Lett. 37: 63-67.

65. Woese, C. R., 1987, Bacterial evolution, Microbiol. Rev. 51: 221-271.

66. Woese, C. R., Stackebrandt, E., Weisburg, W. G., Paster, B. J., Madigan, M. T., Fowler, V. J., Hahn, C. M., Blanz, P., Gupta, R., Nealson, K. H. and Fox, G. E., 1984, The phylogeny of purple bacteria: the alpha subdivision, Syst. Appl. Microbiol. 5: 315-326.

67. Woese, C. R., Stackebrandt, E., Weisburg, W. G., Paster, B. J., Madigan, M. T., Fowler, V. J., Hahn, C. M., Blanz, P., Gupta, R., Nealson, K. H. and Fox, G. E., 1985, The phylogeny of purple bacteria: the gamma subdivision, Syst. Appl. Microbiol. 6: 25-33.

68. Wollenweber, H. W., Schlecht, S., Lüderitz, O. and Rietschel, E., 1983, Fatty acid in lipopolysaccharides of Salmonella species grown at low temperatures, Eur. J. Biochem. 130: 167-171.

69. Wollenweber, H. W., Seydel, U., Lindner, B., Lüderitz, O. and Rietschel, E. Th., 1984, Nature and location of amide-bound (R)3-acyloxyacyl groups in lipid A of lipopolysaccharides from various Gram-negative bacteria, Eur. J. Biochem. 145: 265-272.

70. Yokota, A., Rodriguez, M., Yamada, Y., Imai, K., Borowiak, D. and Mayer, H., 1987a, Lipopolysaccharides of Thiobacillus species containing lipid A with 2,3-diamino-2,3-dideoxyglucose, Arch. Microbiol. 149: 106-111.

71. Yokota, A., Schlecht and Mayer, H., 1987b, Lipopolysaccharides of chemolithotrophic bacteria Thiobacillus versutus and a related Thiobacillus species, FEMS Microbiol. Lett. 44: 197-201.

IMMUNOCHEMISTRY OF LIPID A

N. Kasai, S. Arata, J. Mashimo, T. Hirayama, and M. Ueno

Department of Microbial Chemistry, School of Parmaceutical Sciences, Showa University, Hatanodai, Shinagawa-ku Tokyo 142, Japan

INTRODUCTION

We previously suggested (1, 2, 8-10) that lipid A epitopes are composed of the backbone and acyl groups of the lipid A molecule, and that lipid A has specific and common or cross-reactive epitopes, in which the specificities are derived from the chemical and conformational structures of the backbone and/or acyl groups. In these studies, the in vitro antigenic reactivity of a number of chemically synthesized lipid A analogs with free lipid A preparations from many strains including **E. coli, Salmonella minnesota, Klebsiella pneumoniae, Chromobacterium violaceum, Plesiomonas shigelloides,** and **Pseudomonas diminuta** was analyzed by enzyme-linked immunosorbent assay (ELISA) and ELISA inhibition test with monoclonal and conventional antibodies against the free lipid A from **S. minnesota** R595. During these studies, we found that the development of monoclonal antibodies against lipid A having different backbone and/or hydrophobic structures, and the evaluation of antibody-specificity by various assay systems was important to confirm our hypothesis concerning lipid A epitopes. In the present study, therefore, we examined the in vitro antigenic reactivity of synthetic lipid A analogs and bacterial lipid A with monoclonal and conventional antibodies against the lipid A of **E. coli** F515, **E. coli** J5 and **P. diminuta** JCM 2788, as well as **S. minnesota** R595 by the ELISA, ELISA inhibition test, and the immunodot assay.

MATERIALS AND METHODS

Synthetic Lipid A Analogs

Fig 1, 2 and 3 show the chemical structures of synthetic lipid A analogues. Compounds LA-14-PP (6), LA-15-PP (4, 5), LA-16-PP (10), LA-15-PH (4, 5), LA-16-PH (10), 401 and 408 (15) were obtained through the courtesy of Dr. F. Masumi. Compounds LA-17-PP, LA-18-PP, LA-20-PP, LA-21-PP, LA-23-PP and LA-24-PP, which were synthesized by Imoto et al., (7, 10), were supplied by Drs. T. Shiba and S. Kusumoto. The synthetic monosaccharide analogues (11-14) related to the non-reducing part of lipid A were obtained through the courtesy of Dr. A. Hasegawa (Fig 2 and 3).

Bacterial Lipid A

Free lipid A specimens from **S. minnesota** R595 and **E. coli** F515 were prepared by acid hydrolysis with 1% acetic acid of LPS isolated by the

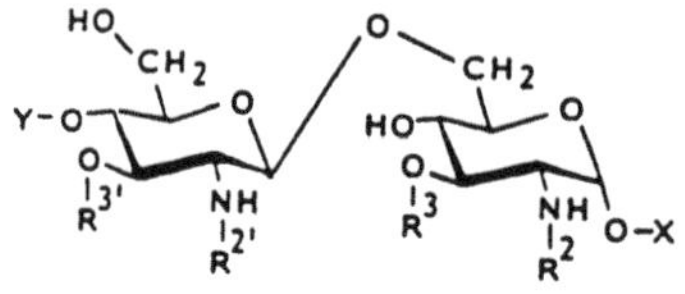

Compound	R3'	R2'	R3	R2	Y	X
LA-23-PP	C10	C10	C10	C10	P	P
LA-24-PP	C10	C14-OH	C10	C14-OH	P	P
LA-17-PP	C14	C14	C14	C14	P	P
LA-18-PP	C14	C14-OH	C14	C14-OH	P	P
LA-14-PP	C14-OH	C14-OH	C14-OH	C14-OH	P	P
LA-20-PP	C14-OH	C14-OH	C14-OH	C14-O-(C16)	P	P
LA-21-PP	C14-OH	C14-O-(C16)	C14-OH	C14-OH	P	P
LA-15-PP	C14-O-(C14)	C14-O-(C12)	C14-OH	C14-OH	P	P
LA-16-PP	C14-O-(C14)	C14-O-(C12)	C14-OH	C14-O-(C16)	P	P
LA-15-PH	C14-O-(C14)	C14-O-(C12)	C14-OH	C14-OH	P	H
LA-16-PH	C14-O-(C14)	C14-O-(C12)	C14-OH	C14-O-(C16)	P	H

Fig 1. Chemical structure of synthetic lipid A analogues. Abbreviations: P, $PO(OH)_2$; C_{10}, decanoyl; C_{14}, tetradecanoyl; C_{14}-OH, (R)-3-hydroxytetradecanoyl; C_{14}-O-(C_{12}), (R)-3-dodecanoyloxytetradecanoyl; C_{14}-O-(C_{14}), (R)-3-tetradecanoyloxytetradecanoyl; C_{14}-O-(C_{16}), (R)-3-hexadecanoyloxytetradecanoyl.

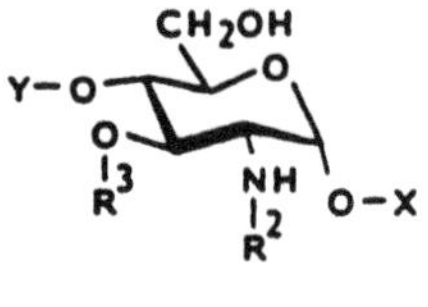

Compound	R^3	R^2	Y	X
401	C14-OH	C14-OH	H	P
408	C14-OH	C14-O-(C16)	H	P
GLA-44	C14	C14-OH	P	H
GLA-46	C14-OH	C14-OH	P	H
GLA-34	H	C14-O-(C14)	P	H
GLA-27	C14	C14-O-(C14)	P	H
GLA-47	C14-O-(C14)	C14-O-(C14)	P	H
GLA-37	C12	C12-O-(C12)	P	H
GLA-38	C16	C16-O-(C16)	P	H
GLA-57	C14	C14-O-(C12)	P	H
GLA-58	C14	C14-O-(C16)	P	H
GLA-61	C14-OH	C14-O-(C12)	P	H
GLA-59	C14-OH	C14-O-(C14)	P	H
GLA-62	C14-OH	C14-O-(C16)	P	H
GLA-63	C14-O-(C12)	C14-OH	P	H
GLA-60	C14-O-(C14)	C14-OH	P	H
GLA-64	C14-O-(C16)	C14-OH	P	H
GLA-67	C14-O-(C12)	C14	P	H
GLA-68	C14-O-(C14)	C14	P	H
GLA-69	C14-O-(C16)	C14	P	H

Fig 2. Chemical structure of synthetic monosaccharide lipid A analogs.

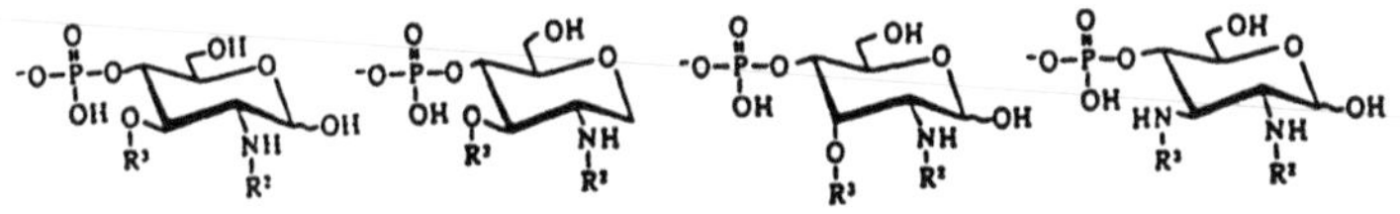

(I) (II)* (III)** (IV)***

Compound	R^3	R^2
GLA-113	2-(C10)-C14	C14-OH
GLA-114	2-(C12)-C14	C14-OH
GLA-115	2-(C14)-C14	C14-OH
GLA-116	2-(C16)-C14	C14-OH
GLA-117	2-(C18)-C14	C14-OH
GLA-78	2-(C14)-C16	C14-OH
GLA-112	2-(C9)-C7	C14-OH
GLA-40 *	C14	C14-O-(C14)
GLA-43 **	C14	C14-O-(C14)
GLA-48 ***	C14	C14-O-(C14)

Fig 3. Chemical structure of synthetic monosaccharide lipid A analogs. Abbreviation: 2-(C_{10})-C_{14}, 2-decanyl-tetradecanoyl. Symbols I, II, III, and IV denote structural groups of the monosaccharide analogues.

phenol/chloroform/petroleum ether method as described previously (16). The purified lipid A preparations of **E. coli** F515, A2, A3 and A7 were prepared by preparative thin-layer chromatography (TLC) as reported previously (16). Free lipid A and purified preparations of **P. diminuta** JCM 2788 and **P. vesicularis** JCM 1477 were prepared as described previously (8, 16).

Conventional and Monoclonal Antibodies (mAb)

Rabbit antisera against **S. minnesota** R595 lipid A, E. coli F515, and **P. diminuta** JCM 2788 lipid A were prepared as previously described (10). Mouse monoclonal antibodies against S. minnesota R595 lipid A derived from the four hybridomas, Sm5G(IgG 2b), Sm36G(IgG 3), Sm161M(IgM) and Sm1-9M(IgM) were as described in (10). Mouse monoclonal antibodies against E. coli F515 lipid A derived from the three hybridomas, Ec3G(IgG 2b), Ec711G(IgG 2b) and Ec14G(IgG 2a) were prepared as in (10). Two monoclonal antibodies against **P. diminuta** lipid A, Pd6G(IgG 2b), and Pd4G(IgG 1) were prepared by Aoki et al., (Japan. J. Med. Sci. Biol. 40: 198-199, 1987) according to the procedure described in (10). Monoclonal antibodies against E. coli J5, 8A1(IgG 1) and 2A6(IgM) were obtained from Dr. R. T. Coughlin.

Serological Assays

Details of the ELISA and ELISA inhibition test were as described in (10). In the ELISA, microtitration plates (Linbro/Titertek, Flow Laboratories, Inc, McLean, Va.) coated with either synthetic or bacterial lipid A preparation of 2ug/0.2ml per well were reacted with serial dilution of conventional or monoclonal antibodies. In the ELISA inhibition test, a fixed dilution of lipid A antibodies was preincubated for 30 min at 37°C with an equal volume of inhibiting ligands in different concentrations. The mixture (0.2ml) was then placed in the wells of microtitration plates, which were precoated with the given lipid A described in each table, and incubated for 2.5 hr at 37°C. After being washed, the standard ELISA procedure (10) was followed. The 50% inhibitory value was expressed as the ug per well of a ligand needed to obtain a 50% decrease in the absorbance at 405 nm as compared with the control well to which no inhibitor was added.

A modified immunodot assay by the method of Hawkes et al., (3) was performed with an ATTO Immunodot apparatus (Type AE-6190, ATTO Corporation, Tokyo). Briefly, the sample dissolved in distilled water containing 0.01 or 0.05% triethylamine was dotted into a nitrocellulose membrane filter (Type TM-2, Toyo Roshi Co., Ltd., Tokyo) through the sample wells. The antigen-dotted filter was treated with a blocking solution containing 5% fetal calf serum, and reacted with serial or fixed dilution of lipid A antibodies at 37°C for 2hr. After washing with 50mM tris-buffer containing 200 mM NaCl (TBS), the membrane filter was incubated with the alkaline phosphatase-conjugated second antibody solution, which was prepared as described in (10), and then developed with 0.1% 5-bromo-4-chloro-3-indolyl phosphate in 0.05 M carbonate buffer (pH 9.8).

RESULTS AND DISCUSSION

1. Epitope Analysis with mAb against S. minnesota R595 Lipid A

The antigenic reactivities of synthetic disaccharide analogs and monosaccharide analogs as determined by the ELISA and ELISA inhibition test with 4 monoclonal antibodies, Sm5G, Sm36G, Sm161M and Sm1-9M, have been shown previously (1, 2, 9, 10). The results suggested that the Sm5G and Sm36G antibodies recognize the structure of **S. minnesota**-type lipid A, compound LA-16-PP, in which the structure including the acyloxyacyl group at the C-2 position rather than those at the C-2' and probably C-3' positions as shown by the strong reactivity of LA-20-PP might be important in the recognition by these antibodies.

The results also suggest that the Sm161M antibody recognizes a common conformational structure widely present in bacterial lipid A including the **P. diminuta** and **P. vesicularis** lipid A, the backbone of which contains a nonglycosidic phosphomonoester of 3-amino-D-glucosamine disaccharide (8). Since the Sm161M antibody cross-reacted strongly with the 1-dephospho-compound of **E. coli** or **S. minnesota**-type lipid A and with monosaccharide analogs of the nonreducing part of lipid A, it was considered that this antibody recognizes the nonreducing part of the lipid A molecule. Hasegawa et al., recently synthesized a new series of monosaccharide lipid A analogs having a branched-chain fatty acyl group of various chain-lengths, in place of an acyloxyacyl group. The results of the ELISA inhibition test with Sm161M antibody showed that there is a suitable combination of chain length to react with this antibody: for example, the antigenic reactivity of GLA-44, which has the structure of 4-phospho-D-glucosamine carrying the 3-hydroxytetradecanoyl group at the C-2 position and tetradecanoyl group at the C-3 position, considerably increased the reactivity when a 2-tetradecanyl-tetradecanoyl group was substituted for the tetradecanoyl residue (data not shown). This supports the previous observation that the chain length of the fatty acid as well as the nature of the linkage might be imporant in the serological reactivity (1).

The Sm1-9M antibody was similar to Sm161M in its strong recognition of the 1-dephospho-compound of **E. coli** or **S. minnesota**-type lipid A. However, its specificity is different from that of Sm161M since it did not cross-react with the **P. diminuta** and **P. vesicularis** lipid A.

Essentially similar results were obtained by the immunodot assay with Sm5G and Sm161M antibodies, but in the immunodot assay, Sm5G hardly recognized the structural difference between the hydrophobic parts of the compounds LA-15-PP and LA-16-PP. On the other hand, the cross-reactivity of Re-type LPS with Sm161M was greater in this assay system that in the ELISA.

This suggests that the lipid A epitopes of Re LPS are more readily exposed on the nitrocellulose membrane surface than on the polystyrene surface in the ELISA.

2. Epitope Analysis with mAb against E. coli F515 Lipid A

Tables 1 and 2 show the results of the ELISA and ELISA inhibition test with monoclonal and conventional antibodies. The conventional antibodies (No. 225) were highly reactive to E. coli F515 Lipid A (A3) and compound LA-15-PP, suggesting that the antibodies contained a specific antibody directed to the E. coli-type lipid A. The similar result has been observed with mouse conventional antibodies (data not shown).

Ec3G and Ec711G reacted strongly with compounds LA-14-PP, LA-21-PP and LA-15-PP, but the reactivity of LA-20-PP and LA-16-PP with these monoclonal antibodies was about 1/10-1/20 that of LA-15-PP. This suggests that the acyloxyacyl groups are not essential for recognition by these monoclonal antibodies, and also that the acyloxyacyl group at the C-2 position might hinder antibody binding. Ec3G and Ec711G did not react with LA-15-PH or LA-16-PH which lacks glycosidic phosphate, which indicates that the phosphate group is important for these antibodies to recognize the compounds. Thus, Ec3G and Ec711G was considered to recognize strongly the backbone containing the 1,4'-bisphosphorylated glucosamine disaccharide structure, and that acylation pattern also affected the reactivity. On the other hand, Ec14G reacted strongly with compounds LA-14-PP, LA-20-PP, LA-21-PP, LA-15-PP, and LA-16-PP. In contrast with Ec3G or Ec711G, this antibody reacted with LA-15-PH and LA-16-PH. Thus, the results show that the specificity of the Ec14G antibody is clearly different from that of Ec3G and Ec711G. In addition, Ec3G and Ec711G reacted strongly with LA-23-PP, LA-24-PP, LA-17-PP and LA-18-PP, whereas Ec14G hardly reacted with these compounds (data not shown). These results support our previous hypothesis that the hydrophobic structure together with the backbone are involved in the epitopes of the lipid A molecule.

3. Epitope Analysis with mAb against E. coli J5

Tables 1 and 3 show the results of the ELISA and ELISA inhibition test with monoclonal antibodies, 8A1 and 2A6. The 8A1 antibody reacted strongly with compounds LA-20-PP, LA-21-PP, LA-15-PP, and LA-16-PP, but LA-14-PP which lacks the acyloxyacyl group exhibited a reactivity of about 1/20 of LA-15-PP. The 8A1 antibody also reacted with **P. diminuta** and **P. vesicularis** lipid A and the monosaccharide analog GLA-27. Thus, 8A1 was considered to be cross-reactive antibody similar to that of Sm161M.

In the immunodot assay with 8A1 and 2A6, a reactivity similar to that in the ELISA and ELISA inhibition test was observed among the tested preparations. Moreover, in these assays, some synthetic analogs and Re-type LPS, which was only slightly active in the ELISA, expressed the reactivity (data not shown). Thus, it was concluded that the exposure of lipid A epitopes depends partly on the reaction system utilized.

The 26A antibody exhibited the highest reactivity with LA-15-PH and LA-16-PH among the tested compounds, whereas the reactivity of bisphosphorylated compounds having acyloxyacyl group(s) was about 1/5 - 1/10 that of LA-15-PH or LA-16-PH, suggesting that the glycosidic phosphate might hinder the antibody binding. The 2A6 antibody also cross-reacted partly with **P. diminuta** and **P. vescularis** lipid A and GLA-27.

Table 1. Reactivity of monoclonal lipid A antibodies as determined by ELISA with lipid A and LPS.

Coating antigen	E.coli F515			E.coli J5		P.diminuta	
	Ec3G (IgG2b)	Ec711G (IgG2b)	Ec14G (IgG2b)	8A1 (IgG1)	2A6 (IgM)	Pd6G (IgG2b)	Pd4G (IgG1)
Lipid A preparation							
E.coli F515	13	9	15	4	398	196	9
S.minnesota R595	49	134	27	4	35	27	13
P.diminuta JCM 2788	>50,000	>50,000	66	6	1,580	3	9
LPS preparation							
E.coli F515	>50,000	>50,000	>1,000	>1,000	5,900	>20,000	>70
P.diminuta JCM 2788	>50,000	>50,000	>1,000	>1,000	>10,000	>20,000	>70

The antibody titer is expressed as the concentration (ng/ml) giving a reaction of 0.1 by determining the optical density at 405nm.

Table 2. Antigenic reactivity of synthetic and bacterial lipid A in ELISA inhibition test with mAb and conventional antibodies against **E. coli** F515 lipid A.

Test antigen	Inhibitory activity (ug/well) of test antigen as determined with the following antibodies:			
	Ec3G	Ec711G	Ec14G	#225(conv.)
LA-14-PP	0.38	0.17	0.02	4.1
LA-20-PP	3.3	3.2	0.02	NT
LA-21-PP	0.42	0.13	0.01	NT
LA-15-PP	0.45	0.16	0.04	0.04
LA-16-PP	9.7	7.3	0.04	0.15
LA-15-PH	>10	>10	0.32	>10
LA-16-PH	>10	>10	0.21	>10
Bacterial lipid A				
E. coli F515	0.28	0.39	0.03	0.11
S. minnesota R595	0.50	0.68	0.05	0.17
P. diminuta JCM 2788	>10	>10	>10	>10
P. vesicularis JCM 1477	>10	>10	>10	>10

Microtitration plates were coated with **E. coli** F515 lipid A of 2 μg/0.2ml per well. NT: Not tested

Table 3. Antigenic reactivity of synthetic and bacterial lipid A ELISA inhibition with mAb against **E. coli** J5.

Test antigen	Inhibitory activity (µg/well) of test antigen as determined with the following mAb:	
	8A1	2A6
LA-14-PP	3.2	>10
LA-20-PP	0.28	0.78
LA-21-PP	0.28	0.62
LA-15-PP	0.15	0.30
LA-16-PP	0.25	0.28
LA-15-PH	2.6	0.07
LA-16-PH	0.90	0.08
401	>10	>10
408	>10	>10
GLA-44	>10	>10
GLA-44	3.1	2.1
Bacterial lipid A		
E. coli F515	0.17	0.83
S. minnesota R595	0.09	0.63
P. diminuta JCM 2788	1.1	15
P. vesicularis JCM 1477	1.3	14

Microtitration plates were coated with compound LA-15-PP of 2 µg/0.2 ml per well.

Table 4. Antigenic reactivity of synthetic and bacterial lipid A in ELISA inhibition test with mAb and conventional antibodies against **P. diminuta** lipid A.

Test antigen	Inhibitory activity (µg/well) of test antigen as determined with the following antibodies:		
	Pd6G	Pd4G	#280(conv.)
LA-14-PP	>10	>10	NT
LA-15-PP	10	0.11	NT
LA-16-PP	8.8	0.29	NT
LA-15-PH	8.8	0.95	NT
LA-16-PH	4.2	1.3	NT
Bacterial lipid A			
P. diminuta JCM 2788	0.01	0.01	0.30
A2	0.01	0.04	0.57
A3	0.05	0.01	0.15
P. vesicuralis JCM 1477	0.01	0.03	0.32
E. coli F515	>10	0.31	>10
S. minnesota R595	>10	0.47	>10

Microtitration plates were coated with **P. diminuta** JCM 2788 lipid A of 2 µg/0.2 ml per well.

4. Epitope Analysis with mAb against **P. diminuta** Lipid A

By the ELISA and ELISA inhibition test with conventional antibody against P. diminuta or P. vesicularis lipid A, the antibodies have been suggested to contain a specific antibody to the lipid A. As shown in Tables 1 and 4, in the ELISA and ELISA inhibition test the Pd6G antibody reacted strongly with the **P. diminuta** and **P. vesicularis** lipid A especially with the A2 fraction. Partial deacylation by a mild hydrazinolysis results in a considerable loss of the antigenic reactivity to this antibody. The Pd6G reacted only slightly with the synthetic **E. coli** or **S. minnesota**-type lipid A analogues so far tested. Pd4G antibody reacted strongly with the **P. diminuta** and **P. vesicularis** lipid A, especially with the main lipid A component, A3. This antibody cross-reacted partially with LA-15-PP and LA-16-PP.

It was concluded that the Pd6G and Pd4G, though the specificities are somewhat different, recognize a specific lipid A structure of **P. diminuta** or **P. vesicularis.**

In summary, in the present study using anti-lipid A monoclonal and conventional antibodies of different origins, we demonstrated that lipid A produces various antibodies carrying similar or different specificities, and that serological specificities are derived from the backbone and/or acyl groups of the lipid A molecule.

ACKNOWLEDGMENTS

We thank Drs. T. Shiba, S. Kusumoto, A. Hasegawa, M. Kiso and F. Masumi for supplying synthetic lipid A analogs, and Dr. R. T. Coughlin for supplying monoclonal antibodies. We also thank Dr. A. Simpson for reviewing and correcting this manuscript.

REFERENCES

1. Arata, S., Mashimo, J., Kasai, N., Okuda, K., Aihara, Y., Hasegawa, A., and Kiso, M., 1987, Analysis of antigenic reactivity of synthetic monosaccharide lipid A analogs with monoclonal antibodies. FEMS Microbiol. Lett. 44: 231.

2. Arata, S., Mashimo, J., Kasai, N., Okuda, K., Aihara, Y., Kotani, S., Takada, H., Shiba, T., Kusumoto, S., Shimamoto, T., and Kusunose, N., 1988, Characterization of monoclonal lipid A antibodies with synthetic lipid A analogs. FEMS Microbiol. Lett. 49: 479.

3. Hawkes, R., Niday, E., and Cordon, J., 1982, A dot-immunobinding assay for monoclonal and other antibodies. Anal. Biochem. 119: 142.

4. Imoto, M., Yoshimura, H., Kusumoto, S., and Shiba, T., 1984, Total synthesis of lipid A, active principle of bacterial endotoxin. Proc. Japan Acad. 60(Ser.B): 285.

5. Imoto, M., Yoshimura, H., Shimamoto, T., Sakaguchi, N., Kusumoto, S., and Shiba, T., 1987, Total synthesis of **Escherichia coli** lipid A, the endotoxically active principle of cell-surface lipopolysaccharide. Bull. Chem. Soc. Jpn. 60: 2205.

6. Imoto, M., Yoshimura, H., Yamamoto, M., Shimamoto, T., Kusumoto, S., and Shiba, T., 1984, Chemical synthesis of phosphorylated tetraacyl disaccharide corresponding to a biosynthetic precursor of lipid A. Tetrahedron. Lett. 25: 2667.

7. Imoto, M., Yoshimura, H., Yamamoto, M., Shimamoto, T., Kusumoto, S., and Shiba, T., 1987, Chemical synthesis of a biosynthetic precursor of lipid A with a phosphorylated tetraacyl disaccharide structure. Bull. Chem. Soc. Jpn. 60: 2197.

8. Kasai, N., Arata, S., Mashimo, J., Akiyama, Y., Tanaka, C., Egawa, K., Tanaka, S., 1987, **Pseudomonas diminuta** LPS with a new endotoxic lipid A structure. Biochem. Biophys. Res. Commun. 142: 972.

9. Kasai, N., Arata, S., Mashimo, J., Okuda, K., Aihara, Y., Kotani, S., Takada, H., Shiba, T., and Kusumoto, S., 1985, In vitro antigenic reactivity of synthetic lipid A analogs as determined by monoclonal and conventional antibodies. Biochem. Biophys. Res. Commun. 128: 607.

10. Kasai, N., Arata, S., Mashimo, J., Okuda, K., Aihara, Y., Kotani, S., Takada, H., Shiba, T., Kusumoto, S., Imoto, M., Yoshimura, H., and Shimamoto, T., 1986, Synthetic **Salmonella**-type lipid A antigen with high serological specificity. Infect. Immun. 51: 43.

11. Kiso, M., Ishida, H., and Hasegawa, A., 1984, Synthesis of biologically active, novel monosaccharide analogs of lipid A. Agric. Biol. Chem. 48: 251.

12. Kiso, M., Tanaka, S., Fujita, M., Fujishima, Y., Ogawa, Y., and Hasegawa, A., 1987, Synthesis of nonreducing-sugar subunit analogs of bacterial lipid A carrying an amide-bound(3**R**)-3-acyloxytetradecanoyl group. Carbohydr. Res. 162: 247.

13. Kiso, M., Tanaka, S., Fujita, M., Fujishima, Y., Ogawa, Y., Ishida, H., and Hasegawa, A., 1987, Synthesis of the optically active 4-**O**-phosphono-D-glucosamine derivatives related to the nonreducing-sugar subunit of bacterial lipid A. Carbohydr. Res. 162: 127.

14. Kiso, M., Tanaka, S., Takahashi, M., Fujishima, Y., Ogawa, Y., and Hasegawa, A., 1986, Synthesis of 2-deoxy-4-**O**-phosphono-3-O-tetradecanoyl-2-[(3R)-and-(3S)-3-tetradecanoyloxytetradecanamido]-D-glucose: a diastereoisomeric pair of 4-O-phosphono-D-glucosamine-derivatives (GLA-27) related to bacterial lipid A. Carbohydr. Res. 148: 221.

15. Kusumoto, S., Yamamoto, M., and Shiba, T., 1984, Chemical synthesis of lipid X and lipid Y, acylglucosamine 1-phosphates isolated from E. coli mutants. Tetrahedron. Lett. 25: 3727.

16. Mashimo, J., Tanaka, C., Arata, S., Akiyama, Y., Hata, S., Hirayama, T., Egawa, K., and Kasai, N., 1988, Structural heterogeneity regarding local shwartzman activity of lipid A. Microbiol. Immun. 32: 653.

BACTERIAL LIPOPOLYSACCHARIDES: RELATIONSHIP OF STRUCTURE AND CONFORMATION TO ENDOTOXIC ACTIVITY, SEROLOGICAL SPECIFICITY AND BIOLOGICAL FUNCTION

E. Th. Rietschel, L. Brade, U. Schade, U. Seydel, U. Zähringer, K. Brandenburg, I. Helander, O. Holst, S. Kondo, H. M. Kuhn, B. Lindner, E. Röhrscheidt, R. Russa, *H. Labischinski, *D. Naumann, and H. Brade

Forschungsinstitut Borstel, Institut fur Experimentelle Biologie und Medizin, D-2061 Borstel, FRG and *Robert-Koch-Institut des Bundesgesundheitsamtes, D-1000 Berlin 65, FRG

INTRODUCTION

Gram-negative bacteria express in their cell envelope various amphiphilic macromolecules among which the lipopolysaccharides (LPS) are of special significance for bacterial viability and the interaction of bacteria with host organisms. Together with phospholipids and proteins, lipopolysaccharides form the outer membrane of gram-negative bacteria. This outer membrane has an asymmetric architecture, i.e., lipopolysaccharides are located exclusively in the outer leaflet through which the bacterial cell interacts with its environment.

As exposed cell surface components, lipopolysaccharides play an important role in the interaction of the bacterial cell with the host, e.g., during infection. Thus, lipopolysaccharides may prevent the engulfment of bacteria by phagocytic cells of the host and they contribute to the resistance of microorganisms against the bactericidal action of serum. On the other hand, contact of gram-negative bacteria with the immune system of higher organisms leads to the production of antibacterial antibodies which are predominantly directed against determinants embedded in the lipopolysaccharide molecule. Accordingly, lipopolysaccharides belong to the principal surface antigens of gram-negative bacteria, a property being expressed by the term O-antigen which is often used instead of the name lipopolysaccharide.

Injection of gram-negative bacteria into experimental animals causes a range of nonspecific pathophysiological reactions. These acute effects include fever, hypotension, changes in white blood cell counts, disseminated intravascular coagulation and, if administered in higher doses, irreversible shock. These pathophysiolgical reactions are equally elicited by isolated and purified lipopolysaccharide. Lipopolysaccharides, therefore, represent potent bacterial toxins and this quality is indicated by the term endotoxin which is also used synonymously for the name lipopolysaccharide.

In view of their manifold pathological and physiological activities, lipopolysaccharides have been studied in many laboratories over the last decades. The goals of these investigations included:

1. Clarification of the mechanisms involved in endotoxin action in vivo and in vitro.
2. Development of strategies to immunologically and pharmacologically control harmful manifestations of endotoxicosis.
3. Elucidation of the genetic determination and biosynthetic pathways of lipopolysaccharide.
4. Definition of biologically active regions of lipopolysaccharides.
5. Analysis of the chemical structure and conformation of such regions.
6. Chemical synthesis of these regions.
7. Establishment of (quantitative) relationships between the chemical as well as the physical structure and biological activity of lipopolysaccharides.
8. Determination of the involvement of lipopolysaccharides in outer membrane architecture and the function of this membrane as a permeation barrier, and thus
9. Elucidation of the role of lipopolysaccharide in bacterial viability (bacterial growth and survival).

The progress made in these fields has been summarized in the "Handbook of Endotoxin" (30). The interest of our group was, during recent years, primarily focused on relationships between the structure and the conformation of lipopolysaccharides to i) endotoxic activity, ii) antigenicity and immunogenicity and iii) outer membrane architecture and permeation-barrier function.

In the present paper some newer results concerning these areas are presented and discussed. Of the considerable literature available on these subjects only recent summarizing reviews and a few original publications are cited.

CHEMISTRY OF LIPOPOLYSACCHARIDES

Lipopolysaccharides, as this term implies, consist chemically of a polysaccharide and a covalently bound lipid component, termed lipid A. The polysaccharide component of enterobacterial lipopolysaccharides consists of two regions which differ in their genetic determination, biosynthesis and architecture. These regions are the O-specific chain and the core oligosaccharide. A variety of nonenterobacterial wild-type strains of photorophic and some human pathogenic gram-negative bacteria including **Neisseria, Acinetobacter, Bordetella, Bacteroides** and **Haemophilus** form lipopolysaccharides which consist only of the core and lipid A region, thus lacking the O-specific chain (11, 34).

O-Specific Chain

The O-specific chain is a polymer of repeating oligosaccharide units which contain up to six sugar residues. A large diversity of the constituent components of repeating units has been revealed within different gram-negative bacteria. The nature, ring form, type of linkage, and type of substitution of the individual monosaccharide residues, as well as their sequence within a repeating unit is characteristic and unique for a given lipopolysaccharide and the parental bacterial strain, i.e., a bacterial species. Thus, the O-specific chain is species-specific (25). Because of the diversity of constituents and their linkages, an enormous number of structures of O-specific chains is conceivable and also verified in Nature. Therefore, an immense structural variability is revealed if the O-specific chains of distinct bacterial origin are compared.

Core Oligosaccharide

The core region of enterobacterial lipopolysaccharides consists of a heterooligosaccharide which can be formally subdivided into the O-chain-proximal outer core and the lipid A-proximal inner core. The outer core contains the common sugars D-glucose, D-galactose, and N-acetyl-D-glucosamine, whereas the inner core region is composed of the unusual sugars heptose, mainly in the L-glycero-D-manno (L,D-heptose) and the D-glycero-D-manno configuration, and 2-keto-3-deoxyoctonic acid (KDO, systematically termed 3-deoxy-D-manno-2-octulosonic acid, dOclA). These residues are, in general, substituted by charged groups such as phosphate, pyrophosphate, phosphorylethanolamine and pyrophosphorylethanolamine, often in nonstoichiometric amounts. Therefore, the inner core region exhibits microheterogeneity and a considerable accumulation of charged residues.

The structural variability of the core within different bacterial species is limited. Thus, in the genus **Salmonella** only one core type (Ra core) exists for all serotypes, and in **Escherichia coli** so far five core types (R1, R2, R3, R4 and K-12) have been described for more than a hundred different serotypes. The structural variability of core types relates primarily to the outer region, while the KDO-containing inner core appears to be structurally more conserved. In the chemical analysis of the KDO-containing inner core, enterobacterial rough-(R)-mutants which synthesize lipopolysaccharides lacking the O-specific chain and parts of the core proved to be most valuable. Using the lipopolysaccharide of a **S. minnesota** Rd1P-mutant (strain R7), the structure of the enterobacterial inner core region could be established as shown in Fig 1 (37).

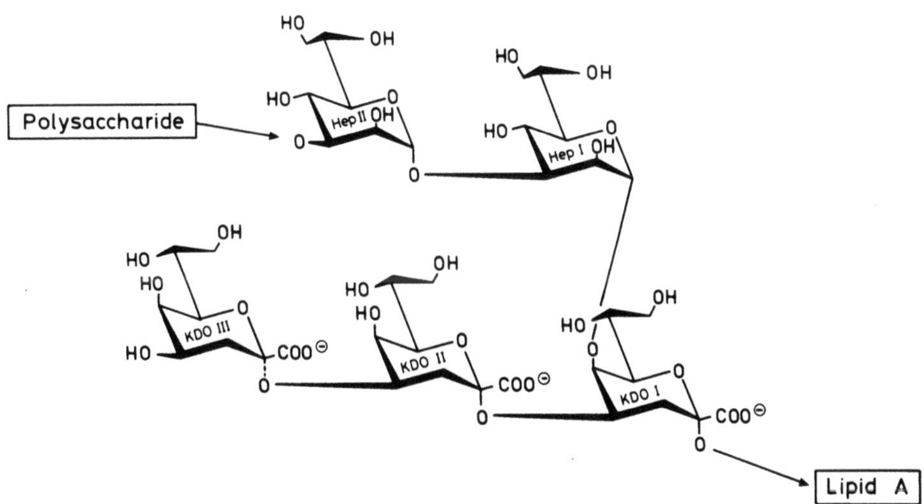

Fig 1. Chemical structure of the core oligosaccharide in the lipopolysaccharide of **S. minnesota** chemotype Rd1P (strain R7). KDO I and KDO II are the only core constituents in Re-type lipopolysaccharide. KDO III is only found in mutants other than Re where it is not always present in stoichiometric amounts (as indicated by the dotted line). KDO-bound phosphorylethanolamine is not shown (1, 37).

Accordingly, one KDO residue is present in the main core oligosaccharide chain (KDO I) being substituted in position 4 by A-linked KDO II, which in turn may carry, at position 4, nonstoichiometric amounts of a further A-linked KDO residue (KDO III). All KDO groups are present as pyranosides. In its position 5, the KDO I residue carries A-bound L,D-heptose (Hep I) to which a second L,D-heptose residue (Hep II) is A-linked (position 3). In lipopolysaccharides of less defective mutants and wild-type bacteria, the saccharide chain extends from the hydroxyl group in position 3 of Hep II. KDO I is A-detosidically linked to the primary hydroxyl group (position 6') of the nonreducing (distal) D-glucosamine residue (GlcN II) of the lipid A backbone (see Fig 2).

The analysis of the inner core architecture of other bacterial groups was, and still is, very difficult (1). This is due to the problems encountered with the analytical chemistry of KDO and the nonavailability of enzymes cleaving the ketosidic linkage of KDO. KDO is a polyfunctional sugar acid with eight carbon atoms harboring carboxyl, keto, deoxy and hydroxyl groups. This accumulation of different functional groups renders KDO extremely sensitive to the action of acid and other chemical reagents. Thus, under the experimental conditions of its isolation, purification or derivatization, KDO undergoes numerous side reactions yielding many artifacts. On the other hand, KDO may carry other residues, a fact which further hampers the elucidation of the inner core structure. In principle, each hydroxyl group of KDO may be substituted (34). Thus, depending on the bacterial origin of lipopolysaccharide, the hydroxyl group in position 4 may be substituted by negatively charged residues such as KDO (Fig 1) or phosphate. Position 5 often carries neutral sugars such as L,D-heptose, D-glucose or D-mannose. At position 7, phosphorylethanolamine may be present and to the primary hydroxyl group in position 8, KDO or 4-amino-4-deoxy-L-arabinopyranose may be bound. A special case was encountered in the lipopolysaccharide of **Acinetobacter calcoaceticus** (strain NCTC 10305) (19). Here KDO I is positionally replaced by an octulosonic acid, which probably has the D-glycero-D-talo configuration and, therefore, is isosteric to KDO. Also in **A. calcoaceticus** lipopolysaccharide, 2-keto-3-deoxy-1,7-dicarboxyheptonic acid (3-deoxy-heptulosonaric acid) and in **Vibrio parahemolyticus** 012 a 2-keto-3-deoxyhexonic acid was identified (21).

Some lipopolysaccharides (e.g., of **Vibrio cholerae**) had previously been claimed to lack KDO, and in **V. cholerae** KDO was postulated to be positionally replaced by D-fructose. It was recently found, however, that in **V. cholerae** KDO phosphate (detected as KDO-5-phosphate) is present and that D-fructose, rather, occupies a branch position (16). Also the lipopolysaccharides of **Bordetella pertussis, Bacteroides** strains, **V. parahemolyticus, Aeromonas salmonicidae,** and **Hemophilus influenzae** contains phosphorylated KDO (for literature see (4, 6, 10, 20, 34). In this context the lipopolysaccharide of a **Haemophilus influenzae** deep rough mutant (strain I-69 Rd /b$^+$) which was genetically constructed by Moxon et al., (27) is of interest. As our chemical analyses show, the lipopolysaccharide contains only one KDO residue which is phosphorylated and A-linked to lipid A (10). The phosphate group is mainly (75%) present at position 4 of KDO, but smaller amounts of KDO 5-phosphate were also detected. This lipopolysaccharide is remarkable in that its core is represented by a single KDO (phosphate) residue. Since this H. influenzae strain is able to multiply it follows that one (phosphorylated) KDO group in the lipopolysaccharide suffices for the growth of a gram-negative bacterium.

According to present knowledge all lipopolysaccharides, independent of their bacterial origin, contain at least one pyranosidic or furanosidic

KDO residue (or a derivative thereof) with a free carboxyl group occupying an internal position in the inner core region. KDO or a derivative, therefore, represents a common and obligatory constituent of lipopolysaccharides. In all cases studied, this KDO group is A-ketosidically bound to the primary hydroxyl group of the distal glucosamine unit (GlcN II) of the lipid A disaccharide backbone (see Fig 2). It is this KDO residue which carries the polysaccharide chain and, thus, mediates the link between the polysaccharide and lipid A components in lipopolysaccharides.

Lipid A

Lipid A represents the covalently linked lipid component of lipopolysaccharides. Polysaccharide-free lipid A does not exist in bacteria, a fact which is related to the biosynthesis of lipid A. Thus, KDO is transferred to a lipid A precursor molecule (tetraacyl precursor Ia) before the completion of the lipid A structure by addition of nonhydroxylated fatty acids (31). Enzymes which cleave the polysaccharide-lipid A bond are not known and hence, polysaccharide-deprived free lipid A can only be prepared by acid catalyzed hydrolysis of lipopolysaccharide.

The primary structure of lipid A of enterobacterial and some nonenterobacterial lipid A's, has been elucidated (34, 35). In Fig 2, two examples of lipid A structures are shown, i.e., those of **E. coli** and **Chromobacterium violaceum** with molecular weights of 1796 Da and 1655 Da (or 1671 Da), respectively. In both cases lipid A is composed of a β-D-glucosaminyl-(1-6)-β-D-glucosamine disaccharide which carries two phosphoryl groups: one in position 4' (of the distal glucosaminyl residue, GlcN II) and one in position 1 (of the reducing glucosaminyl residue, GlcN I). This hydrophilic lipid A backbone is, in both cases, acylated by four residues of (R)-3-hydroxy fatty acids at positions 2, 3, 2', and 3'. As a further common feature both lipid A's contain two free hydroxyl groups at positions 4 and 6'. The latter primary hydroxyl group is only free in polysaccharide-deprived lipid A (termed free lipid A) as obtained on acid treatment of lipopolysaccharide since this hydroxyl group serves as the attachment site of KDO and thus the polysaccharide component.

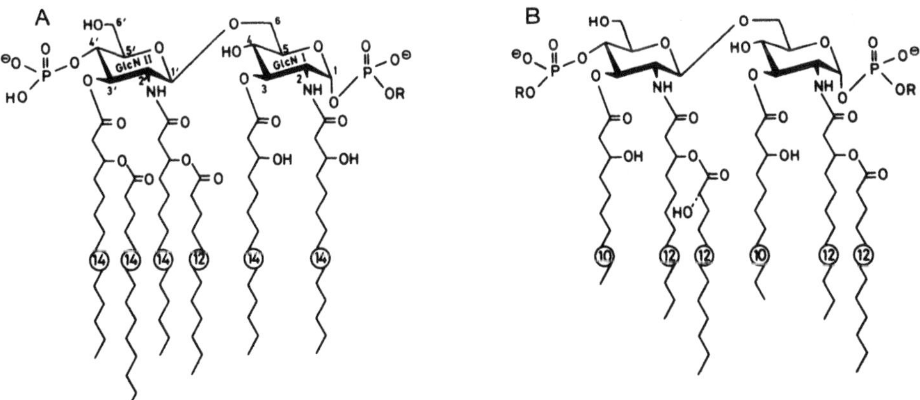

Fig 2. Chemical structure of the lipid A component of (A) **Escherichia coli** and (B) **Chromobacterium violaceum** (34).

Differences between the two lipid A's shown in Fig 2 are noted with regard to the chain length of hydroxylated and nonhydroxylated fatty acids and the location of ester-bound acyl groups. In **E. coli**, (R)-3-hydroxytetradecanoic acid (14:0(3-OH)) is present in ester and amide linkage. The hydroxyl groups of the two 14:0(3-OH) residues bound to GlcN II at positions 2' and 3' carry dodecanoic (12:0) and tetradecanoic acid (14:0), respectively. The two 14:0(3-OH) residues bound to GlcN I are not 3-O-acylated. In **C. violaceum** lipid A, two moles of (R)-3-hydroxydodecanoic acid (12:0(3-OH)) are amide-bound and two moles of (R)-3-hydroxydecanoic acid (10:0(3-OH)) are ester-linked to the lipid A backbone. The latter are not substituted at their 3-hydroxyl group while the amide-bound 12:0(3-OH) residues at positions 2 and 2' each carry 12:0. The 12:0(3-OH) residue at position 2' may carry (S)-2-hydroxydodecanoic acid (2-OH(12:0)) instead of 12:0. Thus, two molecular species of lipid A are revealed differing in the substituion of the amino group of GlcN II by either 3-(dodecanoyloxy)dodecanoic or 3-(2-hydroxydodecanoyloxy)dodecanoic acid. **E. coli** type lipid A with an asymmetrical acylation pattern has been detected in many enterobacterial lipopolysaccharides and e.g., in **Haemophilus** (10), while the C. violaceum type structure was shown to be present in **Neisseria gonorrhoeae** (39), and our analyses suggest that it also occurs in **Pseudomonas, Xanthomonas** and **Bacteroides** strains. As indicated in Fig 2, the phosphoryl groups in positions 1 and 4' may be substituted (symbol R) and phosphate (E. coli), D-glucosamine and 4-amino-4-deoxy-L-arabinopyranose (**C. violaceum**) have been identified as polar headgroups. Since their distribution over phosphoryl groups is presently under investigation and since they are not of major importance for endotoxic activity, these substituents are not shown in Fig 2.

As these analyses show, endotoxically active lipid A's of different bacterial origin are structurally closely related. Characteristic and common to them is the presence of a bisphosphorylated β(1-6)-linked D-glucosamine disaccharide. This structure has so far not been identified in other natural compounds and hence, it is unique to lipid A. The lipid A backbone carries, in general, approximately four mole equivalents of (R)-3-hydroxy fatty acids (carbon numbers 10 to 18), two of which occupy amino functions and two of which are linked to backbone hydroxyl groups. Both amide- and ester-bound (R)-3-hydroxy-fatty acids are, in part, acylated at their 3-hydroxyl group. Such (R)-3-acyloxyacyl residues were found in evolutionary distinct groups of gram-negative bacteria and they are also characteristic of lipid A. It is noteworthy that cyclopropane and unsaturated fatty acids are, in general, absent from lipid A's. The two phosphate groups of the lipid A backbone may be substituted (as in **E. coli** or **C. violaceum**) by nonacylated and, in most cases, amino function carrying residues. Some examples are known, however, in which one or both backbone phosphate groups appear not to be substituted.

It should be mentioned that some components of lipid A (fatty acids, phosphate substituents) are not always present in stoichiometric amounts. Hence, in a lipid A preparation several molecules may be present that possess an identical backbone but differ in the substitution pattern of the backbone. This structural diversity is at least partially responsible for the well-known intrinsic heterogeneity of lipid A and lipopolysaccharide (29).

Despite these variations, the lipid A component is the least variable region of biologically active lipopolysaccharides. Lipid A is an obligatory constitutent of lipopolysaccharides and its structure appears to be highly conserved.

Certain gram-negative microbes, notably photosynthetic bacteria, produce lipopolysaccharides which are less or not endotoxically active. (Thus, not all lipopolysaccharides are endotoxins). Their lipid A component has been shown to differ structurally from those lipid A's described above (26). As an example, **Rhodopseudomonas sphaeroides** lipid A contains the common bisphosphorylated β(1-6)-linked D-glucosamine disaccharide but carries amide-linked 3-oxotetradecanoic and 3-(7-tetradecenoyloxy)tetradecanoic acid. Lipid A of **Rh. palustris** and **Rh. viridis,** on the other hand, lacks the backbone disaccharide and contains instead nonphosphorylated 2,3-diamino-2,3-dideoxy-D-glucose monomers which, like endotoxically active lipid A's carry 14:0(3-OH) residues.

Synthetic Lipid A

Based on the results of these analyses lipid A has been chemically synthesized by Shiba, Kusumoto et al. (13). The first fully synthetic lipid A molecule (preparation 506 or LA-15-PP) corresponds in structure to **E. coli** lipid A (Figs 2 and 3). Later, other lipid A's and lipid A partial structures were prepared which all contain a β(1-6)-linked D-glucosamine disaccharide but which differ in the acylation and phosphorylation pattern (Fig 3). These preparations include the heptaacyl species of **S. minnesota** lipid A (compound 516 or LA-16-PP), the tetraacyl precursor Ia (406 or LA-14-PP), the pentaacyl precursor Ib (LA-20-PP), an isomer of precursor Ib (LA-21-PP), hexaacyl **E. coli** lipid A (506 or LA-15-PP) as well as the 1-dephospho (compound 504 or LA-15-PH) and the 4'dephospho (505 or LA-15-HP) partial structures of **E. coli** lipid A (Fig 3). Also, lipid A disaccharide analogs with an acylation pattern which is distinct from that of bacterial lipid A have been chemically synthesized (36).

Further, a great number of monosaccharide partial structures with a different acylation and phosphorylation pattern have been prepared by several groups (9, 23, 32). These compounds include synthetic counterparts of bacterial products such as lipid X and lipid Y, as well as other partial structures and analogs corresponding to either the reducing or the distal glucosamine unit of lipid A.

PHYSICAL STATE OF LIPOPOLYSACCHARIDE AND LIPID A

It can be assumed that the physical structure of the supramolecular arrangement of lipopolysaccharide and lipid A, being determined by its primary structure, plays an essential role for biological activity. It can also be expected that lipid A, as an amphiphilic molecule, behaves similarly as phospholipids which are known to adopt different physical structures depending on ambient conditions such as temperature, pH and charge state. Between such structures, reversible and non-reversible phase transitions can take place ranging from lamellar to non-lamellar (inverted) systems which can each be subdivided into the non-melted (gel or α) and the melted (liquid- crystalline or β) state of the hydrocarbon chains of the lipid molecule (14). Information on the different phase states and on the transitions between them may be obtained by the application of various physical techniques such as fluorescence (polarization) and IR-spectroscopy, light scattering, differential thermal analysis, X-ray diffraction and ^{31}P-NMR. These techniques provide data on temperatures and enthalpies of the different phase transitions, on states of order and orientations of various functional groups of the lipid molecule within different phases, on the three-dimensional architecture of the molecular assembly, and on cross-sectional areas of single molecules.

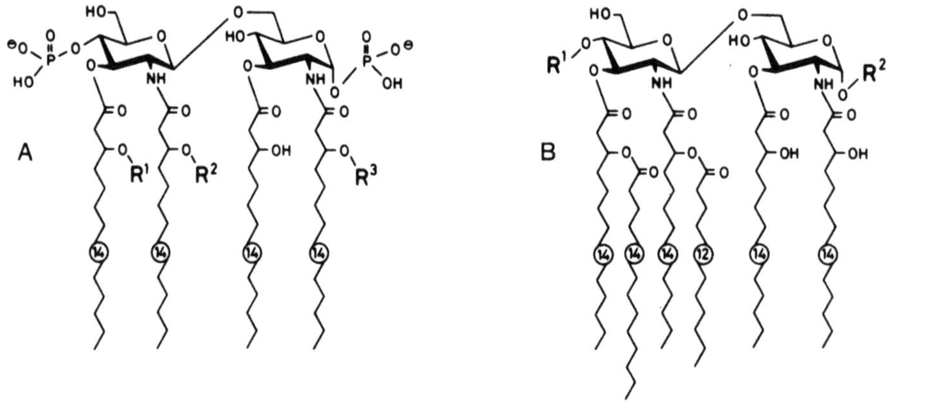

Designation of Preparation		Nature of		
Bacterial	Synthetic	R^1	R^2	R^3
Precursor Ia	LA-14-PP (406)	H	H	H
Precursor Ib	LA-20-PP	H	H	16:0
Isomer of Precursor Ib	LA-21-PP	H	16:0	H
E coli Lipid A	LA-15-PP (506)	14:0	12:0	H
S.minnesota heptaacyl Lipid A	LA-16-PP (516)	14:0	12:0	16:0

12:0, dodecanoic; 14:0, tetradecanoic; 16:0, hexadecanoic acid

Designation of Preparation		Nature of	
Bacterial	Synthetic	R^1	R^2
Lipid A-HCl (Monophosphoryl Lipid A)	LA-15-PH (504)	$PO(OH)_2$	H
——	LA-15-HP (505)	H	$PO(OH)_2$
E coli Lipid A	LA-15-PP (506)	$PO(OH)_2$	$PO(OH)_2$

Fig 3. Chemical structure of natural and synthetic lipid A's and disaccharide-containing partial structures. A: compounds differing in the number and distribution of acyl groups. B: compounds differing in the number and location of phosphoryl groups (34).

By application of some of the above techniques evidence was obtained that, depending on the environmental conditions such as temperature, pH, water content and counter ions, lipid A assemblies can adopt both bilayered lamellar arrangements and inverted phases as depicted in Fig 4. In the case of **E. coli** lipid A and deep rough mutant lipopolysaccharides in physiological conditions (temperature, cation concentrations) even the existence of mixed phases comprising lamellar and non-lamellar states has been proposed (3, 28).

IR-spectroscopy was used, on the other hand, to determine the termperature of the B ↔ A phase transition. Using this technique, the position of the peak maximum and the band intensity (area) of the anti-symmetric stretching vibration v as (CH_2) was plotted vs. temperature for the synthetic preparations 506 and 516 in comparison with free bacterial **E. coli** lipid A and lipopolysaccharide of an **E. coli** Re mutant. As Fig 5 shows, bacterial and synthetic E. coli lipid A exhibit a phase transition at approximately 42°C, while with preparation 516 a phase transition is seen at higher temperature (~ 47°C). The phase transition of **E. coli** Re lipopolysaccharide takes place at significantly lower temperatures (32° ± 2°C) indicating that KDO, i.e., the core-oligosaccharide, greatly influences the phase behavior of lipid A.

In a different approach, dried samples of bacterial and synthetic lipid A (as well as lipopolysaccharide) were examined by X-ray diffraction. It was found that under these conditions bacterial and synthetic lipid A form bilayered lamellar arrangements. In this state the lipid A fatty acids are oriented perpendicularly to the membrane surface and are tightly packed in a dense two-dimensional hexagonal lattice. In such lipid A membrane systems a strong tendency to form domains comprising up to 1200 lipid A molecules was observed in which lipid A units are partly arranged in parallel (24). As suggested by conformational energy calculations, the bisphosphorylated glucosamine disaccharide is oriented approximately 45° relative to the membrane surface.

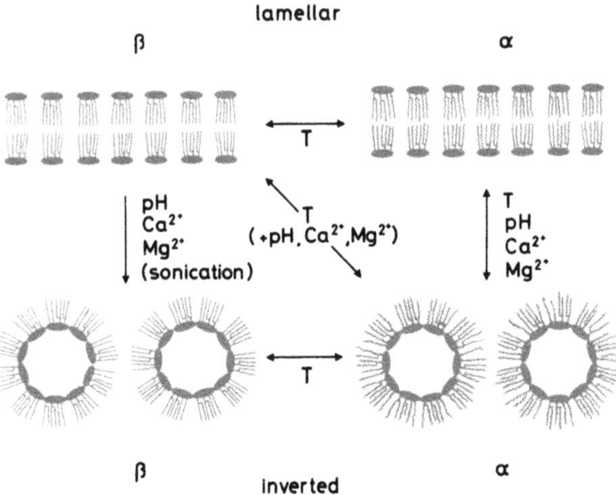

Fig 4. Tentative scheme of the structural polymorphism of lipid A (34). Waved lines indicate melted fatty acids. Not all states have been experimentally defined.

RELATIONSHIP OF STRUCTURE AND CONFORMATION TO BIOLOGICAL ACTIVITY AND FUNCTION

Some selected aspects of the significance of the chemical and physical structure for biological activity and function of lipid A (or lipopolysaccharide) are discussed below.

Endotoxicity

For a long time it had been postulated, and experimental evidence has been provided, that the lipid A component represents the endotoxic principle, being responsible for the induction of the manifold pathophysiological effects of lipopolysaccharides (8, 42). The successful chemical synthesis of lipid A and partial structures then offered the possibility to confirm this concept as well as the structural proposals made for lipid A. Further, the biological analysis of synthetic, i.e., homogenous, lipid A and partial structures should allow to establish relationships of the chemical and physical structure to endotoxic activity at a molecular level. Thus, the synthetic preparations were analyzed in typical in vivo and in vitro endotoxin test systems and compared with the corresponding natural structures (7, 8, 12, 17, 22, 32, 33, 38). The most important results of these investigations can be summarized as follows:

1. Bacterial and synthetic **E. coli** lipid A expressed, with identical effective doses, the same degree of in vivo and in vitro activity in all biological assays employed. This result shows that indeed lipid A represents the endotoxic center of lipopolysaccharides and that of variable substituents bacterial lipid A (e.g., residues R of Fig 2) the expression are not required for endotoxicity. The chemical and physical identity of bacterial and synthetic lipid A proves that the structural proposal made for lipid A, as derived from analytical work, is correct.

2. The in vivo activity of the bisphosphorylated disaccharide-contain ing preparations differing in the acylation pattern (Fig 3A) was, as compared to **E. coli** lipid A, similar (pentaacyl precursor Ib and its isomer) or significantly lower (tetraacyl precursor Ia, and hepta-acyl **S. minnesota** lipid A). The latter two compounds were not cap able of preparing for or of eliciting the dermal Shwartzman reaction. A synthetic analog containing five fatty acids, but in an arrangement different to that in **E. coli** lipid A, exhibited only marginal endotoxicity. Therefore, the location of fatty acids, the number of acyl chains present (and possibly the acyl chain length and configuration of 3-hydroxy fatty acids) are of importance for lipid A endotoxic activity in vivo.

3. The 1- and 4'-monodephospho partial structures such as compounds 504 (LA-15-PH) and 505 (LA-15-HP) (Fig 3B) were, in general, less active in vivo than the bisphosphorylated parent compounds as pyrogens, lethal toxins, and in preparing for or in eliciting the local Shwartzman reaction.

4. Glucosamine monosaccharide partial structures show activity in some in vitro systems. They lack, however, without exception, endotoxic in vivo activity such as pyrogenicity and lethality (23, 32).

Collectively, these data suggest that endotoxin activity is determined by a molecule containing two D-glucosamine residues (which are β (1-6)-interlinked), two phosphoryl groups and at least five, but not more than six, fatty acids including one or two 3-acyloxyacyl groups in a defined location as it is present in **E. coli** lipid A (compound 506). Molecules lacking only one component, irrespective of its chemical nature, or molecules with a different distribution of components are less or not endotoxically active. This shows that slight modifications at any site of the **E. coli** lipid A architecture result in a significant reduction of biological activity, suggesting that endotoxicity is not dependent on one single lipid A constituent. It appears that it is a unique molecular structure and, thus, the supramolecular conformation of lipid A which allows the optimal expression of endotoxic activity. Being in this conformation, lipid A is bioavailable and capable of interacting, perhaps selectively, with humoral factors, or cellular and subcellular targets of the endotoxin-susceptible host. We presently favor the view that for the expression of endotoxic activity, a particular supramolecular structure including at least partial melting of acyl chains at physiological temperature are prerequisites. It seems reasonable to assume that a higher fluidity of the hydrocarbon chains of lipid A should favor the interaction with the host cell membrane, the fluidity of which is higher at the physiological temperature than that of bound or free lipid A. This means that such biological effects which are provoked by a direct incorporation of the lipid A portion into the host cell lipid matrix should proceed at a higher rate. This concept is supported by the fact that the biologically less active compound 516 exhibits a relatively high phase transition temperature (Fig 5), while biologically active preparations have lower phase transition temperatures. It is not known, however, which physical structure of lipid A is involved in endotoxic activity. Based on the acylation pattern of the biologically less active compound 516 leading to an increase of the critical packing parameter, and as suggested by our serological studies (see below), it may be assumed that compound 516 adopts, in aqueous solution, to a larger extent more complex physical structures including inverted phases. On the other hand, preparation 406, which is also less active than lipid A, should be preferentially present in the lamellar or even micellar state. It, therefore, appears that neither of these structures per se is responsible for triggering the initial steps of endotoxic events. Bacterial and synthetic **E. coli** lipid A can, under physiological conditions, adopt both lamellar and inverted structures and it is possible that this ability to express both these supramolecular structures is related to its potent endotoxic activity.

Immunoreactivity

Studies on the reaction of lipid A with antibodies have revealed further structure-activity relationships and have shed new light on the importance of the conformational state of lipid A for biological activity. In recent serological studies we could characterize the reaction pattern of five different lipid A antibody specificities present in polyclonal (rabbit) antisera (2). The antisera were prepared by the immunization of rabbits with liposome-incorporated preparations 506 (**E. coli** lipid A), 505 and 504 (Fig 3B). The specificity of antibodies was determined by using different lipid A-related disaccharide and monosaccharide antigens in the passive hemolysis assay. It was found that the lipid A antibodies recognize epitopes which all reside in the hydrophilic backbone of lipid A. The reaction pattern of anti-lipid A antibodies is schematically displayed in Fig 6. These antibodies are reactive with monosaccharide (specificities D and E) or disaccharide antigens (specificities A, B and C) carrying one or two phosphoryl groups. Antibodies against a defined partial structure cross-react with structurally

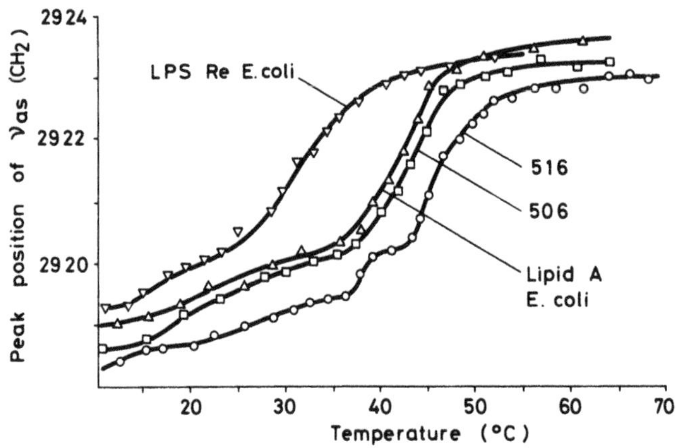

Fig 5. Temperature dependence of the frequency of the peak position of the v as(CH_2)-absorption band. Shown is the phase behavior of synthetic lipid A's (preparations 506 and 516) in comparison with bacterial lipid A and lipopolysaccharide of the **E. coli** Re mutant F515.

more complex antigens containing this partial structure. Thus, antibody specificity D reacts with a 4'-phosphorylated monosaccharide and a 4-phosphorylated disaccharide partial structure as well as with lipid A (Fig 6). In turn, antibody specificity A reacts exclusively with lipid A (compound 506) which shows the broadest reactivity since all five antibodies are detected with this antigen. On the other hand, antibodies recognizing 1-phosphorylated compounds do not cross-react with 4'-phosphorylated antigens and vice versa. The specificity of lipid A antibodies is largely independent of the acylation pattern and, in the case of monosaccharide-reactive antibodies, it is also expressed by preparations differing in the nature of the backbone sugar (D-glucose, D-glucosamine, 2,3-diamino-2,3-dideoxy-D-glucose). Our results (2) show that phosphoryl groups are clearly involved in the expression of the different antigenic determinants (5, 18). However, it cannot be decided at present whether they are integral components of the individual epitopes. It is also possible that phosphoryl groups strongly influence the conformation of vicinal regions within the lipid A backbone leading to different immunoreactivities of the monodephospho partial structures and lipid A.

The expression of the different epitopes was found to greatly depend on the supramolecular structure of lipid A assemblies (2). This became evident when synthetic lipid A antigens having the same hydrophilic backbone structure (1,4'-bishosphorylated β(1-6)-linked D-glucosamine disaccharide), but differing in the number, type and distribution of fatty acids were tested as native, or liposome-incorporated antigens, in the passive hemolysis inhibition assay for their reactivity with anti-506 antiserum. The inhibition values for various native antigens varied from 2 to 500 ng, e.g., preparation 506 exhibiting low and preparation 516 high inhibition values. The inhibitory capacity of these antigens, however, was comparable and significantly better (0.5 to 1 ng) if the preparations were tested after incorporation into liposome membranes. This could mean that under physiological conditions notably those preparations, which in aqueous solution show high inhibition values (e.g., preparation 516) adopt preferentially nonlamellar structures rendering the immunoreactive sites, which are located in the lipid A back-

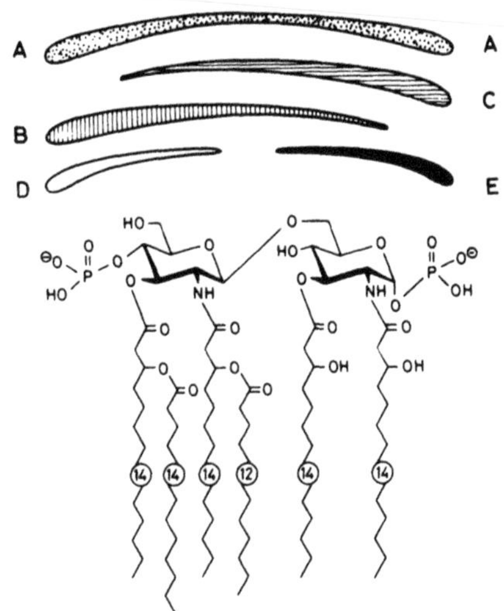

Structure Recognized	Reactivity of Antibody Specificity				
	A	B	C	D	E
GlcN-1-P	–	–	–	–	+
4-P-GlcN	–	–	–	+	–
GlcNβ(1-6) GlcN-1-P	–	–	+	–	+
4'-P-GlcNβ(1-6) GlcN	–	+	–	+	–
4'-P-GlcNβ(1-6) GlcN-1-P	+	+	+	+	+

Fig 6. Schematic display of the epitope specificities of disaccharide (A, B, C) and monosaccharide (D, E)-reactive antibodies (2)

bone, less accessible to recognition by antibody. However, in the liposomal membrane the lipid A preparations are present in a lamellar arrangement in which the lipid A backbone is exposed allowing an optimal expression of its epitopes. It is interesting to note that this exposure is further modulated by the fluidity of the surrounding lipid matrix and the curvature of liposomes. Thus, in the same serological test system, small liposomes (0.1 um) exhibited significantly lower inhibition values than larger liposomes (10 um), and liposomes containing 14:0 in phospholipids were better inhibitors than those containing phospholipid-bound 18:0 (lower fluidity).

Collectively, these results show that the immunoreactive properties of lipid A clearly depend on its conformational state.

Outer Membrane Architecture and Function

The results of physical measurements, notably X-ray diffraction and fluorescence polarization, also provide information as to the role of lipopolysaccharide and lipid A for outer membrane architecture and function. Most remarkable in this context is the high degree of order of lipopolysaccharide. The lipid A fatty acids, because of their compact and ordered arrangement form a comparatively rigid structure (as compared to the phospholipids of the inner leaflet). The dense packing of the hydrophobic region of lipid A, which is favored by the absence of unsaturated fatty acids, causes a high state of order of the outer membrane system. The resulting microviscosity is likely to inhibit hydrophobic molecules from diffusing into or through the outer membrane and it may, therefore, be responsible for the marked impermeability of this membrane to bile acids, detergents and hydrophobic antibiotics (40). Moreover, the anisotropic backbone region favors the formation of domains in which lipid A molecules tend to be packed more or less parallel and which can be preserved for long periods of time (this is in marked contrast to the complete rotational disorder observed for 'natural' phospholipids). It can, therefore, be assumed that the permeation-barrier properties of the outer membrane, restricting the entrance of hydrophobic substances, is related to the comparatively rigid and well-ordered conformation of lipopolysaccharide and lipid A.

Based on these results and considerations, a tentative model of the outer membrane architecture has been proposed (Fig 7) which emphasizes the main structural and conformational properties as obtained experimentally for isolated lipopolysaccharide and free lipid A: 1. lipopolysaccharide exhibits a remarkably highly ordered state (as compared to phospholipids of the inner leaflet at 37°C) which is mediated by its well-ordered lipid A arrangement resulting in a relatively rigid structure; 2. the hydrophilic backbone region of lipid A is oriented 45° to the membrane surface, leading to a sawtooth-like surface structure; 3. lipid A units tend to form domains in which a more or less ordered arrangement of these anisotropic molecules can be preserved for long periods of time; and 4. the O-specific chains assume a heavily coiled conformation.

It is known that in the outer membrane lipid A is associated with proteins (not shown in Fig 7) which are, e.g., involved in the recognition of phages and cells, and it has been shown that the presence of lipid A is essential for the expression of bacteriophage receptor activity (41). It is possible that through hydrophobic and ionic interactions lipid A stabilizes an active conformation of such membrane proteins. This interaction of lipid A with bacterial proteins requires a proper fluidity of the outer membrane system. Membrane fluidity is, in general, regulated by the fatty acid composition of constituting lipids which is greatly influenced by external factors such as temperature. At low growth temperature, in general, higher levels of unsaturated (cis) fatty acids are incorporated into membrane lipids. This is also the case for lipid A. Thus, the incorporation of Δ^9-cis-hexodecenoic acid (at the expense of 12:0) into lipid A was demonstrated when **E. coli** or **Salmonella** bacteria were cultivated at 12°C (41, 43). It, therefore, appears that lipid A is involved in the maintenance of the correct membrane fluidity required for a number of physiological membrane activities.

CONCLUDING REMARKS

As discussed in the present paper, it is now established that the manifold biological properties of lipopolysaccharides are induced by, or dependent on, the lipid A component. The primary structure of lipid A has been elucidated, lipid A has been chemically synthesized, partial structures and analogs have been prepared and the principal structural requirements for defined biological activities are known. It is unknown, however, in which way these structural parameters are important for the expression of biological activity of lipid A.

It is possible that in the humoral or cellular compartment of a susceptible host a particular recognition molecule exists which is able to specifically interact with certain determinants of the lipid A structure, thus initiating the cascade of events leading to endotoxic manifestations. The presence of a lipid A binding protein on host cells has been postulated (15) and very recently strong experimental evidence was provided for its existence (see Lei, Flebbe, Roeder and Morrison, present volume). So far, however, it is unknown whether this protein has the characteristics of a functional receptor molecule which, after binding of lipid A, transmits an activation signal.

On the other hand, in considering the chemical properties of lipid A in relation to bioactivity it has to be taken into account that lipid A is an amphiphilic molecule. The amphiphilic nature of lipid A is due to the simultaneous presence of a hydrophilic region (phosphorylated glucosamine disaccharide) and a lipophilic region (fatty acids). Amphiphiles, in general,

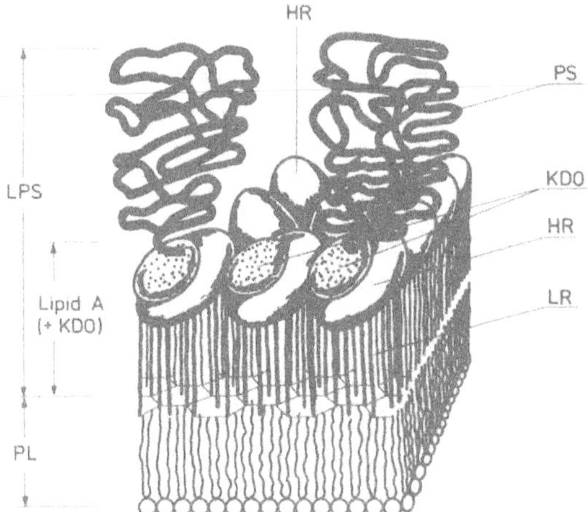

Fig 7. Tentative view of a section of the gram-negative outer membrane (24, 35). Only a small section of the outer membrane, in which proteins and other membrane constituents are omitted, is depicted. HR = hydrophilic region (phosphorylated glucosamine disaccharide), LR = lipophilic region (acyl residues) of lipid A. The hexagonal packing of the schematically drawn acyl residues of lipid A is indicated. The polysaccharide chains (PS), which are drawn schematically, can adopt a heavily coiled conformation, and may, or may not be intermingled. For better clarity only two polysaccharide chains are shown.

tend to form a multiplicity of specific three-dimensional aggregates, and also lipid A or partial structures adopt, depending on intrinsic and extrinsic factors, different supramolecular structures. Thus, particular parameters of the primary structure could determine unique three-dimensional organizations of lipid A which are essential for the expression of biological activity. In the present paper examples are discussed which suggest the importance of the conformational state of lipid A for some of its bioactivities. While it appears that a lamellar arrangement of lipid A is essential for its antigenicity and its contribution to outer membrane barrier function, the nature of the physical structure that is involved in endotoxic activity of lipid A is not yet established. Presently, therefore, our efforts are directed at the charactęrization of lipid A conformation(s) important for its endotoxic properties. These studies are performed in the hope that knowledge of the physical structure of endotoxically active lipid A will enable us to understand the initial steps of the lipid A-host interaction and, thus, the mechanisms involved in endotoxin effects.

ACKNOWLEDGEMENTS

The financial support of the Deutsche Forschungsgemeinschaft (Br 731/4-1, Br 731/7, Scha 402/1-1, Scha 402/1-2), the Bundesministerium fur Foschung und Technologie (HB, 01 Zr 8604), the Kultusminister des Landes Schleswig-Holstein (EThR, 3156.46-7-2), and the Fonds der Chemischen Industrie (EThR) is greatfully acknoweldged. We also thank Mrs. M. Lohs, G. Stegelmann, and B. Kohler for illustrations and photographic work, and Mrs. I. Bendt for typing this manuscript.

REFERENCES

1. Brade, H., Brade, L., and E. Th. Rietschel, 1988, Structure-activity relationships of bacterial lipopolysaccharides (endotoxins). Zbl. Bakt. Hyg. A 268: 151-179.

2. Brade, L., Brandenburg, K., Kuhn, H.-M., Kusumoto, S., Macher, I., Rietschel, E. Th., and Brade, H., 1987, The immunogenicity and antigenicity of lipid A are influenced by its physicochemical state and environment. Infect. Immun. 55: 2636-2644.

3. Brandenburg, K., and Seydel, U., 1984, Physical aspects of structure and function of membranes made from lipopolysaccharides and free lipid A. Biochem. Biophys. Acta 775: 225-238.

4. Caroff, M., Lebbar, S., and Szabo, L., 1987, Detection of 3-deoxy-2-octulosonic acid in thiobarbiturate-negative endotoxins. Carb. Res. 161: C4-C7.

5. Chaby, R., Charon, D., Pedron, T., and Girard, R., 1987, Antigenic determinants of lipid A analyzed with synthetic models and monoclonal antibodies. Biochem. Biophys. Res. Commun. 143: 723-731.

6. Chaby, R. and Szabo, L., 1975, 3-Deoxy-2-octulosonic acid 5-phosphate: a component of the endotoxin of Bordetella pertussis, Eur. J. Biochem. 59: 277-280.

7. Galanos, C., Luderitz, O., Freudenberg, M. A., Brade, L., Schade, U., Rietschel, E. Th., Kusumoto, S., and Shiba, T., 1986, Biological activity of synthetic heptaacyl lipid A representing a component of Salmonella minnesota R595 lipid A. Eur. J. Biochem. 160: 55-59.

8. Galanos, C., Luderitz, O., Rietschel, E. Th., and Westphal, O., 1977, Newer aspects of the chemistry and biology of bacterial lipopolysaccharides, with special reference to their lipid A component, in: "International Review of Biochemistry, Biochemistry of Lipids II," T. W. Goodwin, ed., University Park Press, Baltimore 14: 239-335.

9. Haselberger, A., Hildebrandt, J., Lam, C., Liehl, E., Loibner, H., Macher, I., Rosenwirth, B., Schutze, E., Vyplel, H., and Unger, F. M., 1987, Immunopharmacology of lipopolysaccharides (endotoxins) from gram-negative bacteria. Triangle, Sandoz Journal of Medical Science 26: 33-49.

10. Helander, I., Lindner, B., Brade, H., Altmann, K., Lindberg, A. A., Rietschel, and Zahringer, U., 1988, Chemical structure of the lipopolysaccharide of Haemophilus influenzae strain I-69 $Rd^{-H/b+}$. Description of a novel deep rough chemotype. Eur. J. Biochem. 177: 483-492.

11. Hitchcock, P., Leive, L., Makela, P. H., Rietschel, E. Th., Strittmatter, W., and Morris, D., 1986, Lipopolysaccharide nomenclature - past, present and future. J. Bacteriol. 166: 699-705.

12. Homma, J. Y., Matsuura, M., Kanegasakai, S., Kawakubo, Y., Kojima, Y., Shibukawa, N., Kumazawa, Y., Yamamoto, A., Tanamoto, K., Yasuda, T., Imoto, M., Yoshimura, H., Kusumoto, S., and Shiba, T., 1985, Structural requirements of lipid A responsible for the functions: a study with chemically synthesized lipid A and its analogues. J. Biochem. (Tokyo) 98: 395-406.

13. Imoto, M., Yoshimura, H., Shimamoto, T., Sakaguchi, N., Kusumoto, S., and Shiba, T., 1987, Total synthesis of Escherichia coli lipid A, the endotoxically active principle of cell-surface lipopolysaccharide. Bull. Chem. Soc. Jpn. 60: 2205-2214.

14. Israelachvili, J. N., Marcelja, S., and Horn, R. G., 1980, Physical principles of membrane organization. Quart. Rev. Biophys. 13: 121-200.

15. Jacobs, D., 1984, Structural features of binding of lipopolysaccharides to murine lymphocytes. Rev. Infect. Dis. 6: 501-505.

16. Kaca, W., Brade, L., Rietschel, E. Th., and Brade, H., 1986, The effect of removal of D-fructose on the antigenicity of the lipopolysaccharide from a rough mutant of **Vibrio cholerae** OGAWA. Carb. Res. 149: 293-298.

17. Kanegasaki, S., Tanamoto, K., Yasuda, T., Homma, J. Y., Matsuura, M., Nakatsuka, M., Kumazawa, Y., Yamamoto, A., Shiba, T., Kusumoto, S., Imoto, M., Yoshimura, A., and Shimamoto, T., 1986, Structure-activity relationship of lipid A: Comparison of biological activities of natural and synthetic lipid A's with different fatty acid compositions. J. Biochem. (Tokyo) 99: 1203-1210.

18. Kasai, N., Arata, S., Mashimo, J.-I., Okuda, K., Aihara, Y., Kotani, S., Takada, H., Shiba, T., Kusumoto, S., Imoto, M., Yoshimura, H., and Shimamoto, T., 1986, Synthetic Salmonella-type lipid A with high serological specificity. Infect. Immun. 51: 43-48.

19. Kawahara, K., Brade, H., Rietschel, E. Th., and Zahringer, U., 1987, Studies on the chemical structure of the core-lipid A region of the lipopolysaccharide of Acinetobacter calcoaceticus NCTC 10305. Detection of a new 2-octulosonic acid interlinking the core oligosaccharide and lipid A component. Eur. J. Biochem. 163: 489-495.

20. Kondo, S., Iguchi, T., and Kisatsune, K., 1988, Occurrence of thiobarbituric acid test-positive substances in lipopolysaccharides (LPS) of Vibrionaceae. in: "Adv. Res. Cholera and Related Diarrheas," Vol. 4: 71-76, KTK Scientific Publishers, Tokyo.

21. Kondo, S., Zahringer, U., Rietschel, E. Th., and Hisatsune, K., 1989, Isolation and identification of 3-deoxy-D-threo-hexulosonic acid as a constituent of the lipopolysaccharide of Vibrio parahaemolyticus serotypes 07 and 012. Carb. Res. in press.

22. Kotani, S., Takada, H., Tsujimoto, M., Ogawa, T., Takahashi, I., Ikeda, T., Otsuka, K., Shimanchi, H., Kasai, N., Mashimo, J., Nagao, S., Tanaka, S., Harada, K., Nagaki, K., Kitamura, H., Shiba, T., Kusumoto, S., Imoto, M., and Yoshimura, H., 1985, Synthetic lipid A with endotoxic and related biological activities comparable to those of a natural lipid A from an **Escherichia coli** Re-mutant. Infect. Immun. 49: 225-237.

23. Kumazawa, Y., Nakatsuka, M., Takimoto, H., Furuya, T., Nagumo, T., Yamamoto, A., Homma, J. Y., Inada, K., Yoshida, M., Kiso, M., and Hasegawa, A., 1988, Importance of fatty acid substituents of chemically synthesized lipid A-subunit analogs in the expression of immunopharmacological activity. Infect. Immun. 56: 149-155.

24. Labischinski, H., Barnickel, G., Bradaczek, H., Naumann, D., Rietschel, E. Th., and Giesbrecht, P., 1985, High state of order of isolated bacterial lipopolysaccharide and its possible contribution to the permeation barrier property of the outer membrane. J. Bacteriol. 162: 9-20.

25. Luderitz, O., Freudenberg, M. A., Galanos, C., Lehmann, V., Rietschel, E. Th., and Shaw, D. H., 1982, Lipopolysaccharides of gram-negative bacteria. in: "Membrane Lipids of Procaryotes. Current Topics in Membranes and Transport," S. Razin and S. Rottem, eds. Academic Press, Inc., New York, pp. 79-151.

26. Mayer, H., and Weckesser, J., 1984, Unusual lipid A's: structures taxonomical relevance and potential value for endotoxin research. in: "Handbook of Endotoxins," R. Proctor, ed., Vol. 1, Chemistry of Endotoxin. E. Th. Rietschel, ed., Elsevier/North-Holland Biomedical Press, Amsterdam, pp. 221-247.

27. Moxon, E. R., 1985, Antigen expression influencing tissue invasion of Haemophilus influenza type B, in: "Bayer-Symposium VIII. The pathogenesis of bacterial infections," G. G. Jackson and H. Thomas, eds. Springer Verlag, Berlin/Heidelberg, pp. 17-29.

28. Naumann, D., Schultz, C., Born, J., Labischinski, H., Brandenburg, K., von Busse, Brade, H., and Seydel, U., 1987, Investigations on the polymorphism of lipid A from lipopolysaccharides of **Escherichia coli** and **Salmonella minnesota** by fourier-transform infrared spectroscopy. Eur. J. Biochem. 164: 159-169.

29. Nowotny, A., 1984, Heterogeneity of endotoxins, in: "Handbook of Endotoxins," R. Proctor, ed., "Chemistry of Endotoxin", E. Th. Rietschel, ed. Vol. 1, Elsevier/North-Holland Biomedical Press, Amsterdam, pp. 308-338.

30. Proctor, R. A., ed., "Handbook of Endotoxins," Vol. 1, Chemistry of Endotoxin, 1984; Vol. 2, Pathophysiology of endotoxin, 1985; Vol. 3, Cellular biology of endotoxin, 1985; Vol. 4, Clinical aspects of endotoxin shock, 1986, Elsevier/North-Holland Biomedical Press, Amsterdam.

31. Raetz, C., R., H., 1987, Structure and biosynthesis of lipid A, in: "Escherichia coli and Salmonella typhimurium. Cellular and molecular biology," C. Neidhardt, J. L. Ingraham, K. Brooks Low, B. Magasanik, M. Schaechter, and H. E. Umbarger, eds. Am. Soc. Microbiol., Washington, D.C., pp. 498-503.

32. Rietschel, E. Th., Brade, H., Brade, L., Brandeburg, K., Schade, U. F., Seydel, U., Zahringer, U., Galanos, C., Luderitz, O., Westphal, O., Labischinski, H., Kusumoto, S., and Shiba, T., 1987, Lipid A, the endotoxic center of bacterial lipopolysaccharides: relation of chemical structure to biological activity. Prog. Clin. Biol. Res. 231: 25-53. (Alan R. Liss, New York)

33. Rietschel, E. Th., Brade, L., Schade, U., Galanos, C., Freudenberg, M., Luderitz, O., Kusumoto, S., and Shiba, T., 1987, Endotoxic properties of synthetic petaacyl lipid A precursor Ib and a structural isomer. Eur. J. Biochem. 169: 27-31.

34. Rietschel, E. Th., Brade, L., Schade, U. F., Seydel, U., Zahringer, U., and Brade, H., 1988, Bacterial endotoxins: properties and structure of biologically active domains, in: "Surface structures of microorganisms and their interaction with the mammalian host," E. Schrinner, M. Richmond, G. Seibert, and U. Schwartz, eds. Verlag Chemie, Weinheim, pp. 1-41.

35. Rietschel, E. Th., Wollenweber, H. W., Brade, H., Zahringer, U., Lindner,

B., Seydel, U., Bradaczek, H., Barnickel, G., Labischinski, H., and Giesbrecht, P., 1984, Structure and conformation of the lipid A component of lipopolysaccharides, in: "Handbook of Endotoxins," R. Proctor, ed., Vol. 1, "Chemistry of Endotoxins," E. Th. Rietschel, ed, Elsevier, Amsterdam, New York, Oxford, pp. 187-220.

36. Shiba, T., and Kusumoto, S., 1984, Chemical synthesis and biological activity of lipid A analogs, in: "Handbook of Endotoxins," R. Proctor, ed., Vol. 1, "Chemistry of Endotoxin," E. Th. Rietschel, ed. Elsevier, Amsterdam, New York, Oxford, pp. 284-302.

37. Tacken, A., Rietschel, E. Th., and Brade, H., 1986, Methylation analysis of the heptose/3-deoxy-D-manno-2-octulosonic acid region (inner core) of lipopolysaccharide from **Salmonella minnesota** rough mutants. Carbohydr. Res. 149: 279-291.

38. Takahashi, I., Kotani, S., Takada, H., Tsujimoto, M., Ogawa, T., Shiba, T., Kusumoto, S., Yamamoto, M., Hasegawa, A., Kiso, M., Nishijima, M., Amano, F., Akamatsu, Y., Harada, K., Tanaka, S., Okamura, H., and Tamura, T., 1987, Requirement of a properly acylated (1-6)-D-glucosamine disaccharide bisphosphate structure for efficient manifestation of full endotoxic and associated bioactivities of lipid A. Infect. Immun. 65: 57-68.

39. Takayama, K., Quereshi, N., Hyver, K., Honovich, J., Cotter, R. J., Mascagni, P., and Schneider, H., 1986, Characterization of a structural series of lipid A obtained from the lipopolysaccharides of **Neisseria gonorrhoeae.** J. Biol. Chem. 261: 10624-10631.

40. Vaara, M., and Nikaido, H., 1984, Molecular organization of bacterial outer membrane, in: "Handbook of Endotoxins," R. Proctor, ed., Vol. 1, "Chemistry of Endotoxin," E. Th. Rietschel, ed. Elsevier, Amsterdam, New York, Oxford, pp. 1-45.

41. van Alphen, L., Lugtenberg, B., Rietschel, E. Th., and Mombers, C., 1979, Architecture of the outer membrane of Escherichia coli K12. Phase transitions of the bacteriophage K3 receptor complex. Eur. J. Biochem. 101: 571-579.

42. Westphal, O., and Luderitz, O., 1954, Chemische Erforschung von Lipopolysacchariden Gram-negative Bakterien. Angew. Chem. 66: 407-417.

43. Wollenweber, H.-W., Schlecht, S., Luderitz, O., and Rietschel, E. Th., 1983, Fatty acids in lipopolysaccharides of **Salmonella** species grown at low temperature. Identification and position. Eur. J. Biochem. 130: 167-171.

STRUCTURE-ACTIVITY RELATIONSHIP OF CHEMICALLY SYNTHESIZED NONREDUCING PARTS OF LIPID A ANALOGS

J. Y. Homma, M. Matsuura, and Y. Kumazawa*

The Kitasato Institute and *School of Pharmaceutical Sciences
Kitasato University, Tokyo, Japan

INTRODUCTION

One of the main aims of endotoxin researchers for almost half a century to date has been to discover the intrinsic chemical nature of endotoxin from complicated chemical complexes of enormous molecular weight. The lipopolysaccharide-protein complex which proved to exhibit all the activities of endotoxin was first isolated from the cell wall of gram-negative bacteria. After precise immunochemical studies on endotoxin by several pioneers, the portion called free lipid A was claimed by Westphal and Lüderitz to be responsible for the endotoxin activities. This was in the early 1950's. Much experimental data was collected to prove that free lipid A is the sole structure responsible for endotoxicity (5).

In 1983, chemical synnthesis based on the structure, which had been revised on a few points from the structure proposed earlier, was achieved by Shiba, Kusumoto and their colleagues (8, 18). By biological analysis of the synthesized compounds, it was confirmed without doubt that lipid A with a molecular weight of only ca. 2,000 was the active center of the endotoxin (3, 4, 13).

Meanwhile, in line with Shiba's group, Hasegawa, Kiso and their colleagues began to synthesize lipid A-subunit analogs in 1983 (9, 10). We have been investigating the structure-biological activity relationship of these analogs of the nonreducing part of lipid A. Most of these compounds exert only limited biological activities of endotoxin (19-21). However, these compounds are very valuable in helping us to clarify the structure requirements for expressing a given activity of the endotoxin, whether it be protective or toxic.

In this paper, we would like to discuss biological activities of nonreducing part analogs of lipid A with special reference to structure-activity relationship.

MATERIALS AND METHODS

Synthetic Compounds and Control Lipid A

Lipid A-subunit analogs were synthesized chemically and purified by high-performance liquid chromatography. Natural free lipid A prepared from **E. coli**

F-515 (Re) was kindly donated by Drs. O. Luderitz and C. Galanos, Max-Planck-Institut fur Immunobiologie, Freiburg, and used as a control. The synthetic compounds and control natural free lipid A were solubilized in pyrogen free water by treating with triethylamine, complexing with bovine serum albumin then used for testing biological activities.

Determination of Immunopharmacological Activities

Mitogenic activity was assessed by determining [^{3}H]dThd uptake into C3H/He and C3H/HeJ spleen cells which were incubated in triplicate at 37°C for 48 hr with or without test samples (14). Polyclonal B-cell activation (PBA) activity was assessed by counting as plaque-forming cells against trinitrophenylated horse erythrocytes (14).

Phagocytic activity was assessed by measuring the radioactivity of ^{51}Cr-labeled, antibody-sensitized sheep erythrocytes which were phagocytosed by peritoneal macrophages stimulated **in vivo** with test sample as described previously (16). Cellular lysosomal enzyme (acid phosphatase) activity of peritoneal macrophages was measured by the methods described elsewhere (16). Cytostasis-inducing activity was tested according to the method described previously (16). The activity of peritoneal macrophages stimulated **in vivo** was assessed by measuring the growth inhibitory action against EL-4 cells.

Adjuvant activity was assessed by measuring anti-BSA immunogloblin G (IgG) antibody response in the serum of mice which had been immunized i.p. with 10 μg of BSA and 10 μg of test sample 3 weeks earlier. Anti-BSA IgG antibody titers were determined by an enzyme-linked immunosorbent assay (17).

Tumor necrosis factor (TNF)-inducing activity was tested according to the method described previously (19). Ten ug samples were administered i.v. into **Propionibacterium acnes**-primed ICR mice. The sera were separated from the blood 1.5 hr after administration of the test samples and treated at 56°C for 30 min to reduce nonspecific cytotoxicity against tumor cells. The activity of TNF in the sera was determined as the growth inhibitory action against L929 cells, which was measured as the percent inhibition of [^{3}H]dThd uptake into L929 cells.

Interferon (IFN)-inducing activity was assessed by either of the following methods. (i) A cell suspension derived from spleen, bone marrow and mesenteric lymph node of Japanese white rabbit was mixed with a test sample. IFN released into the culture fluid was assayed by plaque reduction method using RK-13 cell line of rabbit kidney and vesicular stomatitis virus (4). (ii) IFN-inducing activity was assessed by measuring the IFN titer in sera of ICR mice which had been primed i.p. with **P. acnes** 7 days previously then injected i.v. with 10 μg test samples 2 hr earlier. IFN titers in sera were assayed by determining reduction of cytopacy in L929 cells infected with vesicular stomatitis virus (6).

Colony stimulating factor (CSF)-inducing activity was determined by a slight modification of the method of Apte et al. (1). Ten μg of samples were injected i.v. into 8-wk-old mice. After 6 hr, sera were separated to determine CSF activity (17).

Determination of Endotoxic Activities

Lethality was performed according to the method described by Galanos et al. (2), using galactosamine-sensitized 10-week-old male C57BL/6 mice. Pyrogenicity was determined by methods described previously (4). The local Shwartzman reaction was tested as follows. Eighteen hours after preparatory intradermal injection with test samples in 0.1 ml of water, a challenge injection of natural lipid A (20 µg/kg) was made i.v. The intensity of reactions was read 5 hr after the provacative injection.

Limulus Amebocyte Lysate Gelation

Activation of proclotting enzyme of horseshoe crab, Limulus polyphemus by synthetic compounds and control lipid A was assayed by gelation of amebocyte lysate. Detection limit of the reagent of Limulus amebocyte against **E. coli** 0111:B4 endotoxin was 0.030 to 0.015 ng per ml.

RESULTS AND DISCUSSION

Effect of Acyl Substituent and Phosphorylation on Biological Activities of Chemically Synthesized Partial Structure Analogs of Lipid A

Among 14 chemically synthesized compounds having a glucosamine backbone (type I compounds) shown in Fig 1, we found one analog (GLA-27) which exhibits intensive activities such as Limulus, mitogenic, PBA, IFN-inducing and TNF-inducing activities but not pyrogenic activity or Shwartzman reactivity (Table 1). The structure of GLA-27 comprises 4-O-phosphono-D-glucosamine with tetradecanoyl (C_{14}) and 3-tetradecanoyloxytetradecanoyl (C_{14}-O-(C_{14})) groups as the 3-O- and 2-N-substituents, respectively.

Although none of the compounds examined was found to be more active than GLA-27, the requisite structure for expressing biological activities could be analyzed (15, 20, 21).

Substituent				Compound number					
				Type					
R_1 (2-N-)	R_2 (3-O- or N-)	R_3 (4-O-)	R_4 (6-O-)	I	II	III	IV	V	VI
		H	H	GLA-25	GLA-39				
C_{14}-O-(C_{14})	C_{14}	P	H	GLA-27	GLA-40	GLA-43	GLA-48	GLA-51	
		H	P	GLA-35	GLA-41				
		P	P	GLA-36	GLA-42				
C_{14}-O-(C_{14})	H			GLA-34					
C_{14}-O-(C_{14})	C_{14}-O-(C_{14})			GLA-47			GLA-49		GLA-52
C_{14}-OH	C_{14}			GLA-44					
C_{14}-OH	C_{14}-OH	P	H	GLA-46					
C_{14}	C_{14}			GLA-26					
C_{12}-O-(C_{12})	C_{12}			GLA-37					
C_{16}-O-(C_{16})	C_{16}			GLA-38					
C_{14}-O-(C_{14})	H			GLA-45					
C_{14}-OH	C_{14}	P	C_{14}	GLA-29					
C_{12}-OH	C_{14}			GLA-28					

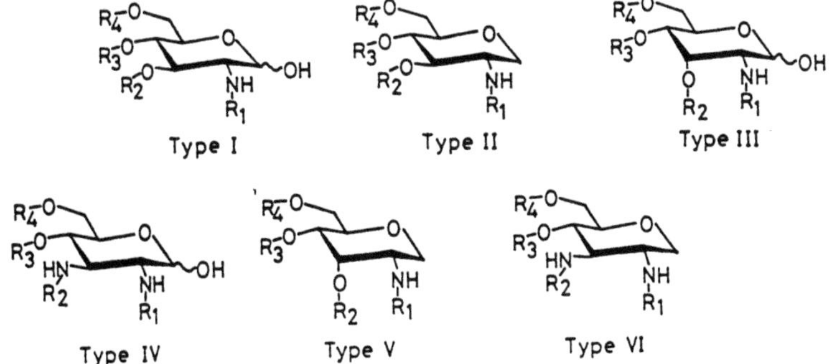

Fig 1. Backbone and substituent structures of chemically synthesized compounds.

Table 1. Biological activities of GLA-27 and lipid A

	GLA-27	Lipid A
Pyrogenicity		
minimum pyrogenic dose (μg)	>10	0.001
Lethality in galactosamine-sensitized mice (LD_{50} μg)	0.54	0.0078
Shwartzman reaction		
minimum preparatory dose (μg)	>50	1.25
TNF-inducing activity (ED_{50} μg)	3.0	0.1
IFN-inducing activity (ED_{50} μg)	0.1	0.001
Mitogenicity (SI)*	11.5	30.6
Macrophage activation		
Phagocytosis (SI)*	2.6	3.5
Adjuvant activity (SI)*	3.4	3.2

*SI (Stimulation Index): relative value to the control.

When the 3-O-acyl (C_{14}) group of GLA-27 was eliminated or transferred to the 6-O- position, the resulting compound, (GLA-34 or GLA-45, respectively), exhibited none of the biological activities examined. When 3-O-acyl group was altered to C_{14}-O-(C_{14}) (GLA-47), only Limulus activity remained unchanged; the other activities were lost (Table 2).

A compound (GLA-44) possessing 3-hydroxytetradecanoyl (C_{14}-OH) group as the 2-N-acyl substituent showed only Limulus activity, which was much weaker than that of GLA-27. A compound, GLA-26, possessing C_{14} as the 2-N-acyl substituent exhibited slightly weaker activities in tests for Limulus amebocyte gelation and TNF induction.

From the biological activities of GLA-37 and GLA-38 it was also found that the chain length of the acyl groups significantly affects biological activities.

As for phosphorylation effect, 4-O-monophosphorylation is more effective for expression of various biological activities than 6-O-mono or 4,6-O-bis-phosphorylation at least when the acylation pattern is the same as that of GLA-27. Dephosphorylation caused most activities of GLA-27 to disappear altogether. Similar phosphorylation effect was observed for compounds with 1-deoxyglucosamine backbone structure (Fig 1, Table 2).

These results indicate that acyl substituents, their acylation positions and phosphorylation positions in the glucosamine backbone structure markedly affect the expression of biological activities.

Table 2. Effects of acyl substituent and phosphorylation on immunopharmacological and Limulus amebocyte gelation activities

	Substituent								
	2-N-	3-O-	4-O-	6-O-	Limulus	Mitogen	PBA	TNF	IFN
GLA-27			P	H	++++	+++	+++	+++	+++
GLA-25	C_{14}-O-(C_{14})	C_{14}	H	H	−	±	+	−	−
GLA-35			H	P	+	++	++	−	−
GLA-36			P	P	±	++	++	−	−
GLA-34	C_{14}-O-(C_{14})	H			−	−	−	−	−
GLA-47	C_{14}-O-(C_{14})	C_{14}-O-(C_{14})			++++	+	+	−	−
GLA-44	C_{14}-OH	C_{14}			±	−	−	−	−
GLA-26	C_{14}	C_{14}	P	H	++	−	−	−	−
GLA-46	C_{14}-OH	C_{14}-OH			±	−	−	−	−
GLA-37	C_{12}-O-(C_{12})	C_{12}			+++	−	+	−	−
GLA-38	C_{16}-O-(C_{16})	C_{16}			++	−	−	−	−
GLA-45	C_{14}-O-(C_{14})	H			−	−	−	−	−
GLA-29	C_{14}-OH	C_{14}	P	C_{14}	−	−	−	−	−
GLA-28	C_{14}-OH	C_{14}			−	−	−	−	−

Toxic activities such as pyrogenicity (10 μg/kg), local Shwartzman reaction (50 μg) and lethal toxicity in galactosamine-sensitized mice were found negative. Limulus: Limulus amebocyte galation. Mitogen: mitogenic activity. PBA: polyclonal B cell activation activity. TNF: tumor necrosis factor inducing activity. IFN: interferon inducing activity. P: phosphoryl. C_{12}: dodecanoyl. C_{14}: tetradecanoyl. C_{12}-O-(C_{12}): 3-dodecanoyloxydodecanoyl. C_{14}-OH: 3-hydroxytetradecanoyl. C_{14}-O-(C_{14}): 3-tetradecanoyloxytetradecanoyl. C_{16}: hexadecanoyl. C_{16}-O-(C_{16}): 3-hexadecanoyloxyhexadecanoyl.

Effects of Backbone Structure and Stereospecificity of Acyl Substituent on Immunopharmacological Activities of Lipid A Subunit Analogs

We then synthesized derivatives of GLA-27 or GLA-47 with the same acyl and phosphoryl substituents but with different backbone structures and examined the relationship between biological activity and chemical structure (15, 20, 21).

Synthetic compounds with six different backbone structures (tentatively designated as types I-VI) are shown in Fig 1. The backbone structure of type I is glucosamine and those of types II, III, IV, V and VI correspond to the 1-deoxy, 3-epimeric (allose form), 3-amino, 1-deoxy-3-epimeric, and 1 deoxy-3-amino types of glucosamine, respectively.

TNF-inducing and mitogenic activities of the compounds possessing the same acylation pattern as that of GLA-27 but different backbone structures are shown in Fig 2. Strong TNF activity was induced in the sera of mice given GLA-27, GLA-43, GLA-51, and GLA-40 (Fig 2(A)). GLA-48, with backbone type IV, was weak.

The mitogenic activity of the compounds is shown in Fig 2(B). GLA-40 exhibited the strongest activity, followed by GLA-27, GLA-51 and GLA-48, which exhibited moderate activities in that order. GLA-43 with backbone type

III showed very weak activity. The TNF-inducing and mitogenic activities of the compounds with C_{14}-O-(C_{14}) as the 3-O-substituent (GLA-49, GLA-52 and GLA-47) were very weak regardless of backbone structure.

PBA activity of the compounds was examined using spleen cells from C3H/HeN mice. Results similar to those obtained for mitogenic activity were obtained. Compounds with C_{14} as the 3-O-substituent but different backbone structure (GLA-27, GLA-40, GLA-43, GLA-48 and GLA-51) exhibited relatively stronger activities compared with those of the compounds with C_{14}-O-(C_{14}) as the 3-O-substituent (GLA-47, GLA-49 and GLA-52) regardless of backbone structure.

None of these compounds exhibited either mitogenic or PBA activity in spleen cells from C3H/HeJ mice.

These results indicate that modification of the backbone structure is less influential than modification of the acyl and phosphoryl substituents for expressing biological activities.

As GLA-27 has an asymmetric carbon at the C-3 position in its acyloxy-acyl substituent (C_{14}-O-(C_{14})), stereospecific isomers of this compound, (R) and (S) forms, were synthesized and their biological activities tested. In addition to these isomers, those of GLA-40 were also examined (16).

TNF-inducing activity of the (S) isomer of GLA-27 was stronger than that of the (R) isomer, while the (R) isomer exhibited stronger mitogenic, PBA and macrophage activation activities than the (S) isomer. Macrophage activation activities of these isomers were investigated by measuring phagocytic, lysosomal enzyme activation and cytostatic activities of peritoneal macrophages obtained from mice administerd i.p. with test samples. Among stereoisomers of GLA-27, the (R) isomer exhibited somewhat stronger phagocytic, lysosomal

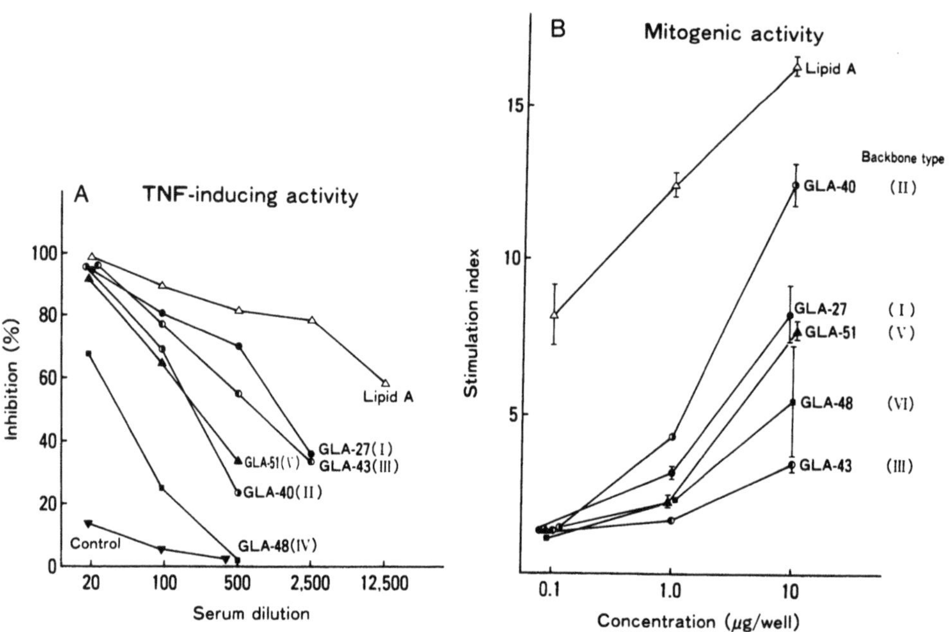

Fig 2. TNF-inducing and mitogenic activities of the compounds possessing the same acylation pattern as that of GLA-27 but with different backbone structures.
(A): TNF-inducing activity (B): mitogenic activity

enzyme and cytostasis-inducing activities than the (S) isomer, while there was no appreciable difference in the activities between the isomers of GLA-40.

These results so far obtained indicate that lipid A subunit analogs tend to express immunopharmacological activities such as B cell and macrophage activation as well as mediator (TNF and IFN)-inducing activities separately from toxic activities such as pyrogenicity and lethality as well as Shwartzman reaction eliciting activity. It was also proved that Limulus amebocyte lysate gelation activity is exhibited independently of immunopharmacological and toxic activities in the case of lipid A subunit analogs.

Effects of Acyl Substituents and their Stereospecificities Linked to 3-O- and 2-N-Positions of 4-O-phosphono-D-glucosamine in the Expression of Immunopharmacological Activities

The above results indicating that alteration of acyl substituents including their configurations affect biological activities of the derivatives more than alteration of backbone structure led us to further more detailed investigations on the manner of altering acyl substituents in glucosamine backbone structures. A dozen 4-O-phosphono-D-glucosamines carrying different combinations of acyl groups at 2-N- and 3-O- positions were chemically synthesized (Fig 3) (1, 11). Immunopharmacological properties of these compounds (GLA-27,

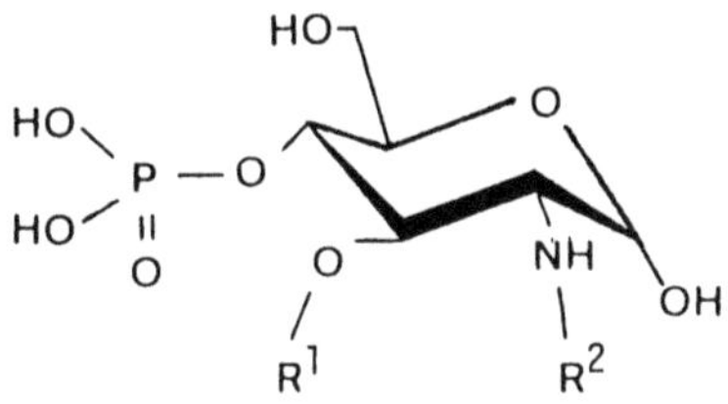

	R^1 (3-O-)	R^2 (2-N-)
GLA-57	C_{14}	C_{14}-O-(C_{12})
GLA-27	C_{14}	C_{14}-O-(C_{14})
GLA-58	C_{14}	C_{14}-O-(C_{16})
GLA-61	C_{14}OH	C_{14}-O-(C_{12})
GLA-59	C_{14}OH	C_{14}-O-(C_{14})
GLA-62	C_{14}OH	C_{14}-O-(C_{16})
GLA-67	C_{14}-O-(C_{12})	C_{14}
GLA-68	C_{14}-O-(C_{14})	C_{14}
GLA-69	C_{14}-O-(C_{16})	C_{14}
GLA-63	C_{14}-O-(C_{12})	C_{14}OH
GLA-60	C_{14}-O-(C_{14})	C_{14}OH
GLA-64	C_{14}-O-(C_{16})	C_{14}OH

Fig 3. 4-O-phosphono-D-glucosamine derivatives carrying different combinations of acyl groups at the 2-N- and 3-O- positions.

GLA-57, GLA-58, GLA-59 and GLA-60) were assayed and compared with each other as follows (17).

GLA-59 and GLA-60 exhibited significant CSF-inducing activity, comparable to that of GLA-27, though weaker than that of natural lipid A. The activity of GLA-57 with an N-linked C_{14}-O-(C_{12}) group was weaker than that of GLA-27. GLA-58 with an N-linked C_{14}-O-(C_{16}) group did not show significant activity.

All the compounds except GLA-58 exhibited similar significant TNF-inducing activity, though the activity was weaker than that of lipid A. Less activity was seen with GLA-58.

GLA-27 exhibited significant IFN-inducing activity in **P. acnes**-primed mice. Among the compounds, GLA-57 showed stronger activity than GLA-27. On the other hand, the activity of GLA-58 was much lower. The activity of GLA-60 was higher than that of GLA-59, which was stronger than that of GLA-27 (Table 3).

Mitogenic and PBA activities of these compounds were investigated with similar results. GLA-60 and GLA-59 showed much higher activity than GLA-27, while GLA-58 did not show detectable activity. GLA-57 showed weaker mitogenic activity than GLA-27, while it showed PBA activity almost equivalent to that of GLA-27.

Strong macrophage activation was induced by i.p. administration of either 20 ug of GLA-27 or GLA-60. The activity of GLA-57 and GLA-59 was significant, whereas GLA-58 did not induce appreciable macrophage activation.

GLA-27 induced significant adjuvant activity, whereas GLA-58 induced very weak response. GLA-57 and GLA-59 were somewhat more active than GLA-27. Among the compounds, GLA-60 showed the strongest adjuvant activity.

Table 3. IFN-inducing activity of synthetic lipid A analogs

Compounds	IFN titer (IU/0.1 ml)
Exp. 1	
Mock control	< 10
GLA-27 (RS)	380
GLA-57 (RS)	640
GLA-58 (RS)	10
GLA-59 (RS)	480
GLA-60 (RS)	640
Lipid A	1,920
Exp. 2	
Mock control	<10
GLA-59 (R)	640
GLA-59 (RS)	320
GLA-59 (S)	160
GLA-60 (R)	640
GLA-60 (RS)	640
GLA-60 (S)	320
Lipid A	1,920

These results showed that newly synthesized comounds possessing C_{14}-OH and C_{14}-O-(C_{14}) as acyl substituents such as GLA-59 and GLA-60 exhibit comparable or higher immunopharmacological activities than GLA-27.

Since acyl substituents such as C_{14}-OH and C_{14}-O-(C_{14}) have asymmetric carbons in their C-3 positions, stereoisomers composed of acyl substituents with the (R) and (S) configurations were compared for their immunopharmacological activities. In all of the immunopharmacological activities tested, (R) isomers of both GLA-59 and GLA-60 showed stronger activities than those of (S) isomers.

This result is easily understood given the fact that natural lipid A's have (R) form acyl substituents.

Endotoxic Activities such as Pyrogenicity, Local Shwartzman Reaction and Lethal Toxicity in Galactosamine-Sensitized Mice

None of the synthetic compounds showed any detectable pyrogenic activity at a dose of 10 µg/kg in Japanese white rabbits, while natural lipid A exhibited remarkable pyrogenicity at a dose of 0.001 µg/kg. Whereas natural lipid A induced local Shwartzman reaction at a dose of 1.25 ug, none of the synthetic compounds showed positive reaction at a dose of 50 ug. Weak lethal toxicity in galactosamine-sensitized mice was detected at a dose of 1 ug per mouse for all compounds except GLA-58, which did not show toxicity at a dose of 10 µg per mouse.

We then investigated whether these compounds exhibit nonspecific protective activity and antitumor activity, and if so, to what extent they preserve them compared with lipid A. All the synthetic compounds tested in the following paragraphs were (R) isomers unless otherwise noted.

Nonspecific Protective Activity against P. aeruginosa Infection

Ten ug synthetic compound per mouse was injected i.p. to 7-wk-old female ICR mice the day before i.p. infection with 5 x 10^7 CFU of **P. aeruginosa** 5E81-1 strain. As a control, 1 µg of **E. coli** lipid A was used. The number of surviving mice was counted 7 days later (22, 23).

All the synthetic compounds with an acyloxyacyl group (C_{14}-O-(C_{12}), C_{14}-O-(C_{14}) or C_{14}-O-C($_{16}$)) at the 2-N- position of the glucosamine exhibited low protective activity under the experimental conditions in which surviving ratio of mice injected 1µg of lipid A was 90% and that of mice without sample injection was 3%, as shown in Table 4.

On the other hand, as shown in the table, compounds possessing an acyloxyacyl group at the 3-O- position of glucosamine, except GLA-69 and GLA-64 which carry C_{14}-O-(C_{16}) as the acyloxyacyl substituent, showed remarkable enhancing effect of nonspecific protective activity to a degree similar to that of lipid A injected at a dose of 1 ug/head.

Dose-potency experiments of four compounds, GLA-60, GLA-63, GLA-67 and GLA-68, were also performed. As shown in Fig 4, GLA-60 and GLA-63 possessing a C_{14}-OH at the 2-N- position of the glucosamine exhibited significant activity at a dose of 1 µg per head, while GLA-67 and GLA-68 carrying a C_{14} at the 2-N- position did not exhibit any activity at the same dose. Potency of GLA-60 and GLA-63 was about one tenth that of natural lipid A by weight.

It is noteworthy that GLA-59 possessing the same acyl components as those of GLA-60 but with reversed binding positions was found to be less active than GLA-60.

Table 4. Enhancement of nonspecific resistance against **P. aeruginosa** infection by synthetic lipid A analogs

Compounds	No. of mice (survived/tested)	% Survival	P value
Mock control	1/35	3	
GLA-57	9/20	45	0.001
GLA-27	8/20	40	0.001
GLA-58	5/20	25	0.05
GLA-61	10/20	50	0.001
GLA-59	7/20	35	0.01
GLA-62	5/20	25	0.05
GLA-67	17/20	85	0.001
GLA-68	20/20	100	0.001
GLA-69	4/20	20	ns*
GLA-63	18/20	90	0.001
GLA-60	18/20	90	0.001
GLA-64	4/20	20	ns*
Lipid A	27/30	90	0.001

Synthetic compounds with (R) configuration and natural lipid A were administered i.p. at a dose of 10 μg and 1 μg per mouse, respectively, 1 day before i.p. infection with 5 x 10^7 CFU of **P. aeruginosa** 5E81-1 strain.
*ns: not significant

These results indicated that the binding sites of the acyl substituents play a role in the manifestation of nonspecific protective activity against **P. aeruginosa** infection. Moreover, compounds with C_{14}-OH at the 2-N- position showed stronger activity than compounds with C_{14}.

Nonspecific Protective Activity to Vaccinia Virus Infection

According to i.v. inoculation with 10^4 pfu of vaccinia virus, discrete dermal vesicles appeared on the tail of ddY mice on day 4, reading maximum size (about 40 lesions) on day 7. Virus titers in tail lesions closely depended on the number of vesicles. A test sample was administered i.v. 1 day before the infection, since the strongest antiviral activity of LPS was observed when mice were intravenously administered LPS 1 day before the infection (6, 7).

The influence of the chain length of the acyloxyacyl group bound to the 2-N- position of GLA-27 was investigated. The activity of compounds (RS) with N-acyloxyacyl groups of differing carbon chain lengths, e.g., C_{14}-O-(C_{12}), C_{14}-O-(C_{14}), C_{14}-O-(C_{16}), termed GLA-57, GLA-27 and GLA-58 respectively, is shown in Table 5. GLA-57 exhibited somewhat stronger protective activity than GLA-27, while GLA-58 completely lost the activity. A compound (GLA-39) with N-C_{14}-OH and 3-O-C_{14}-O-(C_{14}) groups enhanced nonspecific protective activity to the viral infection more than did GLA-57. GLA-60 showed the strongest activity among the compound tested. The antiviral activity of compounds GLA-27 and GLA-60 was compared with lipid A of **E. coli** Re mutant, and N-acetylmuramyl-L-alanyl-D-isoglutamine (MDP) as shown in Fig 5. Lipid A exhibited much stronger antiviral activity than GLA-27, but the activity of GLA-27 was 100 times higher than that of MDP. The activity of GLA-60 was 10 times higher than that of GLA-27.

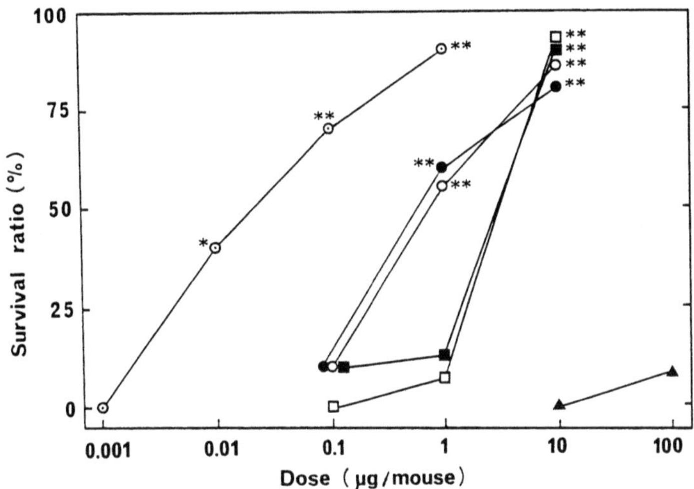

Fig 4. Effects of different acyl groups at the 2-N- and 3-O- positions of glucosamine derivatives on the expression of nonspecific resistance against **P. aeruginosa** infection.

Female ICR mice were administered ip with the indicated dose of test samples, i.e., GLA-60(O), GLA-63(●), GLA-67(■), GLA-68(□), lipid A(⊙), MDP(▲), the day before challenge infection with i.p. injection of 5 x 10^7 **P. aeruginosa.** Surviving ration (%) = (survived mice/tested mice) x 100. *; P<0.01, **; P<0.001.

It was clarified that lipid A-subunit analogs, e.g., GLA-59 and GLA-60, significantly increased nonspecific resistance against vaccinia virus infection by i.v. administration of samples the day before infection, though the activity was weaker than that of lipid A.

We have also shown that the antiviral activity of GLA-27 was much stronger than that of MDP, a well known synthetic immunostimulator. However, the activity of GLA-27 was weaker than that of new synthetic compounds GLA-59 and GLA-60. The only structural difference between GLA-27 and GLA-59 is the 3-O-linked acy substituent (C_{14} and C_{14}-OH groups), suggesting that the co-presence of C_{14}-OH and C_{14}-O-(C_{14}) groups in lipid A-subunit analogs is very important for expression of antiviral activity. GLA-58 carrying an N-C_{14}-O-(C_{16}) group did not show significant activity. On the other hand, GLA-57 carrying an N-C_{14}-O-(C_{12}) group exhibited stronger activity than GLA-27. This suggests that the chain length of the acyloxyacyl groups in lipid A-subunit analogs strongly influences the expression of antiviral activity.

Antitumor Activity

To evaluate the antitumor activity of the compounds, 1 x 10^5 Meth A fibrosarcoma cells for intravenous sample administration and 2 x 10^5 Meth A for intratumoral sample administration were transplanted into the epidermis of the right flank of mice. A test compound was administered either intravenously or intratumorally twice at a dose of 100 μg per mouse days 7 and 9 after transplantation. Natural free lipid A was administered twice at a dose of 10 μg/mouse. Controls were injected with saline. Four weeks after tumor inoculation, mice were sacrificed and the excised tumor weighed. Cured mice

Table 5. Effect of different acyl groups at the 2-N- and 3-O-positions of glucosamine on the expression of antiviral activity

Test sample	Dose (μg)	Number of lesions (mean±SEM)	% inhibition (mean±SEM)
Saline	-	34.8 ± 4.5	-
GLA-27	0.1	36.6 ± 4.5^{ns}	0
	1	19.9 ± 2.1**	43 ± 6
	10	10.2 ± 1.9*	71 ± 5
GLA-57	0.1	34.2 ± 4.7^{ns}	2
	1	17.7 ± 3.4**	49 ± 10
	10	4.3 ± 1.5*	88 ± 4
GLA-58	0.1	33.5 ± 2.4^{ns}	4
	1	39.3 ± 3.3^{ns}	0
	10	29.9 ± 3.6^{ns}	14 ± 10
GLA-59	0.1	25.0 ± 4.3^{ns}	28 ± 12
	1	16.9 ± 3.1***	51 ± 9
	10	6.0 ± 1.4*	83 ± 4
GLA-60	0.1	21.0 ± 2.6***	40 ± 7
	1	12.2 ± 2.7*	65 ± 8
	10	7.0 ± 1.9*	80 ± 5

Female ddy mice were administered i.v. with the indicated dose of test samples the day before challenge with 10^4 pfu of vaccinia virus. The number of lesions formed on the tail were counted on the 7th day after virus infection. Results were expressed as the percent inhibition ± SEM of ten mice per group. Significant difference from control (*, P<0.001; **, P<0.01; ***, P<0.05).

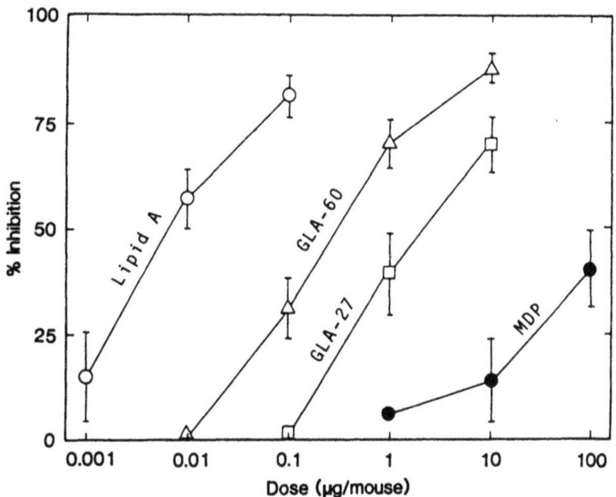

Fig 5. Dose-response curve of lipid A, GLA-60, GLA-27, and MDP on inhibition of lesion formation induced by vaccinia virus infection.

Female ddY mice were administered i.v. with the indicated dose of test samples, the day before challenge with 10^4 pfu of vaccinia virus. The number of lesions formed on the tail were counted on day 7 after virus infection. Results are expressed as the percent inhibition $\pm$ SEM of ten mice per group. Significant difference from the control (*, P<0.001; **, P<0.01; ***, P<0.05).

were rechallenged with 1 x 10^6 Meth A fibrosarcoma cells (22-23) and no tumor growth was observed.

Figure 6 and Table 6 (Exp. 1) show the results of antitumor activity in mice intravenously administered 100 μg of test samples or 10 μg of natural lipid A. GLA-59 and GLA-60 exhibited strong activity comparable to that of 10 ug natural lipid A. Tumor size of mice treated with GLA-59, GLA-60 or free lipid A started to decrease on day 9, 2 days after sample administration and became smallest around day 17. After that tumor size increased gradually. In mice treated with GLA-27 or GLA-68, tumors grew monotonously.

Half the mice were completely cured by the administration of compounds GLA-59 and GLA-60, which were as effective as natural lipid A (P<0.05). Tumor growth was significantly inhibited and size and weight of tumor decreased conspicuously in mice treated with GLA-59 and GLA-60 as well as in those treated with 10 μg natural lipid A (P<0.001). Significant activity of GLA-68 was observed only in the decrement of tumor weight (P<0.05), while GLA-27 did not show detectable antitumor activity at a dose of 100 μg. In mice treated with GLA-27 tumor grew monotonously as it did in the control.

The above experiment was repeated using GLA-59, GLA-60 and natural lipid A injected i.v. as described above. The results are shown in Table 6 (Exp. 2). More than half the mice were completely cured by the administration of compounds GLA-59 and GLA-60, which were as effective as natural lipid A. Size and weight of tumor decreased conspicuously in mice treated with GLA-59 and GLA-60 as well as in those treated with 10 μg natural lipid A.

Since i.v. injection of GLA-59 and GLA-60 induced remarkable regression of tumor growth, both compounds were injected intratumorally on days 7 and 9. As shown in Fig 7 and Table 6 (Exp. 3), GLA-59 and GLA-60 induced remarkable

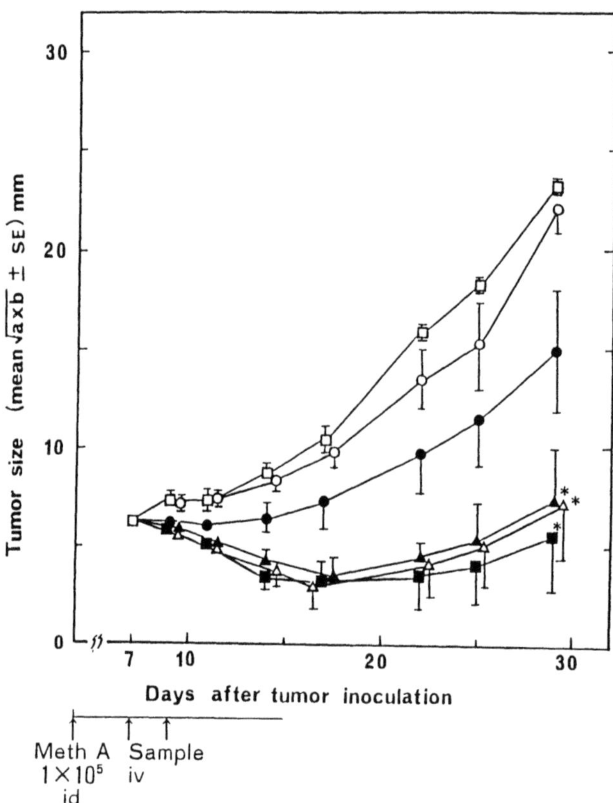

Fig 6. Antitumor activity of intravenously administered 4-O-phosphono-D-glucosamine derivatives carrying different acyl group at the 2-N- and 3-O- positions. Control(□), GLA-27 100 μg x 2(O), GLA-59 100 μg x 2(Δ), GLA-60 100 μg x 2(▲), GLA-68 100 μg x 2(●), lipid A 10 μg x 2(■). *P 0.001.

Table 6. Effect of intravenously or intratumorally administered lipid A-subunit analogs on Meth A fibrosarcoma.

Sample	Dose (μg/mouse)	Route	Tumor size (mm) mean±SE	Tumor weight (mg) mean±SE	Complete regression cured/total
Exp. 1					
Saline		iv	23.2 ± 0.4	2,859 ± 243	0/6
GLA-27	100 x 2	iv	22.1 ± 1.2	2,428 ± 570	1/8
GLA-59	100 x 2	iv	7.1 ± 2.7	399 ± 263	4/8
GLA-67	100 x 2	iv	11.1 ± 3.3	580 ± 278	1/4
GLA-68	100 x 2	iv	15.0 ± 3.3	1,525 ± 420	2/8
GLA-63	100 x 2	iv	7.6 ± 2.9	500 ± 268	4/8
GLA-60	100 x 2	iv	7.3 ± 2.7	355 ± 185	4/8
Lipid A	10 x 2	iv	5.6 ± 2.7	373 ± 231	5/8
Exp. 2					
Saline		iv	18.4 ± 1.4	1,685 ± 433	0/9
GLA-59	100 x 2	iv	5.5 ± 4.6	550 ± 306	6/9
GLA-60	100 x 2	iv	2.8 ± 1.9	176 ± 139	7/9
Lipid A	10 x 2	iv	7.9 ± 3.0	830 ± 439	5/9
Exp. 3					
Saline		itu	23.1 ± 1.1	3,200 ± 408	0/9
GLA-59	100 x 2	itu	4.1 ± 2.7	404 ± 273	7/9
GLA-60	100 x 2	itu	3.2 ± 1.7	81 ± 48	6/9
Lipid A	10 x 2	itu	1.4 ± 1.4	52 ± 52	8/9

reduction of tumor size and tumor weight ($P<0.001$). Also in these cases, tumor size decreased gradually after sample treatment and became smallest around day 22. More than half the mice were cured by these two compounds. Similar results were obtained using natural lipid A.

No detectable tumor growth was observed when 1×10^6 Meth A cells were rechallenged into cured mice. In Winn's assay, significant tumor growth was observed in mice transplanted with Meth A and normal spleen cells but not in mice with Meth A and spleen cells from cured mice.

In 4-O-phosphono-D-glucosamine derivatives carrying 2-N- and 3-O-acyl substituents, the combination of C_{14}-OH and C_{14}-O-(C_{14}) groups plays a criti-

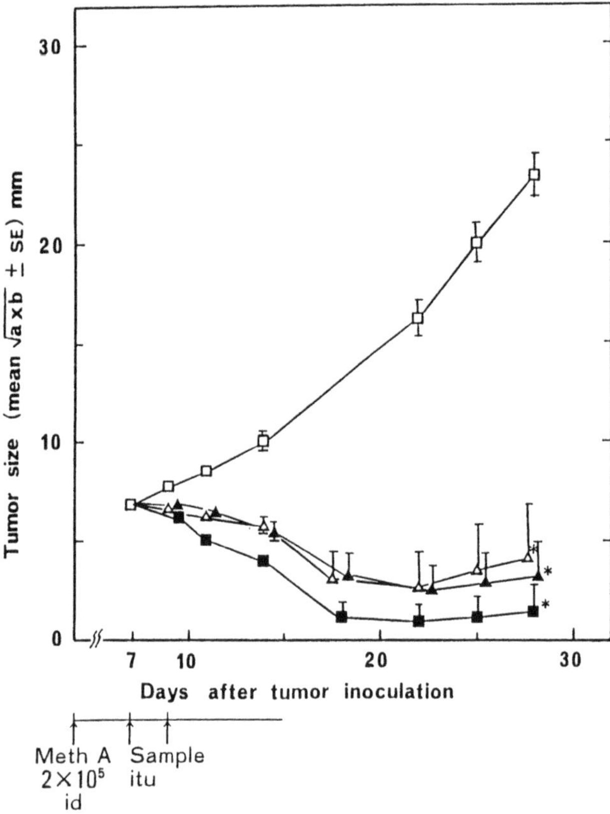

Fig 7. Growth inhibition of Meth A fibrosarcoma by intratumorally administration of 4-O-phosphono-D-glucosanine derivatives, GLA-59 and GLA-60. Control(□), GLA-27 100 µg x 2(O), GLA-59 100 µg x 2(Δ), GLA-60 100 µg x 2(▲), GLA-68 100 µg x 2(●), lipid A 10 µg x 2(■). *P<0.001.

cal role in the manifestation of antitumor activity, since the antitumor activity of compounds GLA-27 and GLA-68 with C_{14} and C_{14}-O-(C_{14}) groups as acyl substituents was far weaker than that of GLA-59 and GLA-60. The former compounds did not exhibit the activity at all at a dose of 100 µg/mouse. GLA 27 showed significant antitumor activity only when injected with 250 ug per mouse as reported elsewhere (22).

Difference in expression of antitumor activity was not affected by the binding position of C_{14}-OH at 2-N- or 3-O-. The binding site of C_{14}-OH at either 2-N- or 3-O-, however, plays a role in the manifestation of nonspecific protective activities against **P. aeruginosa** infection, and in a somewhat lower degree, vaccinia virus infection.

SUMMARY

Some synthetic compounds of the nonreducing part of lipid A were found to preserve significant immunopharmacological activities of the endotoxin, at the same time showing very slight if any endotoxic activity such as pyrogenicity, lethality or Shwartzman reactivity. Thus, divers activities of the endotoxin which had earlier been considered intrinsic and inseparable were shown to be separable when certain synthetic analogs of lipid A-subunit are at work.

The combination of acyl components as well as phosphorylation and acylation positions in these partial structure analogs of lipid A affect the expression of biological activities of the endotoxin. Moreover, stereospecificities of acyl substituents contribute differently to enhance the various biological activities of the endotoxin.

It was remarkable that protective activities of the endotoxin such as enhancing nonspecific resistance against microbial infections and antitumor activity are preserved in lipid A-subunit analogs of small molecular weight of ca. 1,000, which at the same time lose all or most toxic activity such as pyrogenicity, lethality and Shwartzman reactivity.

It is hoped that new derivatives of lipid A and/or lipid A-subunit which exert only limited biological activities of endotoxin, whether they be protective or toxic, can be synthesized in order to clarify the stuctural requirements for expressing a given activity. Such compounds will be useful not only for promoting basic endotoxin research but also for application in clinical medicine. Further detailed experiments on the structure-activity relationships of the newly synthesized 4-O-phosphono-D-glucosamine derivatives binding acyl substituents of varying carbon chain length at the 2-N- and 3-O- positions are in progress.

ACKNOWLEDGMENTS

The authors wish to thank our many colleagues, whose dedicated work generated the results summarized in this review. The authors wish to thank Mr. Hiroaki Takimoto for preparing this manuscript.

REFERENCES

1. Apte, R. N., Galanos, C., Pluznik, D. H., 1976, Lipid A, the active part of bacterial endotoxins in including serum colony stimulating activity and proliferation of splenic granulocyte/macrophage progenitor cells. J. Cell. Physiol. 87: 71.

2. Galanos, C., Freudenberg, M. A., Reutter, W., 1979, Galactosamine-induced sensitization to the lethal effects of endotoxin. Proc. Natl. Acad. Sci. USA. 76: 5939.

3. Galanos, C., Lüderitz, O., Rietschel, E. T., Westphal, O., Brade, H., Brade, L., Freudenberg, M., Schade, U., Imoto, M., Yoshimura, H., Kusumoto, S., and Shiba, T., 1985, Synthetic and natural **Escherichia coli** free lipid A express identical endotoxic activities. Eur. J. Biochem. 148: 1.

4. Homma, J. Y., Matsuura, M., Kanegasaki, S., Kawakubo, Y., Kojima, Y., Shibukawa, N., Kumazawa, Y., Yamamoto, A., Tanamoto, K., Yasuda, T., Imoto, M., Yoshimura, H., Kusumoto, S., Shiba, T., 1985, Structure requirements of lipid A responsible for the functions: a study with chemically synthesized lipid A and its analogues. J. Biochem. 98: 395.

5. Homma, J. Y., 1987, On the threshhold a new era in endotoxin research. EOS: Rivista di Immunologia ed Immunofarmacologia. 7: 142.

6. Ikeda, S., Nishimura, C., Nakatsuka, M., Homma, J. Y., Kiso, M., and Hasegawa, A., 1988, Antiviral and immunomodulating activities of chemically synthesized lipid A-subunit analogues GLA-27 and GLA-60. Antiviral Res. 9: 37.

7. Ikeda, S., Kumazawa, Y., Nishimura, C., Nakatsuka, M., Homma, J. Y., Kiso, M., and Hasegawa, A., 1988, Enhancement of nonspecific resistance

to viral infection by chemically synthesized 4'-O-monophosphoryl lipid A and its subunit analogues with different backbone structures and acyl groups. Antiviral Res. 10: 167.

8. Imoto, M., Yoshimura, H., Kusumoto, S., and Shiba, T., 1984, Total synthesis of lipid A, active principle of bacterial endotoxin. Proc. Japan Acad. 60, Ser. B. 285.

9. Kiso, M., Ishida, H., and Hasegawa, A., 1984, Synthesis of biologically active, novel monosaccharide analogs of lipid A, Agric. Biol. Chem. 48: 251.

10. Kiso, M. and Hasegawa, A., 1984, Synthetic studies on lipid A and related compounds, in: "Bacterial endotoxin: chemical and biological and clinical aspects." J. Y. Homma et al., eds., Verlag Chemie, Weinheim.

11. Kiso, M., Tanaka, S., Fujita, M., Ogawa, Y., Ishida, H., and Hasegawa, A., 1987, Synthesis of the optically active 4-O-phosphono-D-glucosamine derivatives related to the non-reducing sugar subunit of bacterial lipid A. Carbohydr. Res. 162: 127.

12. Kiso, M., Tanaka, S., Fujishima, M., Ogawa, Y., and Hasegawa, A., 1987, Synthesis of nonreducing-sugar subunit analogs of bacterial lipid A carrying an amido-bound (3R)-3-acyloxytetradecanoyl group. Carbohydr. Res. 162: 247.

13. Kotani, S., Takada, H., Tsujimoto, M., Ogawa, T., Takahashi, I., Ikeda, T., Otsuka, K., Shimanouchi, H., Kasai, N., Mashimo, J., Nagao, S., Tanaka, A., Tanaka, S., Harada, K., Nagaki, K., and Kitamura, H., 1985, Synthetic lipid A with endotoxic and related biological activities comparable to those of a natural lipid A from an **Escherichia coli** Re-mutant. Infect. Immun. 49: 225.

14. Kumazawa, Y., Matsuura, M., Homma, J. Y., Nakatsuru, Y., and Hasegawa, A., 1985, B cell activation and adjuvant activities of chemically synthesized analogues of the non-reducing sugar moiety of lipid A. Eur. J. Immunol. 15: 199.

15. Kumazawa, Y., Matsuura, M., Maruyama, T., Homma, J. Y., Kiso, M., and Hasegawa, A., 1986, Structure requirements for inducing in vitro B lymphocyte activation by chemically synthesized derivatives related to the nonreducing D-glucosamine subunit of lipid A. Eur. J. Immunol. 16: 1099.

16. Kumazawa, Y., Ikeda, S., Takimoto, H., Nishimura, C., Nakatsuka, M., Homma, J. Y., Yamamoto, A., Kiso, M., and Hasegawa, A., 1987, Effect of stereospecificity of chemically synthesized lipid A-subunit analogues GLA-27 and GLA-40 in the expression of immunopharmacological activities, Eur. J. Immunol. 17: 663.

17. Kumazawa, Y., Nakatsuka, M., Takimoto, H., Furuya, T., Nagumo, T., Yamamoto, A., Homma, J. Y., Inada, K., Yoshida, M., Kiso, M., Hasegawa, A., 1988, Importance of fatty acid substituents of chemically synthesized lipid A-subunit analogues in the expression of immunopharmacological activity. Infect. Immun. 56: 149.

18. Kusumoto, S., Yoshimura, H., Imoto, M., Shimamoto, T., and Shiba, T., 1985, Chemical synthesis of 1-dephosphono derivative of **Escherichia coli** lipid A. Tetrahedron Lett. 26: 909.

19. Matsuura, M., Kojima, Y., Homma, J. Y., Kubota, Y., Yamamoto, A., Kiso,

M., and Hasegawa, A., 1984, Biological activities of chemically synthesized analogues of the nonreducing sugar moiety of lipid A. FEBS Lett. 167: 226.

20. Matsuura, M., Kojima, Y., Homma, J. Y., Kubota, Y., Yamamoto, A., Kiso, M., and Hasegawa, A., 1985, Biological activities of chemically synthesized partial structure analogues of lipd A. J. Biochem. 98: 1229.

21. Matsuura, M., Kojima, Y., Homma, J. Y., Kumazawa, Y., Yamamoto, A., Kiso, M., and Hasegawa, A., 1986, Effect of backbone structures and stereospecificities of lipid A-subunit analogues on their biological activities. J. Biochem. 99: 1377.

22. Nakatsuka, M., Kumazawa, Y., Ikeda, S., Yamamoto, A., Nishimura, C., Homma, J. Y., Kiso, M., and Hasegwa, A., 1988, Antitumor and antimicrobial activities of lipid A-subunit analogue GLA-27. J. Clin. Lab. Immun. 26: 43.

23. (a) Nakatsuka, M., Kumazawa, Y., Homma, J. Y., Kiso, M., and Hasegawa, A., 1987, Enhancement of nonspecific resistance by chemically synthesized lipid A subunit analogs GLA-60 against **Pseudomonas aeruginosa** infection. Proc. Japan. Cancer Association (46th Annual Meeting, Tokyo) Japan J. Cancer Research, p. 337.

(b) Kumazawa, Y., Nakatsuka, M., Homma, J. Y., Kiso, M., and Hasegawa, A., 1987, Antitumor activity of chemically synthesized lipid A-subunit analogs GLA-59 and GLA-60. Proc. Japan. Cancer Association (46th Annual Meeting, Tokyo) Japan J. Cancer Research, p. 336.

THE CHEMICAL STRUCTURE OF THE LIPOPOLYSACCHARIDE OF A Rc-TYPE MUTANT OF PROTEUS MIRABILIS LACKING 4-AMINO-4-DEOXY-L ARABINOSE AND ITS SUSCEPTIBILITY TOWARDS POLYMYXIN B

J. Radziejewska-Lebrecht, U. R. Bhat*, H. Brade **, W. Kaca, and H. Mayer*

Institute of Microbiology, University of Lodz, PL-90237 Lodz, Poland, *Max-Planck-Institut fur Immunobiologie, D-7800 Freiburg i.Br., and **Forschungsinstitut Borstel, D-2061 Borstel, F.R.G.

The mutant Proteus mirabilis R4 (R4/028) was obtained from the wild-type strain **P. mirabilis** 028 (F87) by ultraviolet irradiation. Isolation of R4/028 lipopolysaccharide (LPS) and the partial elucidation of the glucose-heptose region as a trisaccharide: β-glucosyl-(1→ 3/4)-**L**-glycero-α -**D**-manno-heptosyl-(1 → 4/3)-**L**-glycero-α-**D**-manno-heptosyl-7-phosphate has already been described (11). The linkage region between dOclA and heptose, the terminal and side chain-linked dOclA, the substituents of the phosphate groups and the lipid A structure were the aim of this study. In addition, we examined the effect of polymyxin B on **P. mirabilis** R4/028 mutant, after finding that its LPS is lacking 4-amino-4-deoxy-L-arabinose (Ara4N). The presence of that unusual aminopentose has been suggested by Vaara et al., (15, 16) to be the reason for the resistance of **P. mirabilis** strains towards the action of polymyxin.

Studies on Lipopolysaccharide

The chemical composition of LPS and derived products is shown in Table 1. All fractions were free of galactose, galacturonic acid, 4-amino-4-deoxy--L-arabinose, lysine, glycine which are present in the wild type strain 028. Deoxycholate/PAGE banding pattern of R4/028 LPS against well-defined R and SR lipopolysaccharides of **Salmonella** allowed to classify the strain R4/028 as an Rc mutant with some leakiness, which is in accordance with chemical studies.

Studies of the R-core Oligosaccharide

Previous methylation studies of the R4/028 core oligosaccharide (11) were indicating an incomplete substitution of the terminal heptose at C-7 by phosphate. The status of phosphorus was presently investigated by ^{31}P-NMR. Spectra were taken at different pH values, from 6.0 to 10.0, in order to examine the pH-dependence of respective signals according to the technique of Batley et al. (1), and hence, to determine their character. The main signal resonating at +1.06 ppm was pH-independent and thus recognized as a phosphodiester, originating from Hep-7P-EtN. Three minor signals at +4.8 ppm, +5.6 ppm and +18 ppm where attributed to Hep-6-P and Hep-7-P (as phosphomonoesters; pH-dependent) and the last one (pH-independent) to the cyclic Hep-6,7-P. The two phosphomonoesters originated from phosphate migration in the case where Hep-7-P is not entirely substituted by EtN. The cyclic 6,7 phos-

Table 1. Chemical Composition of Lipopolysaccharide and Derived Products of **P. mirabilis** R4/028 mutant

Component	Amount in		
	Lipopoly-saccharide	Core oligo-saccharide	Lipid A
	% (by mass)		
D-Glucose	4.4	13.3	
LD-Heptose	9.7	22.3	
D-Glucosamine	8.1		19.6
Ethanolamine	0.64	1.6	
Ethanolamine/glucosamine-phosphate			5.6
Phosphorus	2.8	3.4	2.4
dOclA	9.7	8.7	
Dodecanoic acid	0.16		0.3
Tetradecanoic acid	10.17		16.0
3-Hydroxytetradecanoic acid	17.66		28.4
Hexadecanoic acid	1.69		2.8
Hexadecanoic acid	1.09		2.2

phate is the intermediate of the migration process (6, 10, 12). In most core types of **Enterobacteriaceae** heptose is substiuted at C-4 with pyrophosphoryl-ethanolamine (8).

Data of ^{13}C-NMR studies and CrO_3-oxidation together with earlier findings of ^{1}H-NMR (11) revealed that the two residues of heptose were α-linked, whereas the terminal glucose was β-linked. In other Rc mutants of **Salmonella** or **E. coli**, hexoses have α-linkages (8).

Linkage of heptose to dOclA was elucidated with the procedure of Brade et al. (2). LPS was Smith-degraded, mildly hydrolysed at pH 4.4 and dialysed. The liberated core oligosaccharide was reduced, permethylated according to a modified Hakomori procedure (5) and subjected to GC-MS. Results of this procedure revealed the branching heptose being linked to C-5 of the reducing dOclA residue.

Three step hydrolysis with acetate buffer pH 4.4 (Brade et al., 2) was applied to R4/028 LPS in order to determine the linkage between the dOclA residues. Although expected, the α-2- 4-linked dOclA disaccharide was not detected in GC-MS analysis under the condition described, its presence is nevertheless very likely. The quantitative determination of dOclA after hydrolytic release under different conditions showed that R4/028 LPS contains either no or only very small amounts of a third dOclA. The results are in accordance with reports (3) for rough-mutant LPS of **S. minnesota.**

Studies of Lipid A

The isolation and chemical analysis of the lipid A backbone was carried out according to Hase and Rietschel (7) with some modifications described by Bhat et al. (4). Lipid A contained glucosamine and phosphate in a molar ratio of 1:0.90. The reduced lipid A-OH on hydrolysis gave glucosamine and glucosaminitol in a molar ratio of 1:0.75. Only lipid A-OH, but not free

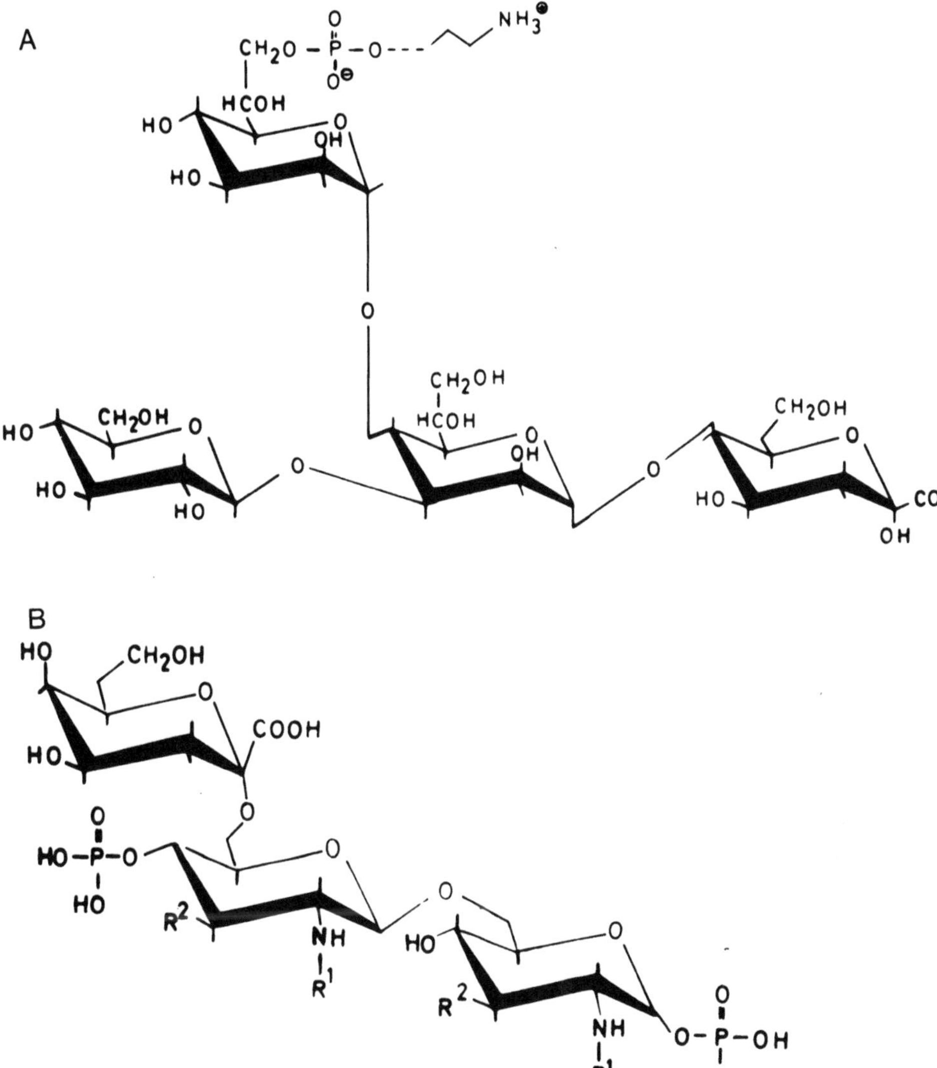

Fig 1. Proposed structure of **P. mirabilis** R4/028 lipopolysaccharide. (A) Glucose-heptose-dOclA region (the linkages of the two non-reducing terminal sugars might be reversed) (11); (B) dOclA-lipid A region.

Table 2. Effect of polymyxin B on <u>Proteus mirabilis</u> wild type strains and their rough mutants

Strain	Type	Polymyxin phenotype	MIC µg/ml	Precipitation of LPS with PMB	PMB bound mol/mol LPS**	Presence of Ara4N in LPS
O28	S	resistant	>1250	+	n.d.	+
R4/O28	Rc	sensitive	9	+	1.5	-
1959	S	resistant	>1250	+	n.d.	+
R45/1959	Re	resistant	>1250	+	1.0	+
R110/1959	Ra	resistant	>1250	+	1.0	+
R13/1959	Ra leaky	resistant	>1250	+	n.d.	+
R14/1959	Rb leaky	resistant	>1250	+	n.d.	+

* - 80 n mol of LPS was precipitated with 200 n mol of polymyxin B (PMB)
** - molar amount of LPS were quantified on the basis of GlcN content (2 moles GlcN = 1 mol LPS of R4/O28 and R45/1959, 3 moles GlcN = 1 mol LPS in case of R110/1959), amount of polymyxin B - on the basis of threonine content (2 mol threonine = 1 mol of polymyxin B)
n.d. - not determined

lipid A could be reduced, indicating the position of phosphate at C-1 of the reducing glucosamine.

Localization of phosphate in the lipid A backbone was also studied by ^{31}P-NMR, using the Batley technique (1). Two signals resonating at +2.5 ppm and +4.63 ppm, were pH-dependent and assigned to the C-1-glycosidic and to the C-4' ester-linked phosphate. A similar phosphate substitution was observed for **Shigella sonnei** lipid A (4).

GC-MS analysis of permethylated and reduced backbone disaccharide revealed glucosaminyl-β (1→ 6) glucosaminitol and glucosaminyl- α (1→ 6) glucosaminitol in a molar ratio of 8:1. The α(1→ 6)-disaccharide was not encountered previously for lipid A's and this result has to be corroborated for other **P. mirabilis** strains.

Significant amounts of 3-0-(14:0-14:0 amide- and ester-linked diesters were found in lipid A of R4/028 mutant, as well as in lipid A of the parental strain 028. In both lipid A's the ester-linked 16:0 seems to be partly replaced by 16:1 or 12:0. These minor fatty acids were not encountered for P. mirabilis lipid A (13).

On the basis of these results the structure shown in Fig 1 is proposed for R4/028 lipopolysaccharide. The core oligosaccharide and lipid A of R4/028 mutant were free of Ara4N. This aminopentose was found in lipid A of the parental strain 028 to be linked to phosphate at C-4' of the glucosamine and additionally, in the core oligosaccharide, linked (probably) to phosphate at dOclA, hence differently than described for R45/1959 mutant (14) and others: R110/1959, R13/1959, R14/1959 (unpublished results).

Sensitivity towards polymyxin B of the Ara4N-lacking mutant R4/028 in comparison with its parental strain as well as with all the above mentioned R mutants of P. mirabilis 1959 was examined (Table 2). All strains were resistant, besides the mutant R4/028. LPS R4/028 binds 50% more polymyxin B than LPS's of two resistant mutants. These results corroborate well with the above mentioned hypothesis of Vaara. We could, however, "sensitize" resistant strains P. mirabilis 028, R45/1959 and R110/1959 towards polymyxin B. Polymyxin B (500 μg/ml), in the presence of N-ethylmaleimide (blocker of SH-groups), totally inhibited the growth of the investigated strains. We assume that this inhibitor may block some enzyme(s) degrading polymyxin B. Hence the action of polymyxin B is not restrcited to a single cell envelope component only (W. Kaca et al. - in preparation).

REFERENCES

1. Batley, M., Packer, N. H., and Redmond, J. W., 1985, Analytical studies of lipopolysaccharide and its derivatives from **Salmonella minnesota** R595. Biochim. Biophys. Acta. 821: 179.

2. Brade, H., Moll, H., and Rietschel, E. Th., 1985, Structural investigation on the inner core region of lipopolysaccharides from **Salmonella minnesota** rough mutants. Biomed. Mass Spectrom 12: 602.

3. Brade, L., Kosma, P., Appelmelk, B. J., Paulsen, H., and Brade, H., 1987, Use of synthetic antigens to determine the epitope specificities of monoclonal antibodies against the 3-deoxy-D-manno-L-octulosonate region of bacterial lipopolysaccharide. Infect. Immun. 55: 462.

4. Bhat, U. R., Kontrohr, T., and Mayer, H., 1987, Structure of **Shigella sonnei** lipid A. FEMS Microbiology Letters 40: 189.

5. Darvill, T. J., McNeil, A. G., and Albersheim, P., 1983, Determination, by methylation analysis, of the glycosyl-linkage compositions of microgram quantities of complex carbohydrates. Carbohydr. Res. 123: 281.

6. Egan, W., Schneerson, R., Werner, K. E., and Zon, G., 1982, Structural studies and chemistry of bacterial capsular polysaccharides. Investigation of phosphodiester-linked capsular polysaccharides isolated from Haemophilus influenzae types a, b, c and f: Spectroscopic identification and chemical modification of end groups and the nature of base-catalyzed hydrolytic depolymerization. J. Am. Chem. Soc. 104: 2898.

7. Hase, S., and Rietschel, E. Th., 1976, Isolation and analysis of the lipid A backbone. Lipid A structure of lipopolysaccharides from various bacterial groups. Eur. J. Biochem. 63: 101.

8. Jann, K., and Jann, B., 1984, Structure and biosynthesis of O-antigens, in: "Handbook of Endotoxins," E. Th. Rietschel, ed., Elsevier Science Publishers, Amsterdam.

9. Jensen, M., Borowiak, D., Paulsen, H., and Rietschel, E. Th., 1979, Analysis of permethylated glucosaminyl-glucosaminitol disaccharides by combined gas-liquid chromatography mass spectrometry. Biomed. Mass Spectrom. 6: 559.

10. Leloir, L. F., and Cardini, C. E., 1963, Sugar phosphates, in: "Comprehensive Biochemistry," Vol. 5, M. Florkin and E. H. Stotz, eds. Elsevier Publishing Company, London, p. 113.

11. Radziejewska-Lebrecht, J., Feige, U., Jensen, M., Kotelko, K., Friebolin, H., and Mayer, H., 1980, Structural studies on the glucose-heptose region of the Proteus mirabilis R core. Eur. J. Biochem. 107: 31.

12. Rietschel, E. Th., Wollenweber, H. W., Sidorczyk, Z., Zähringer, U., and Lüderitz, O., 1983, Analysis of the primary structure of lipid A, in: "Bacterial Lipopolysaccharides: Structure, Synthesis, Biological Activities," L. Anderson and F. Unger, eds. Am. Chem. Soc. Washington, D.C.

13. Sidorczyk, Z., Zähringer, U., and Rietschel, E. Th., 1983, Chemical structure of the lipid A component of the lipopolysaccharide from a Proteus mirabilis Re mutant. Eur. J. Biochem. 137: 15.

14. Sidorczyk, Z., Kaca, W., Rietschel, E. Th., and Zähringer, U., 1987, Isolation and structural characterization of an 8-O-(4-amino-4-deoxy-β-L-arabinopyranosyl)-3-deoxy-D-manno-octulosonic acid disaccharide in the lipopolysaccharide of a **Proteus mirabilis** deep rough mutant. Eur. J. Biochem. 168: 269.

15. Vaara, M., Vaara, T., Jensen, M., Helander, T., Nurminen, M., Rietschel, E. Th. and Mäkelä, P. H., 1981, Characterization of the lipopolysaccharide from the polymyxin-resistant pmrA mutants of **Salmonella typhimurium**. FEBS Lett. 129: 145.

16. Vaara, M., and Viljanen, P., 1985, Binding of polymyxin B nonapeptide to gram-negative bacteria. Antimicrob. Agents Chemother. 27: 548.

THE STRUCTURE OF O-SPECIFIC POLYSACCHARIDE OF **PROTEUS VULGARIS** 019 LIPOPOLYSACCHARIDE

E. V. Vinogradov[1], W. Kaca[2], Y. A. Knirel[1], A. Rozalski[2], K. Kotelko[2], and N. K. Kochetkov[2]

[1]N. D. Zelinsky Institute of Organic Chemistry, Academy of Sciences of the USSR, Moscow, USSR, [2]Institute of Microbiology University of Lodz, Lodz, Poland

INTRODUCTION

The chemical composition of lipopolysaccharides isolated from respective **Proteus vulgaris** and **P. mirabilis** strains belonging to 49 different serotypes (Kauffmann and Perch classification) allowed us to divide the investigated LPS's into 16 chemotypes. The major part of LPS's is clustered in two chemotypes - IX and XV (4). The structure of the O specific part of LPS, isolated from **P. vulgaris** serotype 019 strain, from the chemotype IX, together with some serological data, is presented in this paper.

MATERIALS AND METHODS

Isolation of LPS and its polysaccharide fraction was performed as described in (2). Structural investigations of O-specific fraction from LPS 019 were done according to (3, 5). SDS-, DOC-PAGE were carried out in the system of Laemmli. Gels were colored by silver staining. Western blot analysis was done using routine procedure (1). For serological investigation 019 polyclonal antiserum was used in double immunodiffusion and quantitative precipitation tests.

RESULTS

Immunodiffusion

The LPS, PS and O-specific fraction of **P. vulgaris** 019 react with homologous antiserum in the double immunodiffusion test. Out of 26 different serogroups of **P. vulgaris** only LPS 042 reveals cross reaction with anti 019 serum.

SDS-, DOC-PAGE and Immunoblot of LPS

The lipopolysaccharide isolated from **P. vulgaris** 019 strain shows in electrophoresis the regular step-like band pattern typical for smooth type of LPS containing a varying number of repeating unit in its O-specific chains (Fig 1). Results of DOC-PAGE-Western blotting indicate that homologous anti 019 serum recognizes the O-specific part of LPS and does not react with faster migrating bands which represent core-lipid A fraction not substituted by O-specific chains (Fig 1, lane 6). Additionally, this antiserum gives

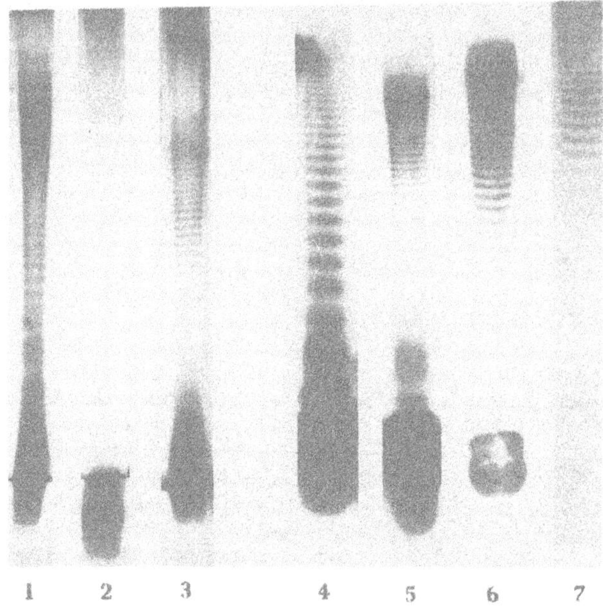

Fig 1. Silver-stained electrophoresis profiles and parallel immunoblot of LPS's from **Proteus vulgaris** and **P. mirabilis** strains.

LPS **P. vulgaris** 019 - SDS-PAGE (lane 3), DOC-PAGE (lane 4) and Western blot with homologous antiserum (lane 6).

LPS **P. vulgaris** 042 - DOC-PAGE (lane 5) and Western blot with **P. vulgaris** 019 antiserum (lane 7).

LPS's **P. mirabilis** S1959 - S form (lane 1), and R110 - Ra mutant (lane 2). On SDS -, DOC-PAGE the 5 µg of LPS's were applied to each lane and in immunoblot the antiserum was diluted 1:500.

weak cross reaction with bands corresponding to high molecular weight fractions of LPS from **P. vulgaris** 042 (Fig 1, lane 7).

Chemical and Structural Investigation of the O-specific Polysaccharide **P. vulgaris** 019

Methylation analysis of O-part of LPS **P. vulgaris** 019 revealed in the polysaccharide the presence of galactose, fucosamine and glucosamine residues substituted at position 3, whereas galactosamine at position 4. The above mentioned constituents are in molar ratio 1:1:1:1. The ^{13}C-NMR spectrum of the 0-19 polysaccharide showed its regular structure built up of tetrasaccharide repeating units. The computerized calculation of the ^{13}C-NMR spectrum of the 019 polysaccharide (Table 1), based on the monosaccharide composition, spectra of free monosaccharides and glycosylation effects, together with the chemical analysis (methylation) and computer assisted evaluation of the specific optical rotation by the Klyne's rule allow to propose the following structure of repeating units of LPS 019:

→3)-α-L-FucNAcp-(1→3)-β-D-GlcNAcp-(1→3)-α-D-Galp-(1→
4)-α-D-GalNAcp-(1→

Table 1. Chemical shifts in the ^{13}C-NMR spectrum of the polysaccharide (the calculated values are given in parentheses)

Monosaccharide residue	Chemical shifts (ppm)					
	C-1	C-2	C-3	C-4	C-5	C-6
-3)-α-D-Galp-(1-	101.9	68.8	79.4	70.0	71.6	62.0
	(101.5)	(68.2)	(79.7)	(70.4)	(71.7)	(62.4)
-4)-α-D-GalNAcp-(1-	99.7	51.3	68.4	79.4	73.2	61.7
	(100.6)	(51.0)	(67.8)	(78.8)	(72.9)	(62.4)
-3)-α-L-FucNAcp-(1-	98.7	49.7	74.4	72.2	67.9	16.4
	(98.9)	(49.9)	(75.0)	(71.9)	(67.5)	(16.7)
-3)-β-D-GlcNAcp-(1-	104.0	56.9	80.3	69.6	76.8	61.7
	(104.0)	(56.4)	(79.9)	(69.8)	(77.2)	(62.1)

DISCUSSION AND CONCLUSIONS

The established structure of O-part of LPS **P. vulgaris** 019 contains N-acetyl-L-fucosamine which was identified for the first time to be a constitutent of **Proteus** lipopolysaccharide. This newly revealed component must be taken into account in the necessary future revision of **Proteus** LPS's chemotypes scheme. **P. vulgaris** 019 O-specific polysaccharide, as well as **Salmonella arizonae** 059 (5) and **Pseudomonas aeruginosa** 07 polysaccharides (5) contain N-acetyl-L-fucosamine residue substituted at position 3. Moreover, the **P. vulgaris** 019 and **S. arizonae** 059 PS's possess a common disaccharide fragment, α-L-FucNAc-(1-3)-β-D-GlcNAc. However, none of two heterologous polysaccharides cross-reacts with anti 019 serum in quantitative precipitation test. These results indicate that N-acetyl-fucosamine does not play an important role in manifesting O-specificity of **P. vulgaris** 019.

REFERENCES

1. Bitter, M., Kupfer, P., and Morris, C. F., 1980, Electrophoresis transfer of proteins and nucleic acids from slab to diazobenzylmethyl cellulose or nitrocellulose sheets. Anal. Biochem. 102: 459-471.

2. Kaca, W., Knirel, Y. A., Vinogradov, E. V., and Kotelko, K., 1987, Structure of the O-specific polysaccharide of **Proteus mirabilis** S1959. Arch. Immunol. Ther. Exp. 35: 431-437.

3. Knirel, Y. A., Vinogradov, E. V., Shaskov, A. S., Dimitrev, B. A., Kochetkov, N. K., Stanislavsky, E. S., and Mashilova, G. M., 1986, Somatic antigens of **Pseudomonas aeruginosa**. The structure of O-specific polysaccharide chains of **P. aeruginosa** O10 (Lanyi) lipopolysaccharides. Eur. J. Biochem. 157: 129-138.

4. Kotelko, K., 1986, **Proteus mirabilis**: taxonomic position, peculiarities of growth, components of cell envelope. Curr. Topics Microbiol. Immunol. 129: 181-215.

5. Vinogradov, E. V., Knirel, Y. A., Lipkind, G. M., Shashkov, A. S., Kochetkov, N. K., Stanislavsky, E. S., and Kholodkova, E. V., 1987, Antigenic polysaccharides of bacteria. 23. The structure of the O-specific polysaccharide chain of the lipopolysaccharide **Salmonella arizonae** 059. Bioorg. Khim. 13: 1275-1281.

ENDOTOXINS OF *PSEUDOMONAS FLUORESCENS*

G.M. Zdorovenko, S.N. Veremeychenko, I. Ya. Zakharova and Yu. A. Knirel

Zabolotny Institute of Microbiology and Virology of the Ukrainian Academy of Sciences, Kiev, USSR

Heterogenous in both phenotype and genotype species, *Pseudomonas fluorescens* is presented by 5 biovars in Bergey's Manual. In spite of their belonging to saprophytic organisms the strains of *Pseudomonas fluorescens* are frequently isolated from clinical specimens (5). The endotoxins (LPS) of microbial cells are responsible for the mechanisms of interaction between micro- and macroorganisms in the infectious process. Therefore, we studied the LPS's of *P. fluorescens*.

The strains under study were obtained from the Collection of the Institute of Microbiology and Virology (IMV) and represented the biovars: I (IMV 4125=ATCC 13525), II (IMV 1602), III (IMV 2125), IV (IMV 2111), V (IMV 2763), and biovar i (IMV 2303) initially described in the USSR (2). Bacteria were grown on nutrient agar media. LPS was extracted from the acetone-dried cells by the Westphal method. All methods of analysis were described (3, 6, 7).

LPS's were active in homologous reactions of immunoprecipitation (approximate titer was 1:100,000) and in the Ouchterlony test (1-3 precipitation lines). Weak crossreactions were observed only between strains of biovars I and i, IV and V.

We studied separately different parts of the LPS macromolecule (O-chain, core, lipid A) obtained after its cleavage by acetic acid hydrolysis. The fraction of O-specific polysaccharide (PS) was serologically active in each strain (approximate immunoprecipitation titer was 1:500,000). Table 1 shows the results of sugar analysis of the O-chain. The following features of sugar compositions were detected:

1. Each strain had its characteristic sugar composition.

2. Rhamnose and amino sugars were the main components in the majority of strains.

3. Inclusion of rarely occurring sugars such as 3-acetamido-3,6-dideoxy-D-galactose, N-acetyl-L-fucosamine, 6-deoxy-L-talose, 2,4-diacetamido-2,4,6-trideoxy-D-glucose.

Table 1. The main sugar components of O-specific PS (wt %). (Sugar composition was estimated using GLC, LC, GC-MS, ^{1}H and ^{13}C NMR-spectroscopy, etc., analysis)

Sugar	4125	1602	2125	2111	2303	2763
Rhamnose	49	41	16	-	52	-
6-deoxy-L talose	-	-	-	-	-	20
Fucose	-	-	22	-	-	-
Mannose	-	-	-	-	-	20
Glucose	-	-	-	54	-	-
N-acetyl-D glucosamine	-	-	-	-	18	-
N-acetyl-D-galactosamine	-	20	-	-	-	19
N-acetyl-L-fucosamine	-	-	21	-	-	-
3-acetamido-3, 6-dideoxy-D-galactose	23	-	-	-	12	-
2,4-diacetamido-2,4,6-trideoxy-D-glucose	-	11	-	-	-	-
Unidentified aminosugar	-	-	-	-	14	-

Studies on the core fractions showed their composition usual for pseudomonas (Table 2). The only exception was the strain 2763. We did not succeed to find in its core rhamnose, alanine, phosphorus and KDO but at the same time it contained too much heptose and glucosamine.

The fatty acids presented in lipid A of type strain 4125 (Fig 1) were also found in lipid A of 2125, 2111 and 2303. Lipid A of 1602 was similar but it contained 2-OH C_{12}:0. Strain 2763 differed from above strains. 3-OH C_{14}:0 was the major component of its lipid A.

Because 2763 was considerably different in its LPS composition from other strains, the structural investigations were performed on its PS. ^{13}C NMR-spectroscopy of intact PS demonstrated its irregularity, but a strictly regular polymer (Fig 2) have been received after O-deacetylation of PS. Using ^{1}H and ^{13}C NMR-spectroscopy, methylation, partial hydrolysis, etc., the repeating unit of PS was found to have the structure:

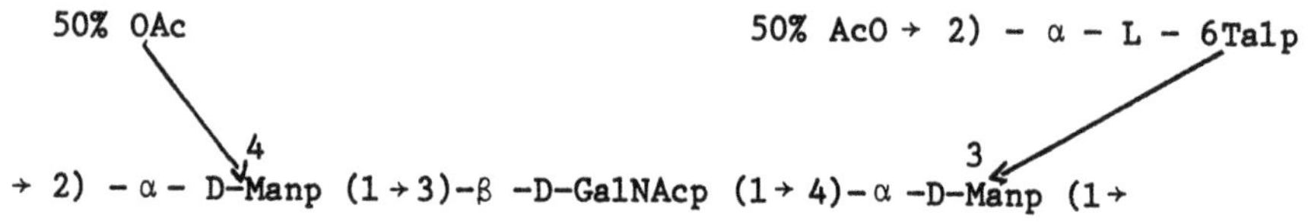

As far as we know only the structure of P. fluorescence LPS was determined earlier (1). The presence of 6-deoxy-L-talose is the only similarity between these structures.

Table 2. Composition of core oligosaccharide

Strain	4125	1602	2125	2111	2303	2763
Rhamnose	19.8	21.0	52.0	3.8	38.0	-
Fucose	-	-	39.0	-	-	-
Arabinose	-	14.8	-	-	-	tr
Mannose	18.0	18.5	1.2	17.3	tr	1.2
Glucose	61.1	33.3	3.6	57.7	41.4	37.6
Galactose	tr	12.3	1.2	19.2	tr	19.5
Heptose	tr	tr	3.0	tr	19.8	41.8
*D-glucosamine	1.0	tr	tr	tr	7.2	14.4
*D-galactosamine	0.5	0.4	6.7	0.7	tr	1.0
*2-keto-3-deoxy-octulosonic acid	0.6	7.5	4.6	2.7	0.2	-
*Alanine	2.0	1.1	1.8	2.8	3.5	-
*Phosphorus	3.6	2.8	3.7	5.2	5.0	-

(Peak area % GLC-analysis) *(wt %)

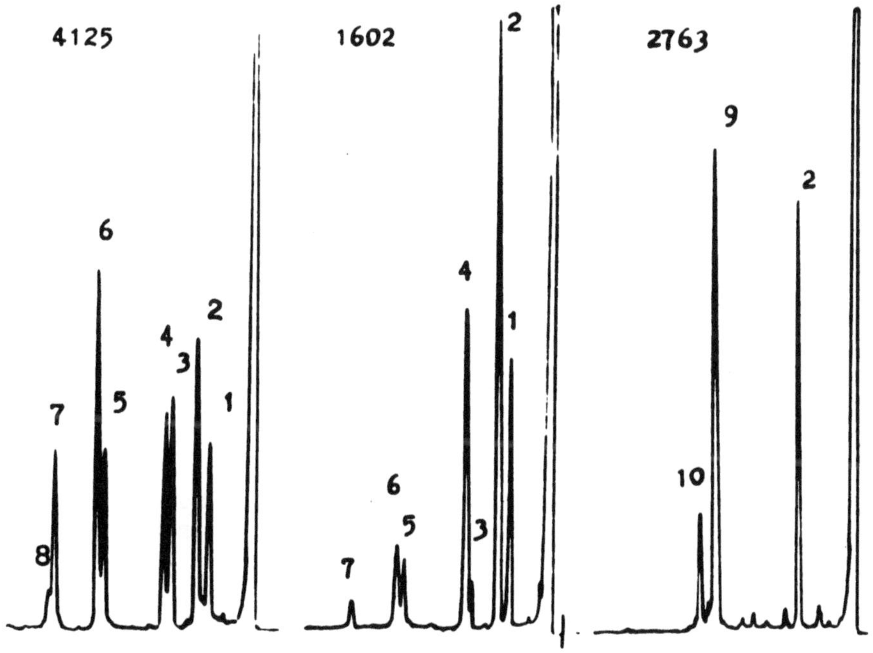

Fig 1. GL chromatograms of fatty acid components of lipid A fractions released by acid (1% CH_3COOH, 100°C, 1.5 hr) hydrolysis from LPS. Methyl esters received by using 1.5N methanolic HCl were separated on column (0.3 x 120 cm) with 5% SE-30 on Chromaton N-AW-DMCS, 80-100 mesh at 130-230°C, 3°C/min. Identification of peaks was made by co-chromatography with authentic standards and by GC-MS. The peaks correspond to: 3-OH C_{10}:0((1), C_{12}:0(2), 2-OH C_{12}:0(3), 3-OH C_{12}:0(4), C_{16}:1(5), C_{16}:0(6), C_{18}:1(7), C_{18}:0(8), 3-OH C_{14}:0(9), 3-OH C_{15}:0(10).

Biovar V is a heterogenous group of bacteria (5) which lack some peculiarities of pseudomonas. We may speculate that unusual compositions of these LPS may provide additional characteristics for this group. There is a correlation between diversity of the strains by biological properties and their LPS composition. By inclusion of 6-deoxyhexoses and aminosugars into the O-chain, as well as lipid A composition of P. fluorescence resembles corresponding products from some serotypes of P. aeruginosa and some enteric bacteria (4).

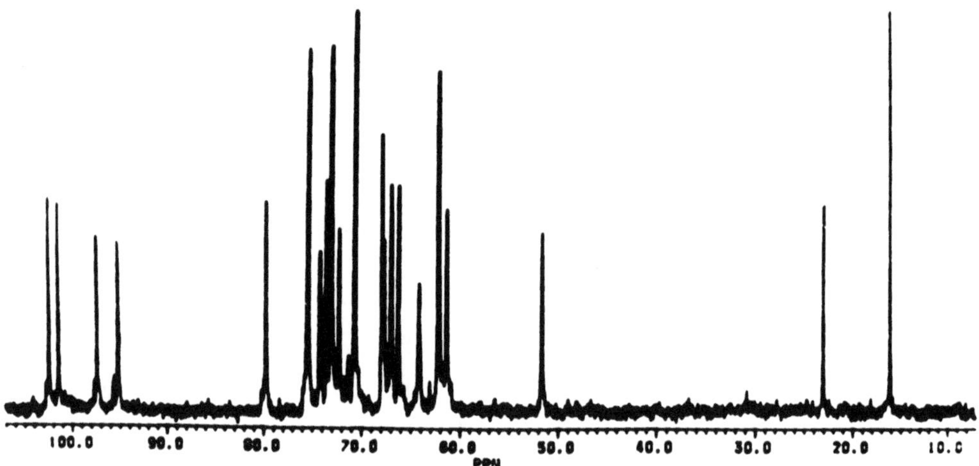

Fig 2. ^{13}C NMR-spectrum of O-specific polysaccharide of P. fluorescence IMV 2763.

REFERENCES

1. Khomenko, V. A., Naberezhnych, G. A., Isakov, V. V., Solov'eva, T. F., Ovodov, Y. S., Knirel, Y. A., Vinogradov, E. V., 1986, Structural study of O-specific polysaccharide chain of Pseudomonas fluorescens lipopolysaccharide. Bioorg. Chem. 12: 1641.

2. Kiprianova, E. A., Panichev, A. V., Boyko, O. I., and Garagulya, A. D., 1979, Numerical taxonomy of bacteria belonging to the genus Pseudomonas. Microbiology, XLVIII: 1023.

3. Knirel, Yu. A., Zdorovenko, G. M., Dashunin, V. M., Yakovleva, L. M., Shashkov, A. S., Zakharova, I. Ya., Gvozdyac, R. I., Kochetkov, N. K., 1986, Antigenic polysaccharides of bacteria. 15. Structure of the repeating unit of O-specific polysaccharide chain of Pseudomonas wieringae lipopolysaccharide. Bioorg. Chem. 12: 1253.

4. Knirel, Yu. A., 1985, Lipopolysaccharides of gram-negative bacteria, in: "Progress in chemistry of carbohydrates," I.V. Torgov, ed., Science, Moskow.

5. Palleroni, N. J., 1984, Family I. Pseudomonadaceae, in: "Bergey's Manual of Systematic Bacteriology," J. G. Holt, ed., Williams & Wilkins, Baltimore, MD.

6. Veremeychenko, S. N., 1986, Core oligosaccharides of Pseudomonas fluorescens. Microbiol. J. 49: 18.

7. Zdorovenko, G. M., Veremeychenko, S. N., Zakharova, I. Ya., 1986, Comparative characteristic of lipopolysaccharides from different Pseudmonas fluorescens strains. Microbiol. J. 49: 12.

CLONING AND EXPRESSION OF **rfe** GENE

M. Ohta, N. Kido, K. Jann*, Y. Arakawa, T. Komatsu, H. Ito and N. Kato

Department of Bacteriology, Nagoya University School of Medicine Tsuramai-cho 65, Showa-ku, Nagoya 466, Japan, and *Max-Planck-Institut für Immunbiologie, Freiburg, FRG

Bacterial **rfe** gene is involved in the synthesis of enterobacterial common antigen (ECA) as well as some kind of endotoxins such as lipopolysaccharides (LPS) from **Escherichia coli** 08, 09, **Salmonella typhimurium**, and other members of the family Enterobacteriaceae (1, 2, 3, 6). The gene **rfe** is located close to **ilv** genes at 84.5 min on the **E. coli** chromosomal map in the gene order **ilv rfe rff uvrD metE** (4). In the recent study, it was suggested that the products of the **rfe** gene(s) function mainly in supporting the coordinated elongation of the 09 mannan chain of **E. coli** (7). Moreover, Lew and coworkers showed that one of the enzymes coded for by the **rfe** gene cluster in group C1 salmonellae is dTDPglucose pyrophosphorylase, the function of which in group C1 is to produce a component of ECA.

In order to study the entire function of **rfe** gene(s) in polysaccharide synthesis, we tried to clone the **rfe** gene(s) from the phage library constructed from K12 chromosomal DNA. Partially digested chromosomal DNA of **E. coli** K12 W3110 with Sau3A were ligated into BamH1 digestion site of γ-phage vector EMBL3. Fragments of DNA were subcloned into plasmid vector pBR322

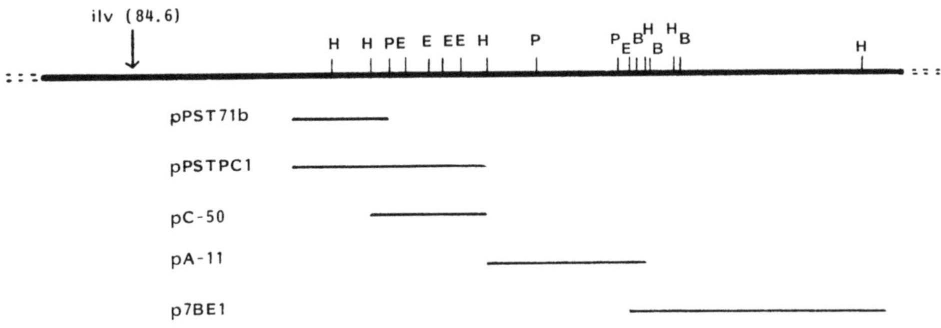

Fig 1. Restriction map of clones
Restriction enzyme map and subclones are illustrated. Restriction endonuclease abbreviations: E, EcoRI; B, BamHI; H, HindIII; P, PstI.

from phage clones which carried DNA fragments of flanking region of ilv (Fig 1).

These clones, designated as pPST71b, pPSTPC1, pC-50, pA-11 and p7BE1, respectively, were physically mapped with restriction enzymes. Subclones were introduced into a **rfe** negative strain F1357p (**rfe, pmi**$^+$:09$^-$, ECA$^-$) and resulting colonies were characterized with anti-09 serum and anti-ECA serum. Anti-09 and anti-ECA sera were prepared by immunization of rabbits with **E. coli** Bi316-42(09) and **E. coli** 014:K7HNM, an ECA immunogenic strain, respectively. Bacteria which carried a clone (designated as pPST71b) of 4 kb DNA fragment were agglutinated with the anti-ECA serum as well as with the anti-09 serum. Other clones containing flanking DNA sequences did not cause any antigenic change in host bacteria (Table 1).

Moreover, the serum obtained from a patient with ulcerative colitis reacted positively with pPST71b/F1357p as well as **E. coli** 014HMN. The LPS preparation extracted from pPST71b/F1357p showed a ladder pattern on the gel after sodium dodecylsulfate-polyacrylamide gel electrophoresis, whereas the LPS preparation from F1357p did not (Fig 2).

After the acid-hydrolysis of this LPS preparation, sugar components were analyzed chromatographically. Interestingly, even a trace amount of mannose, the sole component of polysaccharide side-chain of 09 LPS, was not detected in the hydrolysate of this LPS (data not shown). Since the anti-09 serum contained antibodies to ECA as well (Table 1), and it was reported that sera of patients with ulcerative colitis contain antibodies to ECA at significant levels, the antigenically positive substance produced on the surface of pPST71b/F1357p is considered to be ECA. The agglutination of pPST71b/F1357p with the anti-09 serum was relatively weak and mannose was not detected in the hydrolysate of its LPS preparation. Therefore, 09 polysaccharide is not synthesized in pPST71b/F1357p. Since other clones covering 27 Kb of the flanking region of **ilv** locus of K12 chromosome failed to express 09 polysaccharide synthesis in F1357p too, it is likely that the **rfe** region of K12 is active only partially and does not function to recover the synthesis of 09 polysaccharide of F1357p. The ladder pattern found on the acrylamide gel should be ascribed to the polysaccharide of ECA, although the possibility of the synthesis of other O polysaccharides than 09 can not be excluded. The intact **rfe** gene(s) responsible for the synthesis of both 09 polysaccharide

Table 1. Agglutination Reaction

Bacteria	Phenotype	Antisera Anti-09[a)]	Anti-ECA[b)]	UC serum[c)]
D282S	08	+	+	+
F379	**his,** :09	+	+	
F379(1-4)	**his, rfb**::Tn5	+	+	
014HNM	ECA immunogenic	+	+	+
F1357p	**his, rfe**	-	-	-
pPST71b/F1357p		+	+	+
pC-50/F1357p		-	-	
pA-11/F1357p		-	-	
p7BE1/F1357p		-	-	

a) Prepared by immunization of a rabbit with **E. coli** Bi316-42 (09:ECA$^+$).
b) Prepared by immunization of a rabbit with **E. coli** 014:K7HNM, an ECA immunogenic strain.
c) Obtained from a patient of ulcerative colitis.

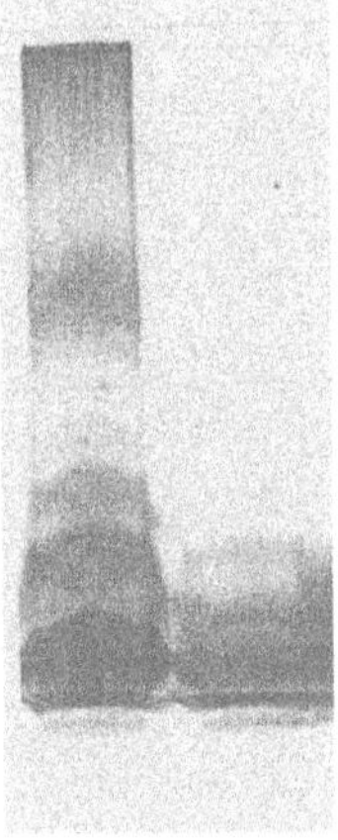

Figure 2. Electrophoresis of LPS preparations
The LPS preparations were electrophoresed with sodium dodecylsulfate polyacrylamide gel and stained with the silver-staining method. Lane A, LPS preparation from pPST71b/F1357b; lane B, LPS preparation from F1357b.

and ECA were already cloned from **E. coli** strains F379 and F719, by using a hybrid plasmid RP4::miniMu. Subcloning and analysis of the gene(s) are currently progressing.

REFERENCES

1. Jann, K., Goldemann, G., Weisgerber, C., Wolf-Ullisch, C., and Kanegasaki, S., 1982, Biosynthesis of the 09 antigen of **Escherichia coli**: Initial reaction and overall mechanism. Eur. J. Biochem. 127: 157.

2. Jann, K. and Jann, B., 1984, Structure and biosynthesis of O-antigens, in: "Handbook of Endotoxin, volume 1, Chemistry of Endotoxin," E. Th. Rietschel, ed., Elsevier, Amsterdam.

3. Lew, H. C., Mäkelä, P. H., Kuhn, H-M., Mayer, H., and Nikaido, H., 1986, Biosynthesis of enterobacterial common antigen requires dTDPglucose pyrophosphorylase determined by a Salmonella montevideo **rfe** gene. J. Bacteriol. 168: 715.

4. Meier, U. and Mayer, H., 1985, Genetic location of genes encoding enterobacterial common antigen. J. Bacteriol. 163: 756.

5. Rick, P. D., Mayer, H., Neumeyer, B. A., Wolski, S., and Bitter-Suermann, D., 1985, Biosynthesis of enterobacterial common antigen. J. Bacteriol. 162: 494.

6. Schmidt, G., Mayer, H., and Mäkelä, P. H., 1976, Presence of **rfe** genes in **Escherichia coli**: their participation in biosynthesis of O antigen and enterobacterial common antigen. J. Bacteriol. 127: 755.

7. Weisgerber, C., Jann, B., and Jann, K., 1984, Biosynthesis of the 09 antigen of **Escherichia coli**: Core structure of **rfe** mutant as indication of assembly mechanism. Eur. J. Biochem. 140: 553.

CLONING AND ANALYSIS OF **rfb** GENE SYNTHESIZING THE MANNAN O SIDE CHAIN OF **ESCHERICHIA COLI** O9 LIPOPOLYSACCHARIDE

N. Kido, M. Ohta, H. Ito, K-I. Iida, Y. Arakawa,
T. Komatsu, K. Jann*, and N. Kato

Department of Bacteriology, Nagoya University School of Medicine, Showa-ku, Nagoy, Aichi 466, Japan, *Max-Planck-Institut fur Immunbiologie, Freiburg, F.R.G.

SUMMARY

The **rfb** gene encoding the proteins responsible for the synthesis of the repeating units (O side-chain) of **Escherichia coli** O9 lipopolysaccharide was cloned into a conjugative plasmid RP4::miniMu and was expressed in **E. coli** K-12.

INTRODUCTION

In our previous studies, it was demonstrated that the lipopolysaccharides (LPSs) possessing mannose-homopolymer (mannan) as their O-side chains showed very strong adjuvant activities in the induction of both antibody response and delayed-type hypersensitivity to protein antigens. **E. coli** O8 and O9, and **Klebsiella pneumoniae** O3 and O5 belong to a group of LPSs possessing the mannan O side-chains. The contribution of the mannan O side-chains to the adjuvant action of these LPSs was confirmed by the facts that the strong adjuvant activity is inhibited by the pretreatment of LPS with concanavalin A and that the R-form LPSs from O side-chain-less mutants lack the strong adjuvant activity (5). However, we have not yet determined the effect of substitution of the lipid A+R core portions on the adjuvant activity of these LPSs. In this study, we tried to produce the hybrid LPS possessing the mannan O side-chain of **E. coli** O9 LPS and the R core+lipid A portions of **E. coli** K-12 LPS. We cloned the **rfb** gene of **E. coli** O9 LPS and the gene introduced into **E. coli** K-12 strains produced the hybrid LPS consisting of the mannan O side-chain of **E. coli** O9 and R core and lipid A of **E. coli** K-12.

MATERIALS AND METHODS

3.1. Strains

E. coli O9 strain F719 (O9:K-:H-, **his**) and the revertant mutant of **his** (F719H) isolated in our laboratory were used as donors of the **rfb** gene. **E. coli** K-12 D21 (**his-51 trp-30 proA23 lac-28 ampA strA173 tsx-81**), D21recA (the **rec A** mutant of D21 isolated in our laboratory), and **E. coli** K-12 JA221 (F^- **leuB6 trpE5 hsdR hsdM recA1 lacY**) were used as recipient strains.

3.2. Media

L broth (4) and Mueller Hinton II agar (BBL, MD, USA) were used routinely. As the minimal medium, the synthetic liquid medium according to the procedures described by Batshon et al., (1) was used. Media were supplemented with ampicillin (50 μg/ml), kanamycin (50 μg/ml), tetracycline (15 μg/ml), and streptomycin (100 μg/ml) when used for the culture of bacteria carrying the R-prime plasmid.

3.3. Matings

A conjugative hybrid plasmid RP4::miniMu was transferred from MXR (pULB113) into **E. coli** F719H in the following way (7). Donor and recipient strains were grown with gentle shaking in L broth supplemented with ampicillin, kanamycin, and tetracycline for MXR, and L broth without antibiotics for **E. coli** F719H. A few drops of the mixture was then placed on the L broth agar plate and incubated at 30°C for 2 hr. The bacterial growth was then streaked on the agar plate of the minimal medium containing ampicillin, kanamycin, and tetracycline. **E. coli** F719H (RP4::miniMu) transconjugants alone grew up on this selection plate and formed colonies. Transconjugants were tested for agglutination in **E. coli** O9-specific antiserum. RP4::miniMu R-prime plasmids carrying **his-rfb** region of **E. coli** F719H were isolated as follows. Donor strain F719H (RP4::miniMu) was grown in L broth containing ampicillin, kanamycin and tetracycline with gentle shaking until the culture reached an absorbance at 600 nm to 0.5. The function of Mu phage was induced at 42°C for 3 hr and then the mating was carried out for 3 hr with the recipient **E. coli** K-12 D21recA in the same way as above. The suspension of bacteria was spread on the minimal agar medium supplemented with tryptophane and proline and with ampicillin, kanamycin, tetracycline, and streptomycin.

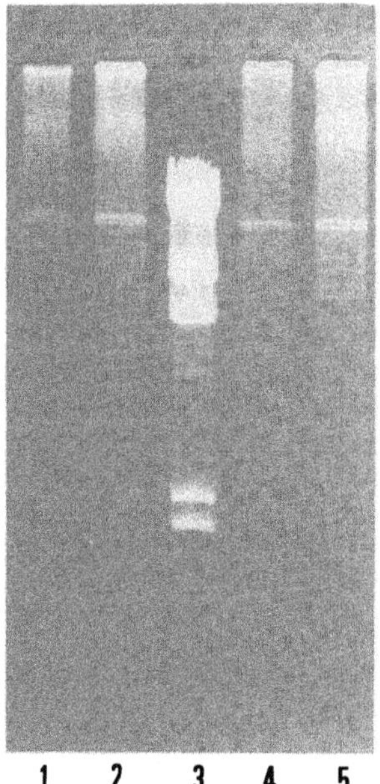

Fig 1. R-prime plasmids DNA extracted from 4 individual R-prime plasmids were digested with the restriction enzyme **PstI** and analyzed by the 1% agarose gel electrophoresis (lane 1,2,4 and 5). **HindIII** digested lambda phage DNA was applied on lane 3 for the molecular weight marker.

RESULTS AND DISCUSSION

We constructed the R-prime plasmids carrying the **his-rfb** region of **E. coli** 09 strain F719H by using conjugative plasmid RP4::miniMu and expressed the **rfb** gene in **E. coli** K-12 (8). The four independent clones were isolated. It was found that **E. coli** K-12 harboring these R-prime plasmids had mannan as the repeating unit of LPS and that anti-**E. coli** 09 rabbit serum resulted in the agglutination of cells carrying these R-prime plasmids. The plasmid DNAs were extracted by the method of Kado et al. (3) and digested with the restriction enzyme **Pst I.** Fig 1 showed the restriction enzyme digestion patterns of four clones that carried the **his-rfb** region of **E. coli** F719H. The 6 fragments found commonly in all four clones were identified as vector plasmid pULB113 origin and other bands were identified as originated from the **his-rfb** DNA region. LPS from **E. coli** K-12 carrying R-prime plasmids was extracted by phenol-water method and analyzed by SDS polyacrylamide gel electrophoresis and immunoblotting on nitrocellulose membrane. The silver-staining of the gel showed the typical ladder patterns of smooth LPS in the lanes of preparations from the **E. coli** K-12 carrying R-prime plasmids (Fig 2, lane 1). However, a LPS preparation from **E. coli** K-12 showed only small molecular weight bands of rough LPS (Fig 2, lane 2). These repeating units reacted positively with anti-**E. coli** 09 rabbit serum when blotted to nitrocellulose membrane electrophoretically and stained with anti-**E. coli** 09 rabbit serum and peroxidase-conjugated anti-rabbit immunoglobulin goat serum, whereas the LPS from **E. coli** K-12 JA221 did not (data not shown).

About one hundred deletion mutants lacking the **rfb** function were isolated from R-prime plasmid R'-6. Using these deletion plasmids and southern hybridization technique, we made restriction enzyme map of R'-6 plasmid (Fig 3). The map of R'-6 revealed that **rfb** gene of **E. coli** 09 located in or around C fragment (about 17kbp) of restriction enzyme **Bgl II.**

Fig 2. LPSs, extracted by phenol-water method, were subjected to electrophoresis on 14% polyacrylamide gels containing 4M urea. LPSs were stained by the method of silver staining. LPSs of JA221 (lane 1) and Ja221 carrying R'-6 (lane 2) were shown.

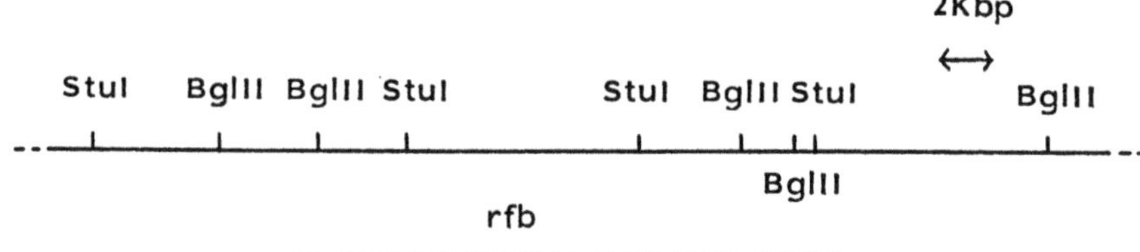

Fig 3. Restriction enzyme map was determined using the restriction enzyme StuI, **Bgl II**. Cleavage sites were determined by the deletion method newly developed in our laboratory (Kido et al., manuscript in preparation).

LPS is one of the major outer membrane constituents of the gram-negative bacteria and is considered as an important virulence factor of **E. coli, Shigella, Salmonella,** etc. LPS is considered as one of the protective factors against the host defense mechanisms. Therefore LPS is a favored antigen as a candidate of vaccines against some of these pathogenic bacteria. For developing LPS vaccines, **rfb** genes derived from **S. dysenteriae** 1 and **S. typhimurium** LT2 were cloned recently and analyzed in detail (6,2). For making safe vaccine strains using gene cloning techniques, it is necessary to express **rfb** genes in non-pathogenic strains such as **E. coli** K-12. However, the **rfb** gene of **S. dysenteriae** required **rfp** gene additional for the expression of its function in **E. coli** K-12. Moreover, the cloned **S. typhimurium** **rfb** gene failed to express in host strains. Unlike these works, we have succeeded in expressing the cloned **rfb** gene in **E. coli** K-12.

The study of the biological activities of the synthetic lipid A is one of the important themes of today's study of endotoxin. The structural modification of lipid A with the residues of phosphate, KDO and other sugars, found in R core or lipid A, is helpful for our understanding the biological activities of LPS. So far we have obtained these modified lipid A preparations only by chemical synthesis. The possibility of structural modification of LPS by gene engineering has been suggested from this study.

REFERENCES

1. Batshon, A. B., Baer, H.. and Sheffer, M.F., 1963, Immunologic paralysis produced in mice by **Klebsiella pneumoniae** type 2 polysaccharide. J. Immunol. 90: 121-126.

2. Brahmbhatt, H. N., Wyk, P., Quigley, N. B. and Reeves, P. R., 1988, Complete physical map of the **rfb** gene cluster encoding biosynthetic enzymes for the O antigen of **Salmonella typhimurium** LT2. J. Bact. 170: 98-102.

3. Kado, C. I. and Liu, S.-T., 1981, Rapid procedure for detection and isolation of large and small plasmids. J. Bact. 145: 1365-1373.

4. Maniatis, T., Fritsch, E. F. and Sambrook, J., 1982, Molecular cloning, Cold Spring Harbor Laboratory.

5. Ohta, M., Kido, N., Hasegawa, T., Ito, H., Fujii, Y., Arakawa, Y., Komatsu, T. and Kato, N., 1987, Contribution of the mannan O side-chains to the adjuvant action of lipopolysaccharides. Immunology 60: 503-507.

6. Sturm, S. and Timmis, K. N., 1986, Cloning of the **rfb** gene region of **Shigella dysenteriae** 1 and construction of an **rfb-rfp** gene cassette for the development of lipopolysaccharide-based live anti-dysentery vaccines. Microbial Pathogenesis 1: 289-287.

7. Timmis, K. N., Clayton, C. L. and Sekizaki, T., 1985, Localization of Shiga toxin gene in the region of **Shigella dysenteriae** 1 chromosome specifying virulence functions. FEMS Microbiol. Lett. 30: 301-305.

8. Weisgerber, C., Jann, B. and Jann, K., 1984, Biosynthesis of the 09 antigen of **Escherichia coli.** Eur. J. Biochem. 140: 553-556.

SECTION II.

ACTIVE SITES, CONTAMINANTS, QUALITATIVE AND QUANTITATIVE ASSAYS

THE ACTIVATION OF C3H/HeJ CELLS BY CERTAIN TYPES OF LIPOPOLYSACCHARIDES

B. M. Sultzer and R. Castagna

Department of Microbiology and Immunology, State University of New York, Health Science Center at Brooklyn, Brooklyn, New York 11203, U.S.A.

INTRODUCTION

Experimentation with the endotoxin non-responder C3H/HeJ mouse has provided considerable insight into the genetic control of the pathophysiological and immunobiological effects induced by lipopolysaccharide endotoxin (LPS); however, the mechanism underlying this deficiency has never been fully elucidated. At the cellular level much of the research has focused on the B-lymphocyte of the C3H/HeJ strain. Although it is known that C3H/HeJ B-cells can respond to protein mitogens (8, 13, 14), there is no conclusive evidence that typical protein-free LPS or lipid A can stimulate DNA synthesis or polyclonal antibody production by these cells equivalent to that seen with normal responder cells. However, recently several reports have appeared indicating that C3H/HeJ spleen cells in culture could be stimulated by certain forms of LPS to proliferate to some extent. By gel filtration chromatography, Vukajlovich and Morrison prepared homogeneous monomeric components of **E. coli** 055:B5 LPS (17). One of these fractions, which was protein-free, enriched in lipid A and contained a trace of O-antigen, induced a significant but limited amount of ^{3}H-thymidine incorporation by C3H/HeJ splenic lymphocytes as compared to responder C3HeB/FeJ cells (17). Vogel et al., (16) reported that a lipid A precursor obtained from a temperature sensitive mutant of **S. typhimurium** was active for C3H/HeJ B-cells and macrophages although the preparation contained a trace of protein. In contrast, the lipid X precursor of Raetz et al., (10) from **E. coli** failed to stimulate C3H/HeJ cells although it is a polyclonal B-cell activator (PBA) for LPS-responder cells. With the advent of synthetic lipid A, studies on its activity and various analogues were initiated with responder and non-responder cells. Kumazawa et al., (3) reported that one non-phosphorylated derivative containing 3-hydroxytetradecanoic acid stimulated ^{3}H-thymidine uptake 3 to 6-fold in C3H/HeJ spleen cells although the net cpms were half that obtained with C3H/HeN responder cells. Synthetic lipid A as well as all of the other derivatives which were monophosphorylated, diphosphorylated, or nonphosphorylated and contained various mixtures of myristic and hydromyristic acids were inactive on C3H/HeJ cells (3). Finally, Girard et al., (2) reported that the LPS from **B. pertussis** was active in stimulating C3H/HeJ splenic lymphocytes to proliferate but the activity was ascribed to the polysaccharide components rather than the lipid A.

In experiments designed to learn about the immunoregulating properties of endotoxin associated proteins (EP) from **B. pertussis,** we found that certain protein-free preparations of LPS from this organism extracted by the phenol-chloroform-petroleum ether method (1) activated C3H/HeJ B-cells and macrophages (11). In addition we have extracted and purified the LPS from the Re mutant of **Salmonella minnesota** R595 to examine its potential to activate C3H/HeJ B-cells, which we will describe in this paper. However, in the process of these studies, we also found unexpectedly that the LPS from **S. typhi** 0-901, which typically does not stimulate C3H/HeJ lymphocytes or macrophages, can actually inhibit the activation of these cells by protein mitogens and the lipopolysaccharides of **B. pertussis** (PLPS) and **S. minnesota** (MLPS).

MATERIALS AND METHODS

Animals

C3H/HeJ and C3H/OuJ mice were obtained from Jackson Laboratories (Bar Harbor, Maine) and subsequently bred in our facilities. Mice of both sexes were used at four to six months of age and maintained on water and Purina mouse chow ad libitum.

Lipopolysaccharides and Endotoxin Protein

LPS was extracted directly from acetone dried cells of **Bordetella pertussis** 3779B-114 by the phenol-chloroform-petroleum ether method (1). In a similar manner, LPS was extracted from **Salmonella minnesota** R595. The lipopolysaccharides so obtained were also re-extracted by the hot phenol-water method to remove any small amounts of residual outer-membrane protein (18). Protein was assayed by a modified Lowry procedure (5). LPS was prepared from **Salmonella typhi** 0-901 by the Westphal method (18). EP from **S. typhi** 0-901 and **B. pertussis** was prepared as previously described (13). Lipid A and polysaccharide fractions of the LPS from **B. pertussis** were prepared by acetic acid hydrolysis at $100^{o}C$ for 1 hr (2). Polymyxin B sulfate was obtained from Sigma Chemical Co. (St. Louis, MO).

Lymphocyte Cultures

Single cell suspensions were prepared from spleens and the cells cultured in RPMI-1640 medium supplemented with 1% fetal calf serum (Gibco Lake, Grand Island, N.Y.), 100U of penicillin and 100 ug of streptomycin as previously described (13). For those experiments involving direct activation of DNA synthesis, lymphocyte cultures were set up in 96 well microtiter plates at 2.5×10^{6} cells per 0.2 ml. For inhibition experiments, tube cultures were used at a cell density of 2.5×10^{6} cells per ml. In cultures depleted of T-cells, monoclonal anti-Thy 1.2 antibody and Low Tox rabbit complement were used (Cedarlane Labs., Ontario, Canada). DNA synthesis was measured by ^{3}H-thymidine incorporation by adding 1μCi of ^{3}H-Tdr in the last 18 hr of a 48 hr culture. All cultures were done in triplicate. Variation about the mean did not exceed ± 10%.

RESULTS

We have previously reported that pertussis LPS extracted by the phenol-chloroform-petroleum ether method has the property of activating C3H/HeJ splenic B-cells to proliferate (11). The LPS was free of protein and did not stimulate T-cells to DNA synthesis. C3H/HeJ B-cells are also stimulated to polyclonal antibody synthesis and their macrophages can be induced to synthesize Interleukin-1 (submitted for publication). When analyzed by SDS-polyacrylamide gel electrophoresis, PLPS produced two major low molecular weight species which were separated by hydroxylapatite chromatography. The slower migrating component was found to be active on C3H/HeJ cells whereas the faster and more abundant species was essentially inactive, although both components were highly active on C3H/OuJ responder cells (11).

Table 1. Stimulation of DNA Synthesis in C3H/HeJ Splenic Lymphocytes by Pertussis Lipopolysaccharide

Mitogen (μg/culture)		Mean Net cpm of $[^3H]$-thymidine Incorporation[f]	
		C3H/HeJ	C3H/OuJ
TLPS[a]	0.1	651	35,931
	1.0	409	46,276
	10.0	490	37,489
TEP[b]	0.1	22,027	17,101
	1.0	41,552	52,250
	10.0	47,406	55,778
PLPS[c]	0.1	6,808	28,624
	1.0	10,554	29,245
	10.0	21,504	33,949
PL[d]	1.0	13,326	35,325
PP[e]	1.0	2,106	13,315

[a]**Salmonella typhi** 0-901 lipopolysaccharide
[b]**Salmonella typhi** 0-901 endotoxin protein
[c]**Bordetella pertussis** lipopolysaccharide
[d]Lipid-enriched fraction from acetic acid hydrolyzed pertussis LPS.
[e]Polysaccharide fraction from acetic acid hydrolyzed pertussis LPS.
[f]Mean of triplicate cultures. Variation about the mean did not exceed + 10%.

Representative results shown in Table 1 indicate that PLPS stimulates proliferation in C3H/HeJ splenic lymphocytes in contrast to TLPS which does not; however, the level of activation achieved is less than that obtained with the endotoxin protein extracted from **Salmonella typhi.** Normal LPS responder C3H/OuJ cells respond to all of the preparations tested. When the PLPS was subjected to acetic acid hydrolysis two fractions were obtained. The lipid-enriched fraction (PL) was active on C3H/HeJ cells although again to a lesser extent than that obtained with C3H/OuJ cells. On the other hand, the polysaccharide fraction (PP) was inactive on C3H/HeJ cells but stimulated C3H/OuJ cells, confirming the results of Girard et al., (2) to the extent that pertussis endotoxin polysaccharides are mitogenic at least for LPS responder cells. When polymyxin B (10 μg) was added to cultures stimulated by the PL (0.1 μg) almost complete inhibition was obtained in the C3H/HeJ cultures indicating that if any trace protein in this system was present, it was not functioning in this system (Table 2).

As a consequence of these results, we extended our studies by extracting a true R-type LPS from **Salmonella minnesota** R595 by the Galanos method (1) followed by re-extraction by the phenol-water method (18). The resulting preparation (MLPS) was active as a mitogen for C3H/HeJ cells as shown in Table 3. A residual of 0.25% protein was detected in this preparation; however, as shown in Table 4 essentially all of its activity in stimulating DNA synthesis was neutralized by polymyxin B. Polymyxin B has no effect on B-cell protein mitogens such as EP or PPD-tuberculin so that the trace amount of outer membrane protein present in the MLPS as determined by a modified

Table 2. Polymyxin B Inhibition of DNA Synthesis in C3H/HeJ Splenic Lymphocytes Stimulated by Pertussis Glycolipid

PL[a] (μg/culture)	Mean Net cpm of $[^3H]$-thymidine Incorporation	
	C3H/HeJ	C3H/OuJ
0.1	8,661	36,429
1.0	14,452	57,016
0.1 + Polymyxin B, 10 g	1,611	10,828
1.0 + " ", 10 g	9,018	37,607

[a]Pertussis glycolipid prepared by acetic acid hydrolysis. See Materials and Methods.

Lowry procedure (5) we believe is not responsible for the activity we have observed. Indeed, as shown in Table 3, MLPS is active at 0.1 g which would mean that if the activity were due to the contaminating protein, it would be active at a level of 0.25 ng, which we have not found to be active with purified endotoxin associated protein from **Salmonella.** Based on the evidence so far, it is our conclusion that both PLPS and MLPS can stimulate C3H/HeJ cells, although not to the same extent as LPS responder cells.

This conclusion, albeit tentative, suggested to us that perhaps the elusive trigger receptor for LPS on responder B-cells may exist on non-responder cells in some altered form which could react with certain types of types of LPS or lipid A. If this were so, it might be possible to block the interaction of PLPS or MLPS with this presumed receptor by the addition of a wild-type LPS. For this purpose, we extracted LPS from **S. typhi** 0-901 (TLPS), which is inactive on C3H/HeJ cells as represented in the data of Table 1. However, when added to lymphocyte cultures at the same time or 1 hr prior to

Table 3. Activation of DNA Synthesis in C3H/HeJ Splenic Lymphocytes by **Salmonella minnesota** R595 Lipopolysaccharide

LPS, μg/culture	Mean Net cpm of $[^3H]$-thymidine Incorporation[a]			
	C3H/HeJ		C3H/OuJ	
	Exp. 1	Exp. 2	Exp. 1	Exp. 2
0.1	3,837	6,361	23,525	39,536
1.0	11,308	23,796	30,840	41,827
10.0	26,168	20,771	42,945	43,421

[a]Mean background control counts for C3H/HeJ cells = 2717 cpm and for C3H/OuJ cells = 7713 cpm.

Table 4. Inhibition of **S. minnesota** R595 LPS Stimulated DNA Synthesis by Polymyxin B in C3H/HeJ Splenic Lymphocytes

LPS (µg/culture)	Polymyxin B (µg/culture)	Mean Net cpm (^{3}H)-thymidine Incorporation	Percent Inhibition
1.0	-	2,077	-
10.0	-	19,379	-
1.0	10.0	- 62	100.0
10.0	10.0	1,628	91.6

[a]Background ^{3}H-Tdr incorporation = 2,907 cpm

the addition of a stimulating mitogen, a marked inhibition of DNA synthesis occurred. This effect is dose dependent (Table 5) when 10 µg of TLPS is used with various concentrations of MLPS but at this concentration of TLPS, insignificant inhibition occurred with the mitogen pertussis endotoxin protein (PEP). At first glance it appeared that the inhibition was specific, suggesting that the LPS mitogen receptor was blocked; however, at higher concentrations of TLPS (50 µg), a comparable degree of inhibition was observed with PEP. PPD-tuberculin activation of DNA synthesis and, polyclonal antibody synthesis induced by MLPS in C3H/HeJ splenic B-cells is similarly inhibited by TLPS (data not shown).

In order to learn something about the mechanism of this inhibitory effect induced by TLPS, we designed a kinetic experiment wherein TLPS and MLPS were added together at the start of the culture. Subsequently the cells were washed after various time periods with RPMI-1640 medium by three centrifugations and reconstituted in medium containing MLPS at the original concentration. The results depicted in Table 6 indicate that the maximum level of inhibition in DNA synthesis occurred at 12 hrs. At 6 hrs, the inhibitory effect was minimal, if at all, suggesting that a critical period occurs during the G1 phase of the cell cycle when the cells are susceptible to the inhibitory effect of the TLPS.

This lag period before the full expression of the inhibitory effect of the TLPS suggested perhaps accessory cells were activated which might suppress the proliferation of the C3H/HeJ B-cells. In a preliminary experiment whereby T-cells were depleted from the spleen cells by monoclonal anti-Thy 1.2 and C', no change in the extent of inhibition was observed (Table 7). Depletion of macrophages by a triple adsorption with carbonyl iron also had no effect on the level of inhibitions induced by TLPS (data not shown) suggesting neither subpopulations of suppressor T-cells nor macrophages of C3H/HeJ mice are activated by TLPS.

DISCUSSION

Recently, Morrison et al., have provided evidence that R-type LPS can activate C3H/HeJ splenic lymphocytes to DNA synthesis (9). Both Ra and Re-LPS from **S. minnesota** were processed by polyacrylamide gel electrophoresis in deoxycholate to remove any protein contamination. The material recovered from the gels stimulated ^{3}H-thymidine uptake to a limited extent in both C3H/HeJ and C3Heb/FeJ splenocytes with stimulation indices of 5 to 7 times background (9). Our results with the MLPS confirm and extend these results. We have shown that the DNA synthesis stimulated by MLPS can be completely neutralized by polymyxin B. Furthermore, as is the case with the pertussis

Table 5. Inhibition of C3H/HeJ Lymphocyte Activation by **Salmonella typhi** Lipopolysaccharide

Stimulant (μg/culture)		Inhibitor (μg/culture)	Mean Net cpm [^{3}H)-thymidine Incorporation		Percent Inhibition
			Exp. 1	Exp. 2	
[a]MLPS,	0.1	-	5,276	7,952	-
"	1.0	-	14,314	17,517	-
"	10.0	-	32,492	34,234	-
[b]PEP	0.1	-	17,596	25,863	-
"	1.0	-	39,317	49,904	-
"	10.0	-	64,321	67,244	-
MLPS	0.1	10	1,775	-	66
"	1.0	"	6,244	-	56
"	10.0	"	24,670	-	24
PEP	0.1	10	15,879	-	10
"	1.0	"	33,078	-	16
"	10.0	"	52,423	-	19
MLPS	0.1	50	-	1,688	79
"	1.0	"	-	2,275	87
"	10.0	"	-	6,288	82
PEP	0.1	50	-	5,884	77
"	1.0	"	-	24,256	51
"	10.0	"	-	40,130	40

[a]**Salmonella minnesota** R595 lipopolysaccharide
[b]**Bordetella pertussis** endotoxin protein

Table 6. Effect of Removing Inhibitory Lipopolysaccharide After Activating C3H/HeJ Splenic Lymphocytes

Time of Wash-out (hr)	Percent Inhibition of Mean cpm (^{3}H) Incorporation
1	7.3
6	19.0
12	84.8
24	86.9
Control[a]	82.5

[a]MLPS (activator) added at 10 g/ml and TLPS (inhibitor) added at 50 μg/ml. In the control cultures, the lipopolysaccharides were not removed. After wash-out, all other cultures were reconstituted with MLPS only at 10 μg/ml.

Table 7. Effect of T-Cell Depletion on the Inhibition of C3H/HeJ Lymphocyte Activation by **S. typhi** Lipopolysaccharide

Stimulant (μg/culture)	Inhibitor (μg/culture)	Percent Inhibition of (^{3}H)-thymidine Incorporation	
MLPS[a]	TLPS[b]	Mixed Cells	T-cell Depleted[c]
10	50	66	71
50	50	51	82

[a]**Salmonella minnesota** R595 LPS
[b]**Salmonella typhi** 0-901 LPS
[c]Depletion by monoclonal anti-Thy 1.2 antibody and complement.

LPS, the MLPS can also stimulate IL-1 production from C3H/HeJ splenic macrophages (data not shown), so that the activity of this LPS is not restricted to B-cells. However, it should be emphasized that the levels of activation achieved, whether they be measured by DNA synthesis, plaque-forming cells or IL-1 production are always less than the stimulation measured with normal LPS responder cell culture. Presumably, C3H/HeJ mice have fewer B-cells and macrophages that can be activated by these types of LPS. Nevertheless, the evidence so far suggests certain forms of LPS or lipid A appear to be able to activate lymphocytes and macrophages which ordinarily cannot be stimulated by the LPS derived from wild-type smooth organisms.

More intriguing is our finding that C3H/HeJ cells that are turned on by protein mitogens or R-type LPS can be turned off by the wild-type smooth LPS. It should be noted that in separate experiments, MLPS can be washed out after 30 min to 1 hr of exposure to spleen cells, but the cells are committed to DNA synthesis as measured 48 hrs later. Consequently, C3H/HeJ B-cells are well into the G1 phase of the cell cycle when they are most susceptible to inhibition by the TLPS.

To date, neither suppressor T-cells or macrophages appear to be necessary for this inhibitory effect; however, further experiments are needed to rigorously exclude these accessory cells as participants in this phenomenon. Melchers has put forth evidence that accessory macrophages are necessary for B-cells to respond to LPS by polyclonal proliferation or maturation to Ig secreting cells (6). Perhaps a subpopulation of macrophages can be activated by LPS to be cytotoxic (7); however, it still is conceivable that certain C3H/HeJ macrophages are responsive to wild-type LPS in a manner we have not detected heretofore.

After this work had been completed, we noted that Tomai et al., (15) very recently reported that lipid X, which is a monosaccharide precursor of lipid A, could inhibit the proliferation of C3H/HeJ spleen cells induced by certain Re-glycolipids; however, unlike our results with TLPS, lipid X did not inhibit the proliferation induced by lipid A-protein suggesting to the authors that their results were compatible with the existence of a spleen cell receptor for lipid A (15). In contrast, the nonspecific nature of the inhibition and the results of the kinetic experiments we have obtained indicate that most likely this effect is not due to a stereospecific blockage of mitogen receptor on C3H/HeJ cells by TLPS. A more intriguing possibility is that the inhibition we have observed is directly the result of a biochemical event(s) in the B-cells that has been activated as a negative feedback mechanism to shut off proliferation. If this interpretation proves to be correct, this system can serve as an interesting model to explore signal transduction in B-cells.

ACKNOWLEDGEMENTS

The authors wish to thank Ms. Janice Howard for her excellent assistance in the preparation of this manuscript.

REFERENCES

1. Galanos, C., Luderitz, O., and Westphal, O., 1969, A new method for the extraction of R lipopolysaccharides. Eur. J. Biochem. 9: 945.

2. Girard, R., Chaby, R., and Bordenava, G., 1981, Mitogenic response of C3H/HeJ mouse lymphocytes to polyanionic polysaccharides obtained from **Bordetella pertussis** endotoxin and from other bacterial species. Infect. Immun. 31: 122.

3. Kumazawa, Y., Matsumura, M., Nakatsuru-Watanabe, Y., Fukumoto, M., Nishimura, C., Homma, J. Y., Inage, M., Kusumoto, S., and Shiba, T., 1984, Mitogenic and polyclonal B cell activation activities of synthetic lipid A analogues. Eur. J. Immunol. 14: 109.

4. LeDur, A., Chaby, R., and Szabo, L., 1980, Isolation of two protein-free and chemically different lipopolysaccharides from **Bordetella pertussis** phenol-extracted endotoxin. J. Bacteriol. 143: 78.

5. Markwell, M. A. K., Haas, S. M., Bieber, L. L., and Tolbert, N. E., 1978, A modification of the Lowry procedure to simplify protein determination in membrane and lipoprotein samples. Analyt. Biochem. 87: 206.

6. Melchers, F., 1986, Regulation of the cell cycle of murine B lymphocytes by lipopolysaccharides, in: "Immunobiology and Immunopharmacology of Bacterial Endotoxins", A. Szentivanyi, H. Friedman, and A. Nowotny, eds., Plenum Press, New York, p. 301.

7. Mergenhagen, S. E. and Pluznik, D. H., 1984, Defective responses to lipid A in C3H/HeJ mice: approaches to an understanding of lipid A-cell interaction. Rev. Inf. Dis. 6: 519.

8. Morrison, D. C., Betz, S. J., and Jacobs, D., 1976, Isolation of a lipid A bound polypeptide responsible for "LPS-initiated" mitogenesis of C3H/HeJ spleen cells. J. Exp. Med. 144: 840.

9. Morrison, D. C., Wollenweber, H-W., Vukajlovich, S. W., and Goodman, S.A., 1986, Biochemical, immunological and functional analysis of lymphocytes from the LPS-non-responder C3H/HeJ mouse, in: "Immunobiology and Immunopharmacology of Bacterial Endotoxins", A. Szentivanyi, H. Friedman and A. Nowotny, eds., Plenum Press, New York, p. 315.

10. Raetz, C. R. H., Purcell, S., and Takayama, K., 1983, Molecular requirements for B lymphocyte activation by **Escherichia coli** lipopolysaccharide. Proc. Natl. Acad. Sci. USA 80: 4624.

11. Sultzer, B. M., Craig, J. P., and Castagna, R., 1987, Immunomodulation by outer-membrane proteins associated with the endotoxin of gram-negative bacteria. Prog. Leuk. Biol. 6: 113.

12. Sultzer, B. M., Craig, J. P., and Castagna, R., 1985, The adjuvant effect of pertussis endotoxin protein in modulating the immune response

to cholera toxoid in mice. Develop. Biol. Standard. 61: 225.

13. Sultzer, B. M. and Goodman, G. W., 1976, Endotoxin protein: A B-cell mitogen and polyclonal activator of C3H/HeJ lymphocytes. J. Exp. Med. 144: 821.

14. Sultzer, B. M. and Nilsson, B. S., 1972, PPD Tuberculin--a B-cell mitogen. Nature New Biology. 240: 198.

15. Tomai, M. A., Johnson, A. G., and Ribi, E., 1988, Glycolipid induced proliferation of lipopolysaccharide hyporesponsive C3H/HeJ splenocytes. J. Leuk. Biol. 43: 11.

16. Vogel, S. N., Madonna, G. S., Wahl, L. M., and Rick, P. D., 1984, Stimulation of spleen cells and macrophages of C3H/HeJ mice by a lipid A precursor derived from **Salmonella typhimurium**. Rev. Inf. Dis. 6: 353.

17. Vukajlovich, S. W. and Morrison, D. C., 1983, Conversion of lipopolysaccharides to molecular aggregates with uniform subunit composition: demonstration of LPS-responsiveness in "endotoxin-unresponsive" C3H/HeJ B-lymphocytes. J. Immunol. 130: 2804.

18. Westphal, O., Luderitz, O., and Bister, F., 1952, Uber die extraktion von bakterien mit phenol-wasser. Z. Naturforsch. (C) 7B: 148.

LIPOAMINO ACIDS WHICH ARE SIMILAR TO BACTERIAL ENDOTOXIN IN BOTH STRUCTURE AND BIOLOGICAL ACTIVITY RELATED TO PHYSIOLOGICAL FUNCTION

Y. Kawai,[*] K. Akagawa[**] and I. Yano[***]

[*]Department of Bacteriology and [*]Department of Cellular Immunology, National Institute of Health, Tokyo and [***]Department of Bacteriology, Osaka City University Medical School, Osaka, Japan

Lipoamino acids are the substances which are present as the constituents of the cell membranes of relatively wide range of bacteria. As shown in Fig 1, the structures possess both hydrophobic lipid moiety and hydrophillic amino acid moiety (Ser or Orn) (3, 4, 5). We have investigated the structures and hemagglutinating activity of some lipoamino acids from Bordetella (3), Flavobacterium (4) and Pseudomonas (5). From these studies, it was resolved that the lipoamino acids possessing the fatty acids of carbon number 16-16 or 17-15 exhibit the higher hemagglutinating activity. Serine-containing lipid was found only in Flavobacterium and was named 'Flavolipin' by us (4). Based on these studies, we used this time the two kinds of lipoamino acids of Flavobacterium shown in Fig 1.

The structures of the lipoamino acids were similar to those of lipid A of the bacterial endotoxin (LPS) in which an amino group of the glucosamine is acylated by an O-acylated 3-hydroxy fatty acid, and further the biological activities of the lipoamino acids were found to be similar to those of LPS. Lipoamino acids augmented the mitogenicity of B-lymphocytes from both LPS-responsive and nonresponsive mice (Fig 2). The lipoamino acids activated the mouse peritoneal macrophages to produce tumor necrosis factor (Table 1), prostaglandin E_2 (Table 2) and interleukin-1 (Fig 3), which are known to play a role as the mediators of endotoxemia (6). Further, as same as the LPS (1, 2), sensitivity of the macrophages to the lipoamino acids was augmented by the treatment of the cells with interferon-γ. In addition, the serine-

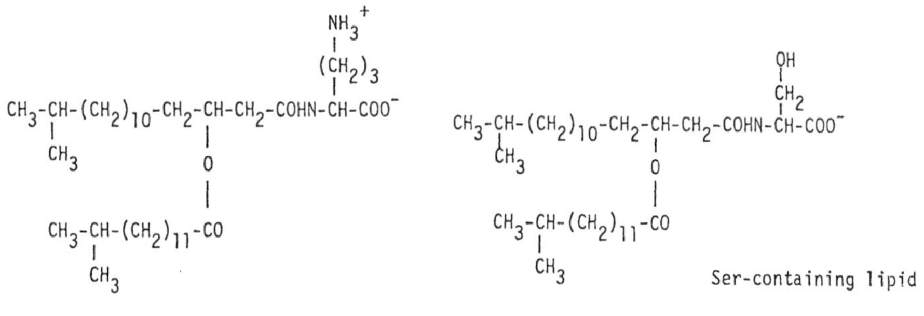

NH_3^+ — $(CH_2)_3$ —
$CH_3\text{-}CH(CH_3)\text{-}(CH_2)_{10}\text{-}CH_2\text{-}CH(O\text{-}CO\text{-}(CH_2)_{11}\text{-}CH(CH_3)\text{-}CH_3)\text{-}CH_2\text{-}COHN\text{-}CH((CH_2)_3NH_3^+)\text{-}COO^-$

Orn-containing lipid

$CH_3\text{-}CH(CH_3)\text{-}(CH_2)_{10}\text{-}CH_2\text{-}CH(O\text{-}CO\text{-}(CH_2)_{11}\text{-}CH(CH_3)\text{-}CH_3)\text{-}CH_2\text{-}COHN\text{-}CH(CH_2OH)\text{-}COO^-$

Ser-containing lipid

Fig 1. The structures of the lipoamino acids.

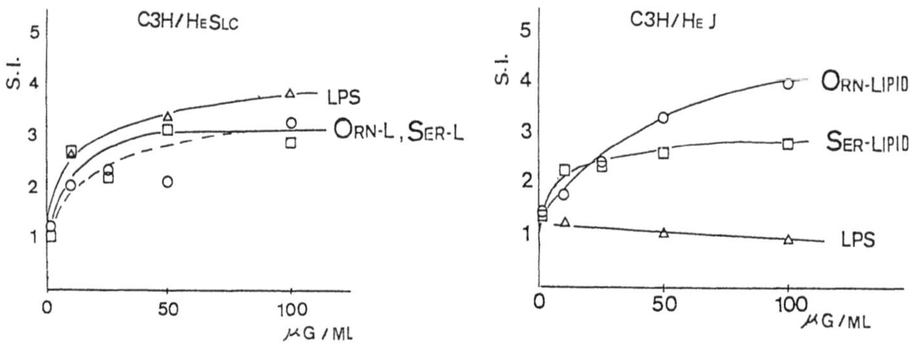

Fig 2. Effect of lipoamino acids on the mitogenicity of B-lymphocytes. S. I. is stimulating index. Abscissa indicates sample concentration.

containing lipid exhibited direct toxic effect on macrophages in vitro, but lethal toxicity was not demonstrated, when 7 mg of the lipoamino acid was injected into a mouse. Ornithine-containing lipid exhibited no toxicity both in vitro and in vivo.

The fact that these activities of the lipoamino acids were similar to those of LPS but were partially different may be based on the structural difference between the lipoamino acids and LPS. From these results, the lipoamino acids were proved to be the substances which were related not only host defense mechanism but also various kinds of physiological functions.

Lipoamino acids will be expected to be a useful immunoactivator.

Table 1. Effect of lipoamino acids on the TNF production from thioglycolate-induced macrophages

		TNF activity (Units)	
		C3H/HeSlc	
		IFN −	IFN +
Ser-Lipid	200 g/ml	<2	256
	100	37	>> 256
	50	18	>> 256
	25	<2	20
Orn-Lipid	200	5	158
	100	13	256
	50	9	315
	25	9	158
LPS	10	26	208
	1	14	>> 256
	0.1	55	> 256

Table 2. Effect of lipoamino acids on the release of PGE_2 from peptone-induced macrophages (C3H/HeSlc)

		Released PGE_2 (ng/106 cells)	
		IFN -	IFN +
Ser Lipid	100 ug/ml	90	110
	50	45	130
	25	60	150
Orn-Lipid	100	60	160
	50	35	140
	25	55	130
LPS	10	49	130
	1	90	130
	0.1	45	85
Medium		1	4

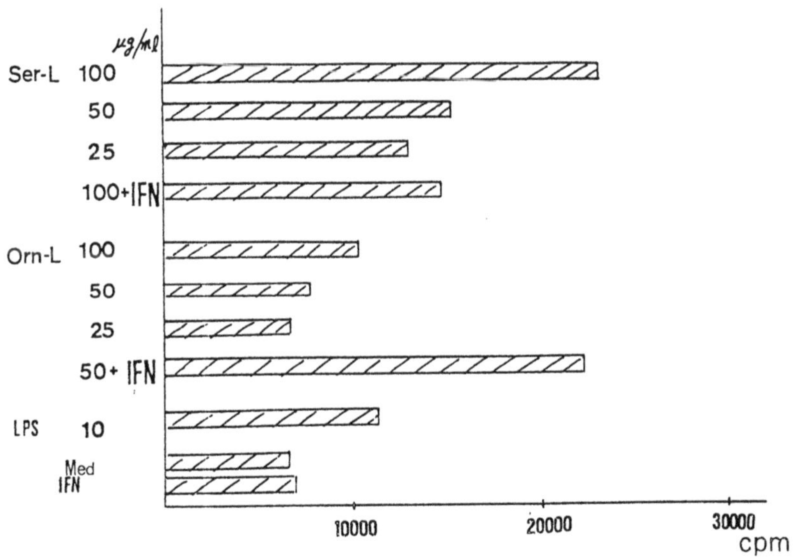

Fig 3. Effect of lipoamino acids on the IL-1 production from thioglycolate-induced macrophages.
IFN, interferon-γ; Med, only medium. Abscissa indicates radioisotope intensity of ^{3}H-TdR incorporated into thymocytes.

REFERENCES

1. Akagawa, K. and Tokunaga, T., 1985, Lack of binding of bacterial lipopolysaccharide to mouse lung macrophages and restoration of binding by γ interferon. J. Exp. Med. 162: 1444.

2. Akagawa, K., Kamoshita, K., Onodera, S. and Tokunaga, T., 1987, Restoration of lipopolysaccharide-mediated cytotoxic macrophage induction in C3H/HeJ mice by interferon- or a calcium ionophore. Jpn. J. Cancer Res. (Gann) 78: 279.

3. Kawai, Y. and Yano, I., 1983, Ornithine-containing lipid of Bordetella, a new type of hemagglutinin. Eur. J. Biochem. 136: 531.

4. Kawai, Y., Yano, I. and Kaneda, K., 1988, Various kinds of lipoamino acids including a novel serine-containing lipid in an opportunistic pathogen Flavobacterium. Their structures and biological activities on erythrocytes. Eur. J. Biochem. 171: 73.

5. Kawai, Y., Yano, I., Kaneda, K., and Yabuuchi, E., 1988, Ornithine-containing lipids of some Pseudomonas species. Eur. J. Biochem. 175: 633.

6. Rietschel, E. Th., Shade, U., Jensen, M., Wollenweber, H. W., Luderitz, O. and Greisman, S. G., 1982, Bacterial endotoxins: chemical structure, biological activity and role in septicaemia. Scan. J. Infect. Dis., Suppl., 31: 8.

CHEMISTRY AND BIOLOGY OF A NOVEL LIPID CONTAMINANT OF SOME ENDOTOXIN PREPARATIONS WITH SELECTIVE CYTOTOXICITY TO TRANSFORMED CELLS

T. Keler[1], C. A. D. Smith[2], and A. Nowotny[1]

[1]The Thomas W. Evans Museum and Dental Institute, University of Pennsylvania, Philadelphia PA 19104, USA, and [2]National Cancer Institute, Bethesda MD 20892, USA

The heterogeneity of various endotoxin (ET) preparations, should they be extracted by the trichloroacetic acid method of Boivin and co-workers, or by the phenol-water procedure of Westphal and Luderitz, has been well documented (26, 27). Several papers from our laboratory elaborated on the experimental details and emphasized the significance of this observation from both chemical and biological viewpoints (23, 24, 25, 29).

ET components can be separated by preparative column chromatography on weak anion exchangers, and the biological activity of the fractions showed the presence of several endotoxic components, even in the most purified ET samples (27). Not only do smooth (or wild type) gram negative bacteria produce chromatographically distinct ET-active components, but the so-called rough mutants also synthesize several endotoxic glycolipids which can be separated by thin-layer chromatography (5, 7, 22, 33).

In ET preparations from smooth or rough bacteria, but particularly in crude ET extracts, many components are present which are not toxic in conventional assays, but manifest beneficial reactions, such as enhancement of the nonspecific resistance to infection with viable bacteria or the induction of colony-stimulating factor (CSF). Similar activities have been observed in crude bacterial extracts such as the White-type polysaccharides (WPS) also known as Freeman polysaccharide, which contains incompletely degraded O-antigens and other components of the bacterium (12, 32). We found that several of these non-endotoxic components can induce the regression of Meth A-induced sarcoma in mice (30) or enhance the resistance of mice to L 1210 leukemia (28).

During the attempts to isolate components from WPS and crude ET preparations we tested the capacity of various fractions for their ability to induce macrophage cytotoxicity, as determined by the destruction of ^{51}Cr labeled P815 mastocytoma cells in vitro. T. Keler in our laboratory found that some WPS or crude ET preparations were cytotoxic to P815 cells, in the absence of macrophages. Purified ET samples did not show this effect. The contaminating cytotoxic activity could be removed from the ET samples by extraction with pure ethanol. The cytotoxic compound is soluble in several organic solvents, such as chloroform, ketones, esters, and alcohols.

ET or WPS preparations contained only very small amounts of this component named DCX (for direct cytotoxicity), however, intact **Serratia marcescens**

08 bacteria contained greater quantities. Chloroform:methanol= 4:1 (CM41) extracts of the lyophilized bacteria were used to obtain DCX. Fractionation of the extracts made it possible to isolate DCX in a chromatographically pure form and test its action on various normal and transformed cells in vitro. DCX was also subjected to various analytical and chemical tests. Some of the early results have been reported in a short paper (16). A more complete summary of our understanding of the biological and chemical nature of DCX is presented here.

MATERIALS AND METHODS

Bacteria

Serratia marcescens 08 was grown by the Merck Sharp and Dohme Co., Rahway, NJ, as a generous contribution to our research efforts. The exact identification of this strain is in process. Other Serratia strains were obtained from the American Type Culture Collection (Rockville, MD).

Bacterial Cultivation

Growth media: 20 g/1 NZ-amine type E (Sheffield Products, Norwich, NY), 5 g/1 sodium chloride, 1 g/1 glycerol, beef extract 3 g/1 adjusted to pH 7.3. One loopful of **Serratia marcenscens** 08 grown on slants was transferred to 200 ml of media and grown overnight in a 28°C waterbath while shaking. The entire content was then transferred to a 20 liter glass jug containing 6 liters of media. Polypropylene glycol (Sigma) was added to prevent excessive foaming. The jug was placed in 28°C waterbath and rocked gently with aeration for 72 hr. The bacteria were harvested by centrifugation and then freeze dried.

Isolation of DCX

Lyophilized (3 g) bacteria were placed into a Soxhlet thimble, and extracted using 100 ml chloroform:methanol=4:1 mixture. The dark purple extract was filtered on a 1 x 3 cm silicic acid 60 (Baker Co., Phillipsburg, NJ) layer and washed with freshly distilled anhydrous ethanol. The filtrate was fractionated by silicic acid column chromatography or preparative thin layer chromatography (TLC). Isolation by TLC was done using the procedure we developed for the fractionation of rough mutant glycolipid ET (6). The solvent system used for the separation and isolation of DCX was ethylacetate:-cyclohexane=1:1. The hydrophobic DCX band was made visible by a fine water spray and scraped off. Scrapings were extracted with pure ethanol and the concentration was adjusted to 1 milligram/ml. The cytotoxic band was identified by the assay described below. For analytical purposes the TLC plates could be sprayed with a modified Schultz and Strauss reagent consisting of 0.2 g ceric (IV) sulfate and 0.5 g phosphomolybdic acid dissolved in 18.8 ml water and 1.2 ml conc. sulfuric acid. The sprayed plates were developed at 115°C for 15 min. Dark blue spots were visible on white background (33). Column chromatography was performed on a commercial Lobar prepacked Si60 (E. Merck) column, size 240 x 10 mm. The column was connected to a Pharmacia FPLC system, and eluted with cyclohexane:ethylacetate=1:1 solvent. The effluent was monitored by a Waters refractive index monitoring instrument and recorded by the Pharmacia FLPC system's recorder. Fractions (2 ml) were collected and tested for cytotoxicity on P815 cells.

Established Cell Lines and Maintenance

P815 mastocytoma cells were a generous gift from Dr. Dolph Adams, Duke University, NC. P388D1 cells were purchased from ATCC, Rockville MD. TA-3 adenocarcinoma cells were donated by Dr. S. Friberg, Karolinska Instituttet,

Stockholm Sweden, the murine L929 cells by Dr. J. Gentsch, the normal human gingival fibroblasts by Dr. R. Stevens, Univ. of Pennsylvania, Philadelphia, PA. Cells were grown in H-MEM: Eagle modified minimum essential medium (Flow Lab Inc. Mclean, VA) supplemented with 2mM glutamine, 15mM Hepes, 2mg/ml sodium bicarbonate, 100 units/ml streptomycin, 100 μg/ml penicillin, pH 7.4 and 10% fetal bovine serum (FBS) (HyClone, Logan, UT). The cells are kept at 37°C in 5% CO_2.

Generation and Maintenance of Murine Fibroblast Cell Lines

10 day Balb/c mice embryos were disrupted and a post-crisis mass cell line was established from the homogenate which grew in an anchorage-dependent manner in vitro (20). From this mass cell culture a fibroblast cell line was cloned and denoted as #802c by a method previously published (39). A subculture of #802c was transformed with SV40 and cloned as described elsewhere (20) and the transformed cell clone was designated as #804csc. Cells were maintained in Dulbecco's modified essential medium (DMEM) containing 4.5 g/1 glucose (Gibco Laboratories, Grand Island, NY), and supplemented with 10% fetal bovine serum. The cells were maintained in a 5% CO_2 incubator at 37°C.

Coulter Counting

At the designated time the plate was removed from the incubator and the media was suctioned off. After 2 washes with cold PBS, 1 ml of 0.25% trypsin/EDTA (Sigma) was added to each well and the cells were suspended by the addition of 1 ml of media. The cells were pipetted gently to insure single cell suspensions. The cells (0.1 to 0.4 ml) were diluted to 10 mls with Isoton II (Curtis Matheson Inc.) for counting with a Coulter cell counter.

Viability Assay

At the designated time the cells were removed from tissue culture plates with trypsin/EDTA and counted with a hemocytometer. Cells excluding the dye after 5 min were counted by diluting the cell suspension 1:10 in 0.4% Trypan Blue stain. Each measurement was the average of duplicate wells.

Chromium Release Assay

6×10^6 P815 cells were labelled with 0.275 mCi ^{51}Cr (Amersham Corp., Arlington Heights, IL) for 90 min. The cells were washed, resuspended and allowed to release excess chromium for 60 minutes before they were washed again. The cells were then plated in 96 well tissue culture plates at 3×10^4 cells per well in 100 μl of H-MEM containing 10% FBS. Cytotoxic samples were diluted in the same medium and added to cells in an additional 100 μl. All values represent the average of triplicate wells. At the designated time 100 μl was removed from each well to quantitate the radioactivity released. Toxicity was calculated by the formula:

$$\%^{51}\text{Cr released} = \frac{\text{experimental release} - \text{spontaneous release}}{\text{freeze thaw release} - \text{spontaneous release}} \times 100\%$$

TD50 is calculated as the dose of DCX which causes the lysis of 50% of the cells.

DNA Synthesis

DNA synthesis was determined by the incorporation of ^{3}H-thymidine (ICN Biochemicals Inc., Costa Mesa, CA). At the designated time 1 uCi/ml ^{3}H-thymidine was added to cultures in 2 mls of media and replaced in the incubator for either 4 hr (804csc cells) or overnight (802c cells). Following incubation the monolayers were washed and trypsinized. 1 ml cell suspension was added to 9 ml cold 10% TCA and vortexed. After 1 hr on ice the samples were filtered through GF/C filters and washed with 10 ml 10% TCA followed by 5 ml ethanol. Filters were dried in scintillation vials before addition of 10 ml Ecolume scintillation fluid (ICN Biochem. Inc., Costa Mesa, CA).

Measurement of Glucose Uptake

5×10^4 cells were seeded in 6-well tissue culture plates with or without DCX in 4 ml DMEM with 4.5 g/1 glucose and 10% serum. 16 hr later the plates were washed once with DMEM with 1.0 g/1 glucose and 10% serum. 2 ml of the same media is then added to each well suplemented with 5 uCi/ml ^{3}H-2-deoxy-D-glucose (ICN) and allowed to accumulate in the cells for 60 min at 37°C. After incubation the plates were washed two times with PBS before 500 µl of 0.4 N NaOH was added to each well to dissolve the cells. 100 µl from each well was used for protein determination by the BIO-RAD kit. The remaining content of each well was added to 10 mls of Ecolume scintillation fluid and counted.

Chemical Studies

Elemental analysis was carried out by MicAnal Lab, Tucson, AZ. Infrared spectroscopy of DCX was done using Fourrier transfer IR analysis. The sample

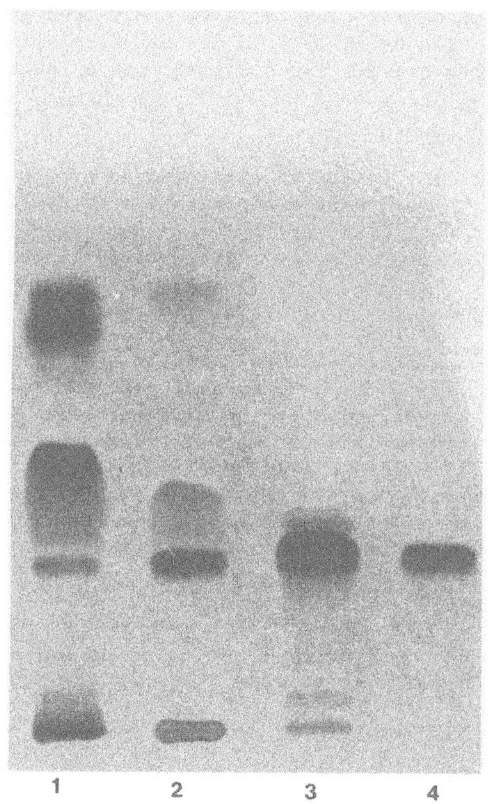

Fig 1. Thin layer chromatography of four purification steps during the isolation of DCX. A: chloroform : methanol = 4:1 extract of dried bacteria. B: ethylacetate : cyclohexane = 1:1 soluble components of A. C: Fractions after Si 60 column filtration of B. D: DCX isolated by preparative thin layer chromatography of C.

was prepared as a film dried from chloroform on KBr crystal, in a Digilab FTS-15 IR spectrophotometer. Fast atom bombardment mass spectroscopy was carried out on deuterated thioglycerol-DCX sample. NMR analysis was carried out by Dr. T. Inubushi (Univ. of Pennsylvania, School of Medicine). The following NMR studies were carried out on a 500 MHerz high-field instrument: One dimensional proton and ^{13}C NMR. In two dimensions: a) ^{1}H COSY (proton-proton connectivity via ^{1}H-^{1}H spin-spin coupling. b) ^{1}H Phase sensitive NOESY (proton-proton through space connectivity. c) Proton-detected ^{1}H-^{13}C chemical shift correlation 2-D (^{1}H-^{13}C) connectivity. d) Proton-detected INADQUET 2-D (^{13}C connectivity).

RESULTS

Isolation and Purification of DCX

The solubility of the DCX in various esters, ketones, alcohols or other lipid-solvents made it relatively easy to obtain sufficient quantities of DCX from lyophilized bacteria for chemical and biological tests. The good stability of DCX in warm organic solvents was another factor which facilitated its quantitative extraction by the Soxhlet procedure.

The preparative TLC procedure was the simplest and most efficient way to obtain chromatographically pure DCX in milligram quantities. The column chromatographic method for preparative isolation was less simple and the DCX containing fractions were slightly contaminated by other non-cytotoxic components which were not even related structurally to DCX, as shown by NMR studies. Therefore, the preparative TLC so far is the best method for isolation, and Fig 1 shows the purity of the fractions after the various purification steps. Fig 2 shows the column chromatographic profile obtained by a refractive index monitoring system.

Crystallization of DCX was attempted, and partially crystalline DCX preparations could be obtained from the amorphous but pure DCX samples in hot 50% ethanol. Such preparations were used for all chemical assays and physicochemical studies of its structure.

Chemical Analysis of DCX

The exact chemical structure of DCX is not fully clarified. The data presented here give our current understanding of the chemical structure of DCX. The melting point was determined in a electrothermal instrument. We

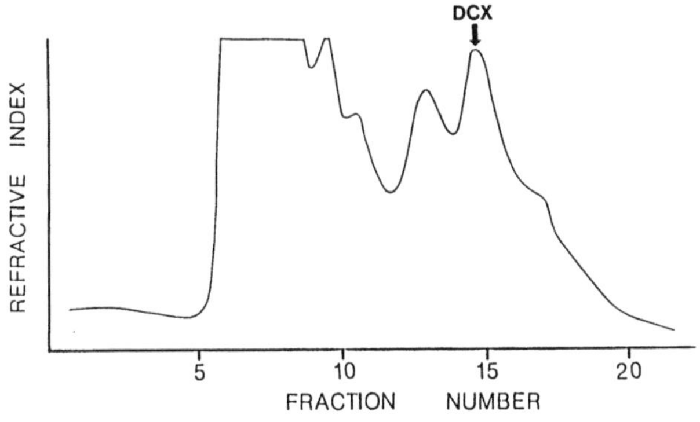

Fig 2. Elution profile of ethylacetate:cyclohexane = 1:1 soluble lipids of **Serratia marcescens** 08. The peak corresponding to the cytotoxic activity is labelled DCX.

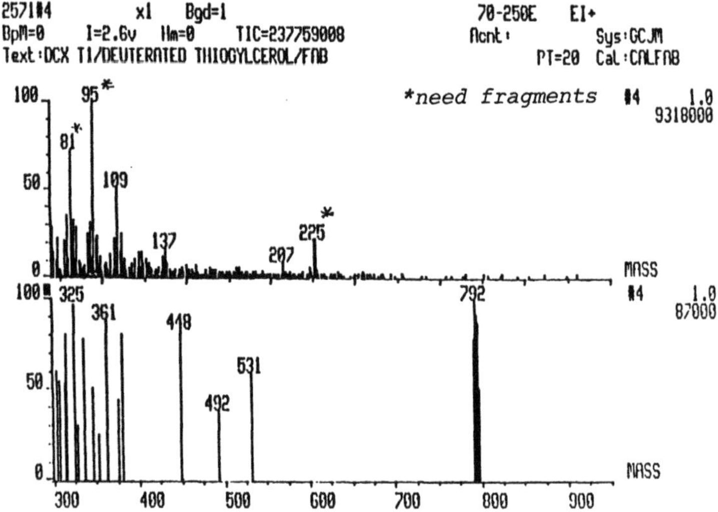

Fig 3. Chart of fragments produced by DCX analyzed by fast atom bombardment mass spectroscopy.

found that melting started at 99°C and was complete at 101°C. No decomposition of the substance was evident during this determination.

The C, H and O percentage determination was repeated on two separate batches of pure DCX samples and the values were: C = 66.11-66.18%, H = 9.11-9.12%, O = 24.51-24.76%. P or N were not detected in DCX samples after digestion.

FAB Mass spectroscopy was carried out by McNeil laboratories (Springhouse, PA). Fig 3 shows the spectrum. Accordingly the molecular weight of DCX is 792 Daltons.

Fourrier transform IR spectroscopy was done and a representative spectrum is shown in Fig 4. Characteristic functional groups detected were OH-, =CO and conjugated double bonds. The aliphatic hydrocarbon nature of the molecule was also evident.

The most important information we obtained came from the NMR studies. Figs 5, 6a and 6b show one and two dimensional NMR spectra. Careful analysis included connectivity possibilities. Of interest is a possible connectivity between distant carbon atoms forming a ring structure containing 17 carbons.

Using all above data, we have concluded that the empirical formula of DCX is most likely to be $C_{44}H_{72}O_{12}$. Although the structural studies are not yet complete, we summarize our present assumptions on the chemical structure of DCX in Fig 7.

DCX shows great chemical similarities with some of the antibiotics produced by Streptomyces, particularly the polyenes which have large lactone rings containing similar functional groups as DCX (19). Furthermore, polyenes are generally not inhibitory to bacteria, but are cytotoxic to fungi and various eucaryotic cells including tumor cells (17). Thus far we have not found any bacteria which are sensitive to DCX, yet DCX does inhibit the growth of several fungi (data not shown).

Effect of DCX Dose, Incubation Time and Temperature on P815 Cells

Due to the high sensitivity of P815 mastocytoma cells to DCX, cytotoxi-

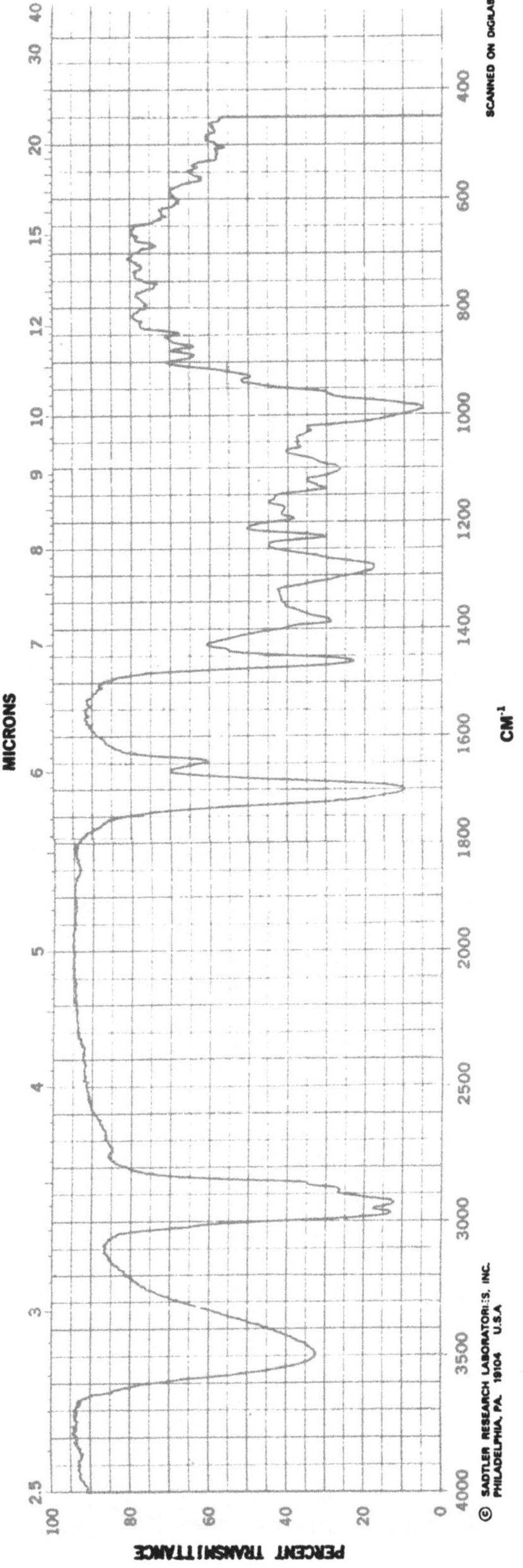

Fig 4. Infrared spectrum of DCX. (Permission granted from Sadtler Research Laboratories, Inc.)

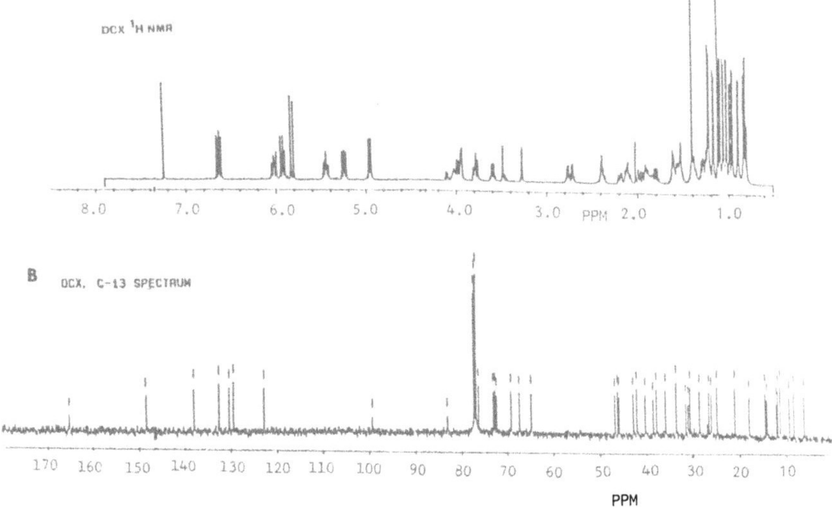

Fig 5. Proton (A) and carbon (B) NMR of DCX.

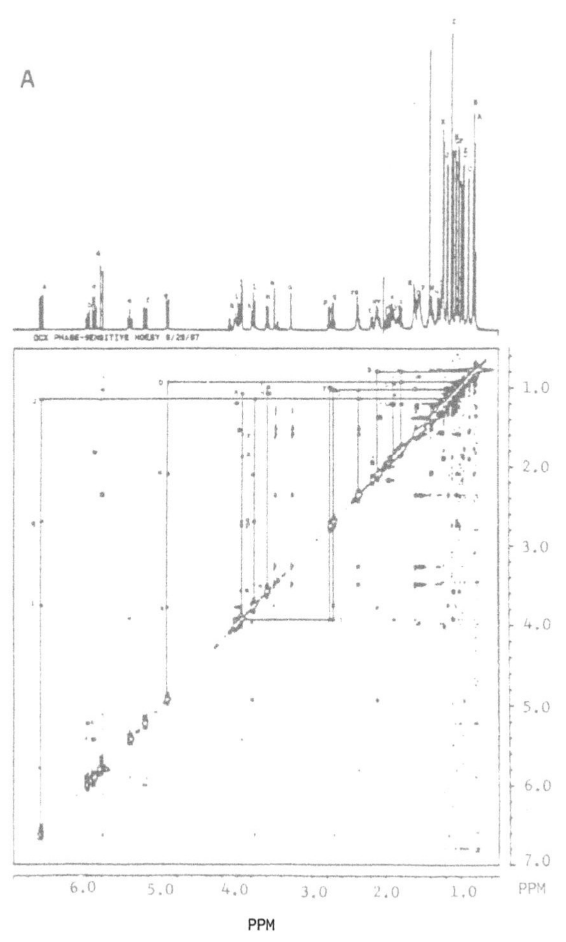

Fig 6a. Two-dimensional NMR of DCX by ^{1}H-NOESY showing proton-proton connectivity through space.

city measurements could be done with the use of the chromium release assay. For this reason the initial characterization of DCX mediated cytotoxicity was carried out on this cell line. The DCX TD50 for P815 cells is approximately 75 pg/ml as determined from the dose response curve shown in Fig 8. The sensitivity to DCX lysis is temperature dependent as shown in the same figure. The time required to initiate lysis varied with the dose of DCX used. At higher concentrations (100 ng/ml) killing is evident in 3 hr, and is nearly completed in 7.5 hr. However, lower concentrations require longer incubation time before lysis of cells is seen.

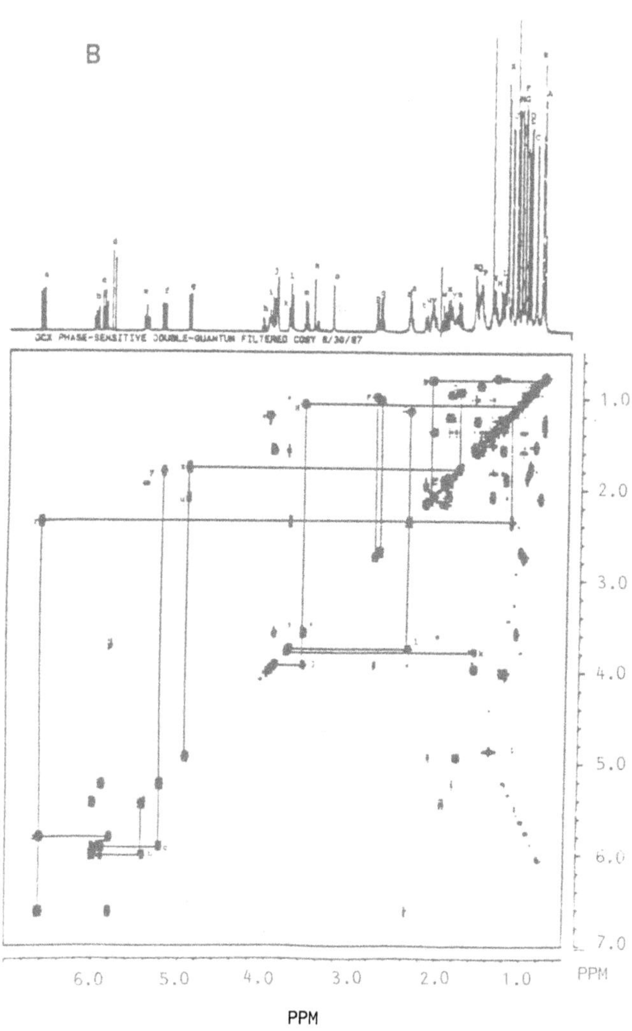

Fig 6b. Two-dimensional NMR of DCX by ^{1}H-COSY showing proton-proton connectivity.

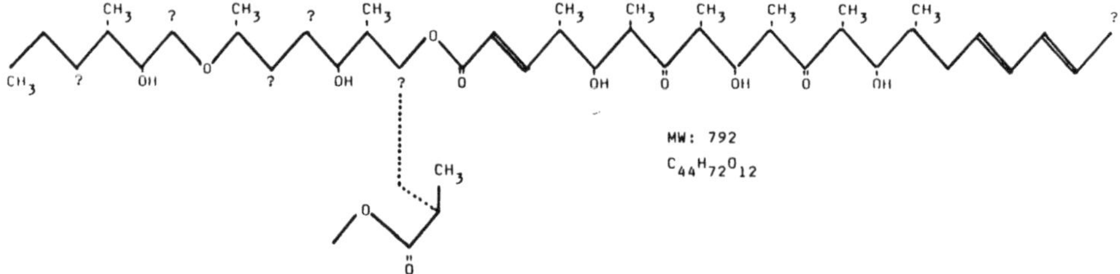

Fig 7. Hypothetical structure of DCX based on our current knowledge of its chemical nature.

Cytotoxicity of DCX to Three Transformed Cell Lines

DCX cytotoxicity studies were extended by testing the effects on three other transformed cell lines available in our laboratory. These include a fibroblast cell line L929 (spontaneously transformed), a macrophage-like cell line P388D1 (methylcholanthrene induced lymphoid neoplasm), and a highly tumorigenic adenocarcinoma cell line TA3 (spontaneous adenocarcinoma) (14). The effect of DCX on these cell lines is presented in Table 1. All three cell types show less sensitivity to DCX than P815 cells, in that more time and larger dose is required for death of the culture. However, 10 ng/ml DCX is sufficient for death of the cultures within 5-7 days.

Effect of DCX on Normal Human Fibroblasts

The effect of DCX on two normal cell cultures was tested to see if the cytotoxic action of DCX may be selective for transformed cells. Human fibroblasts were obtained from surgical explant cultures of synovial and gingival tissues. These cells have been maintained in tissue culture for 8-10 passages before experiments. Fig 9 shows the effect of 10 ng/ml DCX on the two cell types. Both cell cultures were resistant to the cytotoxicity of DCX up to six days, although their growth rate was retarded.

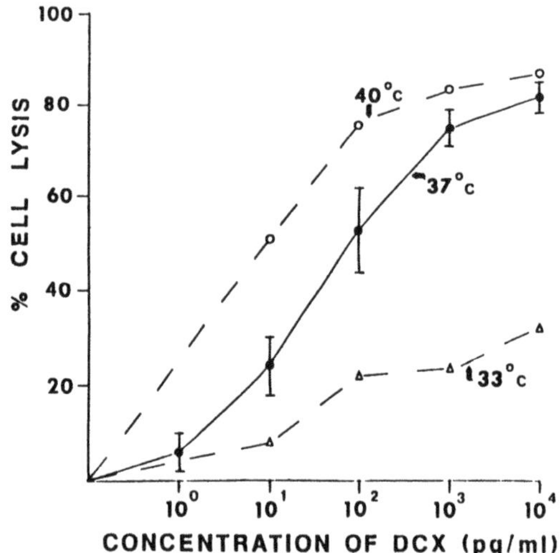

Fig 8. Dose and temperature dependent lysis of P815 cells by DCX in a 16 hr chromium release assay. Error bars represent variation from the mean in five separate experiments. Experimental conditions are described under materials and methods.

Table 1. Effect of DCX on Three Murine Cell Lines

CELL TYPE	DCX ng/ml	% GROWTH INHIBITION
P388D1	0.1	10 %
	1.0	48 %
	10.0	64 %
TA3	0.1	15 %
	1.0	28 %
	10.0	68 %
L929	0.1	6 %
	1.0	11 %
	10.0	41 %

% Growth inhibition was determined at 30 hr by the formula:

$$\% \text{ G.I.} = 100\% - \frac{\text{\# of live cells in treated culture}}{\text{\# of live cells in control culture}} \times 100\%$$

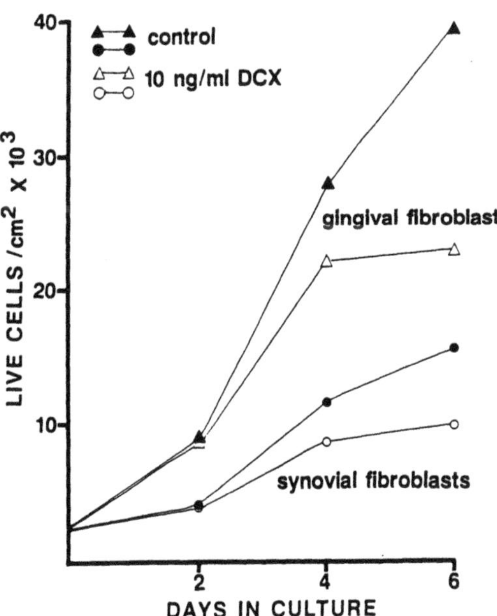

Fig 9. Effect of DCX on two human fibroblast cultures. Human fibroblasts were seeded at 2.5×10^4 in six well plates and cultured in H-MEM supplemented with 10% FBS. 10 ng/ml DCX was added to half of the cultures. Live cells were counted as described under Materials and Methods. The points represent the average of three determinations.

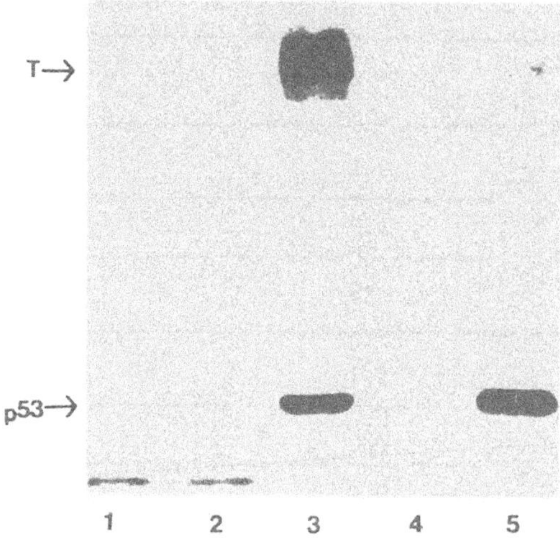

Fig 10. Immunoprecipitation of ^{35}S-methionine labelled cell lysates. pAb 416: anti-TAg monoclonal antibody lanes 1 and 3. pAb 421: anti-p53 monoclonal antibody lanes 2 and 5. Lane 4 control no antibody. Subconfluent monolayers were labelled for 3 hr in methionine free DMEM supplemented with 2% dialyzed FBS, 50 uCi/ml ^{35}S-methionine. Cell lysates were precipitated with the appropriate antibody and run on a polyacrylamine gel, which was dried and detected by autoradiography.

Effect of DCX on Normal (Untransformed) and SV40 Transformed Murine Fibroblasts

In order to further examine the selectivity of DCX cytotoxicity, it was necessary to use clonally related cell lines. Transformation of cells with SV40 has been shown to be a model for malignancy and transformation (4, 38). Therefore, the effect of DCX was tested on a balb/c embryonal fibroblast cell line (denoted 802c) and a clonal derivative obtained after transformation

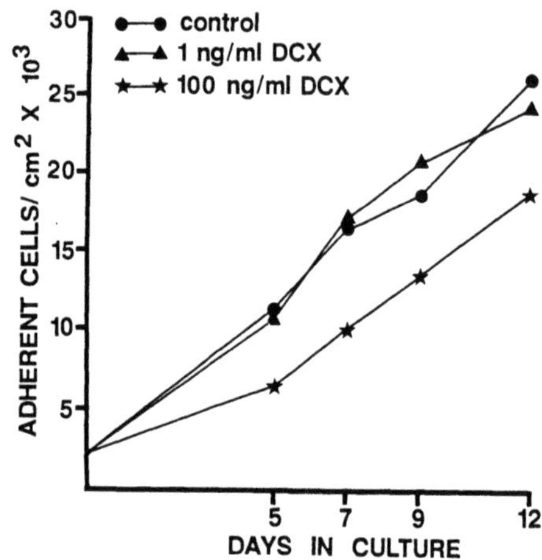

Fig 11. Effect of DCX on growth of 802c cells. 802c cells were seeded at 2×10^4 cells/well in six well plates in DMEM HG with 10% FBS. At the times indicated adherent cells were counted by the use of a coulter counter as described under Materials and Methods. The points represent the average of three separate determinations.

with SV40 (denoted 804csc). The transformation was confirmed by detection of Large T antigen (Tag). Fig 10 shows the presence of Tag in 804csc cell lysates immunoprecipitated with anti-Tag monoclonal antibody PAb-416 and anti-P53 monoclonal antibody PAb-421. The cellular phosphoprotein denoted p53 is known to complex and coprecipitate with Tag in SV40 transformed murine cell extracts (4). Transformation of 802c with SV40 dramatically altered its growth properties. The doubling time for the cells decreased from 40-50 hr to 9-12 hr while the maximum saturation density increased from 3-7 x 10^3 to 2-5 x 10^5 per cm^2.

The effect of DCX on 802c cell growth was studied by two parameters, cell number and DNA synthesis. Fig 11 shows the growth curves of 802c cells cultured with three concentrations of DCX. Treatment of 802c cells with 1 ng/ml DCX did not significantly alter cell growth. 10 ng/ml and 100 ng/ml DCX do inhibit 802c cell growth followed over a 12 day period. However, the

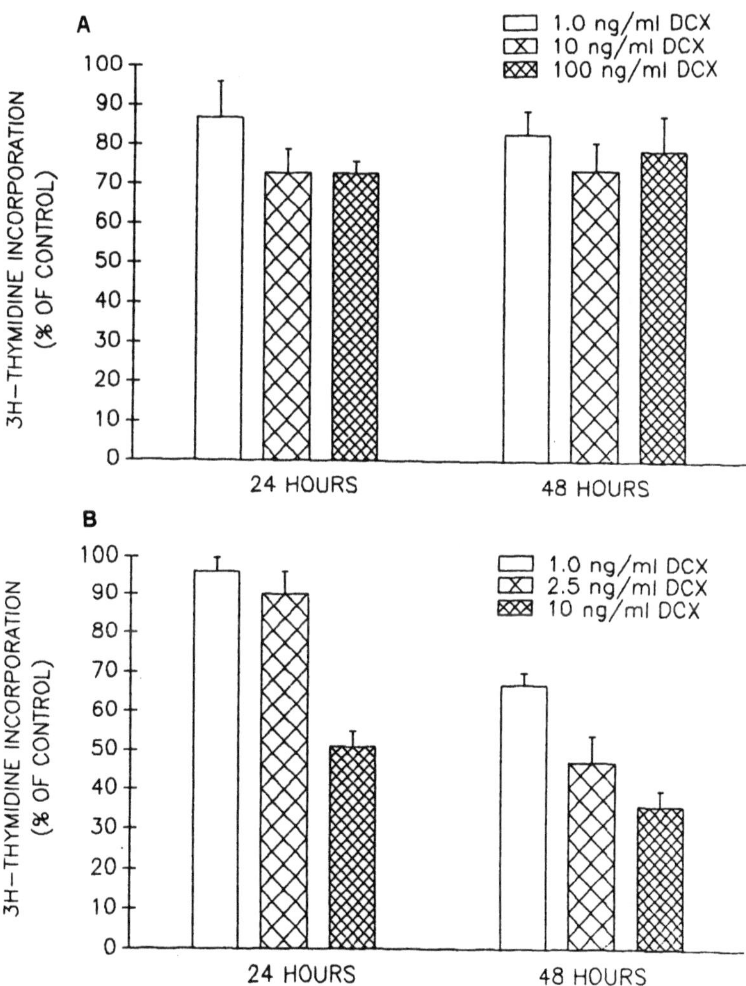

Fig 12. Effect of DCX on DNA synthesis in 802c cells (a) and 804csc cells (b), as measured by the incorporation of ^{3}H-thymidine into acid precipitable material. 802c cells were plated in six well plates in DMEM HG with 10% FBS at 5 x 10^4 per well. DNA synthesis was measured as described under Materials and Methods.

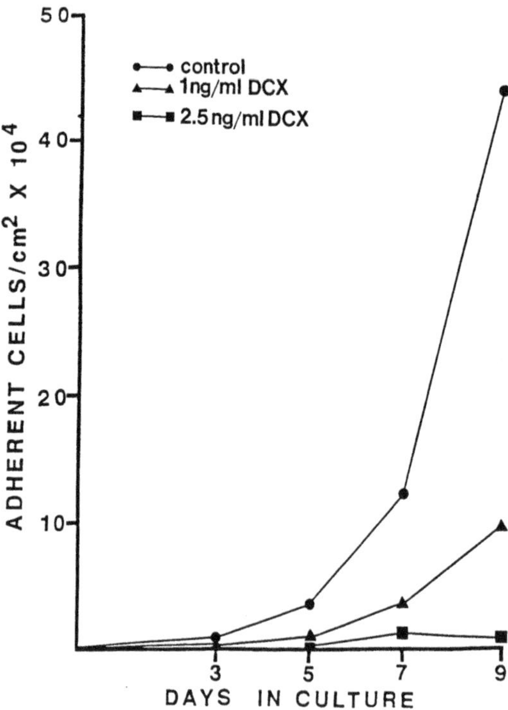

Fig 13. Effect of DCX on the growth of 804csc cells. 804csc cells were seeded at 2×10^4 cells/well in six well plates in DMEM HG with 10% FBS. At the times indicated adherent cells were counted by the use of a coulter counter as described under Materials and Methods. The points represent the average of three separate determinations.

Table 2. Effect of Sub-Toxic Doses of DCX on 804csc Cell Growth

DCX ng/ml	^{3}H-Thymidine Uptake[a]	^{3}H-Thymidine Incorporation[b]	Cell Number[c]
0	100 ± 2.2 %	100 ± 0.5 %	2.03×10^6 .27
0.1	122 ± 3.7 %	119 ± 1.2 %	3.11×10^6 .38
0.5	126 ± 7.0 %	127 ± 1.1 %	2.92×10^6 .37
1.0	72 ± 6.2 %	75 ± 12.1 %	2.07×10^6 .18

^{3}H-thymidine uptake and incorporation experiments were done using 804csc cells seeded at 1×10^5/ 25cm^2 flask in 5ml of DME media with 10% FCS and appropriate concentrations of DCX. After 48 hr incubation, cells are pulse labelled with ^{3}H-thymidine (1 uCi/ml) for 2 hr before harvesting.

[a]Total uptake is determined by counting the ^{3}H-thymidine in cell lysate. Values are expressed as % of control.

[b]Incorporation is determined by counting the ^{3}H-thymidine win TCA precipitable material. Values are expressed as % of control.

[c]Cell number was determined by Coulter counting of cells after trypsinization. The values represent the mean and standard error of five individual determinations.

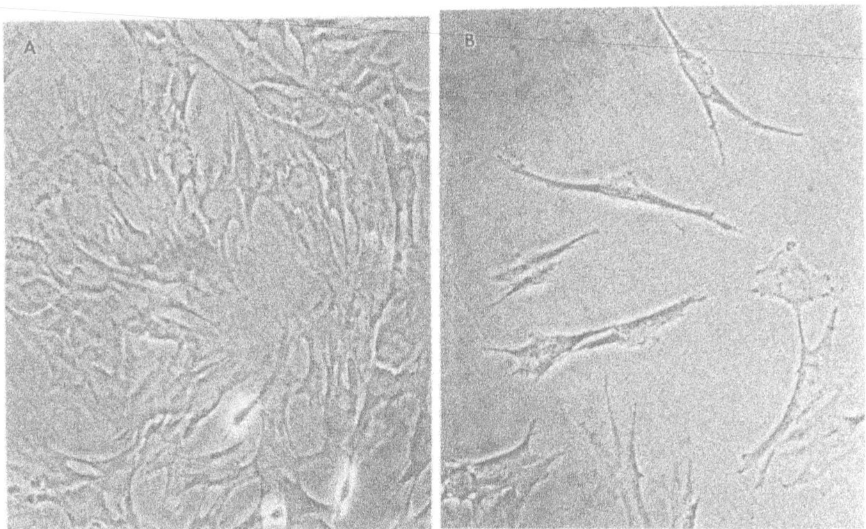

Fig 14. Phase-contrast microscopy showing the effect of DCX on 804csc cells. Panel A: control cells 72 hr, panel B: cells treated with 10 ng/ml DCX for 72 hr. 16 x magnification.

cells continue to grow to confluency. 802c cells treated under these conditions with 10 ng/ml DCX remained viable for five weeks (as determined by replating and trypan blue staining). The effect of DCX on 802c cell DNA synthesis shows a similar response as determined by cell counting. After 48 hr the inhibition by 100 ng/ml DCX is about 25%, as seen in Fig 12a.

The effect of DCX on 804csc cell growth was studied under identical conditions as for the 802c cells. Fig 13 shows the effect on cell number when 804csc cells are cultured in the presence of three concentrations of DCX over a 12 day period. Cell growth is significantly inhibited with as little as 1 ng/ml DCX, and concentrations of 2.5 ng/ml or higher are cytotoxic. Under these assay conditions, increasing the concentration of DCX above 10 ng/ml does not significantly enhance the cytotoxic effect. The cytotoxicity of DCX to 804csc cells is also evident when examining DNA synthesis. Fig 12b shows that cells treated with 10 ng/ml DCX have a 50% reduction in DNA synthesis within 24 hr. It is interesting to note that when the dose of DCX is reduced below cytotoxic levels, an enhancement of DNA synthesis and cell number is seen. Table 2 shows that incubation of 804csc cells with 0.1 -0.5 ng/ml DCX results in a significant increase in ^{3}H-thymidine incorporation and cell number.

Fig 14 shows the effect of DCX on 804csc cells in culture was observed by phase-contrast microscopy. The initial effects were evident 24-48 hr after treatment, and are characterized by very long extensions of processes which often interconnect the cells. By 72 hr vesicle-like formations and lipid droplets appear which are followed by further distortion of the membrane including membrane blebbing. These events continue to progress until the cells die. Fig 15 shows that 802c cells do not show any physical alteration detectable by these means.

Effect of Media on DCX Cytotoxicity

804csc cells were grown with and without 10 ng/ml DCX in media supplemented with varying concentrations of serum. When the cells are treated in media supplemented with 20% serum no significant change is observed in growth

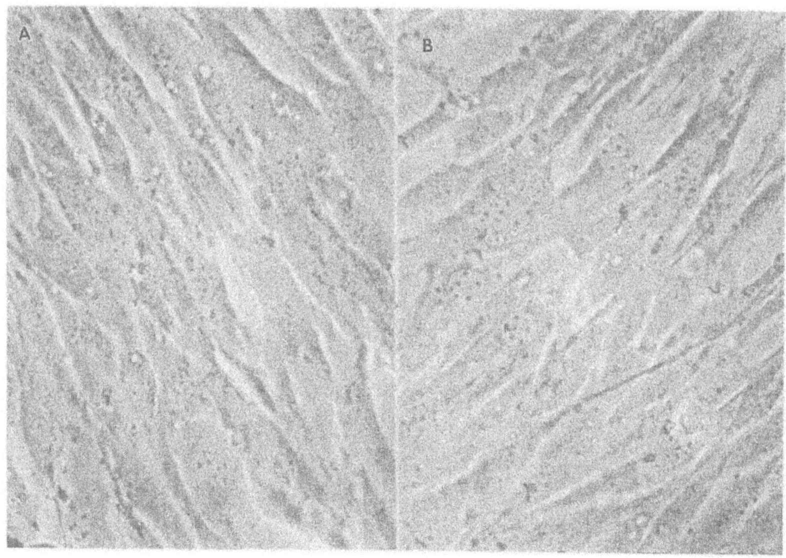

Fig 15. Phase-contrast microscopy of 802c cells without (panel A) and with 10 ng/ml DCX (panel B) after seven days in culture. 16 x magnification.

rate or viability of the control or treated culture compared to treatment in 10% serum. When cells are grown in 2% serum both control and treated cultures grow significantly slower than at the higher serum concentrations. However, expressing the growth inhibition as percent of control, the effect of DCX in 2% serum is similar to that which is seen at 10 and 20% serum. There was no significant difference in length of time the cultures remained viable at the three serum concentrations.

The effect of 10 ng/ml DCX on 804csc cell growth was also tested at two glucose concentrations: low = 1.0g/l and high = 4.5g/l. Treatment of cells in low glucose media accelerated the death of the cultures from 10-12 days to 5 days. The supernatants of the treated cultures were tested for glucose (at 5 days) and found to be negative. Supernatants of treated cultures grown in high glucose still contained in excess of 1 g/l glucose at 12 days, and therefore are not assumed to be dying of glucose starvation.

The increased utilization of glucose after DCX treatment was not restricted to the transformed cells. Deoxy-glucose uptake measurements with 802c and 804csc cells show that both cell types show a dose dependent increase in glucose uptake (Table 3). This is the first evidence that the 802c cells are affected by low concentrations of DCX.

DISCUSSION

The cytotoxicity of DCX was first described on the mastocytoma cell line P815 and various other unrelated murine cell lines. To carefully examine the selectivity of DCX between normal (untransformed) and transformed cells it was necessary to use clonally related cell lines. The initial observation that DCX was not toxic to 802c cells, a Balb/c embryonal fibroblastic cell line with normal characteristics, prompted us to transform them to obtain a transformed clonal derivative of 802c. SV40 transformation is a well studied model, and employing this virus we were able to select a transformed derivative of 802c by clonal selection. With the availability of the clonally

Table 3. Effect of DCX on 2-deoxy-D-glucose Uptake

Cells	DCX ng/ml	2-Deoxy-D-Glucose Uptake CPM/mg Protein/hr	% Increase From Control
802c	0.0	856 ± 36	0.0
	2.5	1258 ± 76	47.0
	10.0	1394 ± 87	63.0
	25.0	1613 ± 69	88.6
804csc	0.0	1794 ± 68	0.0
	2.5	2199 ± 69	22.6
	10.0	2434 ± 248	35.7
	25.0	3043 ± 103	69.6

^{3}H-2-deoxy-D-glucose uptake was measured as a tracer for glucose uptake in DMEM with 1 g/l glucose. Experimental details are given under Materials and Methods.

related cell lines we could attempt a thorough investigation of the selective cytotoxicity of DCX, the initial findings have been reported here.

Transformation of 802c cells with SV40 (804csc cells) renders them sensitive to the cytotoxicity of DCX. DCX at a concentration of 2.5 ng/ml (3×10^{-9}M) is able to kill 804csc cultures whereas, under the same conditions 100 ng/ml DCX is unable to kill 802c cells. DCX cytotoxicity to 804csc cells is characterized by an inhibition in DNA synthesis within the first 24 hr (approximately 50% of control at 10 ng/ml DCX), followed by a period of very retarded growth. During this stage the cells show increasing cytopathological signs. Morphological distortion, membrane blebbing, lipid droplets, and vesicle-like formation are the prominent features visualized by phase-contrast microscopy. After 10-12 days in culture with DCX the cells disintegrate. Treatment of 802c cells with DCX up to 100 ng/ml does not lead to the effects described for 804csc cells. DNA synthesis and growth is inhibited to some extent at the high concentrations of DCX (approximately 70% of control at 100 ng/ml), however, the cells continue to grow to confluency and remain viable for at least 5 weeks.

To gain some insight into the mechanism by which DCX kills 804csc cells, the cytotoxicity of DCX was examined with regard to the media components. Increasing the serum concentration of the media to 20% did not significantly alter the effects of DCX on cell growth. This result indicates that the cytotoxicity of DCX is not due to an expiration of the serum in the media. Lowering the serum concentration to sub-optimal levels for growth, also did not significantly alter the effect of DCX with respect to controls. The fact that cells growing slowly are equally affected as the more quickly dividing cells, implies that the selectivity of DCX mediated cytotoxicity is more complex than a simple correlation with doubling time.

The level of glucose in the media can dramatically alter the cytotoxic response to DCX. When 804csc cells are grown in low-glucose media (1 g/l) with 10 ng/ml DCX, the cultures die within 5 days (in contrast to 12 days in media with 4.5 g/1 glucose). Testing the media of such cultures for glucose showed that the cells had abnormal glucose utilization, and the more rapid death was probably due to glucose starvation. 2-deoxy-D-glucose uptake experiments showed that DCX increases glucose uptake for both 802c cells and 804csc cells. An important implication of this observation is that the 802c cells are affected by very low doses of DCX. In fact, at 2.5 ng/ml DCX, 802c cells showed a greater stimulation in deoxy-glucose uptake (47%) than the 804csc cells (22.6%). This implies that selective cytotoxicity of DCX to 804csc cells is most likely not due to a difference in the binding of DCX to the two cell types. This is further supported by the hydrophobic nature of DCX which is likely to be able to bind any membrane nonspecifically.

An increase of glucose uptake in cells which have a decreased growth rate may indicate an interference with cellular energy production. This phenomena has been reported for other antibiotics (1), specifically those which uncouple oxidative phosphorylation and thus induce the "Pasteur effect" i.e. an increase in glycolysis in response to a decrease in oxidative phosphorylation (18). The Pasteur effect may be occurring in cells treated with DCX. However, many other possibilities still exist. Metabolic interference may come from more general damage by perturbing the integrity of membranes causing permeability changes (17). The structural and biological similarities between DCX and other bacterial compounds which interfere with membrane function and permeability indicate that the plasma membrane is also likely to be a site of DCX action. It is not yet clear why the untransformed cells are able to survive in the presence of DCX, but the data we have so far imply that the resistance of 802c cells is due to their ability to adapt and cope with the harm induced by DCX. This theory is in line with the fact that many transformed cells, especially those transformed by DNA viruses, are unable to survive conditions which arrest proliferation (34).

The production of DCX has not yet been optimized under our own laboratory conditions. Our efforts in cultivation of **Serratia marcescens** 08 have yielded 50-100 fold less DCX than the batch grown for us by Merck, Sharp, and Dohme, determined by percent of dry weight. We believe this discrepancy is most likely due to the differences in culture conditions. The production of DCX by bacteria grown by us was determined by Rf values in two different TLC systems and by the chromium release assay with P815 cells. Four other **Serratia marcescens** strains (ATCC # 60, 13477, 14223, 27857) grown under our conditions have not produced quantities of DCX identifiable by TLC, however, some extracts contained cytotoxic activity which may be due to related compounds or minute levels of DCX. However, the dose needed for TD50 was at least 3-4 magnitudes higher than for the extracts from **Serratia marcescens** 08 strain. The production of DCX in other strains is also likely to vary with respect to culture conditions, and requires further evaluation. The production of DCX appears to be dependent on cultivation conditions as well as the strain of bacteria. This implies that the occurrence of DCX as a contaminant in crude ET preparations is likely to vary greatly.

The renewed interest of experimental as well as clinical scientists in the use of biological response modifiers (see Science 237: 848-850, 1987) as antitumor agents revives the attention which was paid to bacterial products several decades ago. Going even further back in history, one has to recall the results of W. Coley, published in 1895 describing the curative effect of a "mixed bacterial toxin" (MBT) consisting of **B. prodigiosus (Serratia marcescens)** and **B. erysipelatos (Streptococcus pyogenes)** bacteria and their products (9). Coley and his followers reported excellent results in the treatment of lymphosarcoma with MBT (for review see Ref. 21). Shear and coworkers at the NCI started experimental studies as a continuation of Coley's pioneering trials and isolated a polysaccharide from another Serratia strain (35). This preparation had antitumor effects in mice, but the efforts to put this to clinical use brought disappointing results. It was determined later that Shear's polysaccharide consisted mostly of ET (36, 37).

We discovered the heterogeneity of ET in 1966 (25, 29). It was later found that not only are the TCA or phenol-water extracted smooth ET preparations highly heterogeneous but rough mutant ET samples also consist of a number of endotoxic and nonendotoxic components (29). We found that there are components among these which are not toxic, but show other biological activities. The significance of the heterogeneity was repeatedly emphasized by us but remained largely ignored by the scientific community until, in 1975, several papers appeared reporting on the intrinsic heterogeneity of various ETs (3, 8, 13, 15).

These studies of the heterogeneity of ET preparations resulted in the discovery of two non-endotoxic components present in some but not all ET preparations. These two compounds have quite divergent chemical compositions and they manifest their antitumor effects by different mechansims. One compound can activate murine NK cells, induce bone marrow cell colony formation (CSF) and the complete regression of Meth A sarcoma in mice (30). This has been named NK activator or NKA. The other compound DCX, excelled as a cytotoxic agent on P815 mastocytoma cells in a picogram/ml range in vitro (16). Normal fibroblasts are much less sensitive to this cytotoxic agent which we call DCX.

There are numerous reports in the literature which describe the cumulative or even synergistic antitumor effect of various chemotherapeutic agents (2, 10, 31). Coley's "mixed bacterial toxin" (MBT) is a combination of several bacterial products. In the toxin **Serratia marcescens** was co-cultured with **Streptococcus pyogenes.** The bacterial products released into the supernatant formed the preparation named MBT. Coley and his followers reported excellent results in the treatment of lymphosarcoma with MBT, but Shear, who used a different strain of Serratia for experimental as well as clinical trials, could not reproduce the high curative rate reported by Coley. Our results, as they stand today, may offer some possible explanation of the discrepancy. It is possible that Coley had the proper Serratia isolate (this strain is no longer available) and Shear did not. It is tempting to speculate that Coley's Serratia strain produced DCX and NKA (in addition to ET), which made it particularly potent as a source of antitumor preparations. Carrying this speculation a step further, it is possible that the Serratia used by Coley produced DCX and NKA, and the Streptococcus he used had the same components as Picibanil, a preparation marketed today by the Japanese Chugay Pharmaceutical Co. Ltd., for cancer therapy. Picibanil (or OK-432) is an unfractionated freeze-dried suspension of an undisclosed **Streptococcus pyogenes** strain. The two bacterial strains used by Coley are not available anymore and that may be the reason why the excellent results obtained by using the old MBT could not be reproduced by the application of recent MBT preparations.

ACKNOWLEDGEMENTS

This work was supported by N.I.H. grants # CA-24628 and # 5T32-DE07085.

REFERENCES

1. Blum, S. T., Shohet, S. B., Nathan, D. G., and Gardner, F. H., 1969, The effect of amphotericin B on erythrocyte membrane cation permeability: its relation to in vivo erythrocyte survival. J. Lab. Clin. Med. 73: 980.

2. Butler, R. C., and Nowotny, A., 1979, Combined immunostimulation in the prevention of tumor take in mice using endotoxins, their derivatives and other immune adjuvants. Cancer Immunol. Immunotherapy. 6: 255.

3. Buttke, T. M., and Ingram, L. O., 1975, Comparison of lipopolysaccharides from **Agmenellus quadriplicatum** to **Escherichia coli** and **Salmonella typhimurium** by using thin-layer chromatography. J. Bacteriol. 124: 1566.

4. Chang, C., Simmons, D. T., Martin, M. A., and Mora, P. T., 1979, Identification and partial characterization of new antigens from simian virus 40-transformed mouse cells. J. Virol. 31: 463.

5. Chang, C. M., and Nowotny, A., 1975, Relation of structure to function in bacterial O-antigens VII. Endotoxicity of 'Lipid A'. Immunochem. 12: 19.

6. Chen, C. H., Chang, C. M., Nowotny, A. M., and Nowotny, A., 1975, Rapid biological and chemical analysis of bacterial endotoxins separated by preparative thin-layer chromatography. Anal. Biochem. 63: 183.

7. Chen, C. H., Johnson, A. G., Kasai, N., Key, B. A., Levin, J., and Nowotny, A., 1973, Heterogeneity and biological activity of endotoxin glycolipid from **Salmonella minnesota** R595. J. Infect. Dis. 128: s43.

8. Chester, I. R., and Meadow, P. M., 1975, Heterogeneity of lipopolysaccharide from **Psuedomonas aeruginosa**. Eur. J. Biochem. 58: 621.

9. Coley, W. B., 1985, The treatment of inoperable malignant tumors with the toxins of erysipelas and **Bacillus prodigiosus**. Med. Rec. 47: 65.

10. Dye, E. S., and North, R. J., 1980, Macrophage accumulation in murine ascites tumors. I. Cytoxan-induced dominance of macrophages over tumor cells and the antitumor effect of endotoxin. J. Immunol. 125: 1650.

11. Freid, M., and Prives, C., 1986, The biology of simian virus 40 and polyomer virus, in: "Cancer cells IV. DNA tumor viruses", M. Botchan, E. Grubzicker, P. A. Sharp, eds., Cold Spring Harbor Laboratory, NY.

12. Friedman, H., Blanchard, D. K., Newton, C., Klein, T., Stewart II, W., Keler, T., and Nowotny, A., 1987, Distinctive immunomodulatory effects of endotoxin and nontoxic lipopolysaccharide derivatives in lymphoid cell cultures. J. Biol. Response Mod. 6: 664.

13. Gmeiner, J., 1975, The isolation of two different lipopolysaccharide fractions from various **Proteus mitabilis** strains. Eur. J. Biochem. 58: 621.

14. Grohsman, J., and Nowotny, A., 1972, The immune recognition of TA3 tumors, its facilitation by endotoxin and abrogation by ascites fluid. J. Immunol. 109: 1090.

15. Jann, B., Reske, K., and Kann, J., 1975, Heterogeneity of lipopolysaccharides. Analysis of polysaccharide chain lengths by sodium dodecylsulfate-polyacrylamide gel electrophoresis. Eur. J. Biochem. 60: 239.

16. Keler, T., Kovats, E., Nguyen, V., Samu, J., Sanavi, F., Somlyo, B., and Nowotny, A., 1987, Cytotoxicity of a novel lipid-like bacterial product. Biochem. Biophys. Res. Comm. 149: 1033.

17. Kinsky, S. C., 1970, Antibiotic interaction with model membranes. Annu. Rev. Pharmacol. 10: 119.

18. Krebs, H. A., 1972, The Pasteur effect and the relations between respiration and fermentation, in: "Essays in Biochemistry", P. N. Campbell and F. Dickens, eds., Academic Press, Vol. 8.

19. Lampen, J. O., 1966, Interference by antifungal antibiotics (especially nysstatin and filipin) with specific membrane functions, in: "Biochemical studies of antimcrobial drugs", B. A. Newton, P. E. Reynolds, eds., Cambridge Univ. Press.

20. McFarland, V. W., Mora, P. T., Schultz, A., and Pancake, S., 1975, Cell properties after repeated transplantation of spontaneously and of SV40 virus transformed mouse cell lines. I. Growth in culture. J. Cell Physiol. 85: 101.

21. Nauts, H. C., Swift, W. E., and Coley, B. L., 1946, The treatment of malignant tumors by bacterial toxins as developed by the late William B. Coley, M.D., reviewed in the light of modern research. Cancer Res. 1: 731.

22. Ng, A. K., Butler, C., Chen, C. H., and Nowotny, A., 1976, Relationship of structure to function in bacterial endotoxins IX. Differences in the lipid moiety of endotoxic glycolipids. J. Bacteriol. 126: 511.

23. Nowotny, A., 1961, Chemical structure of a phosphomucolipid and its occurrence in some strains of Salmonella. J. Am. Chem. Soc. 83: 501.

24. Nowotny, A., 1963, Relations of structure to function in bacterial O-antigens II. Fractionation of lipids present in Boivin-type endotoxin of **Serratia marcescens**. J. Bacteriol. 85: 127.

25. Nowotny, A., 1966, Heterogeneity of endotoxic bacterial lipopolysaccharides revealed by ion-exchange chromatography. Nature 210: 278.

26. Nowotny, A., 1971, Chemical and biological heterogeneity of endotoxins, in: "Microbial Toxins, Vol. 4: Bacterial Endotoxins", G. Weinbaum, S. Kadis, S. J. Ajl, eds., Academic Press, New York-London.

27. Nowotny, A., 1984, Heterogeneity of endotoxins, in: "Handbook of Endotoxins, Vol. I", E. T. Rietschel, ed., Elsevier Science Publishers, Amsterdam.

28. Nowotny, A., Abdelnoor, A., Behling, U. H., Butler, R. C., Johnson, A. G., and Nowotny, A. M., 1982, Molecular aspects of the adjuvant and other beneficial effects of endotoxins, in: "Immunomodulation by microbial products and related synthetic compounds", Y. Yamura, S. Kotani, eds., Elsevier Science Publishing Co., Amsterdam.

29. Nowotny, A., Cundy, K. R., Neale, N. L., Nowotny, A. M., Radvany, R., Thomas, S. P., and Tripodi, D. J., 1966, Relationship of structure to function in bacterial O-antigens IV. Fractionation of the components. Ann. N.Y. Acad. Sci. 133: 586.

30. Nowotny, A., Keler, T., Pham, P.H., Kovats, E., Aiello, A., Shonekan, O., Friedman, H., and Johnson, A. G., 1988, Isolation of a nonendotoxic antitumor preparation from **Serratia marcescens**. J. Biol. Response Mod. 7: 296.

31. Ribi, E., Parker, R., Strain, S. M., Mizuno, Y., Nowotny, A., von Eschen, K. B., Cantrell, J. L., McLaughlin, C. A., Hwand, K. M., and Goren, M. B., 1979, Peptides as requirements for immunotherapy of the guinea-pig line- 10 tumor with endotoxins. Cancer Immunol. Immunotherapy. 7: 43.

32. Rothman, Y., Johnson, A. G., Friedman, H., Kovats, E., Pham, P. H., Sanavi, F., Nowotny, A. M., and Nowotny, A., 1985, Biological effects of White-type polysaccharide of Gram-negative bacteria. J. Biol. Response Mod. 4: 169.

33. Samu, J., Kovats, E., Nguyen, V., Keler, T., and Nowotny, A., 1988, Thin-layer chromatography of endotoxins, their derivatives and contaminants. J. Chromatog. 435: 167.

34. Schiaffonati, L., and Baserga, R., 1977, Different survival of normal and transformed cells exposed to nutritional conditions nonpermissive for growth. Cancer Res. 37: 541.

35. Shear, M. J., 1941, Effect of a concentrate from **B. prodigiosus** filtrate on subcutaneous primary induced mouse tumors. Cancer Res. 1: 731.

36. Shear, M. J., and Andervont, H. B., 1936, Chemical treatment of tumors. III Separation of hemorrhage-producing fraction of B. coli filtrate. Proc. Soc. Exp. Biol. Med. 34: 323.

37. Shear, M. J., and Turner, F. C., 1943, Chemical treatment of tumors. V. Isolation of hemorrhage-producing fraction from **Serratia marcescens** (**Bacillus prodigiosus**) culture filtrate. J. Natl. Cancer Inst. 4: 81.

38. Tooze, J., 1980, DNA tumor viruses, in: "Molecular Biology of Tumor Viruses, 2nd ed.", J. Tooze, ed., Cold Spring Harbor Laboratory, NY.

39. Winterbourne, D. J., and Mora, P. T., 1978, Altered metabolism of heparan sulfate in simian virus 40 transformed clonal mouse cells. J. Biol. Chem. 253: 5109.

PORIN AS A COMPONENT OF YERSINIA PSEUDOTUBERCULOSIS ENDOTOXIN

Yu. S. Ovodov, T. F. Solovjeva, V. A. Khomenko, O. D. Novikova, G. M. Frolova, I. M. Yermak, and G. A. Naberezhnykh

Pacific Institute of Bioorganic Chemistry, Far-Eastern Branch of USSR Academy of Sciences, Vladivostok-22, U.S.S.R.

Lipopolysaccharide-protein complexes isolated from the cell walls of gram-negative bacteria are known as endotoxins. Lipopolysaccharide (LPS) plays a critical role in the host response to a bacterial endotoxin. There is an experimental evidence for independent biological activity of the protein component of endotoxin itself. However, its contribution to the biological activity of endotoxin has not been sufficiently appreciated. The structure and properties of the endotoxin protein component have been poorly investigated. It may be partly explained by the complex composition of the protein moiety: it consists of a number of distinct proteins, which probably differ between individual endotoxin preparations. It was only recently shown, that the LPS-protein complex containing a single protein can be prepared (8). Owing to its simple protein composition, the endotoxin from Yersinia pseudotuberculosis is suitable to investigate the protein component.

The endotoxin was extracted from whole cells of Y. pseudotuberculosis with a cold trichloroacetic acid (TCA) and purified by Sepharose 2B chromatography. The endotoxin was covered as a relatively homogeneous LPS-protein complex with a density of 1.40 g/ml which was determined by CsCl density gradient ultracentrifugation. The protein component of endotoxin consisted of two polypeptides with an apparent molecular weights of 40 kDa and 14.5 kDa (9:1 w/w, respectively). Electrophoretic mobility in SDS-PAGE and N-terminal amino acid of the major protein (40 kDa) coincided with those of porin from Y. pseudotuberculosis. A comparison of the amino acid composition of this protein (40 kDa) with published data on porin of Y. pseudotuberculosis (5) revealed striking similarity. In addition, the peptide maps of the trypsinolysed products of the fully denatured forms of both proteins were also similar. From the data presented above, it may be concluded that the major protein of Y. pseudotuberculosis endotoxin appears to be porin.

Porins are known to exist in the outer bacterial membrane as trimeric complexes with three identical subunits (4). It is not clear whether the porin maintains its native form during the procedure of isolation of endotoxin from bacterial cells. As has earlier been established, irreversible conformational changes of porin occurred at low pH (3). On the other hand, specific LPS-protein interactions could be expected to increase pH stability of porin. So, it was shown that the B-octylglucoside-porin complexes in solution can protect the protein structure against the denaturing conditions of low pH (3).

To detect the porin form in Y. pseudotuberculosis endotoxin, the following experiments were carried out. The porin with 10% LPS was isolated from the endotoxin by preparative SDS-PAGE under conditions described earlier (7). This procedure removed LPS from porin without loss of protein structure. This crude protein was sedimented in the cesium chloride gradient as a single band with a density of 1.36 g/ml and migrated in SDS-PAGE as a single protein band with apparent molecular weight of about 110 kDa. The above characteristics of the porin component of endotoxin were similar to those of porin trimers of Y. pseudotuberculosis prepared according to the procedure described by Reithmeier and Bragg (6) and purified on Sephacryl in the presence of SDS. The porin component of endotoxin and the isolated porin showed identical properties in planar lipid bilayer membranes (BLM). As shown by analysis of conductance fluctuations of BLM, the most frequent conductance steps were 160 and 240 pS.

Chemical cross-linking provides a useful tool for the study of protein organization. When endotoxin, its porin component and the porin were treated with dimethylsuberimidate in the presence of SDS, a new protein band was observed in all samples in SDS-PAGE. This band corresponded in molecular weight to the trimer of porin and was resistant to boiling in SDS solution. These results suggest the presence of oligomeric protein, trimer, in the initial samples.

By using serological analyses, it was shown that the antigenic determinants specific for porin trimer were expressed on the protein component of endotoxin. Indeed, when rabbit anti-porin trimer serum was pre-adsorbed with LPS and active porin monomer (33.5 kDa) obtained by method (9), a residual population of antibodies remained, which could be detected with porin trimer and protein component of endotoxin.

Taking all these facts together, it may be concluded that at least in part the porin is present as a trimer in endotoxin of Y. pseudotuberculosis. Associated LPS appears to protect the porin from acid denaturation.

Effect of the porin on the physicochemical properties of the LPS in endotoxin of Y. pseudotuberculosis seems to be revealed. Investigations of hydrodynamic properties of pure LPS and endotoxin showed that both formed large polydisperse aggregates in aqueous solution, their molecular weights being dependent on the solution's concentration. At equal concentrations of both compounds, molecular weight of LPS was nearly twice the value found for endotoxin. It should be noted that the content of divalent cations and the average size of O-polysaccharide chains in these compounds were essentially similar. Interactions between the particles in solution were significantly stronger for pure endotoxin than for LPS. The aggregates of LPS and these of endotoxin had a different morphology also (10).

Variations in physical behavior of O-polysaccharide chains between LPS and endotoxin were detected. The carbohydrate chains mobility in endotoxin was higher than that in LPS. As a result, ^{13}C-NMR spectrum signal lines of LPS carbohydrate chains were essentially broader in comparison with those of endotoxin ones (2). In addition, the accessibility of the antigenic determinants expressed on O-polysaccharide chains of both LPS and endotoxin to antibodies was different. At the equal concentrations, the endotoxin bound 1.7 times more Fab-fragments of specific antibodies per one repeating unit of O-polysaccharide chain than LPS did. These data appear to support a previous suggestion that the protein when associated with LPS, disorders its carbohydrate region (1).

Thus, the protein component of endotoxin affecting physical state of LPS may probably modify its biological properties and contribute this way to the biological activity of endotoxin.

REFERENCES

1. Coughlin, R. T., Haug, A. and McGroarty, E. J., 1983, Electron spin resonance probing of lipopolysaccharide domains in the outer membrane of Escherichia coli. Biochim. Biophys. Acta. 729: 161.

2. Krasikova, I. N., Isakov, V. V., Fedoreeva, L. I., Solovjeva, T. F. and Ovodov, Yu. S., 1988, Application of lipopolysaccharide-protein complexes ^{13}C-NMR spectra for establishement of O-specific polysaccharide structure. Bioorgan. Khim. (USSR) 14:419.

3. Markovic-Housley, Z. and Garavito, R., 1986, Effect of temperature and low pH on structure and stability of matrix porin in micellar detergent solutions. Biochim. Biophys. Acta. 869: 158.

4. Nakae, T., Ishii, J. and Tokunaga, M., 1979, Subunit structure of functional porin oligomers that form channels in the outer membrane of Escherichia coli. J. Biol. Chem. 154: 1457.

5. Novikova, O., Zykova, T., Yadykina, G., Glazunov, V., Solovjeva, T. and Ovodov, Yu., 1985, Study of yersinin, a major protein from outer membrane of Yersinia pseudotuberculosis. Biol. Membrany (USSR) 2: 714.

6. Reithmeier, R. and Bragg, P., 1974, Purification and characterization of a heat-modifiable protein from the outer membrane of Escherichia coli. FEBS Lett. 44: 195.

7. Rocque, W., Coughlin, R. T. and McGroarty, E. J., 1987, Lipopolysaccharide tightly bound to porin monomers and trimers from Escherichia coli k-12. J. Bacteriol. 169: 4003.

8. Strittmatter, W. and Galanos, C., 1987, Characterization of protein coextracted together with LPS in Escherichia coli, Salmonella minnesota and Yersinia enterocolitica. Microb. Pathogen. 2: 29.

9. Weckesser, J., Zalman, L. and Nikaido, H., 1984, Porin from Rhodo pseudomonas sphaeroides. J. Bacteriol. 159: 199.

10. Yermak, I. M., Drozdov, A. P., Solovjeva, T. F. and Ovodov, Yu. S., 1986, Lipopolysaccharide-protein complex from Yersinia pseudotuberculosis outer membranes. Physicochemical properties and morphology. Biol. Membrany (USSR) 3: 52.

LIPOPOLYSACCHARIDES OF NON-CHOLERA VIBRIOS POSSESSING COMMON ANTIGEN FACTOR TO 01 **VIBRIO CHOLERAE**

K. Hisatsune, Y. Haishima, T. Iguchi and S. Kondo

Department of Microbiology, School of Pharmaceutical Sciences
Josai University, Sakado, Saitama 350-02, Japan

INTRODUCTION

01 **Vibrio cholerae** is divided into two major serological types, Ogawa and Inaba, on the basis of their heat stable somatic antigen (or O antigen). These two serotypes share group somatic antigen A, but can be separated by Ogawa factor B and Inaba factor C. This is generally accepted as so-called ABC concept for the O-antigenic structure of 01 **V. cholerae** (4, 11). Recently, three groups of non-cholera vibrios possessing common antigen factors of 01 **V. cholerae** have been isolated in Japan. First, a marine vibrio, **Vibrio** bio-serogroup 1875 Original was isolated from sea water in Osaka Bay. Besides its Inaba antigenic variant, so called **Vibrio** bio-serogroup 1875 Variant was isolated (13). Second, **Vibrio fluvialis** Kobe was isolated from imported squid in Kobe (14). Third, **Vibrio cholerae** bio-serogroup Hakata was isolated from sea water in Hakata Bay, Kyushu island (12). The last group, Hakata strain, has now become of current importance in Japan from the public health point of view, in particular, in quarantine administration. At least 31 strains of this group have already been isolated in Japan; 9 of them from imported squid and shrimp, and 22 from the environment. This will probably become a more important public health problem soon, because they may be misdiagnosed as 01 **V. cholerae** unless a polyclonal absorbed antiserum or monoclonal antibody for the single factor A of 01 **V. cholerae** is used. As long as present commercial diagnostic sera for 01 V. cholerae are used in practical bacteriological examination, it is impossible to distinguish 01 **V. cholerae** from this group. Antigenic formulae for their O-antigenic structures were recently elucidated by Shimada and Sakazaki, National Institute of Health, Tokyo, Japan, by cross-agglutination and cross- agglutinin absorption test as shown in Fig 1.

They were found to possess either Ogawa factor B or Inaba factor C, or both B and C of 01 **V. cholerae** but they all lack its group antigenic factor A. In addition, factor D was recognized which is shared in common with all the three groups, factor E shared with 1875 Original, Variant and Kobe strain, and factor F in Hakata strain alone. Therefore, Kobe strain possesses factors C, D and E, thus its antigenic structure is identical to that of 1875 Variant while Hakata srain possesses C, D and F. The presence of B and C, and the lack of A were confirmed by using both factor sera and monoclonal antibodies against each of these three antigen factors.

In the present study, a comparative chemical and serological study, in

Antigenic structure							
01 Vibrio cholerae							
	Ogawa	A	B	(c)			
	Inaba	A		C			
Vibrio bio-serogroup 1875							
	Original		B	(c)	D	E	
	Variant			C	D	E	
Vibrio fluvialis 181-86 (Kobe)				C	D	E	
Vibrio cholerae "Hakata"				C	D		F

Fig 1. O-antigenic structure of 01 **Vibrio cholerae** and the related vibrios.

particular, compositional sugar analysis, was carried out on O-antigenic lipopolysaccharides (LPS) isolated from **Vibrio** bio-serogroup 1875 Original and Variant, **V. fluvialis** Kobe and **V. cholerae** Hakata, and the results were compared with those obtained with LPS from 01 V. cholerae.

MATERIALS AND METHODS

Strains of the groups 1875, Kobe and Hakata employed in the present study were provided from Drs. T. Shimada and R. Sakazaki, National Institute of Health, Tokyo. Strains of the group Hakata were provided from Drs. H. Abe, Osaka Quarantine Office and H. Shimodori, School of Medicine, Kyushu University. Hakata strains were cultivated in nutrient broth (pH 7.8) at 37°C for 16 hr. 1875 and Kobe strains were cultivated in nutrient broth (pH 7.2) containing 1.5% NaCl at 28°C for 16 hr. After killing by heating at 120°C for 20 min, cells were harvested and washed with distilled water by centrifugation, and then acetone dried. The acetone dried cells were at first extracted by Galanos's phenol-chloroform-petroleum ether (PCP) method (5) which is generally used for the extraction of LPS or glycolipid from R-form gram-negative bacteria. The residual cells were then extracted by Westphal's phenol-water method (16) for the extraction of LPS from S-form gram-negative bacteria. LPS were purified by repeated ultracentrifugation and RNase treatment. Neutral sugars except for fructose were analysed by gas-liquid chromatography (column; 3% ECNSS-M, 3 mm x 2 m) as alditol acetate derivatives after hydrolysis in 2 N trifluoroacetic acid at 120°C for 1 hr. Fructose was analyzed by gas-liquid chromatography using the same column as mentioned above as O-acetyl-O-methyl oxime derivative after hydrolysis in 5% acetic acid at 100°C for 2 hr. For the analyses of neutral sugars, xylose was used as internal standard. Amino sugars except perosamine were analysed by gas-liquid chromatography (column; TABSORB, 3 mm x 2 m) as N-acetylated-O-acetylalditol acetate derivatives after hydrolysis in 4N HCL at 100°C for 8 hr. For the analysis of perosamine, samples were hydrolysed in 10M HCl at 90°C for 15 min, and then analysed by the same way as mentioned above. Neutral and amino sugars were identified based on their retention time values in gas-liquid chromatographic analysis and mass spectrum in GC/MS analysis compared with those of the authentic standards. Heptose was determined either by the method of Osborn (10) or by gas-liquid chromatography. Standard **L**-glycero- and **D**-glycero-**D**-mannoheptose were prepared as described by Bagdian et al. (1). KDO was analysed by Weissbach's periodate-thiobarbituric acid test (15). KDO (ammonium salt) used as standard and alkaline phosphatase (Type III-R) were purchased from Sigma Chemical Co. (St. Louis, MO). High-voltage paper electrophoresis was performed using the solvent system pyridine/acetic acid/water (10:4:86), at 50 v/cm for 45 min. Gel-chromatography of degraded polysaccharide (DPS) was performed with Sephadex G-50 column (1.6 x 100 cm) using the solvent system pyridine/ acetic acid/water (10:4:1000) as an effluent at a flow rate of 1.3 ml/hr.

RESULTS AND DISCUSSION

Of particular interest was that S-type LPS of Hakata strains were isolated from phenol-phase but not from water-phase in the Westphal's phenol-water technique in contrast to usual gram-negative bacterial LPS.

The results of sugar analysis of S-type LPS from 1875, Kobe and Hakata strains are presented in Table 1 in comparison with those of 01 **V. cholerae.** These LPS contained all the component sugars present in LPS of 01 **V. cholerae** except for the absense of fructose in Kobe LPS. Glucose, heptose, (that is L-glycero-D-mannoheptose), and glucosamine were found as common component sugar in all LPS of these 4 groups of vibrios examined. Of the three sugars, in general, glucose and L-glycero-D-manno-heptose are considered to be the regular components of the core region of the usual gram-negative bacterial LPS, while glucosamine is considered to be the basic structural unit of their lipid A diglucosaminide backbone. In fact, this was also the case with all LPS of these 4 vibrios as shown later. Galactose present in Hakata LPS was also found to be derived from their core region. On the other hand, it is noticed that, as additional component sugars, galactose, mannose, two unknown neutral sugars NS I and II, and relatively large amounts of uronic acid were found in Kobe LPS, and galactose, mannose and an unknown amino sugar (AS) in Hakata LPS. With respect to uronic acid contained in Kobe LPS, two kinds of uronic acid were identified; one is glucuronic acid of strongly bound type and the other is galacturonic acid that is easily released from LPS by heating in 5% acetic acid at 100°C.

2-Keto-3-deoxyoctonate (KDO), a regular component sugar of the usual gram-negative bacterial LPS, was not detected by the conventional Weissbach's periodate-thiobarbituric acid test under the conventional hydrolysis conditions in LPS of the three groups of vibrios. This apparent undetectability of KDO in LPS was already observed with those isolated from the other members of family Vibrionaceae (8).

However, after treatment of these LPS with strong acid (4N HCl, at 100°C, for 45 min), the hydrolysate released a Weissbach's reaction-positive substance designated as X, yielding a color with maximal absorption at 549 nm, which is identical to that yielded by standard KDO.

Table 1. Sugar composition of LPS isolated from **V. cholerae, Vibrio** Bio-Serogroup 1875 and **V. Fluvialis** 181-86 (KOBE) (Molar Ratio)

	Glc	Gal	Man	Fru	unknown NS[a)] I	unknown NS[a)] II	Hep	GlcN	GalN	QuiN	PerN	unknown[b)] AS	Uronic acid	KDO
P1418 (Ogawa)	1.0	–	–	0.8	–	–	3.0	1.6	–	0.6	8.4	–	–	nd[c)]
P1418-UV601 (Inaba)	0.9	–	–	0.8	–	–	3.0	1.4	–	1.1	12.0	–	–	nd
1875 Original	1.6	–	0.1	1.9	+	+	3.0	2.0	–	0.4	1.2	–	–	nd
1875 Variant	1.9	–	0.2	2.1	+	+	3.0	2.0	–	0.4	1.2	–	–	nd
V. fluvialis 181-86														
water phase LPS	3.0	0.1	0.1	–	+	+	3.0	2.0	0.1	0.4	0.6	–	4.5	nd
Hakata 487-85														
phenol phase LPS	2.8	1.4	0.7	1.5	–	–	3.0	2.1	–	1.3	0.8	6.7	–	nd

molar ratio; Heptose=3.0, a) NS; neutral sugar, b) AS; amino sugar, c) nd; not detectable by Weissbach's periodate-thiobarbituric acid test

X was isolated from the strong acid hydrolysates by Dowex 50 and Dowex 1 ion-exchange chromatography. Although the absorption spectrum of the reaction mixture of the partially purified X in Weissbach's test was the same as that of standard KDO, X was not identical to KDO with respect to stability in strong acid hydrolysis and behavior in high-voltage paper electrophoresis, as shown in Fig 2.

Furthermore, in high-voltage paper electrophoresis, X isolated from Hakata LPS was further separated into two Weissbach's reaction positive substances. A slow-moving substance with RKDO (mobility relative to KDO) value of 1.54 was identical to X1 and a fast-moving substance with RKDO value of 1.80 was identical to X2 both from 01 **V. cholerae** LPS. With regard to the occurrence of these thiobarbituric acid-test positive substances, X1 and X2, in the strong-acid hydrolysates of 01 **V. cholerae** LPS, we already reported them in the 20th U.S-Japan Joint Conference on Cholera in Nara, Japan, three years ago (9).

In contrast to X from Hakata LPS, that from either 1875 or Kobe LPS was not separated into two components, but it was identical to the slow-moving substance X1. As shown in Fig. 2, it was further found that both the slow-moving components are identical, in the paper electrophoresis, to 5-O-phosphoryl-KDO isolated from **Bordetella pertussis** (3).

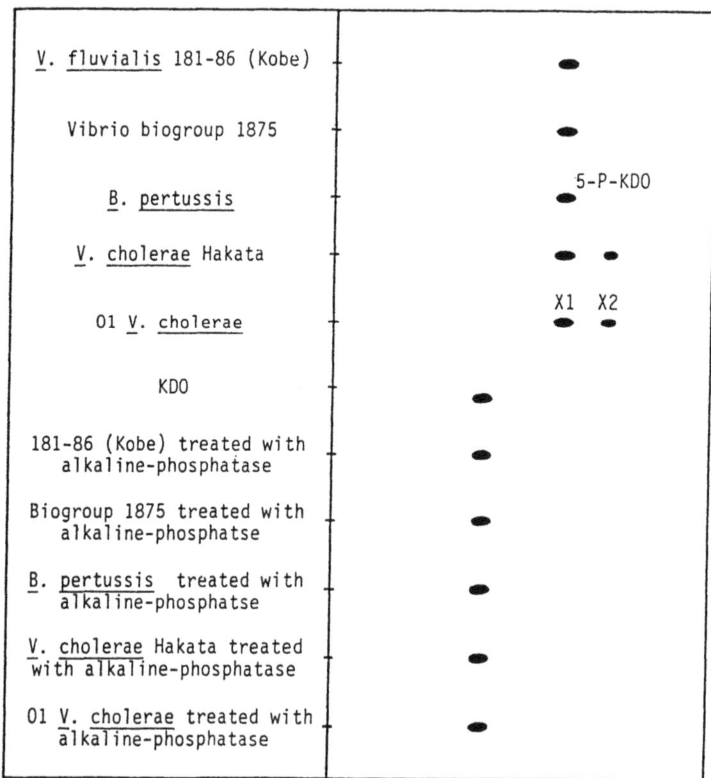

Spots were colorizated with periodate-thiobarbituric acid reagent for KDO

Fig 2. High voltage paper electrophoretic behaviors of 5-O-phosphorylated KDO from **B. pertussis** LPS and the unknown substances (X) present in the strong acid hydrolysate of **V. fluvialis**, **Vibrio** bio-serogroup 1875, **V. cholerae** Hakata and 01 **V. cholerae** LPS before and after treatment with alkaline-phosphatase.

The strong acid hydrolysates of these LPS were treated with alkaline phosphatase at 37°C for 16 hr, and then subjected to high-voltage paper electrophoresis. As shown in the lower part of Fig 2, the spots corresponding to X1 and X2 disappeared, and concomitantly a spot which had the same mobility as that of standard KDO appeared. These results probably support our contention that X1 and X2 are some kind of phosphorylated derivatives of KDO, and that, as far as the results of the high-voltage paper electrophoresis experiment show, X1 is likely 5-O-phosphoryl KDO. In this respect, it is relevant that Brade recently reported the isolation of 5-O- phosphoryl KDO from 01 **V. cholerae** LPS (2). The place of possible localization of X1 and X2 in LPS molecules of these vibrios is considered to be likely their core region, in particular, the inner core region, unless they are artifacts produced by the strong acid treatment of LPS.

The distribution of the component sugars between the core and O-specific side chain regions in LPS can often be determined by gel-filtration fractionation of degraded polysaccharide (DPS) isolated from LPS by mild acid hydrolysis. Typically, the elution profile from Sephadex G-50 gel-chromatography shows three peaks for Salmonella and E. coli. Fraction I, eluted in the void volume, corresponds to a polymeric O-specific side chain with attached core: Fraction III, to core oligosaccharide alone and Fraction IV to low-molecular-weight fragment, predominantly inorganic orthophosphate and KDO. Three peaks are also observed in the elution profile for DPS of 01 **V. cholerae**, Bio-serogroup 1875, Kobe water-phase and Hakata phenol phase LPS; Fraction II corresponds to the polymeric O-specific side chain with attached core, Fraction III to core oligosaccharide and Fraction IV to a monosaccharide fraction that contains fructose instead of KDO. Thus, the elution profiles of DPS of these 4 vibrios were found to be almost identical.

The results of compositional analysis of the three fractions obtained from DPS prepared from 1875, Kobe and Hakata LPS are presented in Table 2. As mentioned before, Fraction II corresponds to a polymeric O-antigenic side-chain plus the core oligosaccharide. Therefore, we can know the composition of the O-side chain by subtraction of the value of Fraction III from that of Fraction II; namely, the difference between Fraction II and III in the sugar composition represents that of the O-side chain of each vibrio.

The sugar composition of Fraction II from these 4 vibrios showed characteristic features of chemotaxonomic and antigenic interest. Mannose was found in common in three vibrios, bio-serogroup 1875, Kobe and Hakata, but not in 01 **V. cholerae.** The unknown neutral sugars NS I and II were found in both 1875 and Kobe, and the unknown amino sugar AS in Hakata. On the basis of this compositional pattern of Fraction II and the antigenic relationship among these 4 vibrios elucidated by Shimada and Sakazaki, it was indicated that mannose is probably associated with O-antigen factor D shared with bio-serogroup 1875, Original as well as Variant, Kobe and Hakata, the neutral sugars NS I and II with factor E shared with 1875 and Kobe, and factor F specifically with bio-serogroup Hakata.

With regard to the rarely occurring amino sugars perosamine and quinovosamine, they were demonstrated by us before to be substantially associated with 01-specificity of LPS from cholera vibrios. S-R mutation of cholera vibrios involves total elimination of these two component amino sugars of S-form LPS. This elimination results in the loss of O-specificity of S-form LPS and concomitant appearance of strong serological cross-reactivity among R-form LPS regardless of the serotype (Inaba or Ogawa) of their S parent strain (6). In the present study, the pair perosamine and quinovosamine was also found in common in Fraction II of all the 3 vibrios other than 01 **V. cholerae**, indicating that the same perosamine homopolymer is present in their LPS. However, the present analytical data indicated that its chain length in these three vibrios, in particular, Kobe and Hakata, is very short in con-

Table 2. Sugar composition of DPS fraction separated by sephadez G-50 gel-chromatography from **V. cholerae, V. fluvialis** and **Vibrio** bio-serogroup 1875 (molar ratio)

		Glc	Gal	Man	Fru	unknown NS[a] I	unknown NS[a] II	Hep	GlcN	GalN	PerN	QuiN	unknown[b] AS
Frc.II	P1418 (Ogawa)	0.9	–	–	–	–	–	3.0	–	–	18.0	1.7	–
	P1418-UV601 (Inaba)	0.7	–	–	–	–	–	3.0	–	–	18.0	1.7	–
	1875 Original	1.2	–	0.7	–	+	+	3.0	1.0	–	3.2	1.3	–
	1875 Variant	1.2	–	0.7	–	+	+	3.0	1.0	–	3.2	1.3	–
	Kobe water phase	2.8	–	0.7	–	+	+	3.0	0.1	0.1	2.1	1.2	–
	Hakata phenol phase	2.5	1.3	0.5	–	–	–	3.0	0.3	–	0.5	1.2	7.1
Frc.III	P1418 (Ogawa)	0.9	–	–	–	–	–	3.0	0.1	–	–	–	–
	P1418-UV601 (Inaba)	0.9	–	–	–	–	–	3.0	0.1	–	–	–	–
	1875 Original	1.2	–	–	–	–	–	3.0	1.2	–	–	–	–
	1875 Variant	1.2	–	–	–	–	–	3.0	1.2	–	–	–	–
	Kobe water phase	1.8	–	–	–	–	–	3.0	0.1	0.1	–	–	–
	Hakata phenol phase	2.5	1.1	–	–	–	–	3.0	0.3	–	–	–	–
Frc.IV	P1418 (Ogawa)	–	–	–	+++	–	–	–	–	–	–	–	–
	P1418-UV601 (Inaba)	–	–	–	+++	–	–	–	–	–	–	–	–
	1875 Original	–	–	–	+++	–	–	–	–	–	–	–	–
	1875 Variant	–	–	–	+++	–	–	–	–	–	–	–	–
	Kobe water phase	–	+	–	–	–	–	–	–	–	–	–	–
	Hakata phenol phase	–	–	–	+++	–	–	–	–	–	–	–	–

molar ratio; Heptose=3.0, a) NS; neutral sugar, b) AS; amino sugar

trast to that of the same homopolymer present in 01 **V. cholerae** P1418 LPS because the former two consist of, on average, only 2 and 0.5 repeating units, respectively, while the latter consists of 18 repeating units. As mentioned above, it is certain that the pair perosamine and quinovosamine is involved in the O-specificity of 01 **V. cholerae,** however, it is not yet known whether the pair is substantially associated with all or part of the antigenic factors A, B and C. Of particular interest was the occurrence of the amino sugar AS in considerable amounts in the O-side chain of Hakata LPS. Our preliminary chemical characterization indicates that this component is probably an N-acylated derivative of perosamine, but interestingly this N-acyl linkage is quite stable in contrast to the usual N-acyl-amino sugars under the usual acid hydrolysis conditions for sugar analysis where free perosamine is released from the linear perosamine homopolymer of at least 01 **V. cholerae** LPS.

Five years ago, we reported a simple and rapid method to prepare the sample for the compositional sugar analysis of the polysaccharide portion of LPS directly from **V. cholerae** cells without separating LPS (7). By using this method, 31 strains of bio-serogroup Hakata were examined for the sugar composition of the polysaccharide portion of their LPS; 22 of them were isolated from the environment and the other 9 from foods imported from the Phillipines, Bangladesh, India and Vietnam. They were isolated in Japan during the past 8 years in different places, and identified by using monoclonal antibodies against each of factor A, B and C, and also factor sera for them, in particular, anti-F factor serum prepared by Shimada and Sakazaki. Our results presented in Table 3 and 4 show that these Hakata strains are quite homogeneous in the sugar composition of their LPS. All strains contained mannose, the amino sugar AS characteristic of Hakata LPS, and small amounts of perosamine and quinovosamine in addition to the core sugar components, glucose and heptose. As an exception, only three of the 22 strains contained two additional sugar components, galactose and a trace of galactosamine. Thus, the strains isolated from the environment were separated into two groups, one possessing galactose and a trace of galactosamine, and the other lacking these sugars. All the strains isolated form imported foods

Table 3. Sugar composition of the polysaccharide portion of **V. cholerae** hakata LPS isolated by simple and rapid method (μg/g wet cell)

	Glc	Gal	Man	Fru	L-D Hep	GlcN	GalN	PerN	QuiN	unknown[a) AS
Isolated from environment										
NQ-1 (Estuarine water)	282.6	–	47.7	334.8	210.8	21.6	–	29.4	61.8	402.4
NQ-2 (")	249.1	–	47.7	316.8	173.2	25.0	–	28.8	68.2	343.3
NQ-3 (")	362.1	–	38.1	211.0	242.2	31.6	–	13.9	47.6	663.0
NQ-4 (")	256.9	–	39.9	212.5	239.2	42.6	–	23.0	82.0	633.5
NQ-5 (")	197.0	–	30.6	238.0	174.1	25.4	–	27.0	57.8	328.8
NQ-6 (")	261.9	–	32.8	230.0	177.9	22.2	–	26.2	54.2	340.7
NQ-7 (")	209.6	–	36.9	268.0	189.2	27.7	–	31.2	66.6	455.7
NQ-8 (")	251.1	–	42.5	258.8	220.6	33.9	–	33.7	78.9	455.8
NQ-9 (")	339.7	–	30.4	261.1	214.5	24.8	–	19.5	57.5	522.6
NQ-10 (")	297.7	–	41.7	231.6	250.2	22.2	–	30.2	95.1	588.0
NQ-11 (")	342.4	–	39.4	265.9	262.9	18.2	–	21.1	68.2	674.0
NQ-12 (")	442.7	–	46.4	274.2	249.6	31.6	–	30.4	93.6	569.4
NQ-13 (")	245.0	–	34.3	256.8	190.4	23.5	–	32.4	59.4	379.1
NQ-14 (")	235.9	–	39.2	264.0	211.3	26.5	–	32.8	64.5	408.2
NQ-15 (")	251.8	–	42.7	277.6	214.0	33.6	–	37.5	82.5	473.4
NQ-16 (")	223.7	–	35.7	264.4	181.4	28.4	–	33.1	69.9	476.3
NAHA-1 (River water)	274.6	–	46.5	286.0	241.9	28.9	–	36.6	83.1	559.0
683-85 (")	276.4	–	41.7	243.2	196.5	21.1	–	24.5	64.3	369.4
F-C1 (Sea water)	222.2	–	35.5	202.4	181.2	25.4	–	34.0	63.0	400.3
OQ-C1 (Sea water)	323.1	152.8	46.9	272.0	215.5	33.8	8.2	37.5	79.6	470.2
OQ-C3 (")	330.0	155.5	47.7	212.8	204.0	51.9	7.8	42.7	102.5	466.6
487-85 (")	377.9	177.8	47.5	234.0	218.4	39.9	9.3	35.7	81.3	453.2

a) unknown AS, unknown amino sugar determined as perosamine.

belonged to the second group. The values in the Table represent μg by weight per gram wet cells.

Phenotypically, bioserogroup Hakata is precisely **V. cholerae**, and as long as we use the present commercial anti-01 **V. cholerae** antisera in the practical bacteriological examination, as mentioned before, this group is diagnosed as 01 group. In the present study, the chemical properties of Hakata LPS were investigated for the first time, and it was demonstrated that this group is distinguishable from 01 group by the presence of mannose and the amino sugar AS in their LPS. We think we have come to the point where we should think about a redefinition of 01 V. cholerae and consider whether or not we should classify such **V. cholerae** as bio-serogroup Hakata possessing antigen factor C but lacking major common antigen factor A of 01 **V. cholerae** into non-01 group of **Vibrio cholerae.**

Table 4. Sugar composition of the polysaccharide portion of **V. cholerae** Hakata LPS isolated by the simple and rapid method (μg/g wet cell)

	Glc	Gal	Man	Fru	L-D Hep	GlcN	GalN	PerN	QuiN	unknown[a) AS
Isolated from imported foods										
772-82 (Shrimp)	228.6	–	39.9	268.0	174.6	25.2	–	29.4	72.4	309.1
TQ-C1 (")	199.2	–	33.0	248.8	192.1	25.6	–	25.1	55.4	317.1
TQ-C2 (Cuttlefish)	197.8	–	31.7	201.6	171.7	18.6	–	25.7	46.7	431.6
TQ-C3 (")	346.1	–	45.1	181.7	242.5	16.3	–	17.9	70.9	682.6
TQ-C4 (")	328.0	–	43.8	159.6	242.0	31.4	–	18.0	73.6	627.8
TQ-C5 (")	204.0	–	28.6	193.6	202.3	18.7	–	37.6	56.5	423.1
KQ-C1 (")	137.8	–	21.5	171.0	142.1	20.7	–	24.5	60.3	237.2
KQ-C2 (")	236.8	–	30.9	218.0	169.6	24.6	–	26.3	63.3	352.4
OQ-C2 (")	205.5	–	37.6	172.8	199.5	12.1	–	21.4	42.2	429.1

a) unknown AS, unknown amino sugar determined as perosamine.

ACKNOWLEDGMENT

Drs. T. Shimada and R. Sakazaki (National Institute of Health, Tokyo, Japan) are particularly acknowledged for their courtesy in providing us with the strains of **Vibrio** bioserogroup 1875, **V. fluvialis** 181-86 Kobe. We are also grateful to Drs. H. Abe (Osaka Quarantine Office) and H. Shimodori (School of Medicine, Kyushu University) for their courtesy in providing us with the strains of **V. cholerae** bio-serogroup Hakata.

REFERENCES

1. Bagdian, G., Droge, W., Kotelko, K., Luderitz, O., and Westphal, O., 1966, Vorkommen zweier Heptosen in Lipopolysacchariden entero-bacterieller Zellwande: **L**-glycero- and **D**-glycero-**D**-mannoheptose. Biochem. Z. 344: 197-211.

2. Brade, H., 1985, Occurrence of 2-keto-3-deoxy-octonic acid 5-phosphate in lipopolysaccharides of **Vibrio cholerae** Ogawa and Inaba. J. Bacteriol. 161: 795-798.

3. Chaby, R., and Szabo, L., 1975, 3-Deoxy-2-octulosonic acid 5-phosphate: a component of the endotoxin of **Bordetella pertussis.** Eur. J. Biochem. 59: 277-280.

4. Finkelstein, R. A., 1973, Cholera, C.R.C. Critical Reviews in Microbiology, 2: 553-623.

5. Galanos, C., Luderitz, O., and Westphal, O., 1969, A new method for the extraction of R lipopolysaccharides. Eur. J. Biochem. 9: 245-249.

6. Hisatsune, K., and Kondo, S., 1980, Lipopolysaccharides of R mutants isolated from **Vibrio cholerae.** Biochem. J. 185: 77-81.

7. Hisatsune, K., Yamamoto, F., and Kondo, S., 1985, Lipopolysaccaride of **Vibrio cholerae.** -Chemical and serological properties- , in: "Advances in Research on Cholera and Related Diarrheas", S. Kuwahara, and N. F. Pierce, eds., KTK Scientific Publishers, Tokyo, p. 17-24,

8. Hisatsune, K., Kondo, S., Iguchi, T., Yamamoto, F., Inaguma, M., Kokubo, S., and Arai, S, 1984, Lipopolysaccharides of the family Vibrionaceae, in: "Bacterial Endotoxin: Chemical, Biological and Clinical Aspects", J. Y. Homma, S. Kanegasaki, O. Luderitz, T. Shiba and O. Westphal, eds, Verlag Chemie, Basel, p. 187-201.

9. Kondo, S., Haishima, Y., and Hisatsune, K., 1988, Occurrence of thiobartiburic acid test-positive substance in lipopolysaccharides (LPS) of Vibrionaceae, in: "Advances in Research on Cholera and Related Diarrheas", S. Kuwahara, and N. F. Pierce, eds., KTK Scientific Publishers, Tokyo, p. 71-76.

10. Osborn, M. J., 1963, Studies on the gram-negative cell walls. I. Evidence for the role of 2-keto-3-deoxyoctonate in the lipopolysaccharide of **Salmonella typhimurium.** Proceedings of National Academy of Sciences of U.S.A. 50: 499-506.

11. Sakazaki, R., and Tamura, K., 1971, Somatic antigen variation in **Vibrio cholerae,** Japan. J. Med. Sci. Biol. 24: 93-100.

12. Shimada, T., and Sakazaki, R., 1988, A serogroup of non-01 **Vibrio cholerae** possessing the Inaba antigen of Vibrio cholerae 01. J. Appl. Bacteriol. 64: (in press).

13. Shimada, T., Sakazaki, R., and Oue, M., 1987, A bioserogroup of marine vibrios possessing somatic antigen factors in common with **Vibrio cholerae** 01. J. Appl. Bacteriol. 62: 453-456.

14. Shimada, T., Sakazaki, R., and Tobita, K., 1987, **Vibrio fluvialis:** A new serogroup (19) possessing the Inaba antigen of **Vibrio cholerae** 01. Japan. J. Med. Sci. Biol. 40: 153-157.

15. Weissbach, A., and Hurwitz, J., 1959, The formation of 2-keto-3-deoxyheptonic acid in extracts of Escherichia coli B. J. Biol. Chem. 234: 705-709.

16. Westphal, O., Luderitz, O., and Bister, R., 1952, Uber die Extraction von Bakterien mit Phenol/Wasser. Z. Naturforsch. 7b: 148-155.

IMMUNOCYTOCHEMICAL LOCALIZATION OF BACTERIAL LIPOPOLYSACCHARIDE WITH COLLOIDAL-GOLD PROBES IN DIFFERENT TARGET CELLS

A. M. Municio, S. Abarca, J. L. Carrascosa,* R. Garcia, I. Diaz-Laviada, M. J. Ainaga, M. T. Portoles, R. Pagani, C. Risco and M. A. Bosch

Department of Biochemistry & Molecular Biology, Faculty of Chemistry, Universidad Complutense, 28040-Madrid, Spain
*Centro de Biologia Molecular, Universidad Autonoma, 28049-Madrid, Spain

INTRODUCTION

The precise mechanisms involved in the endotoxin-induced shock are not yet clearly understood. A biphasic behaviour has been observed due to a direct interaction of bacterial lipopolysaccharide (LPS) with the membrane of target cells and an indirect activation of multiple homeostatic regulatory mechanisms (3).

Cytotoxic lesions as well as functional and metabolic disturbances occur mainly in adrenal glands, liver and lung of infected animals and we have previously shown that endotoxin binds to the membrane of adrenocortical cells, hepatocytes and type II pneumocytes. This binding results in alterations of the membrane properties and functional activities of these cells (1, 6, 8, 9).

In order to get additional information about the kinetic, distribution and ultrastructural localization of LPS (*E. coli* 0111:B4) in these target cells, we have used the immunocytochemical protein A-gold technique.

MATERIALS AND METHODS

Isolation of Adrenocortical Cells, Hepatocytes and Type II Pneumocytes

Male Wistar rats weighing 200-250g were used to isolate adrenocortical cells by trypsin digestion (5), hepatocytes by the collagenase perfusion method (2) and type II pneumocytes by elastase digestion and Percoll-gradient centrifugation (1). Cell viability, tested by the Trypan blue exclusion assay, was 80-90%. Cells were incubated with LPS (0.5 mg/ml, previously sonicated 5 min in an Ultrason bath), at 37°C for 15, 25, 40 and 60 min.

Fixation and Embedding of Cells

After LPS treatment, cells were washed in phosphate buffered saline (PBS) at 4°C, fixed in 0.5% glutaraldehyde (1% for adrenal cells) and 2% tannic acid in PBS during 10 min. Then, fixative was removed and cells were resuspended in 2 ml PBS and centrifuged 5 sec at 900 g. Pellet was incubated 10 min at 4°C in NH_4Cl 0.4M.

Pellet dehydration was carried out in ethanol at -20°C and embedded in Lowicryl K4M.

Preparation of the pA-Gold Complex

Colloidal gold (5nm) was prepared by the method of Faulk and Taylor (4) as modified by Romano et al. (10). The minimal amount of pA for full stabilization of the colloidal gold was determined by the technique of Horisberger (7) with the modification of Roth and Binder (11).

Immunocytochemical Labelling

Thin sections of the samples, mounted on nickel grids, were sequentially incubated with: 1) 1% insuline/PBS (15 min), 2) LPS antiserum (1/100) (24 hr at 4°C) and 3) pA-gold complex (1/20) (1 hr at room temperature). Staining with uranylacetate was performed before examination in a JEOL 100 B electron microscope.

RESULTS AND DISCUSSION

Binding, localization and distribution of E. coli 0111:B4 lipopolysaccharide in adrenocortical cells, hepatocytes and type II pneumocytes have been studied by the protein A-gold immunolabelling technique. Morphological and ultrastructural studies were previously done in all these cell types as it is shown in Fig 1a, 1b, 2a, 3a and 3b.

From the immunocytochemical labelling a time-dependent endotoxin uptake can be observed at 15-60 min. After 15-25 min of endotoxin treatment, LPS is bound to plasma membrane of each cell observed, mainly associated to microvilli (Fig 1c, 2b and 3c).

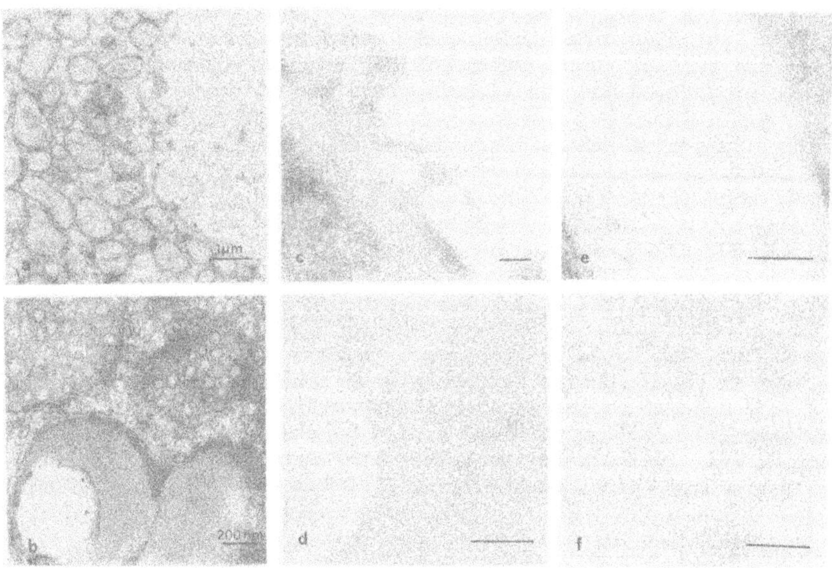

Fig 1. Electron micrograph of zona fasciculata cells isolated from rat adrenal gland. A, B: Morphologic control showing mitochondria with vesicular cristae and lipid droplets. C-F: Ultrastructural localization of LPS by immunogold technique. At 25 min, gold particles are associated to plasma membrane, mainly to microvilli (C). At 40 min, LPS is localized in the cytoplasm either concentrated (D), dispersed (F) or in lipid vesicles (E).

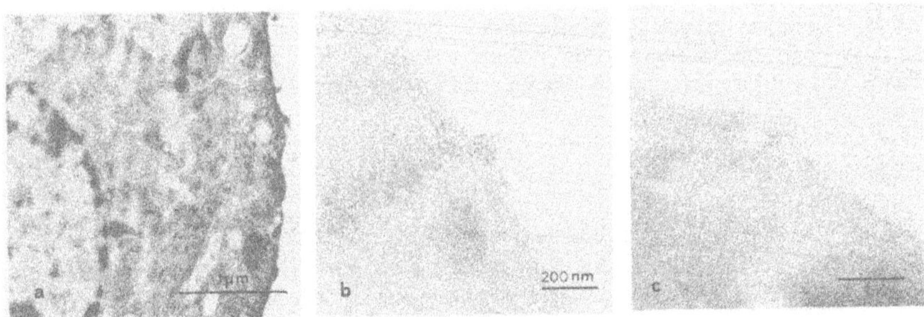

Fig 2. Electron micrographs of hepatocytes isolated from rat liver. A: morphologic control. B, C: Ultrastructural localization of LPS by immunogold technique. LPS is bound to plasma membrane, mainly to microvilli, after 15 min incubation (2B) and it is dispersed through the cytoplasma at 60 min (2C).

These results agree with the binding results previously obtained with [^{14}C] LPS and isolated cells, showing a rapid and non specific interaction between endotoxin and the cell surfaces (1, 6, 8).

The LPS binding increases at 25 min and a progressive internalization is also observed (Fig 3D). The endotoxin uptake can not be related to any receptor-mediated endocytic process. At longer times (40-60 min) the endotoxin is dispersed through the cellular cytoplasm (Fig 1D, 1F, 2C and 3E) showing a higher affinity to lipid domains, mainly in adrenocortical cells (Fig 1E) and type II pneumocytes. The label is rarely seen inside the nucleus (Fig 3F).

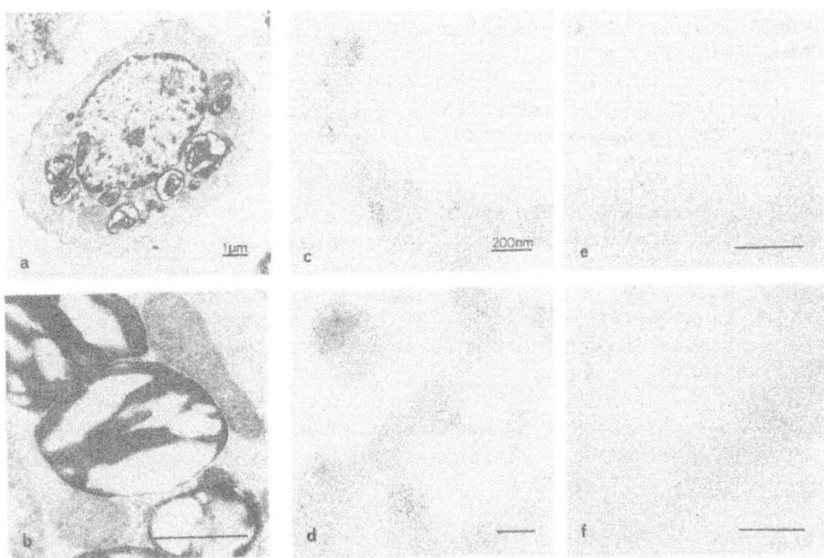

Fig 3. Electron micrographs of type II pneumocytes isolated from rat lung. A, B: Morphologic control showing osmiophilic lamellar bodies. C-F: Ultrastructural localization of LPS by immunogold technique. At 25 min, gold particles are associated to plasma membrane, mainly to microvilli (C). An internalization of LPS is also observed at this time (D). At 40 min, LPS is dispersed through the cytoplasm (E) and the label can be seen rarely inside the nucleus (F).

Although further studies are needed for a precise understanding of the mechanism involved in the endotoxin behaviour in vivo, these results may be an important molecular approach to clarify the primary steps of the endotoxin activity.

ACKNOWLEDGEMENTS

This study was supported by research grants: 84/1001 from "Fondo de Investigaciones Sanitarias de la Seguridad Social" (Spain) and PR84-0506-C02-02 from "Comision Asesora de Investigacion Cientifica y Tecnica del Ministerio de Educacion y Ciencia" (Spain).

REFERENCES

1. Aracil, F. M., Bosch, M. A., and Municio, A. M., 1985, Influence of E. coli lipopolysaccharide binding to rat alveolar type II cells on their functional properties. Mol. Cell Biochem. 68: 59.

2. Berry, M. N. and Friend, D. S., 1969, High-yield preparation of isolated rat liver parenchymal cells. J. Cell Biol. 43: 506.

3. Bradley, S. G., 1979, Cellular and molecular mechanisms of action of bacterial endotoxins. Ann. Rev. Microbiol. 33: 67.

4. Faulk, W. P. and Taylor, G. M., 1971, An immunocolloidal method for the electron microscope. Immunochem. 8: 1081.

5. Garcia, R., Laychock, S. G. and Rubin, R. P., 1982, Inhibition by dibutyryl cyclic AMP induced steroidogenesis in rat adrenocortical cells by the putative calcium antagonist TMB-8. J. Steroid Biochem. 16: 317.

6. Garcia, R., Viloria, M. D. and Municio, A. M., 1985, Influence of E. - coli endotoxin on ACTH induced adrenal cell steroidogenesis. J. Steroid Biochem. 22: 377.

7. Horisberger, M., 1979, Evaluation of colloidal gold as a cytochemical marker for transmission and scanning electron microscopy. Biol. Cell. 36: 253.

8. Pagani, R., Portoles, M. T. and Municio, A. M., 1981, The binding of E. coli endotoxin to isolated rat hepatocytes. FEBS Lett. 131: 103.

9. Portoles, M. T., Pagani, R., Diaz-Laviada, I. and Municio, A. M., 1987, Effect of E. coli lipopolysaccharide on the microviscosity of liver plasma membranes and hepatocyte suspensions and monolayers. Cell. Biochem. & Funct. 5: 54.

10. Romano, E. L., Stolinski, C. and Huges-Jones, N. C., 1974, An antiglobulin reagent labelled with colloidal gold for use in electron microscopy. Immunocytochem. 11: 521.

11. Roth, J. and Binder, M., 1978, Colloidal gold, ferritin and peroxidase as markers for electron microscopic double labelling lectin technique. J. Histochem. Cytochem. 26: 163.

DEVELOPMENT OF A NEW QUANTITATIVE METHOD FOR DETECTION OF ENDOTOXIN BY FLUORESCENCE LABELING OF 3-HYDROXY FATTY ACID

K. Tanamoto

National Institute of Hygienic Sciences, Setagayaku, Tokyo 158, Japan

ABSTRACT

New quantitative method for the detection of minute amounts of endotoxin has been developed using 3-hydroxytetradecanoic acid as a chemical marker. After converting 3-hydroxyteatradecanoic acid to methyl ester, it was coupled with a fluorescent probe, anthracene-9-carboxyl chloride, obtained by chlorization of 9-anthroic acid with oxalyl chloride. The resulting ester was isolated by HPLC on silica column. The purified product, methyl-3-0-(9-carboxy-anthracenyl) tetradecanoate (M/Z 462), was highly responsive to a fluorescence spectrophotometer, showing maximum emission with excitation wavelength at 257 nm and emission wavelength at 458 nm in dichloromethane, the limit of detection being as little as 10 f mol. Using this method it is currently possible to detect **Salmonella abortus equi** endotoxin in aqueous solution at a level of 100 pg.

INTRODUCTION

Gram negative bacillary sepsis is an important clinical entity responsible for a high mortality rate (1). As the result of accumulated findings in clinical and experimental studies (2), endotoxin, which is located in the cell wall of gram-negative bacteria, is thought to be closely related to death or shock in severe septic digestive disorders.

Endotoxin is chemically a lipopolysaccharide (LPS) composed of a polysaccharide portion and a lipid moiety called lipid A (14). Extensive studies using chemically synthesized preparations proved lipid A to be the active center of LPS for almost all biological activities exerted by endotoxin (4, 7, 18), and confirmed its chemical structure (8, 9). According to the results, lipid A has a molecular weight of approximately 1800 (**E. coli** type), its major constituents being D-glucosamine, phosphate and fatty acids. Among the fatty acids, 3-hydroxy fatty acids are so far known to be unique and ubiquitous constituents of endotoxin and may, hence, serve as chemical markers of endotoxin.

Limulus amoebocyte lysate assay is currently the common method for the detection of endotoxin because of its high sensitivity (10). However, it involves several problems, especially when it is applied to biological samples. As in other biological assays, the reaction of **Limulus** lysate also differs depending on the chemical and physicochemical structure of differs depending on the chemical and physicochemical structure of the endotoxin. Thus a new chemical method for direct detection of endotoxin is highly desirable.

Based on the chemical structure of lipid A, the author has developed a new method for detecting endotoxin using 3-hydroxy-fatty acid as a marker by means of fluorescence labeling of the hydroxy group.

The method described here is highly specific and sensitive, determining accurately as little as hundred picograms of **S. abortus** equi LPS in aqueous solution.

MATERIALS AND METHODS

Materials

Chemically synthesized (R)-3-hydroxytetradecanoic acid was a gift from Dr. S. Kusumoto, Osaka University. Oxalyl chloride was purchased from Aldrich Chemical Co., Inc., Milwaukee, and distilled before use. Anthracene-9--carboxylic acid was obtained from Tokyo Kasei Co. and recrystallized with ethanol. Both **S. abortus equi** and **S. minnesota** R595 LPS were the gift of Drs. O. Lüderitz and C. Galanos, Max-Planck-Institut für Immunobiologie, Freiburg. Synthetic lipid A LA-15-PP (506) (**E. coli** type) was purchased from Daiichi Kagaku Co., Tokyo. All solvents were purchased from Kanto Kagaku Co., Tokyo as liquid chromatograph grade.

Glassware was washed well, sonicated and further rinsed with distilled water and methanol before being heated at 300°C for 15 hr. By these treatments, contaminated 3-hydroxy tetradecanoic acid, anthracene-9-carboxylic acid and their derivatives were completely decomposed.

Synthesis of Anthracene-9-carboxyl Chloride (5)

Two ml of oxalyl chloride was added to a suspension of anthracene-9-carboxylic acid (200 mg) in anhydrous dichloromethane (10 ml) and the solution was refluxed for 3 hr. The resulting solution was dried under nitrogen and kept dry in the dark.

High Performance Liquid Chromatography (HPLC)

The instrument used was a Hitachi 655 liquid chromatograph equipped with a Model 655-0020 UV monitor and Model 655-0208 injector, all obtained from Hitachi Ltd. The Hibar column RT 259-4 (25 cm x 4 mm) (Merck, Darmstadt) was used.

Fatty Acid Determination

Fatty acids were determined as a methyl ester by gas chromatography using an instrument of Model GC 6A (Shimadzu Co., Ltd., Kyoto) equipped with 3% OV-1 column.

Methyl esters were prepared by heating LPS or 3-hydroxytetradecanoic acid at 100°C for 3 hr in 5% concentrated hydrochloric acid solution in methanol. The methylated fatty acids of the hydrolysate were extracted five times with hexane. The hexane extracts were pooled, washed with pyrogen free water and dried under nitrogen.

Mass Spectral Analysis

Fast atom bombardment (FAB) mass spectrometry was performed on a JMS-DX-300 mass spectrometer (JEOL Co., Tokyo) utilizing a neutral beam of xenon

$$\text{Anthracene-9-COCl} + CH_3(CH_2)_{10}\overset{OH}{C}HCH_2\overset{O}{\overset{\|}{C}}OCH_3 \longrightarrow \text{Anthracene-9-}\overset{O}{C}\text{-O-}CH_3(CH_2)_{10}CHCH_2\overset{O}{\overset{\|}{C}}OCH_3$$

Fig 1. Transformation of methyl-3-hydroxytetradecanoate with anthracene-9-carboxyl chloride into methyl-3-0-(9-carboxy anthracenyl) tetradecanoate (CAT).

atoms with a translational energy of 8 Kev and a discharge current of 20μ A. The mass range of 50 to 800 was scanned at a rate of 10 s/decade.

RESULTS

Derivatization of Methyl-3-hydroxytetradecanoate with Anthracene-9-carboxylChloride

Reaction conditions for coupling methyl-3-hydroxytetradecanoate with anthracene-9-carboxyl chloride as a fluorescence labeling agent were investigated (Fig 1).

Since condensation of the hydroxy group with acid chloride to form an ester is usually catalyzed in the presence of an organic base, the effect of some bases was studied. The reaction was performed in solutions containing 10 μg of methyl-3-hydroxytetradecanoate, 10 μg of methyltetradecanoate and 100 μg of anthracene-9-carboxyl chloride in 100 μl of solvent. An aliquot of the solution was applied directly to gas chromatograph at different reaction times. The yield of the anthroyl derivative was calculated as the rate of consumption of methyl-3-hydroxytetradecanoate compared with the peak area of methyl-tetradecanoate used as an internal standard since it does not react with the reagent and remains unchanged. The reaction did not proceed at all in the presence of any organic solvent such as pyridine, 2-6-dimethylpyridine or 0.1% triethylamine/acetonitrile even after 60 min at 60°C (Fig 2).

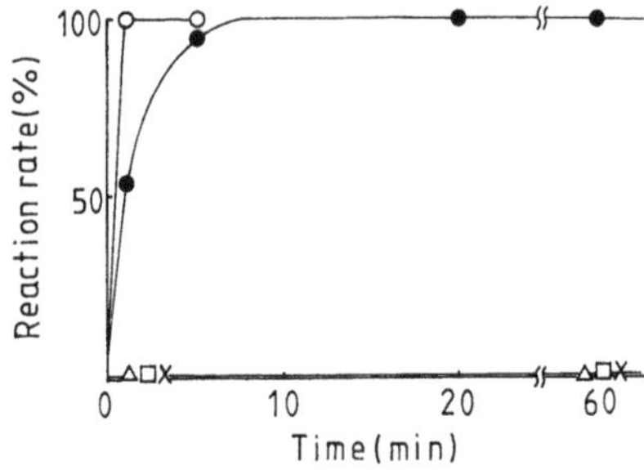

Fig 2. Time course for derivatization of methyl-3-hydroxytetradecanoate with anthracene-9-carboxyl chloride. The reaction rate was calculated as the rate of consumption of methyl-3-hydroxytetradecanoate detected by gas chromatography. Reaction in ; (O) acetonitrile, (●) dichloromethane, (Δ) pyridine, (□) 2-6-dimethylpyridine, (X) 0.1% triethylamine in acetonitrile.

On the other hand, very rapid consumption of methyl-3-hydroxytetradecanoate occurred in acetonitrile or dichloromethane at room temperature in the absence of base. The reaction was completed within one minute in the case of acetonitrile and in 20 min in the case of dichloromethane (Fig 2), resulting in the quantitative formation of methyl-3-O-(9-carboxy-anthracenyl) tetradecanoate (CAT). When the solution was heated at 50°C in a sealed tube, the reaction in dichloromethane was accelerated and completed in one minute. On the basis of these data, condensation was performed in acetonitrile at room temperature.

Isolation and Characterization of CAT

After the condensation of methyl-3-hydroxytetradecanoate with anthracene-9-carboxyl chloride, the new product was visually observed under ultraviolet light as a single spot on silica gel TLC separated using a solvent system of dichloromethane: hexane = 1 : 1 (Fig 3).

The new product was isolated by HPLC on silica column eluted with the solvent system of dichloromethane: hexane = 4:1 and detected by absorption at 257 nm. A typical chromatogram of the eluent of the reaction mixture is shown in Fig 4.

The fraction of new product was collected and applied to FAB mass spectrometer in order to confirm the formation of CAT. The ionization was effectively performed using triethanolamine (TEA) as a matrix. Mass peaks were recognized at M/Z 462 and 612 corresponding to CAT and $(CAT + TEA + H)^+$, respectively (Fig. 5). These results proved the actual formation of CAT. The material purified by HPLC was then used as a standard CAT.

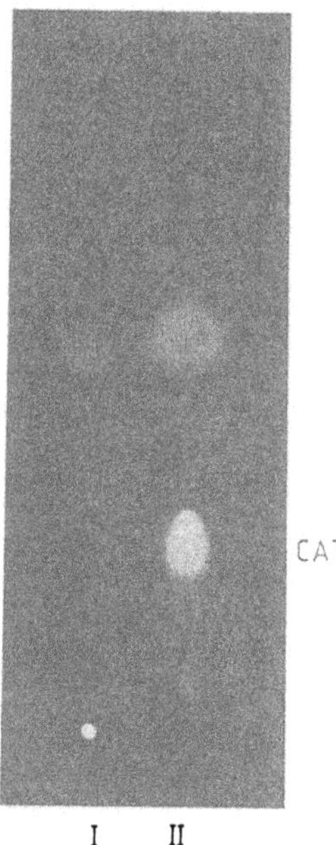

Fig 3. Thin layer chromatograph of CAT.
I, Antracene-9-carboxyl chloride; II, reaction mixture after derivatization

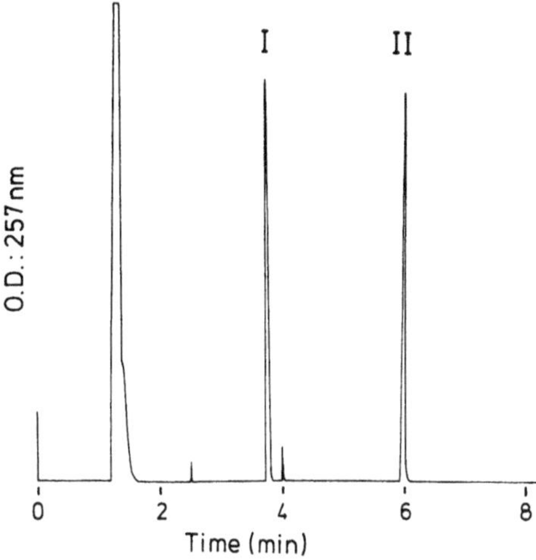

Fig 4. Purification of CAT by high performance liquid chromatography. Dichloromethane: hexane = 4:1 was used as the eluate at a flow rate of 2 ml/min. Other conditions are described in the text. Peaks: I, anthracene-9-carboxyl chloride; 2. CAT.

Standard Curve of Fluorescence of CAT

The fluorescence intensity of the purified CAT was measured in several organic solvents including methanol, acetonitrile, ethylacetate, hexane and dichloromethane. Among these, CAT emitted the highest fluorescence in dichloromethane with the maximum excitation wavelength at 257 nm and emission wavelength at 458 nm. Maximum fluorescence of anthracene-9-carboxyl chloride was obtained with excitation wavelength at 344 nm and emission wavelength at 460 nm.

A known concentration of CAT was prepared and the fluorescence intensity measured in dichloromethane. The standard curve was linear in the range of 1 pg to 100 ng tested. Fig 6 shows that fluorescence intensity is dose dependent on CAT. The intensity with 10 pg of CAT was about 10 in 0.5 ml of dichloromethane. The background of the solvent under this condition was about 10.

Dose Dependency of Methyl-3-hydroxytetradecanoate and Fluorescence Intensity after Derivatization.

One μg of anthracene-9-carboxyl chloride in acetonitrile was added to varying amounts (5-10^4 pg) of methyl-3-hydroxytetradecanoate. In one minute the solution was dried under nitrogen, dissolved with dichloromethane and injected directly into HPLC. The fraction corresponding to CAT was collected and concentrated and the fluorescence measured in dichloromethane. A linear relationship was obtained between fluorescence and increasing amount of methyl-3-hydroxytetradecanoate (Fig 7). The results also showed good quantitative agreement with the standard curve shown in Fig 6.

3-Hydroxytetradecanoic Acid Content of LPS and Synthetic Lipid A

The general scheme for the detection of 3-hydroxytetradecanoic acid is shown in Fig 8.

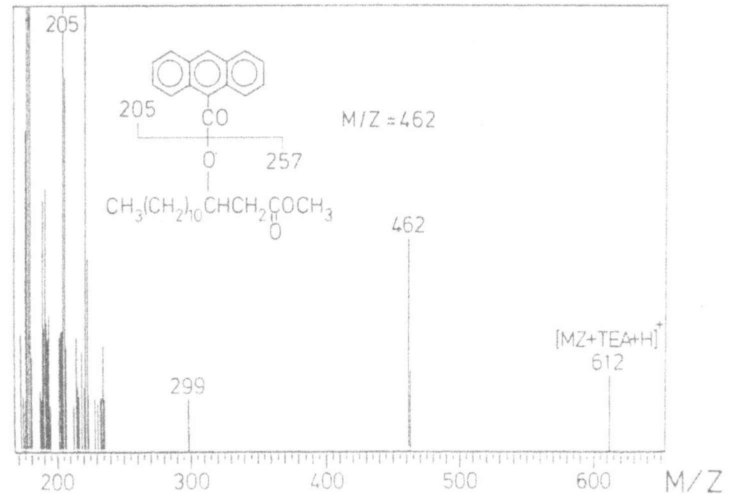

Fig 5. Mass spectrum of CAT.

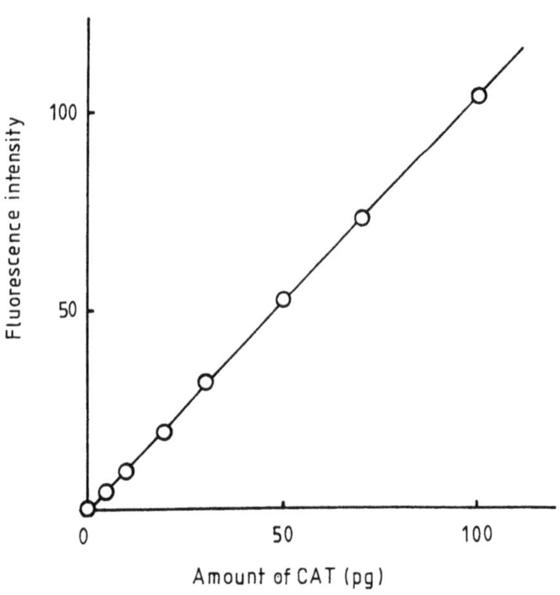

Fig 6. Standard curve of fluorescence of CAT.
Fluorescence was measured in 0.5 ml of dichloromethane with the excitation wavelength at 257 nm and emission wavelength at 458 nm.

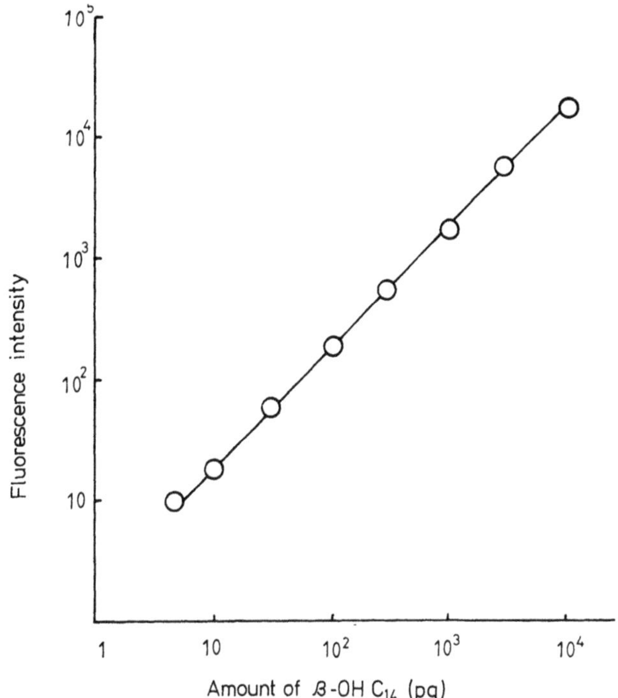

Fig 7. Dose dependency of methyl-3-hydroxytetradecanoate and fluorescence intensity after derivatization.
Varying amounts of methyl-3-hydroxytetradecanoate were derivatized and the fluorescence of the CAT produced was measured as described in Fig 6.

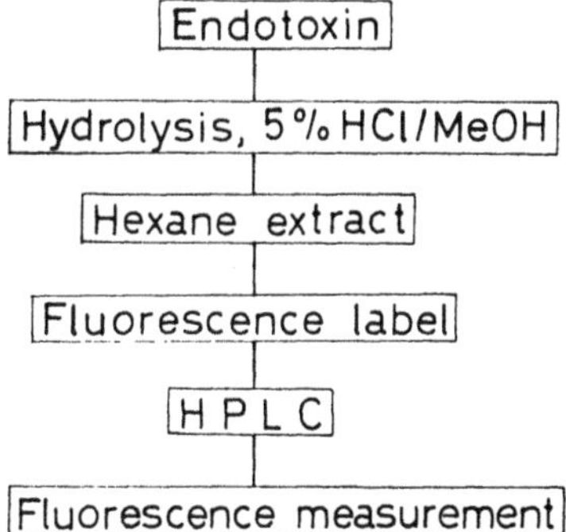

Fig 8. General scheme for determination of 3-hydroxy-tetradecanoate in endotoxin.

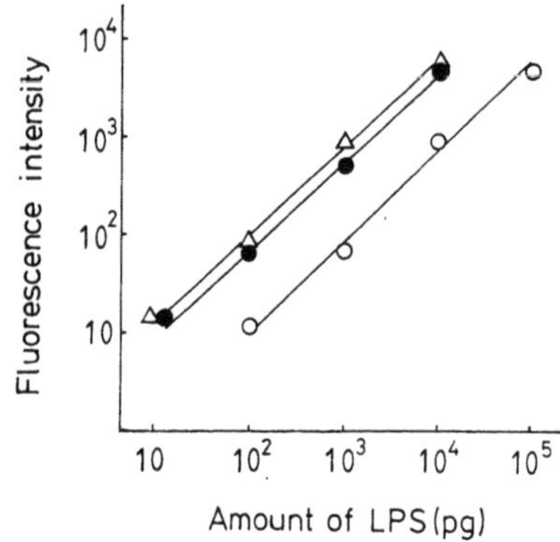

Fig 9. 3-hydroxytetradecanoic acid content of lipid A and lipopolysaccharides.
Varying amounts of lipid A and lipopolysaccharides were hydrolyzed and derivatized. The fluorescence of the CAT produced was measured in the condition described in Fig 6. (O), **S. abortus equi** LPS; (●) **S. minnesota** R 595 LPS; (Δ), synthetic lipid A LA-15-PP (506).

LPS from **S. abortus equi** and **S. minnesota** R595, and synthetic lipid A LA-15-PP (506) were used for the test. Methylated fatty acids from varying amounts of LPS or lipid A were prepared as described in Materials and Methods. Among the methylated fatty acids liberated from the samples, methyl-3-hydroxytetradecannoate was specifically labeled with the fluorescence probe, as confirmed by the disappearance of the corresponding peak on gas chromatogram after the reaction. After purification, fluorescence of the CAT produced was measured. As shown in Fig 9, a linear relationship was observed on double logarithmic graph between fluorescence and increasing amounts of LPS and lipid A. These results also demonstrate that the contents of 3-hydroxytetradecanoic acid of the LPS and lipid A determined by this procedure show a good quantitative coincidence with those obtained by gas chromatography using heptadecanoic acid as an internal standard (data not shown).

DISCUSSION

A new strategy for the direct chemical detection of minute amounts of endotoxin is proposed in this report.

The determination is based on the analysis of 3-hydroxy fatty acid, which is a characteristic and universal component of endotoxin and may, hence, serve as a chemical marker of endotoxin. The 3-hydroxytetradecanoate was specifically and effectively labeled by the fluorescence probe, anthracene-9-carboxyl chloride, producing a coupled ester, methyl-3-O-(9-carboxyanthracenyl) tetradecanoate (CAT). The product was highly sensitive to fluorescence spectrometry and 3-hydroxytetradecanoate was measurable by this technique at the picogram level. A linear relationship was obtained between fluorescence and increasing amounts of LPS or lipid A, showing feasibility of direct chemical measurement of endotoxin chemically. At present 100 pg of **S. abortus equi** LPS in aqueous solution can be accurately determined.

The **Limulus** lysate assay is currently in wide use in most cases concerning quantitization of endotoxin because of its high sensitivity. The assay is, however, not specific to endotoxin (11, 15), and is modified drastically by the presence of inhibitors (13) or activators (20) of the enzymes included in the cascade reaction of the Limulus assay. In addition, endotoxin undergoes the chemical enzymatic degradation (3, 6, 17) or modification by some factors in the host, such as lipoprotein (22). These chemical or physicochemical changes also influence the **Limulus** test greatly as was shown previously using synthetic lipid A analogues (7, 12, 21) or by (22). Considering these points, as in other biological assays, the determination of endotoxin by **Limulus** test does not always reflect the real amount of endotoxin. The establishment of a chemical method for direct detection of endotoxin is, therefore, necessary as an alternative or to confirm the reliability of the **Limulus** test.

Other approaches for the chemical determination of endotoxin have been reported using 3-hydroxytetradecanoic acid as an endotoxin marker, but employed gas chromatography with selected ion monitoring (SIM) detection and electron-ionization mass spectrometry (16), or electron-capture and negative ion chemical ionization mass spectrometry (19). These methods, however, are not sensitive enough to detect physiological amounts of endotoxin so far reported using the Limulus test. Compared with these chemical determinations of endotoxin, the fluorescence labeling method described herein demonstrates a great advantage with regarding to sensitivity.

This method can be used for the determination of endotoxin in a variety of environmental and biological samples. The method also seems to be promising for the analysis of clinical samples, such as serum, if a suitable preparation technique is established. It may also be used to clarify the ambiguous results obtained by biological assay.

REFERENCES

1. Blair, E., Wise, A., and Mackay, A.G., 1969, Gram-negative bacteremic shock. J. Am. Med. Assoc. 207: 333.

2. Cheim, S., Chen, C., Dellenback, J., Usami, S., and Gregerson, M. I., 1966, Hemodynamic changes in endotoxin shock. Am. J. Physiol. 210: 1401.

3. Freudenberg, M. and Galanos, C., 1985, Alteration in rats **in vivo** of the chemical structure of lipopolysaccharide from **Salmonella abortus equi**. Eur. J. Biochem. 152: 353.

4. Galanos, C., Lehmann, V., Lüderitz, O., Rietschel, E. T., Westphal, O., Brade, H., Brade, L., Freudenberg, M. A., Hansen-Hagge, T., Lüderitz, T., McKenzie, G., Shade, U., Strittmatter, W., Tanamoto, K., Zähringer, U., Imoto, M., Yoshimura, H., Yamamoto, M., Shimamoto, T., Kusumoto, S., and Shiba, T., 1984, Endotoxic properties of chemically synthesized lipid A part structures. Eur. J. Biochem. 140: 221.

5. Goto, J., Goto, N., Shamsa, F., Saito, M., Komatsu, S., Suzaki, K., and Nambara, T., 1983, New sensitive derivatization of hydrosteroids for high-performance liquid chromatography with fluorescence detection. Analitica Chimica Acta 147: 397.

6. Hall, C. L. and Munford, R. S., 1983, Enzymatic deacylation of the lipid A moiety of Salmonella typhimurium lipopolysaccharides by human neutrophils. Proc. Natl. Acad. Sci. 80: 6671.

7. Homma, J. Y., Matsuura, M., Kanegasaki, S., Kawakubo, Y., Shibukawa, N., Kumazawa, Y., Yamamoto, A., Tanamoto, K., Yasuda, T., Imoto, M., Yoshimura, H., Kusumoto, S., and Shiba, T., 1985, Structural requirement of lipid A responsible for the function: A study with chemically synthesized lipid A and its analogues. J. Biochem. 98: 395.

8. Imoto, M., Yoshimura, H., Yamamoto, M., Shimamoto, T., Kusumoto, S., and Shiba, T., 1984, Chemical synthesis of phosphorylated tetraacyl disaccharide corresponding to a biosynthetic precursor of lipid A. Tetrahedron Lett. 25: 2667.

9. Imoto, M., Yoshimura, H., Sakaguchi, N., Kusumoto, S., and Shiba, T., 1985, Total synthesis of **Escherichia coli** lipid A. Tetrahedron Lett. 26: 1545.

10. Iwanaga, S., Morita, T., Harada, T., Nakamura, S., Niwa, N., Tanaka, K., Kimura, T., and Sakakibara, S., 1978, Chromogenic substrates for horseshoe crab clotting enzyme. Its application for the assay of bacterial endotoxins. Hameostasis 7: 183.

11. Kakinuma, A., Asano, T., Torii, and Sugini, Y., 1981, Gelation of **Limulus** amoebocyte lysate by an antitumor (1-3)- β-D-glucan. Biochem. Biophys. Res. Commun. 101:434.

12. Kanagasaki, S., Tanamoto, K., Yasuda, T., Homma, J. Y., Matsuura, M., Nakatsuka, M., Kumazawa, Y., Yamamoto, A., Shiba, T., Kusumoto, S., Imoto, M., Yoshimura, H., and Shimamoto, T., 1986, Structure-activity relationship of lipid A: Comparison of biological activities of natural and synthetic lipid A's with different fatty acid compositions. J. Biochem. 99: 1203.

13. Levin, J., Tomasulo, P. A., and Oser, R. S., 1970, Detecton of endotoxin in human blood and demonstration of an inhibitor. J. Lab. Clin. Med. 75: 903.

14. Lüderitz, O., Freudenberg, M., Galanos, C., Lehmann, V., Rietschel, E. T., and Show, D. W., 1982, Lipopolysaccharides of gram-negative bacteria. in: "Microbial membrane lipids," Vol. 17, pp 79-151, C. Razin and S. Rottem, eds. Academic Press, London, New York.

15. Morita, T., Tanaka, S., Nakamura, T., and Iwanaga, S., 1981, A new (1-3)- β -D-glucan mediates coagulation pathway found in Limulus amoebocytes. FEBS Lett. 129: 318.

16. Maitra, S. K., Schotz, M. C., Yoshikawa, T. T., and Guze, A. B., 1978, Determination of lipid A and endotoxin in serum by mass spectroscopy. Proc. Natl. Acad. Sci. 8: 3993.

17. Peterson, A. A. and Munford, R. S., 1987, Dephosphorylation of the lipid A moiety of Escherichia coli lipopolysaccharides by mouse macrophages. Infect. Immun. 55: 974.

18. Rietschel, E. T., Brade, H., Brade, L., Brandeburg, K., Shade, U., Seydel, U., Zähringer, U., Galanos, C., Lüderitz, O., Westphal, O., Labischinski, H., Kusumoto, S., and Shiba, T., 1987, Lipid A, the endotoxic center of bacterial lipopolysaccharides: Relation of chemical structure to biological activity. in: Progr. Clin. Biol.. Res. Vol. 231, pp 25-53. Alan R. Liss, Inc. New York.

19. Soneson, A., Larsson, L., Westerdahl, G., and Odham, G., 1987, Determination of endotoxins by gas chromatography: Evaluation of electron-capture and negative-ion chemical-ionization mass spectrometric detection of halogenated derivates of β - hydroxymyristic acid. J. Chromatography 417: 11.

20. Takagi, K., Moriya, A., Tamura, H., Nakahara, C., Tanaka, S., Fujita, Y., and Kawai, T., 1981, Quantitative measurement of endotoxin in human blood using synthetic chromogenic substrate for horseshoe crab clotting enzyme. A comparison of methods of blood sampling and treatment. Thromb. Res. 23: 51.

21. Tanamoto, K., Zähringer, U., McKenzie, G. R., Galanos, C., Rietschel, E. T., Lüderitz, O., Kusumoto, S., and Shiba, T., 1984, Biological activities of synthetic lipid A analogues: Pyrogenicity, lethal toxicity, anticomplemental activity, and induction of gelation of **Limulus** amoebocyte lysate. Infect. Immun. 44: 421.

22. Ulevitch, R. J., 1985, Interaction of bacterial lipopolysaccharide and plasma high density lipoproteins, in: Handbook of Endotoxin. L. J. Berry, ed., Vol. 3, pp. 372-388, Elsevier, Amsterdam.

A NEW ENDOTOXIN-SPECIFIC ASSAY

T. Obayashi

Department of Clinical Pathology, Jichi Medical School
Minamikawachi-machi, Tochigi, 329-04, Japan

INTRODUCTION

After its development by Levin and Bang in 1968 (4), the limulus amebocyte lysate test had been considered specific for endotoxin until Kakinuma et al., found that carboxymethylated (1→3) - β -D-glucan also activates limulus coagulation enzymes (3). Morita et al., showed that amebocyte lysate contains, in addition to endotoxin-sensitive factor C, a factor G that is sensitive for a trace amount of (1→3)- β -D-glucan (Fig 1a) (5). Thus the author and his colleagues attempted to remove this factor from the lysate to establish an endotoxin-specific assay (Fig 1b)

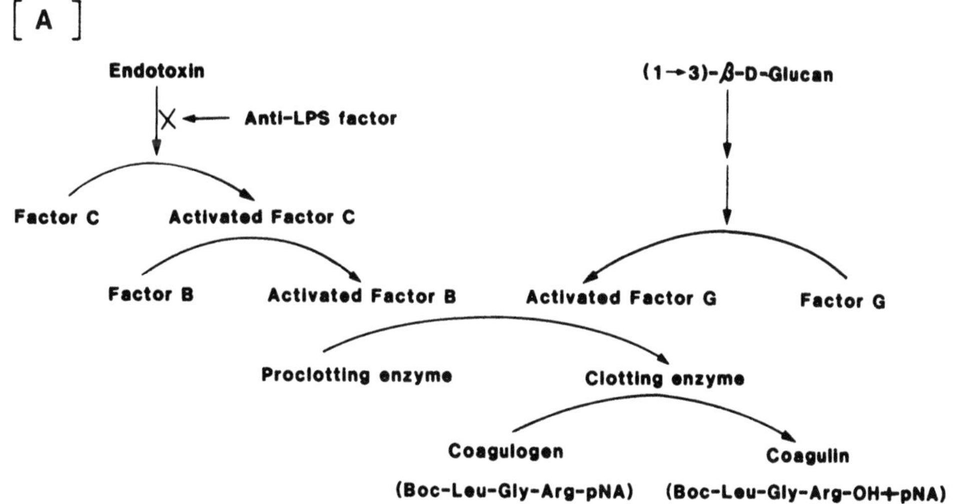

Fig 1a. Coagulation pathways of horseshoe crab

[B]

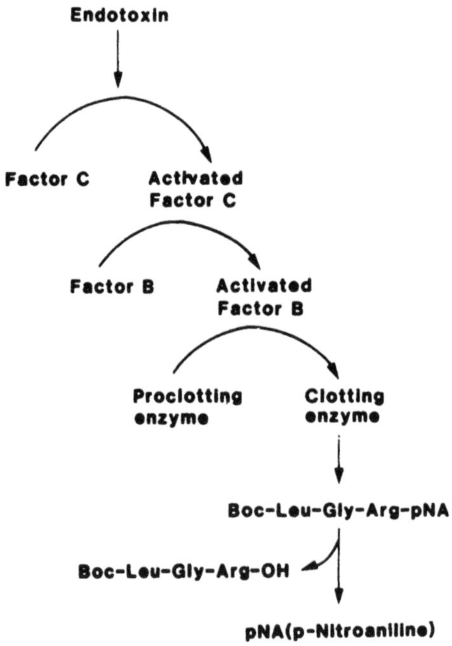

Fig 1b. Principle of Endospecy

[C]

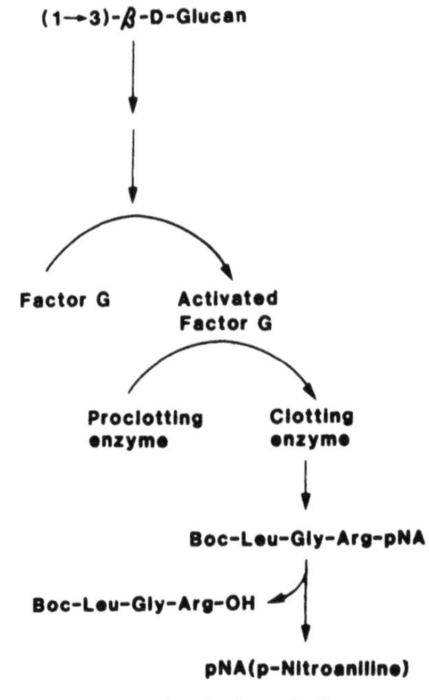

Fig 1c. Principle of G test

MATERIALS AND METHODS

All glassware was dry-heated at 250°C for 2 hr, and reagents autoclaved at 121°C until they proved negative with a chromogenic limulus test (Toxicolor; Seikagaku Kogyo Co., Ltd., Tokyo)

Endotoxins

Eleven endotoxins of Westphal-type were used: Escherichia coli 0111:B4, E. coli 055:B5, and Shigella flexneri endotoxins (Difco Laboratories, Detroit, Mich.); Serratia marcescens, Salmonella typhosa, S. enteritidis, S. abortus equi, and S. typhimurium endotoxins (Sigma Chemical Co., St. Louis, MO); Pseudomonas aeruginosa endotoxin (Biological Laboratories, Campbell, CA); USP reference standard endotoxin (E. coli 0113; US Pharmacopeial Convention) and Novo-Pyrexal endotoxin standard NP1 S. abortus equi; Pyroquant Diagnostik GmbH, Walldorf, FRG).

(1→3)- β-D-glucan (Curdlan; Wako Pure Chemical Industries, Ltd., Osaka, Japan) was made endotoxin-free by dissolving 10 mg of the material in 10 ml of 0.05 mol/1 NaOH, stirring the solution for 30 min with 0.2 g of activated charcoal which had been baked in an oven at 250°C for 2 hr, and filtering the mixture through a Millex-GS sterilizing filter (0.22 m; Millipore Corporation, Bedford, MA).

Preparation of Endotoxin-specific Reagent

According to the method of Iwanaga, amebocyte lysate from Japanese horseshoe crabs, Tachypleus tridentatus, was applied to dextran sulfate-Sepharose CL-6B column (5.0 x 23.0 cm) equilibrated with 0.02 mol/1 Tris-HCl buffer (pH 8.0) containing 0.05 mol/1 NaCl. Stepwise elution was carried out at 4°C, first with the equilibration buffer, secondly with the buffer containing 0.2 mol/1 NaCl, thirdly with the buffer containing 0.45 mol/1 NaCl, and lastly with the buffer containing 2.0 mol/1 NaCl. Fractions were collected at a flow rate of 130 ml/hr. As is shown in the chromatogram (Fig 2), proclotting enzyme was eluted in the breakthrough fraction, factor G and coguloge in the second fraction, factors B and C in the third, and anti-LPS factor in the last fraction. The first and the third fraction were combined with a chromogenic substrate, Boc-Leu-Gly-Arg-p-nitroanilide, and then lyophilized to prepare an endotoxin-specific reagent (Endospecy; Seikagaku Kogyo). As a byproduct, a glucan assay system was constituted by combining the first and second fractions and the chromogenic substrate (G test; Fig 1c).

Assay Procedures of Endospecy, Toxicolor, and G Test

Sample (0.1 ml) was added to 0.1 ml of Endospecy, Toxicolor, or G test dissolved in 0.2 mol/1 Tris-HCl buffer, pH 8.0, and the mixture was incubated at 37°C for 30 min. After diazo-coupling, absorbance was measured at 545 nm (Fig 3).

Specificity of Endospecy

Two-fold serial dilutions of E. coli 0111:B4 endotoxin and of (1→3)-β-D-glucan were assayed with Endospecy. For comparison, the same series of dilutions were assayed with Toxicolor and G test.

Intra-assay Reproducibility of Endospecy

The two fold serial dilutions of E. coli 0111:B4 endotoxin (6.25, 12.5, 25, 50 pg/ml) were assayed six times.

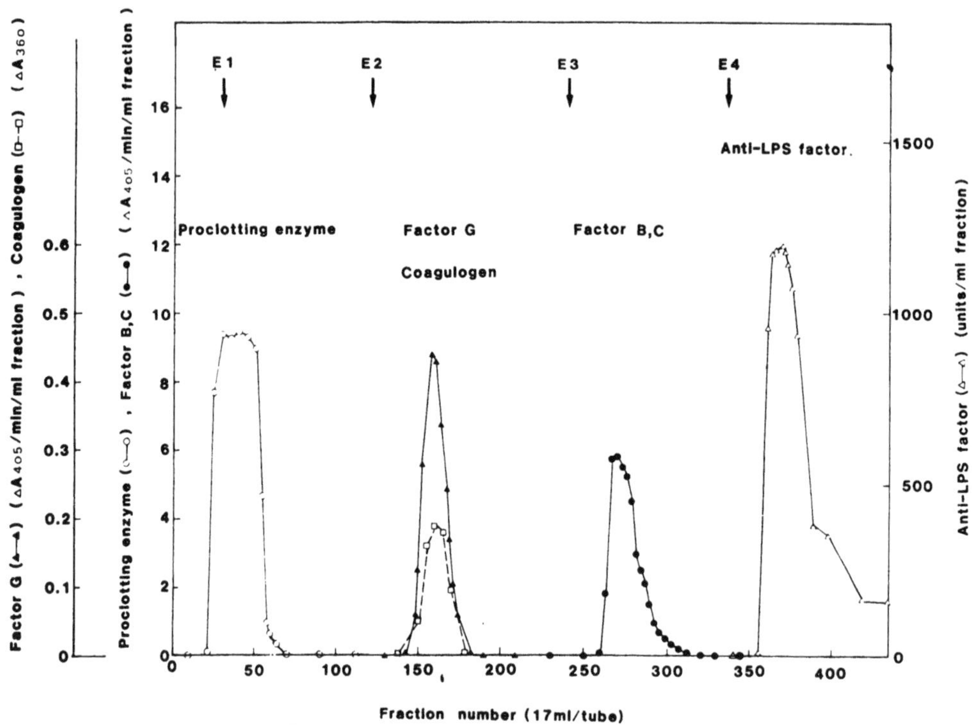

Fig 2. Dextran sulfate-Sepharose CL-6B column chromatogram of amebocyte lysate from Japanese horseshoe crab, Tachypleus tridentatus.

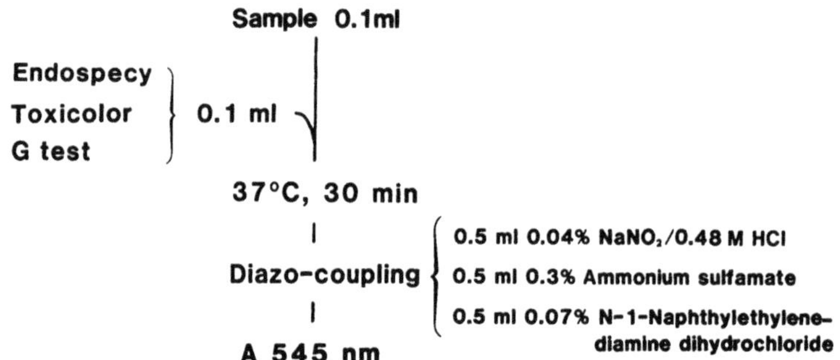

Fig 3. Assay procedures of Endospecy, Toxicolor, and G test.

Regression Lines of Endospecy against Various Endotoxins

A serial dilution of 11 different endotoxins were assayed with Endospecy, and the regression lines were plotted on a bilogarithmic scale to ensure that the test is applicable to diffferent endotoxins.

Clinical Evaluation of Endospecy

Platelet-rich plasmas from septic patients and from patients with chronic renal failure receiving hemodialysis with cellulose membrane were assayed with Endospecy, and the results were compared with those of Toxicolor. Samples were treated with perchloric acid before assay as described elsewhere (6).

RESULTS

Specificity

Endospecy showed a nice linear standard curve without response to (1→3)-β-D-glucan, whereas Toxicolor reacted with either of the substances (Fig 4). G test reacted only with (1→3)-β-D-glucan.

Intra-assay Reproducibility

The co-efficient of variation was less than 4% over the endotoxin concentration from 0 to 50 pg/ml (Fig 5).

Regression Lines Against Different Endotoxins

The regression lines against 11 different endotoxins were all parallel to one another (Fig 6).

Clinical Evaluation

Of 12 samples that showed high levels of endotoxin with a conventional method (Toxicolor), 7 were abnormal, and the remaining 5 were normal with Endospecy. The normal 5 cases were all systemic fungal infections. Dialyzed samples were also normal with Endospecy in spite of abnormally high values with Toxicolor (Table 1)

DISCUSSION

Limulus gelation test, developed by Levin and Bag (4), is highly sensitive for endotoxin. Its chromogenic version (1) is even more sensitive, and permits an objective determination of endotoxin concentrations as low as 1 pg/ml. Having been considered specific for endotoxin for years, the test proved to be not so when Iwanaga and his coworkers revealed that the amebocyte lysate contains a factor G that is sensitive to a minute amount of (1→3)-β-D-glucan.

Thus we removed this factor from the lysate to restore the specificity of the test. The new test, which is now commercially available (Endospecy, Seikagaku Kogyo), reacts only with endotoxin. A conventional method, on the other hand, will yield positive results with fungal polysaccharides and rinses from cellulosic membrane as well (Table 2). Endospecy is acceptable as a laboratory test, since it has a good linear relationship between dose

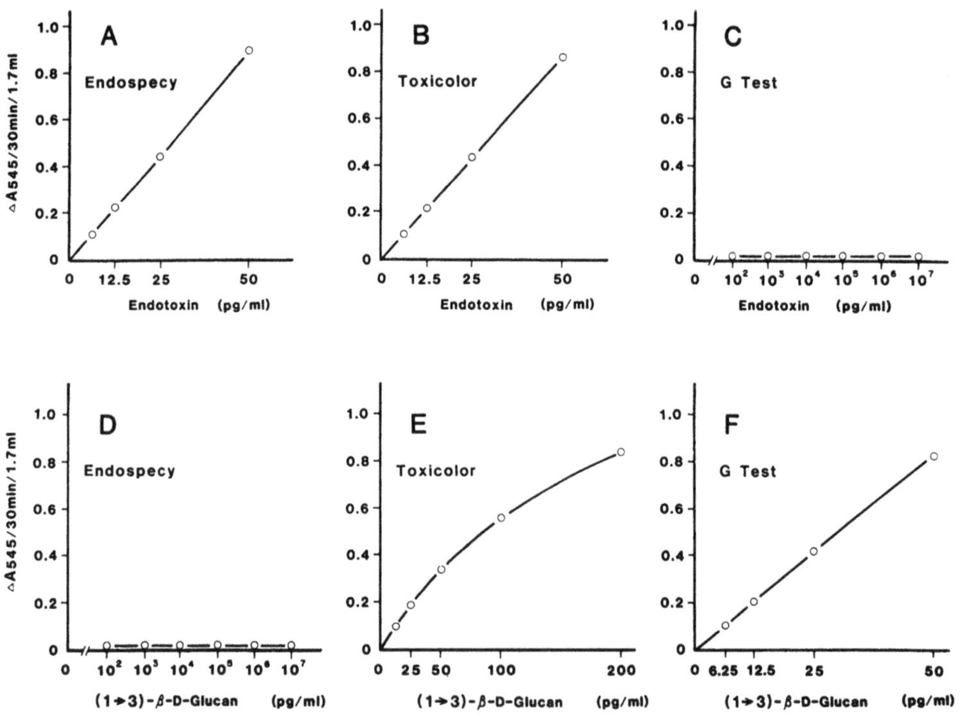

Fig 4. Standard curves of Endospecy, Toxicolor, and G test. The upper row is against endotoxin, the lower against (1→ 3)-β -D-glucan.

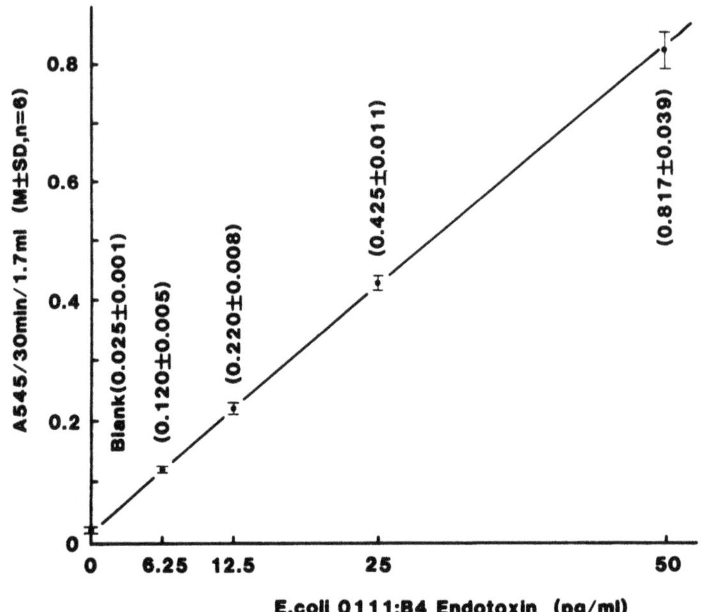

Fig 5. Intra-assay reproducibility of Endospecy.

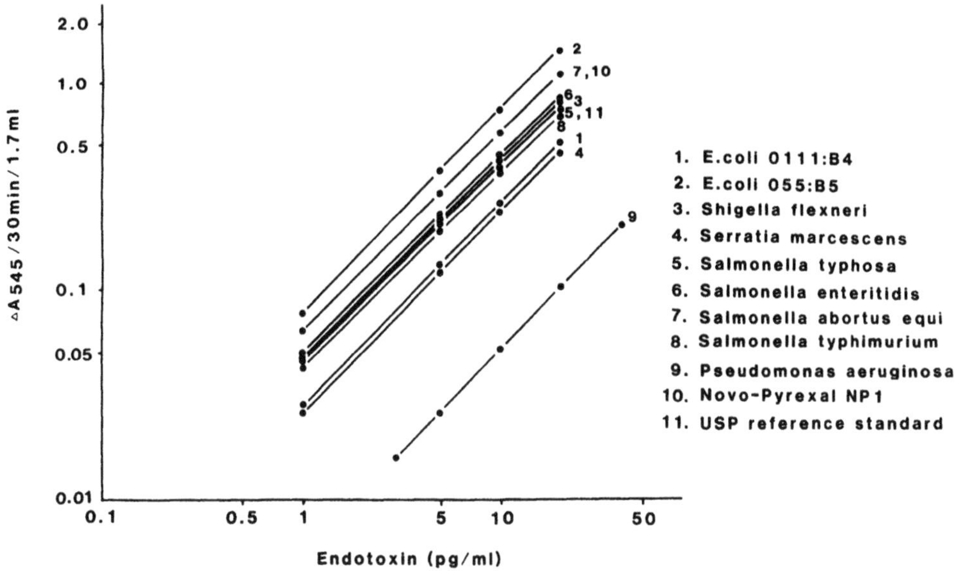

Fig 6. Regression lines of Endospecy against 11 different endotoxins.

Table 1. Endotoxin Determination with Toxicolor and Endospecy in Septic and Dialyzed Blood Samples

Sample (PRP)		Toxicolor	Endospecy	G Test
Normal (Mean ± SD, n=20)		2.2 ± 1.5 pg/ml	0.8 ± 0.6 pg/ml	0.2 ± 0.3 pg/ml
Endotoxemia	a	255.9	87.8	1.4
	b	88.5	86.9	0.6
	c	162.8	68.6	1.2
	d	75.5	61.2	0.2
	e*	119.8	59.7	0.8
	f	112.6	57.2	0.9
	g	46.9	40.1	0.2
Systemic Fungal Infections	h	68.6	0.3	268.9
	i	395.9	0.0	1733.1
	j*	103.0	1.2	328.7
	k*	308.8	0.0	1719.0
	l	52.9	2.5	167.3
Hemodialyzed	m	1107.7	2.2	4628.0
	n	685.2	1.6	2753.6
	o	1198.4	2.5	4635.5
	p	552.4	1.8	2052.1
	q	1080.1	1.2	4104.5
	r	1275.3	2.5	5321.4

E. coli 0111:B4 endotoxin is a reference in Toxicolor and Endospecy; (1→3)-β-D-glucan is a reference in G test. Asterisks indicate positive blood cultures for Pseudomonas aeruginosa (e), Candida guilliermondii (j), and C. albicans (k).

and response with a small co-efficient of intra-assay variation; the parallel regression lines against different endotoxins allow us to take up any one endotoxin as a standard and determine endotoxin concentrations of unknown species.

Table 2. Comparison of the Reactivity of Toxicolor and Endospecy to Various Substances

	Limulus test	Endospecy
Lipopolysaccharides	+	+
Lipid A	+	+
Synthetic lipid A analogs	+	+
(1→3)-β-D-Glucans		
Curdlan	+	-
Pachyman	+	-
Fungal polysaccharides		
Candida albicans	+	-
Microsporum canis	+	-
Trichophyton mentagrophytes	+	-
Trichophyton rubrum	+	-
Aspergillus flavus	+	-
Aspergillus fumigatus	+	-
Saccharomyces cerevisiae	+	-
Lentinan	+	-
Schizophyllan	+	-
Rinses from cellulosic dialyzer	+	-
Phospholipids		
Phosphatidic acid	-	-
Phosphatidylglycerol	-	-
Phosphatidylinositol	-	-
Phosphatidylserine	-	-
Phosphatidylcholine	-	-
Phosphatidylethanolamine	-	-
Gram-positive bacterial polysaccharides		
Staphylococcus epidermidis	-	-
Staphylococcus aureus	-	-
α-*Streptococcus hemolyticus*	-	-

The major advantage of Endospecy with high specificity for endotoxin is evident from the results of the present clinical evaluation. It can avoid false-positive reactions seen with a conventional method in fungemic and hemodialyzed patients. The false-positive reactions in those conditions appear to be brought about by the activation of factor G. This suggests that the diagnosis of systemic fungal infections may be possible by the G test.

ACKNOWLEDGEMENTS

The author thanks Mr. Tanaka and Mr. Tamura for their cooperation in conducting this study.

REFERENCES

1. Iwanaga, S., Morita, T., Harada, T., et al., 1978, Chromogenic substrates for horseshoe crab clotting enzyme. Its application for the assay of bacterial endotoxins. Haemostasis 7: 183-188.

2. Iwanaga, S., Morita, T., Miyata, T., et al., 1984, The limulus coagulation system sensitive to bacterial endotoxins. in: "Bacterial endotoxin: chemical, biological, and clinical aspects. J. Y. Homma et al., eds. Weinheim: Verlag Chemie GmbH, 365-382.

3. Kakinuma, A., Asano, T., Torii, H., and Sugino, Y., 1981, Gelation of Limulus amebocyte lysate by an antitumor (1→3)-β-D-glucan. Biochem. Biophys. Res. Commun. 101: 434-439.

4. Levin, J., and Bang, F. B., 1968, Clottable protein in Limulus: its localization and kinetics of its coagulation by endotoxin. Thromb. Diath. Haemorrh. 19: 186-197.

5. Morita, T., Tanaka, S., Nakamura, T., and Iwanaga, S., 1981, A new (1→3)-β-D-glucan-mediated coagulation pathway found in Limulus amebocytes. FEBS Lett 129: 318-321.

6. Obayashi, T., 1984, Addition of perchloric acid to blood samples for colorimetric limulus test using chromogenic substrate: comparison with conventional procedures and clinical applications. J. Lab. Clin. Med. 104: 321-330.

A NEW PERCHLORIC ACID TREATMENT OF HUMAN PLASMA FOR DETECTION OF ENDOTOXIN BY AN ENDOTOXIN-SPECIFIC CHROMOGENIC TEST

K. Inada[1], M. Yoshida[1], T. Takahashi[1], S. Tamura[2], S. Tanaka[2], S. Endo[3], T. Yoshida[4], H. Suda[5] and T. Komuro[6].

Department of Bacteriology[1], Critical Care and Emergency Center[3], 1st Department of Internal Medicine[4] and Department of Pediatrics[5], School of Medicine, Iwate Medical University, Morioka 020; Tokyo Research Institute[2], Seikagaku Kogyo Co. Ltd., Tokyo 189; and National Institute of Hygiene (Osaka)[6], 520 Osaka, Japan

Recently, an endotoxin-specific colorimetric assay method, using synthetic chromogenic substrate, was developed using factor G-depleted lysate (Endospecy, Seikagaku Kogyo)(3). Since many interfering factors and inhibitors of Limulus amebocyte lysate test are present in human plasma, it became necessary to remove these prior to the detection of endotoxin. Perchloric acid (PCA) treatment of human plasma has been used to inactivate or remove the interfering factors (2). In this method, PCA is added to test plasma and the mixture is incubated. The precipitate is discarded after centrifugation. The supernantant is employed for detection of endotoxin using Endospecy. We have found, however, that a large amount of endospecy activity was recovered from the precipitate, and we developed an improved method of PCA treatment by which endotoxin content in both the precipitate and supernatant could be measured.

Colorimetric Endotoxin-Specific Limulus Test (3)

Endospecy consists of factor G-free amebocyte lysate from **Tachypleus tridentatas** and a chromogenic substrate, Boc-Leu-Gly-Arg-pNA dissolved in 0.2 M tris-HCl buffer (pH 8.0). A 100 μl aliquot of Endospecy was added to 100 μl of plasma treated by the method described below. The contents were mixed thoroughly and incubated at 37°C for 30 min, thereafter, diazo-coupled. The absorbance was measured at 545 nm. Standard curve was plotted using **E. coli** 0111:B4 LPS (W, Difco) in distilled water, on a bilogarithmic scale.

PCA Method for Treatment of Plasma (PCA Treatment)

PCA (100 μl, 0.32 N) was added to 100 μl of test plasma (either PRP or PPP) and incubated at 37°C for 20 min, then centrifuged at 1,000 x g for 15 min. The precipitate was discarded and the supernatant was neutralized with 0.18 N NaOH. The resulting sample, diluted six times, was assayed by Endospecy.

Table 1. Endotoxin levels in the patients plasmas and LPS-spiked plasmas after PCA- and new PCA-treatments

Patient or LPS-spiked plasmas	PCA-treatment			New PCA-treatment
	Supernatant	Precipitate	Supernatant + Precipitate	
T 374	9.9 pg/ml	66.0	75.9	123.0
T 368	8.7	45.6	54.3	103.0
T 369	9.0	108.0	117.0	152.0
50 pg/ml*	0.7	38.5	39.2	45.3
500 pg/ml	38.4	354.3	392.8	476.7

* LPS was added to normal human plasma and incubated for 10 min at 37°C. Thereafter, the plasma was submitted to both treatments.

Detection of Endospecy Activity in the Precipitate of PCA-Treatment

We attempted to detect endotoxin in the precipitate of endotoxin-spiked plasma and patient plasma. The precipitate was dissolved with NaOH, neutralized with HCl, and endotoxin content was measured by Endospecy. Large amounts of endotoxin were found in the precipitates of the plasma of patients suspected of having endotoxemia and of endotoxin-spiked plasmas, as shown in Table 1. It is noteworthy that the endotoxin levels in patient plasmas detected after PCA-treatment were low.

Development of New PCA-Treatment

Therefore, we developed an improved PCA-treatment to detect endotoxin levels in the precipitate and supernatant (Fig 1). To prevent formation of intensive turbidity by PCA, NaOH was added to the test plasma and incubated for 5 min, thereafter, one-half amount of PCA was added. The plasma endotoxin levels determined by Endospecy, of the same patients mentioned above, are shown in Table 1. The endotoxin levels found by the new method were higher than those of the supernatant plus the precipitate.

Furthermore, we confirmed that the precipitate had endotoxin activity from the lethal toxicity and pyrogen test.

Lethal Toxicity of Endotoxin in the Precipitate in Galactosamine-Sensitized Mice

Twenty μg of LPS (**E. coli** 0111:B4) was added to 1 ml of plasma and incubated at 37°C for 10 min. Then the plasma was subjected to the old PCA-treatment. Almost all Endospecy activity and toxicity in galactosame-sensitized mice (1) were found to be retained in the precipitate (Table 2).

Pyrogenic Activity of Endotoxin of the Precipitate

Pyrogenic activity of the precipitate was also observed. Furthermore, rabbits injected with the precipitate developed a tolerant state similar to LPS-injected rabbits (data not shown).

Heparinized plasma 100 µl

↓ + 0.18N NaOH 100 µl

37°C, 5 min

↓ + 0.32N PCA 100 µl

37°C, 10 min

↓ + 0.18N NaOH 200 µl

50 µl aliquot

↓ + 0.2M Tris-HCl buffer, pH 8.0 50 µl

(1:10 diluted)

↓ + Endospecy 100 µl

37°C, 30 min

↓

Diazotization

↓

3,000 rpm, 10 min

↓

Absorbance at 545 nm

Fig 1. Procedures of new PCA-treatment and endospecy assay. Centrifugation at 3,000 rpm for 10 min is recommended when the solution became turbid after the last incubation.

Table 2. Recovery of endotoxin activity in the precipitate and the supernatant of PCA-treatment of LPS-spiked normal human plasma

		LPS was added to		LPS was added to plasma and submitted to PCA-treatment	
		Saline	Plasma	Precipitate	Supernatant
Recovery of Endospecy activity		100%	95%	89%	20%
Lethal Toxicity#	1:10*	2/2**	6/6	4/4	4/4
	1:100	1/2	3/6	3/6	2/6
	1:1000	0/2	0/6	0/6	0/6

* 100 µl of the dilution was injected i.p.

** death/total

galactosamine 8 mg i.p., simultaneously

Mice survived by samples only without galactosamine injection.

Table 3. Endotoxin levels in plasmas of patients with sepsis or liver diseases

#Patients	Diagnosis	Date	New PCA-treatment	PCA-treatment	
31(9d)[1]	Septic shock(DCD VE-2)[2]		2599.4 pg/ml	248.2	
38(3d)	Sepsis (**E. coli**)	7/13	119.5	11.9	CRP3+
		7/15	8.4	3.1	CRP3+
61(63)	Burn(8/29), DIC	9/7	20.5	0	
		9/14	468.7	15.1	
		9/21	467.8	6.9	
		9/25	604.8	118.8	
		10/1	16.9	2.7	
95(58)	Liver cirrhosis	10/26	9.6	0	
		10/28	10.8	0	
		11/2	34.1	0	
		11/4 +	441.7	0	
109(51)	Fluminant hepatitis	11/4	241.7	0	
		11/7	549.1	0	
		11/9 +	0.9	0	
114(60)	Liver cirrhosis	11/4	193.7	0	
		11/6	591.7	0	
		11/9 +	9.6	0	
118(20)	Fluminant hepatitis	11/6	567.0	0	
		11/13	1.6	0	
187(29)	Sepsis (**S. epidermidis**)	12/7	23.9	0.5	
		12/23	5.1	5.0	
	(**Acinetobacter**)	1/2	191.3	16.8	
		1/5	581.5	131.4	
		1/11	12.7	0	
322(58)	Liver cirrhosis, sepsis		558.9	163.5	
Normal range			< 12	< 3	

[1]Age

[2]Bacteria isolated from blood specimen

The mean endotoxin content of normal human plasma, measured by the new PCA-treatment, was 6.1 ± 3.0 (S.D. n=20), whereas, after the old PCA-treatment of the same samples it was only 1.6 ± 1.4. The mean level of endotoxin of plasma (n=175) by the new PCA-treatment was on the average 10 times higher than that by the old PCA-treatment.

As shown in Table 3, endotoxin levels of patient plasmas after PCA- and new PCA-treatment were compared. The endotoxin levels of plasmas treated with PCA, in patients with liver diseases, were almost negligible, however, that of new PCA-treatment were extremely high. Thus, it is necessary to use the new PCA-treatment for measurement of endotoxin levels in cases of liver disease. In the case of a neonate, CRP (C-reactive protein) remained at a high level, although the endotoxin level was reduced to normal range. Thus, the measurement of endotoxin level seems to be available for rapid diagnosis and prognosis of sepsis.

These results indicate that the improved new PCA-treatment of plasma is preferable for endotoxin determination.

REFERENCES

1. Galanos, C., Freudenberg, M. and Reutter, W., 1979, Galactosamine-induced sensitization to the lethal effects of endotoxin. Proc. Natl. Acad. Sci. USA. 76: 5939-5943.

2. Obayashi, T., 1984, Addition of perchloric acid to blood samples for colorimetric Limulus test using chromogenic substrate. J. Lab. Clin. Med. 104: 321-330.

3. Obayashi, T., Tamura, H., Tanaka, S., Ohki, M., Takahashi, S., Arai, M., Masuda, M. and Kawai, T., 1985, A new chromogenic endotoxin-specific assay using recombined Limulus coagulation enzymes and its clinical applications. Clin. Chim. Acta 149: 55-65.

SECTION III.

MOLECULAR INTERACTIONS

FLUORESCENT DETECTION OF LIPOPOLYSACCHARIDE INTERACTIONS WITH MODEL MEMBRANES

D. M. Jacobs, H. Yeh and R. M. Price

Department of Microbiology, School of Medicine and Biomedical Sciences, State University of New York at Buffalo, Buffalo, New York 14214

SUMMARY

The critical importance of the lipid A moiety of LPS in resistance and pathogenesis in gram negative infections has led to the assumption that LPS interaction with target cells is due to hydrophobic interaction with plasma membranes. However, work from several laboratories, including our own, is consistent with the presence of a cell membrane structure with characterstics of a "receptor". We have proposed a two-step model for LPS-membrane interaction which resolves the two views, and have developed a model system to control the first step (binding to membrane protein) and study the second step (intercalation into lipid bilayer). We examined the interaction of LPS with small unilamellar phosphatidylcholine vesicles labeled in the hydrophobic portion of the bilayer with the fluorescent probe diphenylhexatrine (DPH) and detected changes in the physical properties of the bilayer by measuring DPH fluorescence anisotropy (Δr). We have found that purified, phenol-extracted **S. typhimurium** LPS interacts with the bilayer as measured by an increase in Δr and conclude that the LPS aggregate coalesced with the lipid bilayer. The greatest change in Δr was achieved with lipid A, Ra-Re glycolipids and diphosphoryl lipid A. Monophosphoryl lipid A and lipid X were less effective. Preparations of wild-type LPS fractionated according to the length of the O-antigen side chain and unfractionated LPS had least effect on Δr. Thus other factors such as serum components or membrane proteins may be necessary to enhance the interaction of LPS with target cells.

INTRODUCTION

Lipopolysaccharide (LPS) interacts with many types of mammalian cells to induce metabolic and cellular changes which mediate both pathogenesis and host defenses. Although these processes have been well studied, there is little information on the molecular basis of LPS interaction with cells or their membranes. The importance of the lipid A moiety in biological activities of LPS has led to the assumption that the macromolecule interacts hydrophobically with the plasma membrane of target cells via the lipid A region. However, since the prototype monomer of LPS is an amphiphile, LPS exists as bilayer of vesicular aggregates in solution, arrangements in which the hydrophobic lipid A is not exposed to the aqueous environment. In addition, there is scant direct evidence in the literature that LPS interaction with cell membranes is hydrophobic. Furthermore, this approach does not include a role for the polysaccharide portion of LPS in the interaction with mammalian cell membranes, although this region of LPS is clearly important for the solubility of LPS and pathogenicity of Gram-negative organisms in an aqueous environment.

Some studies have examined the physical properties of membranes after interaction with LPS. Fluorescence anisotropy of a probe in macrophages exposed to LPS has been examined; however, the time and temperature used did not preclude the possibility that the measurements reflected the behavior of internal membranes after physiological activation by LPS (16). Some studies have demonstrated an interaction between LPS and phospholipid monolayer or bilayer films as detected by changes in surface pressure and surface potential (1, 6). In other studies, vesicles composed of mixtures of LPS and various phospholipids were examined by NMR, ESR, fluorescence, and microelectrophoresis as models for bacterial outer membranes (17, 18, 21, 28, 33). LPS was found to affect the structural order of the hydrophobic portion of the bilayer, and interactions were dependent on charge and cation concentration.

A quite different concept of the nature of LPS-plasma membrane interaction has developed in cellular immunology. The existence of a "mitogen receptor" or "LPS receptor" has been proposed and is a useful part of models of B cell activation. Within the lymphoid system, the major lymphocyte targets for LPS are bone marrow-derived lymphocytes (B cells) which are activated to DNA synthesis and immunoglobulin synthesis and secretion without the necessity for T cell help. Preferential binding to B cells has been demonstrated at the single cell level in this (10) and other laboratories (2, 8) although attempts to demonstrate selectivity of binding using radiobinding techniques and mass cultures have yielded contradictory results (2, 13, 19, 31, 35). The preference of LPS for activation of B cells would suggest that these cells have a specific LPS binding site or receptor. However, there is no direct evidence for the presence of a stereochemically specific plasma membrane receptor by which the ligand transduces a signal to a target cell, although the binding data from our laboratory is consistent with this possibility.

Recently, the results from studies of LPS binding to murine lymphocytes led us to conclude that LPS association with cell membranes is a two-step process (9, 11). This model proposes that the first step is reversible, is inhibited by polyions, and is temperature independent. The second step is irreversible within the time-scale of the experiment, is not inhibited by polyions, and is not detectable at low temperatures. We have suggested that the two steps are equivalent to (1) the association of the LPS aggregate with the cell surface (adherence) and (2) the incorporation of individual LPS molecules into the cell membrane (coalescence). This two-step model is based on biological data but it addresses physicochemical constraints of LPS-membrane interactions and reconciles otherwise conflicting observations. The model recognizes that ionic interactions are involved in overcoming the electrostatic and hydration repulsion of the two aggregates of amphiphiles with hydrophilic surfaces so that adherence can occur. Adherence is followed by the rearrangement of phospholipids so that acyl chains of LPS subunits are integrated into the phospholipid bilayer. According to our model, many cells bind LPS by this mechanism, and this binding is characterized as non-saturable and non-inhibitable and is detected at high doses of LPS. We further suggest that some cells have membrane structures, presumably proteins, which facilitate ionic interactions characteristic of Step 1. The presence of this facilitator results in the appearance of binding with characteristics usually attributed to a specific receptor: detectable at low doses of LPS; saturable and inhibitable; selective for cells bearing the facilitator; and specifically inhibitable. Cell activation would be a consequence of integration of the lipid A region of LPS with the lipid bilayer and not of LPS interaction with the facilitator site.

Further testing of this model is dependent of a simple system with fewer variables than are found in systems using intact cells. We have used small, unilamellar phospholipid vesicles (SUVs) as models for cell membranes and labeled them with the fluorescent probe diphenylhexatriene (DPH). This probe preferentially partitions into the hydrophobic environment of the acyl chains of the phospholipid bilayer and emits fluorescence only from that environment. (Its fluorescence is quenched in an aqueous environment.) Changes in some optical properties for the probe (anisotropy) thus reflect changes in the physical property of the interior of the bilayer, the order of the acyl chains. We have measured the interaction of LPS with SUVs by detecting the fluorescence anisotropy of DPH. We have found that LPS interaction with the SUVs affected the physical properties of the lipid bilayer so that the measured anisotropy of DPH was increased. We have also found that such a change could not be attributed to transfer of the probe between LPS aggregates and SUVs (24). Using changes in fluorescence anistoropy as an indication that the acyl chains of the lipid A moiety of LPS have partitioned into the bilayer, we have found that this activity can be modulated by the attached carbohydrate side chain.

MATERIALS AND METHODS

Lipopolysaccharide

Escherichia coli 055:B5 lipopolysaccharide (LPS) (List Biologicals, Campbell, CA, USA) was used after extraction of free lipid by hexane:2-propanol (3:2) for the experiments reported in Tables 1-5. Tables 6 and 7 contain data obtained using LPS from wild-type **Salmonella typhimurium** and **Salmonella minnesota** rough mutants R60 (Ra), R345 (Rb2), R5 (Rc), R7 (Rd), and R595 (Re), as well as lipid A (from R595) purchased from List Biologicals, Campbell, CA, USA. Purified monophosphoryl lipid A (MPLA) and diphosphoryl lipid A (DPLA) were a generous gift from Dr. K. Takayama (Madison, WI, USA). Lipid X was kindly supplied by Dr. C. Raetz, (West Point, NJ, USA). LPS, glycolipids and lipids were all dissolved in 150 mM NaCl, 5 mM Hepes*, pH 7.4, and sonicated before use.

S. typhimurium

It was fractionated by size as described by Peterson and McGroarty (23). Briefly, LPS was dissolved in a buffer of 200 mM NaCl, 0.25% sodium deoxycholate, 1 mM EDTA, 0.02% sodium azide and 10 mM Tris-HCl, pH 8.0, passed through a Sephadex G-200 (Pharmacia Fine Chemicals) column (95 x 2.5 cm) at $37^{\circ}C$, and eluted with the same buffer. Fractions were collected and assayed by the thiobarbituric acid assay (4). Three fractions were identified, pooled, exhaustively dialyzed to remove detergent and buffer, and lyophiliz ed. By a variety of analyses (Jacobs and Yeh, unpublished) Fraction 1 appears to contain LPS with an average of 55 repeating units in the O-antigen; Fraction 2, 26 repeating units; and Fraction 3, an average of 2 repeating units.

Vesicles

Small, unilamellar vesicles (SUVs) were prepared from egg phosphatidylcholine (PC) (Avanti Polar Lipids, Birmingham, AL, USA) and were prepared as described (32). The appropriate amount of PC solubilized in chloroform was lyophilized, and multilamellar vesicles were formed by suspending the lipid in an aqueous buffer of 150 mM NaCl, 5 mM Hepes, pH 7.4. SUVs were formed by sonicating the multilamellar vesicle suspension in a bath-type sonicator at

*4-(2-hydroxyethyl)-1-piperazineethanesulphonic acid.

room temperature until it was clear. Any remaining multilamellar vesicles were removed by centrifugation (100,000 x g, 30 min, 4°C), and the supernatant was used as the SUV suspension. Lipid quantitation was by assay of inorganic phosphate by the malachite green method (3). Greater than 95% of the starting lipid was recovered in the SUV preparation. All fluorescence assays were carried out at 20 μM lipid.

Fluorescent Labeling

1,5-diphenyl-hexa-1,3,5-triene (Molecular Probes, Junction City, OR, USA) was dissolved in acetonitrile, and the appropriate amount was added to SUV suspensions to obtain a final lipid to probe molar ratio of 200:1, a ratio previously determined to give acceptable fluorescence with minimal interference by diphenylhexatriene (DPH) itself. The added DPH was incubated with the aqueous SUV suspensions for 90 min at room temperature.

Fluorescence Anisotropy Measurements

PC vesicles labeled with DPH were incubated for 10 min at 37° before reading the baseline anisotropy. Additions were made and samples incubated for a further 10 min at 37° before taking a second set of readings. Each measurement was carried out in triplicate. A Perkin-Elmer (LS5 Luminescence Spectrometer equipped with excitation and emission monochromators and Polaroid film-type polarizers was used to measure DPH anisotropies. The excitation/emission wavelengths were 357/430 nm with slit widths of 3 and 5 nm, respectively. Samples were illuminated for 5s before a signal integration of 4s. DPH anisotropy (r) was calculated from the poralization ratios (P) using an instrumental correction factor (14) for DPH of G = 1.006, i.e., P = IVV/-IVH G), where IVV and IVH are the intensities of vertically polarized excitation with vertically and horizontally polarized emissions, respectively. Anistoropy was then calculated from P as r = (P-1)/(P+2). Lipid bilayer microviscosities were not estimated from r since this approach has been shown to be invalid when using DPH as the fluorescent probe (15). Data is shown as Δr, the anistoropy of DPH in vesicles after addition of LPS or lipids minus the baseline anistropy of DPH before additions. In all the experiments reported here, anistropy was increased and Δr is positive.

RESULTS

We first determined the optimum concentrations of wild type LPS and phospholipid at which to examine their interactions. Phosphatidylcholine SUVs were titrated against a concentration of LPS which had previously shown optimum binding to plasma membranes of intact cells (25 μg/ml) (9) using changes in DPH anisotropy to indicate the extent of the interaction. Increasing the amount of lipid decreased the magnitude of the change in DPH anisotropy to a point where the LPS-SUV interaction was no longer detectable (Table 1). Therefore, for further studies 20 μM lipid was selected because it gave significant changes in DPH anistropy when reacted with LPS and had sufficient fluorescence intensity at the level of labeling used (lipid:probe molar ratio 200:1) so that usable fluorescence intensities were obtained.

When LPS was titrated against 20 μM lipid, the changes in DPH anisotropy between 0 and 50 μg/ml were indicative of a first-order interaction between LPS and the SUVs (Table 2). At 100 μg/ml, however, the observed change in DPH anisotropy fell distinctly out of the pattern formed by the lower concentration of LPS (Table 2). The reason for this deviation has not yet been determined, but may be due to a change in the phase state of LPS induced by its interaction with phospholipids (34).

Table 1. Changes in Small Unilamellar Vesicles Induced by Lipopolysaccharide at Different Concentrations of Lipid

	Lipid (μM)			
	10	20	40	80
r (SUVs alone)	0.064	0.062	0.063	0.063
r (+ lipopolysaccharide)	0.091	0.071	0.065	0.064
% change in r	+42	+14	+3	+1.5

Lipopolysaccharide (25 μg/ml, reaction volume = 2 ml. T = 37°C. Diphenylhexatriene anisotropies are the average of 2 separate determinations.

These results are consistent with an interaction between LPS and SUVs that changes the structure of the acyl region of the SUVs and, thereby, changes the constraints on the motion of the fluorescent probe in that region. However, the observed increase in DPH anisotropy could also be explained by a transfer of DPH from the hydrophobic region of the SUV to the hydrophobic region of free LPS. In this case, the resultant DPH anisotropy would be the weighted sum of the anisotropies of DPH in the SUVs and in the LPS aggregates (14). This possibility was evaluated using two different methods.

First, we examined a system in which DPH could not be transferred between aggregates. LPS (20 μg/ml) was added to PC vesicles (20 μM lipid) containing DPH covalently bound to PC. LPS also induced an increase in DPH anisotropy (SUVs alone, r = 0.131; SUV + LPS, r = 0.143) although the extent of the increase (9%) was less than that observed in systems using free DPH (14%, Tables 1 and 2). Since DPH transfer was not possible in this system, the observed increase in DPH anisotropy must have been due to the interaction between the SUVs and LPS.

The results from the latter experiments suggested that DPH transfer could account for a portion of the observed increase in anisotropy. To determine the extent to which this mechanism affected our results, LPS-SUV interaction was examined in SUVs containing brominated PC (Br-PC) which would quench DPH. The fractional fluorescence intensities of DPH in the SUVs and LPS could be estimated from the fluorescence intensities in the presence and absence of quencher (Table 3). The fraction of fluorescence that was inaccessible to quenching was estimated from a linear regression calculation of the reciprocal of the fractional decrease in fluorescence versus the reciprocal of the concentration of quencher (Br-PC) (14). Thus, if DPH were able to transfer between SUV (quenched) and LPS aggregate (unquenched), a decrease in the proportion of fluorescence susceptible to quenching should have been observed. The results from such calculations are seen in Table 4. As the amount of LPS present increased from 25 to 125 μg/ml, the percentage of fluorescence transfer increased from 2.8 to 3.4%.

Table 2. Changes in Small Unilamellar Vesicles Induced by Lipopolysaccharide at Different Lipopolysaccharide Concentrations

	Lipopolysaccharide (μg/ml)					
	0	5	10	25	50	100
R (SUVs alone)	0.062	0.062	0.063	0.064	0.063	0.063
r (+ lipopoly saccharide)	0.062	0.065	0.070	0.073	0.074	0.089
% change in r	0	+5	+11	+14	+17	+41

SUV lipid 20 μM, reaction volume = 2 ml. T = 37°C. Diphenylhexatriene anistropies are the average of 2 separate determinations.

If the SUVs and LPS were not interacting, then the average anisotropy (r) of the system (SUVs + LPS) would be the linear sum of their individual anisotropies (ri) multiplied by their fractional fluorescence intensities (fi), i.e., r = f(SUV)r(SUV) = f(LPS)r(LPS). The data from Table 4 were used to calculate the anisotropies expected if the results (Table 2) were to reflect the simple transfer of DPH between the non-interacting aggregates (Table 5). Since the measured anisotropies are greater than that due to the individual components, transfer of DPH between aggregates could not account for the magnitude of DPH anisotropy change observed, and these changes should reflect changes induced by LPS interaction with SUVs.

The experiments presented above indicated that this model system could provide useful information in evaluating the factors governing the control of LPS interaction with cell membranes, as both the lipid composition of the SUVs and the LPS could be varied. The use of wild-type LPS poses limitations in interpretation because it is heterogenous in composition by many criteria, including length of the O-antigen side chain and degree of microsubstitution of groups such as phosphates. Concentrations can only be expressed in molar units by making assumptions about an average molecular weight and assuming all monomer subunits interact to the same degree. We therefore systematically examined the behavior of a number of preparations which were more homogeneous than the initial material in order to determine whether they had similar activities on a molar basis. These experiments are summarized in Tables 6 and 7.

We first compared the activities of three fractions of **S. typhimurium** which differed from each other by the length of the O-antigen side chain. Work in this laboratory and others has demonstrated that each fraction contains a population of LPS molecules with a different average O-antigen side chain length as indicated by differences in the number (n) of repeating subunits (7, 12, 22, 23). In our hands, Fraction 1 has an average n of 55; Fraction 2, an average n of 26; Fraction 3, an average n of 2. By assuming an average composition for each fraction, changes in DPH-anisotropy induced by these fractions in PC-SUVs can be evaluated on a molar basis. Both Fractions 2 and 3 have similar activities which are very low, Fraction 1 is somewhat higher. By comparison, all rough LPS examined have a more pronounced effect on the DPH anisotropy of the SUVs. Within the rough LPS there is no reproducible pattern over the dose range tested.

Table 3. Fluorescence Intensities of Diphenylhextriene in Presence of Br-PC and Lipopolysaccharide

	Lipopolysaccharide (μg/ml)		
mol % Br-PC	0	25	125
0	106.1	110.2	111.3
33	62.1	60.0	64.8
66	31.1	32.6	35.4
100	1.8	2.7	4.2

Reaction volume = 2 ml. T = 37°C. Fluorescence intensity values are the average of 2 separate determinations.

Further experiments were carried out to compare different preparations of Lipid A and its biosynthetic precursor, Lipid X. These results are presented in Table 7. Highly purified lipid A (obtained from a commercial source) has the most pronounced effect of any member of the LPS family of molecules. However, it too is likely to sustain microheterogeneity. Fortunately, we were able to obtain HPLC-purified diphosphoryl Lipid A (DPLA) and monophosphoryl lipid A (MPLA) for testing. Both materials were less active than unfractionated Lipid A, but DPLA appeared to have twice the activity of MPLA. Furthermore, Lipid X has an activity similar to MPLA. It should be noted that the smaller molecules can be tested at higher molar concentrations than the larger, wild-type LPS, since light scattering in concentrated solutions of the latter interfere with fluorescence measurements.

Table 4. Percent of Fluorescence Intensity Due to Transfer of Diphenylhextriene between Hydrophobic Regions

	Lipopolysaccharide (μg/ml)		
	0	25	125
correlation coefficient	0.999	0.995	0.997
% fluorescence quenchable	96.0	93.2	92.6
% fluorescence transfer	0	2.8	3.4

Calculated from data in Table 3. See text for details.

Table 5. Calculated Anisotropies of SUV + Lipopolysaccharide System if They do not Interact

	Lipopolysaccharide (μg/ml)	
	25	125
f(SUV)	0.972	0.966
f(lipopolysaccharide)	0.028	0.034
r	0.066	0.067
measured r	0.073	0.089*

*Value from 100 μg/ml lipopolysaccharide, Table 2. Values used for other numbers: r(SUV) = 0.064; r(LPS) = 0.140 (T = 37°C, determined separately).

DISCUSSION

The nature of the association between LPS and the plasma membrane which initiates cell activation poses difficulties when examined in whole cells and has led to two opposing models. We have previously shown that the conditions under which LPS binds to cells is suggestive of a two-step process in which the first step is ionic in nature (9, 11). It is not clear that such charge-mediated interactions on the surface of the plasma membrane are sufficient to activate cells, and there is at least one example of a charge-mediated association of macromolecules with cell surfaces which inactivates cells (25). The second step, the intercalation of the hydrophobic Lipid A portion of LPS into the membrane lipid bilayer, has been assumed to occur on the basis of the Lipid A structure, and LPS has been shown to interact with phospholipid monolayers (6, 27) the intrusion of a large lipid would be expected to alter the order of "fluidity" of the membrane lipid bilayer, and indeed lipid bilayers that are reconstituted with LPS or Lipid A are more ordered (less fluid) than reconstituted bilayers consisting of the lipid alone (5, 18, 20). Therefore, we designed a test system to examine the changes in membrane bilayers which occur upon addition of exogenous LPS. We found that LPS interaction with the lipid bilayer results in increased order of the lipid acyl chains or decreased "fluidity" of that bilayer. Since cell activation is associated with changes in cell membrane fluidity (26, 29), LPS-induced alterations in plasma membrane fluidity may modulate cell responses. We suggest that the association of the LPS aggregate with the cell surface, mediated by the charge on the LPS and some cell surface structure(s) (adherence), increases the thermodynamic probability of the intercalation of LPS monomers into the cell membrane lipid bilayer (coalescence, the second step). This intercalation of the hydrophobic Lipid A portion of LPS decreases the fluidity of that region of the cell membrane, and this change may play a role in cell activation. We have presented evidence elsewhere that the cell attempts to rid itself of this exogenous signalling substance by cytoskeleton-mediated capping of the LPS (30).

If the fatty acids of the Lipid A region of LPS interact with lipid bilayers in the same manner regardless of the structure of the remainder of the molecule and the composition of the material studied, the same changes in anisotropy would be expected for all LPS with identical Lipid A structures. The data in Tables 6 and 7 suggest that this assumption is incorrect. Differences in activity of MPLA and DPLA are apparently attributable to one phosphate on the diglucosamine backbone (Table 7). This could affect the

Table 6. Changes Induced in Small Unilamellar Vesicles by Lipopolysaccharides of Varying Carbohydrate Composition

	0.5 μM	1.0 μM	2.5 μM	5.0 μM	10 μM	25 μM
Fr.1	-	0.016	0.027	0.031	-	-
Fr.2	-	0.011	0.013	0.017	0.024	-
Fr.3	-	0.007	0.013	0.017	0.024	-
Ra	0.013	-	0.030	0.052	-	0.100
Rb2	0.012	-	0.027	0.043	-	0.078
Rc	0.018	-	0.051	0.067	-	0.103
Rd	0.016	-	0.047	0.075	-	0.111
Re	0.030	-	0.043	0.064	-	0.083

Data shown are changes in diphenylhexatriene anistoropy (Δ r) after additions at indicated concentrations. For unfractionated LPS, 25 μg/ml, $\Delta r = 0.024$; 50 μg/ml, $\Delta r = 0.046$. Baseline SUVs, r = 0.072 for 20 mM lipid.

efficiency of the initial ionic interaction of Lipid A aggregates (step 1) or the subseqent interaction of Lipid A either with other Lipid A molecules or with the acyl chains of the bilayer. Lipid X, which is a smaller molecule containing fewer fatty acids than Lipid A, has the same activity on a molar basis as MPLA, indicating that some factor other than or in addition to the number of fatty acids available for intercalation into the bilayer is responsible for the changes observed in the bilayer.

The large differences between anisotropy increases in the presence of commercially prepared Lipid A and the DPLA and MPLA purified by HPLC should also be noted. This Lipid A, derived from R595, is said to be predominantly MPLA. Since it has a much greater activity than HPLC purified material, it must be assumed that components present in trace amounts in the commercial material but absent from the HPLC-purified material have a very strong effect on the ability of Lipid A to interact with the bilayer. These materials may be "impurities" such as free phospholipid, and we have observed that delipidated smooth LPS increases anisotropy to a lesser degree than untreated LPS (Price and Jacobs, unpublished observations). These materials could simply be cations which are normally associated with LPS and remain throughout the purification procedures. Divalent cations are known to enhance vesicle fusion, probably by forming cation bridges between negatively charged groups in apposition. The data reported here therefore suggest that this system is very sensitive to small variations in composition of the materials tested, and definitive interpretation of the results may require exquisite attention to these issues.

The LPS from rough mutants contains core polysaccharide in addition to Lipid A, but their effect on the behavior of the lipid bilayer is no different than that of Lipid A alone (Table 6). There is enough overlap in the data so that no clear pattern of reactivity emerges to suggest the importance of any particular component of these LPS's. Each of the rough LPS was more active than DPLA but less effective than commercial Lipid A. It is not

Table 7. Changes Induced in Small Unilamellar Vesicles by Lipid A's and Lipid X

	0.5 μM	2.5 μM	5.0 μM	10 μM	25 μM	50 μM
Lipid A	0.004	0.037	0.059	-	0.158	0.208
Diphosphoryl lipid A	-	-	0.020	-	0.067	0.103
Monophophoryl lipid A	-	-	0.009	-	0.022	0.059
Lipid X	0.002	0.007	0.005	0.018	0.035	0.052

Data shown are changes in diphenylhexatriene anistropy (Δ r) after additions at indicated concentrations.

possible to know whether the carbohydrate of the intact macromolecule or possible trace amounts of other materials are more important in modulating the interaction of these materials with SUVs.

Results obtained with fractions of **S. typhimurium** LPS differing in the length of the O-antigen side chain are also interesting. These fractions, initially separated in the presence of detergent, contain no detectable detergent, phospholipids or protein. At a concentration of 5 μM, DPLA and Fractions 2 and 3 induce similar changes in anisotropy. However, the change in anisotropy induced by Fraction 1 is almost twice that induced by the other fractions. The degree of difference between Fraction 1 and Fractions 2 and 3 has been observed several times and with different fraction preparations. One interpretation of these results, and the one we consider most likely, is that this LPS preparation with very long O-antigen side chains, self-associates to form microdomains in the bilayer; and this self-association has a greater effect on the order of the bilayer than similar molecules which do not self-associate. The presence of microdomains of LPS in LPS-phospholipid vesicles has been inferred from the NMR and ESR studies of Nikaido et al., (20).

The data presented here indicate that highly purified DPLA and smooth LPS are relatively inefficient in interacting with pure lipid bilayers in an aqueous environment as measured by a change in the order of the hydrophobic region of the bilayer. This is consistent with predictions based on the physicochemical properties of LPS in solution and different from the prediction based solely on the chemical structure of monomer subunits. It is thus likely that the potent biological activity of LPS rests on the in vivo participation of factors which enhance LPS interaction with plasma membranes. Other bacterial outer membrane components and serum lipoproteins are two types of materials which are found to associate with LPS, and they could be important in modulating LPS activities. Cell membrane receptors or binding sites such as those we have noted on lymphocytes (10) may also facilitate localization of low concentrations of LPS on selected cell populations. The system we have developed can be exploited to facilitate the identification and characterization of those other factors which are important for LPS activation of target cells.

ACKNOWLEDGEMENTS

Supported by PHS research grant AI18506 and research development funds from SUNY-Buffalo. Dr. Price was the receipient of a SUNY-Buffalo Presidential Postdoctoral Fellowship.

REFERENCES

1. Benedetto, D. A., Shands, J. W., Jr. and Shah, D.O., 1973, The interaction of bacterial lipopolysaccharide with phospholipid bilayers and monolayers. Biochim. Biophys. Acta. 298: 145.

2. Bona, C., Juy, D., Truffa-Bachi, P., and Kaplan, G. J., 1976, Binding, capping and internalization of lipopolysaccharide in thymic and non-thymic lymphocytes of the mouse. Biological and autoradiographic study. J. Microscopie Biol. Cell. 25: 47.

3. Carter, S. G., and Karl, D. W., 1982, Inorganic phosphate assay with malachite green: An improvement and evaluation. J. Biochem. Biophys. Methods 7: 7.

4. Cynkin, M. A., and Ashwell, G., 1960, Estimation of 3-deoxy sugars by means of the malonaldehydethiobarbituric acid reaction. Nature 186: 155.

5. Emmerling, G., Henning, U., and Gulik-Kryzwicki, T., 1977, Order disorder conformational transition of hydrocarbon chains in lipopolysaccharide from **Escherichia coli**, Eur. J. Biochem. 78: 503.

6. Fried, V. A., and Rothfield, L. I., 1978, Interactions between lipopolysaccharide and phosphatidylethanolamine in molecular monolayers. Biochim. Biphys. Acta. 514: 69.

7. Goldman, R. C., and Leive, L., 1980, Heterogeneity of antigenic-side-chain length in lipolysaccharide from **Escherichia coli** 0111 and **Salmonella typhimurium** LT2. Eur. J. Biochem. 107: 145.

8. Gregory, S. H., Zimmerman, D. H., and Kern, M., 1980, The Lipid A moiety of lipolysaccharide is specificaly bound to B cell subpopulations of responder and nonresponder animals. J. Immunol. 125: 102.

9. Jacobs, D. M., 1984, Structural features of binding of lipopolysaccharide to murine lymphocytes. Rev. Infect. Dis. 6: 501.

10. Jacobs, D. M., and Eldridge, J. H., 1984, Surface phenotype of LPS-binding murine lymphocytes. Proc. Soc. Exp. Biol. Med. 175: 458.

11. Jacobs, D. M. and Price, R. M., 1987, A model for lipopolysaccharide-membrane interaction. in: "Recent Advances in Mucosal Immunology, Part A," J. Mestecky, J. R. McGhee, J. Bienestock, P. L. Ogra, eds. Plenum Publishing Corp.

12. Jann, B., Reske, K., and Jann, K., 1975, Heterogeneity of lipopolysaccharides. Analysis of polysaccharide chain lengths by sodium dodecylsulfate-polyacrylamide gel electrophoresis. Eur. J. Biochem. 60: 239.

13. Kabir, S., and Rosenstreich, D., 1977, Binding of bacterial endotoxin to murine spleen lymphocytes. Infect. Immun. 15: 156.

14. Lakowicz, J. R., 1983, in: "Principles of Fluorescence Spectroscopy," Plenum Press, New York pp. 111-153 and 258-296.

15. Lakowicz, J. R., Prendergast, F. G., and Hogen, D., 1979, Fluorescence anisotropy measurements under oxygen quenching conditions as a method to quantify the depolarizing rotations of fluorophores. Application to diphenylhexatrine in istoropic solvents and in lipid bilayers. Biochem. 18: 520.

16. Larsen, N. E., Enelow, R. I., Simmons, E. R., and Sullivan, R., 1985, Effect of bacterial endotoxin on the transmembrane electrical potential and plasma membrane fluidity of human monocytes. Biochim. Biophys. Acta. 815: 1.

17. Liu, M. S., Onji, T., and Snelgrove, N. E., 1982, Changes in the phase transition temperature of phospholipids induced by endotoxin. Biochim. Biophys. Acta. 710: 248.

18. MacKay, A. L., Nichol, C. P., Weeks, G., and Davis, J. H., 1984, A proton and deuterium nuclear magnetic resonance study of orientational order in aqueous dispersons of lipopolysaccharide and lipopolysaccharide/dipalmitoylphosphatidylcholine mixtures. Biochim. Biophys. Acta. 774: 181.

19. Moller, G., Anderson, J., Pohlit, H., and Sjoberg, O., 1973, Quantitation of the number of mitogen molecules activating DNA synthesis in T and B lymphocytes. Clin. Exp. Immunol. 13: 89.

20. Nikaido, H., Takeuchi, Y., Ohnishi, S. T., and Nakae, T., 1977, Outer membrane of **Salmonella typhimurium**. Electron spin resonance studies. Biochim. Biophys. Acta. 465: 152.

21. Onji, T., and Liu, M. S., 1979, Changes in the surface charge density of liposomes induced by **Escherichia coli** endotoxin. Biochim. Biophys. Acta. 558: 320.

22. Palva, E. T., and Makela, P. H., 1980, Lipopolysaccharide heterogeneity in **Salmonella typhimurium** analyzed by sodium dodecylsulfate/polyacrylamide gel electrophoresis. Eur. J. Biochem. 107: 137.

23. Peterson, A. A. and McGoarty, E. J., 1985, High-molecular-weight components in lipopolysaccharides of **Salmonella typhimurium**, **Salmonella minnesota**, and **Escherichia coli**. J. Bacteriol. 162: 738.

24. Price, R. M. and Jacobs, D. M., 1986, Fluorescent detection of lipopolysaccharide interactions with model membranes. Biochem. Biophys. Acta. 859: 26.

25. Price, R. M., Gersten, D. M. and Ramwell, P. W., 1985, Macromolecules mediate prostacyclin release from human umbilical artery. Biochim. Biophys. Acta. 836: 246.

26. Quinn, P. J., 1981, The fluidity of cell membranes and its regulation. Prog. Biophys. Molec. Biol. 38: 1.

27. Rothfield, L., and Horne, R. W., 1967, Reassociation of purified lipopolysaccharide and phospholipid of the bacterial cell envelope: Electron microscopic and monolayer studies. J. Bacteriol. 93: 1705.

28. Rottem, S., 1978, The effect of Lipid A on the fluidity and permeability properties of phospholipid dispersons. FEBS Letter 95: 121.

29. Salesse, R., and Garnier, J., 1984, Adenylate cyclase and membrane fluidity. Molec. Cell Biochem. 60: 17.

30. Swartzwelder, F. and Jacobs, D. M., 1984, Lipopolysaccharide capping on murine lymphocytes. Rev. Infect. Dis. 6: 578.

31. Symond, D. B. A., and Clarkson, C. A., 1979, The binding of LPS to the lymphocyte surface. Immunology 38: 503.

32. Szoka, F., and Papahadjopoulos, D., 1980, Comparative properties and methods of preparation of lipid vesicles (liposomes). Ann. Rev. Biophys. Bioeng. 9: 467.

33. Takeuchi, Y. and Nikaido, H., 1981, Persistence of segregated phospholipid domains in phospholipid-lipopolysaccharide mixed bilayers: Studies with spin-labeled phospholipids. Biochemistry 20: 523.

34. Van Alphen, L., Verkleij, A., Burnell, E., and Lugtenberg, B., 1980, ^{31}P nuclear magnetic resonance and freeze-fracture electron microscopy studies on **Escherichia coli**. II. Lipopolysaccharide and lipopolysaccharide-phospholipid complexes. Biochim. Biophys. Acta. 597: 502.

35. Zimmerman, D. H., Gregory, S., and Kern, M., 1977, Differentiation of lymphoid cells: The preferential binding of the Lipid A moiety of lipopolysaccharide to B lymphocyte populations. J. Immunol. 119: 1018.

INTERACTION OF Mg^{2+} AND Ca^{2+} IN IN VITRO HEXAGONAL ASSEMBLY OF R-FORM LIPOPOLYSACCHARIDES

N. Kato, M. Ohta, N. Kido, H. Ito, and S. Naito

Department of Bacteriology, Nagoya University School of Medicine, Showa-ku, Nagoya, Aichi 466, Japan

SUMMARY

The R-form lipopolysaccharide (LPS) from **Klebsiella pneumoniae** strain LEN-111 (03-:K1-), from which cationic material had been removed by electrodialysis, formed an orderly hexagonal lattice structure when suspended in 50 mM Tris buffer at pH 8.5 containing $MgCl_2$. The center-to-center distance (lattice constant) of the hexagonal lattice structure depended upon the concentration of $MgCl_2$ and reached the shortest value (15 nm) at 10 mM. In contrast, $CaCl_2$ could not produce the orderly hexagonal lattice structure but produced an irregular network structure with a center to center distance of 19 to 20 nm. When the LPS was suspended in Tris buffer containing 10 mM $MgCl_2$ mixed with 1 or 10 mM $CaCl_2$, formation of the orderly hexagonal lattice structure of the magnesium salt type was inhibited and the LPS showed the structure of the calcium salt type. When 1 or 10 mM $CaCl_2$ was mixed with 10 mM $MgCl_2$, the binding of Mg to the LPS was significantly inhibited compared with when 10 mM $MgCl_2$ was added alone. On the contrary, when 10 mM $CaCl_2$ was mixed with 10 mM $MgCl_2$, the binding of Ca to the LPS was enhanced compared with when 10 mM $CaCl_2$ was added alone. It was therefore concluded that the inhibition of formation of the hexagonal lattice structure of the magnesium salt type by addition of $CaCl_2$ is due to the inhibition of the binding of Mg to the LPS. Such a competitive interaction of Mg^{2+} and Ca^{2+} was also observed with the electrodialyzed LPS of **Escherichia coli** K-12.

INTRODUCTION

Previously we showed that an R-form lipopolysaccharide (LPS) from **Klebsiella pneumoniae** strain LEN-111 (03-:K1-), a mutant lacking O-specific polysaccharide chain of LPS, formed a hexagonal lattice structure with a center to center distance (lattice constant) of 14 to 15 nm when it was precipitated by addition of two volumes of 10 mM $MgCl_2$- ethanol or was converted to the magnesium salt after electrodialysis (2, 3). The LPS from **Escherichia coli** K-12 strain JE1011 also formed the hexagonal lattice structure with the lattice constant of 15 nm when converted to the magnesium salt after electrodialysis (5). Moreover, we found that the R-form LPS of **K. pneumoniae** and **E. coli** K-12, from which cationic material was removed by electrodialysis, formed the hexagonal lattice structure with the lattice constant of 14 to 15 nm when suspended in 50 mM tris (hydroxymethyl) aminomethane (Tris) buffer at pH 8.5 containing 10 mM $MgCl_2$ (4, 6). The optimal pH range for formation of the densest hexagonal lattice structure (lattice constant, 14 to 15 nm) of the electrodialyzed LPS suspended in 50 mM Tris buffer containing 10 mM $MgCl_2$ was 8.3 to 8.8 (6). These findings indicate that the simplest procedure by which the hexagonal lattice structure with the lattice constant of 14 to 15 nm can be formed is that the electrodialyzed LPS is added into 50 mM Tris buffer at pH 8.5 containing 10 mM $MgCl_2$. In our previous study under this experimental condition (7), effects of other divalent metal cations on the hexagonal assembly of the electrodialyzed LPS of **K. pneumoniae** were compared with that of Mg^{2+}. The Zn^{2+}, Hg^{2+}, Cu^{2+}, and Ni^{2+} could produce essentially the same hexagonal lattice structure with the lattice constant of 14.5 to 15.0 nm as that formed with Mg^{2+}. The Cd^{2+}, Co^{2+}, and Fe^{2+} produced the hexagonal lattice structure with the lattice constant of 15.5 to 16.0 nm. However, Ba^{2+}, Sr^{2+}, and Ca^{2+} produced less orderly network structure with the center to center distance of 18 to 20 nm than the hexagonal lattice structure formed with the other divalent cations. In the present study, we investigated the effect of coexistence of Mg^{2+} and Ca^{2+} on in vitro hexagonal assembly of the R-form LPS.

MATERIALS AND METHODS

LPS

LPS was extracted by the phenol-water method (14) from the bacterial cells of **K. pneumoniae** LEN-111 (O3-:K1-) (9), a mutant lacking the O-specific polysaccharide chain derived from strain LEN-1 (O3:K1-) (10) and from the cells of E. coli K-12 strain JE1011 (13). **E. coli** K-12 LPS has been chemically characterized and it has been shown that the K-12 LPS is an R-form LPS lacking the O-specific polysaccharide chain (8, 11, 12). **K. pneumoniae** LEN-111 LPS has been shown to be an R-form LPS (9). The procedure of extraction and purification of LPS was the same as described previously (3). Unless otherwise stated, the experimental results with the electrodialyzed LPS of **K. pneumoniae** LEN-111 are described in the present report.

Electrodialysis of LPS

The procedure was essentially the same as described previously (2, 3). LPS (20 mg) suspended in 10 ml of distilled water was added into an appropriate cellulose tubing and the cellulose tubing was placed in a glass beaker containing 1 liter of distilled water. The anode was inserted into the tubing and the cathode into water outside the tubing. The electrodialysis was carried out for 4 hr with a constant current of 20 mA. The water outside the dialysis tubing was changed every 30 min. At the end of electrodialysis, the pH of the content of the tubing had fallen to 3.4 from the original value of 5.6.

Examination of Interaction of Mg^{2+} and Ca^{2+} in Formation of the Hexagonal Lattice Structure of the Electrodialyzed LPS

The solutions of 100 mM Tris buffer (pH 8.5 at 4°C) containing 20 mM $MgCl_2$ and various concentrations of $CaCl_2$ were prepared. The electrodialyzed LPS (2 mg/ml) was mixed with equal volumes of these solutions. The mixtures were placed in a refrigerator at 4°C overnight and then subjected to electron microscopy and elemental analyses.

Electron Microscopy

For electron microscopy, a drop of the preparation to be tested was negatively stained with ammonium molybdate as described previously (2). The materials were examined with a Hitachi H500 electron microscope operating at 100 kV. The center to center distances of lattice structures were estimated directly from electron micrographs and expressed as the mean ± standard error.

Quantitation of Mg and Ca Bound to the LPS

The quantities of Mg and Ca bound to the LPS were determined with a Hitachi H800 electron microscope fitted with Kevex 7000-Q energy disperse X-ray detector. The materials to be tested were prepared as described previously (6). Analyses were carried out at 100 kV with a beam current of 0.3 to 0.5 nA.

RESULTS

Structure of the Electrodialyzed LPS Suspended in Tris Buffer Containing Various Concentrations of $MgCl_2$ or $CaCl_2$

The electrodialyzed LPS suspended in 50 mM Tris buffer at pH 8.5 without

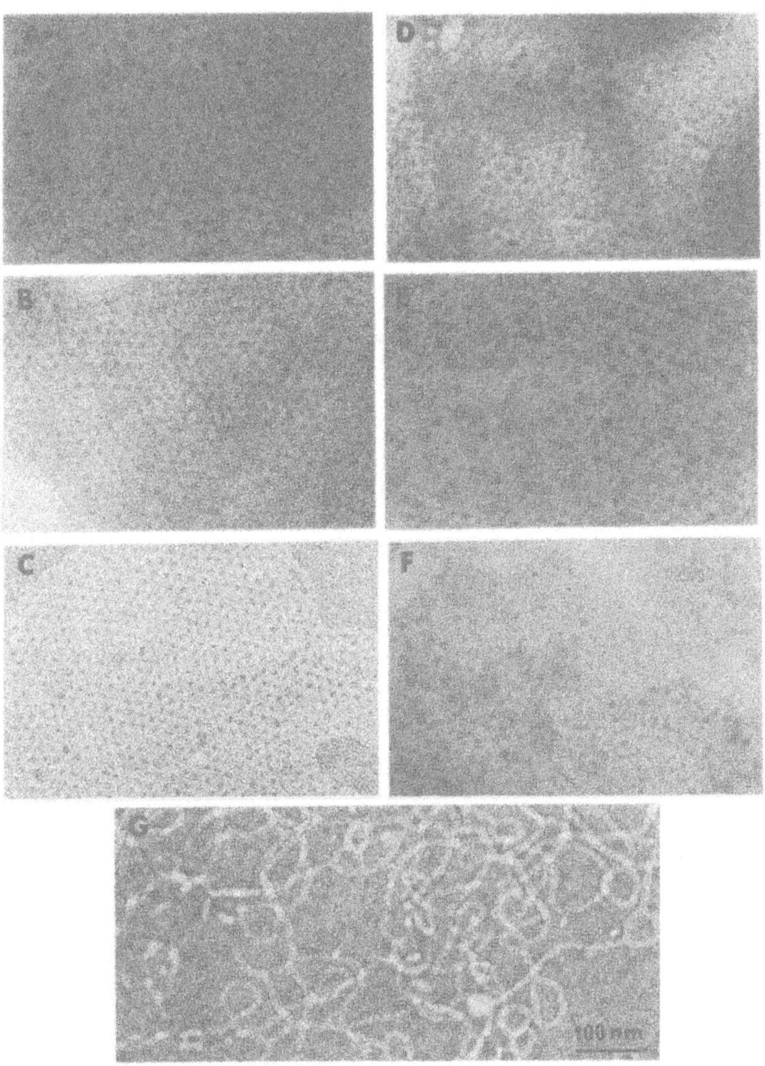

Fig 1. Ultrastructures of the electrodialyzed LPS of **K. pneumoniae** LEN-111 suspended in 50 mM Tris buffer at pH 8.5 (G), Tris buffer containing 10 mM $MgCl_2$ (A), 1 mM $MgCl_2$ (B), 0.1 mM $MgCl_2$ (C), 10 mM $CaCl_2$ (D), 1 mM $CaCl_2$ (E), and 0.1 mM $CaCl_2$ (F).

divalent cations showed ribbon-like structures branching freely and forming loops, the width of which averaged 10 nm (Fig 1G). The structures of the electrodialyzed LPS suspended in Tris buffer containing 0.1, 1, and 10 mM $MgCl_2$ or $CaCl_2$ were compared (Fig 1A-F). The LPS showed the orderly hexagonal lattice structure when suspended in Tris buffer containing 0.1 to 10 mM $MgCl_2$. The center to center distance (lattice constant) of the hexagonal lattice structure correlated with the concentration of $MgCl_2$, and at 10 mM $MgCl_2$ it reached the value (15 nm) of the magnesium salt of the LPS (2, 3) (Table 1). On the other hand, the LPS suspended in Tris buffer containing 0.1 to 10 mM $CaCl_2$ showed irregular network structures compared with the hexagonal lattice structures formed with $MgCl_2$. The center to center distances of the network structures formed with $CaCl_2$ were longer than those of the hexagonal lattice structures formed with $MgCl_2$ throughout the concentrations of 0.1 to 10 mM (Table 1).

Effect of Mixtures of $MgCl_2$ and $CaCl_2$ on Formation of the Hexagonal Lattice Structure of the Electrodialyzed LPS

To determine the effect of addition of $CaCl_2$ to Tris buffer containing 10 mM $MgCl_2$ on formation of the hexagonal lattice structure of the electrodialyzed LPS, the suspension of the electrodialyzed LPS (2 mg/ml) was mixed with an equal volume of 100 mM Tris buffer at pH 8.5 containing 20 mM $MgCl_2$ and various concentrations of $CaCl_2$ and tested for electron microscopy. The electron micrographs of the LPS preparations thus treated are shown in Fig 2 and the center to center distances of the lattice structures are shown in Fig 3. When the LPS was suspended in Tris buffer containing 10 mM $MgCl_2$ mixed with 1 or 10 mM $CaCl_2$, formation of the hexagonal lattice structure of the LPS with the feature of the magnesium salt type was inhibited and the network structure with the feature of the calcium salty type was formed. When 0.1 mM $CaCl_2$ was mixed with 10 mM $MgCl_2$, the LPS showed a hexagonal lattice structure with a longer lattice constant than that of the hexagonal lattice structure formed with 10 mM $MgCl_2$. Addition of 0.01 mM $CaCl_2$ into 10 mM $MgCl_2$ did not affect formation of the hexagonal lattice structure of the magnesium salt type.

Table 1. The center to center distances of the lattice structures of the electrodialyzed LPS of **K. pneumoniae** LEN-111 formed with various concentrations of $MgCl_2$ or $CaCl_2$

Compound	Concentration(mM)	Shape of lattice	Center-to-center distance $\pm$ standard error (nm)
$MgCl_2$	10	Hexagonal	14.7 ± 0.3
	1	Hexagonal	16.6 ± 0.2
	0.1	Hexagonal	17.4 ± 0.3
$CaCl_2$	10	Irregular	19.0 ± 0.4
	1	Irregular	19.5 ± 0.5
	0.1	Irregular	19.9 ± 0.5

a) The electrodialyzed LPS was suspended in 50 mM Tris buffer at pH 8.5 containing 0.1, 1, and 10 mM $MgCl_2$ or $CaCl_2$. The center to center distances were calculated from the electron micrographs shown in Fig 1.

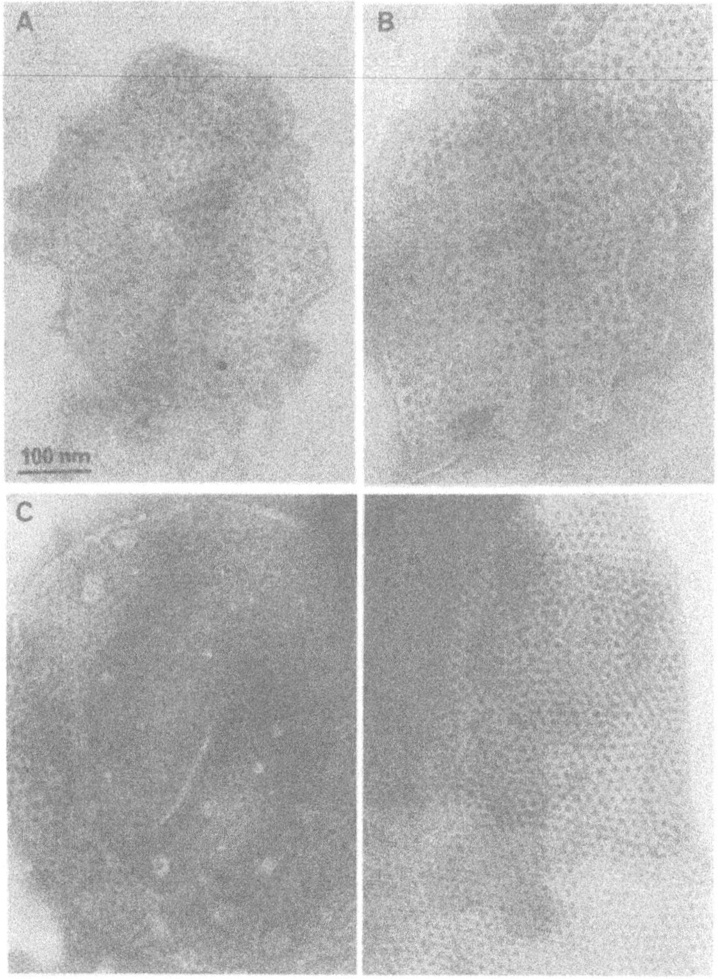

Fig 2. Ultrastructures of the electrodialyzed LPS of **K. pneumoniae** LEN-111 suspended in 50 mM Tris buffer at pH 8.5 containing 10 mM $MgCl_2$ + 10 mM $CaCl_2$ (A), 10 mM $MgCl_2$ + 1 mM $CaCl_2$ (B), 10 mM $MgCl_2$ + 0.1 mM $CaCl_2$ (C), and 10 mM $MgCl_2$ + 0.01 mM $CaCl_2$ (D).

Quantity of Mg and Ca Bound to the Electrodialyzed LPS

An experiment was carried out to determine whether the effect of addition of $CaCl_2$ into $MgCl_2$ on formation of the hexagonal lattice structure of the LPS is due to the change in the quantity of Mg and Ca bound to the LPS. The experimental conditions employed in this experiment were the same as those of the experiment shown in Fig 2. The results are shown in Fig 4. When 1 or 10 mM $CaCl_2$ was mixed with 10 mM $MgCl_2$, the binding of Mg to the LPS was significantly inhibited and the degree of inhibition was more marked at 10 mM $CaCl_2$ than that at 1 mM $CaCl_2$. On the other hand, when 10 mM $CaCl_2$ was mixed with 10 mM $MgCl_2$, the binding of Ca to the LPS was enhanced compared with when 10 mM $CaCl_2$ alone was added.

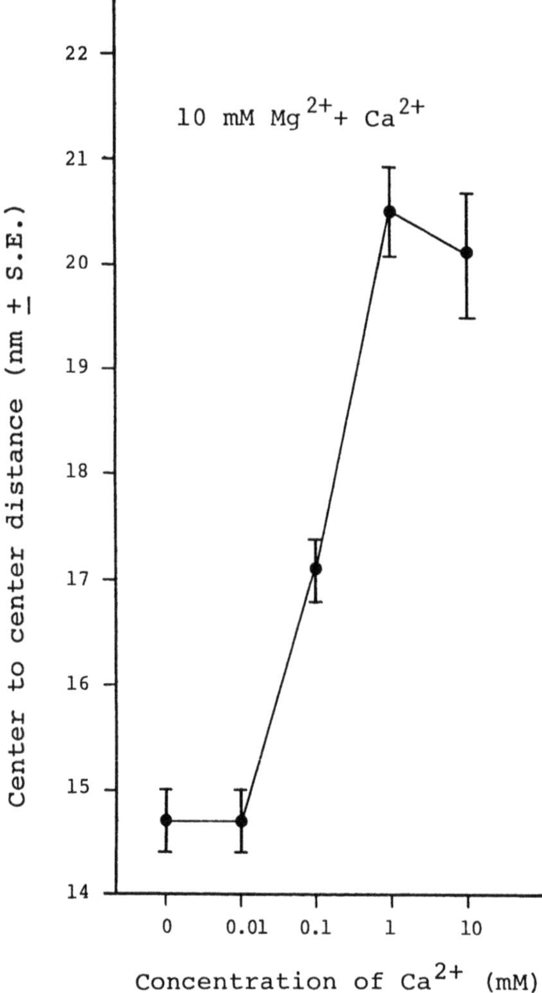

Fig 3. The center-to-center distances of the lattice structures of the electrodialyzed LPS of **K. pneumoniae** LEN-111 formed in 50 mM Tris buffer containing 10 mM $MgCl_2$ + the indicated concentrations of $CaCl_2$. The center to center distances were calculated from the electron micrographs shown in Figs 1 and 2.

Effect of Mixture of $MgCl_2$ and CaCl on Formation of the Hexagonal Lattice Structure of the Electrodialyzed LPS of **E. coli** K-12

An experiment was carried out to determine whether formation of the hexagonal lattice structure of the electrodialyzed LPS of **E. coli** K-12 in the presence of Mg^{2+} is also inhibited by addition of Ca^{2+}. The experimental conditions employed were the same as those of the experiment shown in Fig 2. The results obtained were very similar to those with the electrodialyzed LPS of **K. pneumoniae** LEN-111. The structural features of the electrodialyzed K-12 LPS suspended in Tris buffer containing $MgCl_2$ alone or $CaCl_2$ alone were very similar to those of the electrodialyzed LPS of **K. pneumoniae** LEN-111, respectively. When 1 or 10 mM $CaCl_2$ was added into Tris buffer containing 10 mM $MgCl_2$, formation of the hexagonal lattice structure of the magnesium salt type was inhibited and the K-12 LPS showed the loose network structure of the calcium salt type (data not shown).

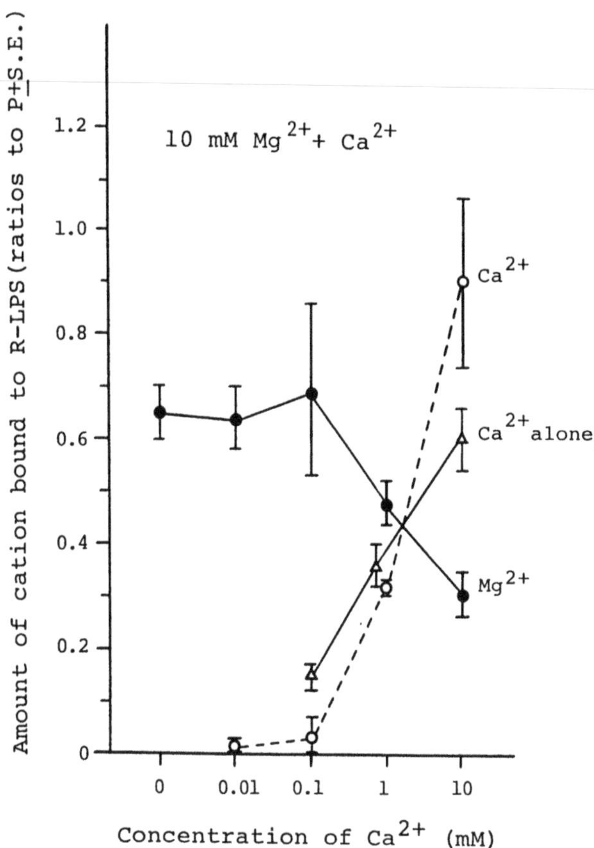

Fig 4. The quantities of Mg and Ca bound to the electrodialyzed LPS of **K. pneumoniae** LEN-111 suspended in 50 mM Tris buffer containing 10 mM $MgCl_2$ + the indicated concentrations of $CaCl_2$. Quantities of Mg and Ca are expressed as the atomic ratios to P. As control, the quantities of Ca bound to the LPS suspended in Tris buffer containing various concentrations of $CaCl_2$ alone were also determined ( ).

DISCUSSION

The R-form LPS of **K. pneumoniae** LEN-111 or **E. coli** K-12, from which cationic material was removed by electrodialysis, formed an irregular network structure with a center to center distance of 19 to 20 nm when suspended in Tris buffer containing 0.1 to 10 mM $CaCl_2$, whereas the LPS formed an orderly hexagonal lattice structure with the lattice constant of 15 nm in Tris buffer containing 10 mM $MgCl_2$. The present study demonstrated that, when the LPS was suspended in Tris buffer containing 10 mM $MgCl_2$ mixed with 1 or 10 mM $CaCl_2$, formation of the hexagonal lattice structure of the magnesium salt type was inhibited and the LPS showed the structural feature of the calcium salt type. Based on the results of quantitation of Mg and Ca bound to the LPS, it was concluded that the inhibition of formation of the hexagonal lattice structure of the magnesium salt type by addition of $CaCl_2$ is due to the inhibition of binding of Mg to the LPS. It is also noteworthy that addition of 1 mM $CaCl_2$ can inhibit significantly the effect of the tenfold higher concentration of $MgCl_2$ on the hexagonal assembly of the LPS. On the contrary, coexistence with 10 mM $MgCl_2$ enhanced the binding of Ca to the LPS. These findings indicate that the ability of Ca to bind to the LPS is significantly stronger than that of Mg. The ionic radii of Mg^{2+} and Ca^{2+} are 0.66

and 0.99 Å, respectively. Coughlin et al. (1), assumed from their analytical data that the LPS from **E. coli** K-12 wild type strains preferentially binds cations of small ionic radius. Our present results are not consistent with their assumption. In our previous study in which the abilities of various divalent metal cations to produce the orderly hexagonal lattice structure were compared with those to bind to the LPS, there was no obvious correlation between their quantities bound to the LPS and their ionic radii (7).

Physiological significance of the competitive interaction of Mg^{2+} and Ca^{2+} in in vitro hexagonal assembly of the LPS must await further investigation.

ACKNOWLEDGEMENTS

We thank T. Kuno for his assistance in the use of the electron microscope.

REFERENCES

1. Coughlin, R. T., Tonsager, S., and McGroarty, E. J., 1981, Quantitation of metal cations bound to membranes and extracted lipopolysaccharide of **Escherichia coli**. Biochemistry 22: 2002.

2. Kato, N., Ohta, M., Kido, N., Ito, H., Naito, S., and Kuno, T., 1985, Formation of a hexagonal lattice structure by an R-form lipopolysaccharide of **Klebsiella** sp. J. Bacteriol. 162: 1142.

3. Kato, N., Ohta, M., Kido, N., Ito, H., Naito, S., and Kuno, T., 1985, Formation of a hexagonal lattice structure by an R-form lipopolysaccharide of **Klebsiella**: relationship between lattice formation and uniform salt forms. Microbiol. Immunol. 29: 1059.

4. Kato, N., Ohta, M., Kido, N., Ito, H., Naito, S., and Kuno, T., 1986, Stability of the hexagonal lattice structure formed by an R-form lipopolysaccharide of **Klebsiella**: decrease in the stability by electrodialysis and recovery by addition of the magnesium. Microbiol. Immunol. 30: 13.

5. Kato, N., Ohta, M., Kido, N., Ito, H., Naito, S., and Kuno, T., 1986, In vitro hexagonal assembly of lipopolysaccharide of **Escherichia coli** K-12. Microbiol. Immunol. 30: 1105.

6. Kato, N., Ohta, M., Kido, N., Ito, H., and Naito, S., 1988, In vitro hexagonal assembly of R-form lipopolysaccharides: effect of pH on the Mg^{2+}-mediated hexagonal assembly. Microbiol. Immunol. 32: 151.

7. Kato, N., Ohta, M., Kido, N., Ito, H., and Naito, S., 1988, Formation of a hexagonal lattice structure by an R-form lipopolysaccharide of **Klebsiella**: effect of various divalent cations on the lattice formation. Microbiol. Immunol. 32: 481.

8. Mayer, H., Rapin, A. M. C., Schmidt, G., and Boman, H. G., 1976, Immunochemical studies on lipopolysaccharides from wild-type and mutants of **Escherichia coli** K-12. Eur. J. Biochem. 66: 357.

9. Ohta, M., Kido, N., Hasegawa, T., Ito, H., Fujii, Y., Arakawa, Y., Komatsu, T., and Kato, N., 1987, Contribution of the mannan O side-chain to the adjuvant action of lipopolysaccharides. Immunology 60: 503.

10. Ohta, M., Mori, M., Hasegawa, T., Nagse, F., Nakashima, I., Naito, S., and Kato, N., 1981, Further studies of the polysaccharide of **Klebsiella pneumoniae** possessing strong adjuvanticity. I. Production of the adjuvant polysaccharide by noncapsulated mutant. Microbiol. Immunol. 25: 939.

11. Prehm, P., Schmidt, G., Jann, B., and Jann, K., 1976, The cell-wall lipopolysaccharide of **Escherichia coli** K-12. Structure and acceptor site for O-antigen and other substituents. Eur. J. Biochem. 70: 171.

12. Prehm, P., Stirm, B., Jann, B., Jann, K., and Boman, H. G., 1976, Cell-wall lipopolysaccharides of ampicillin-resistant mutants of **Escherichia coli** K-12. Eur. J. Biochem. 66: 369.

13. Tamaki, S., Sato, T., and Mitsuhashi, S., 1971, Role of lipopolysaccharides in antibiotic resistance and bacteriophage absorption of **Escherichia coli** K-12. J. Bacteriol. 105: 968.

14. Westphal, O., and Jann, K., 1965, Bacterial lipopolysaccharides - extraction with phenol water and further application of the procedure, in: "Methods in Carbohydrate Chemistry, Vol. 5", R. L. Whistler, ed., Academic Press, New York, p. 83.

BIOLOGICAL ACTIVITIES OF ANTI-LPS FACTOR AND LPS BINDING PEPTIDE FROM HORSESHOE CRAB AMOEBOCYTES

M. Niwa[1], He Hua[1], S. Iwanaga[2], T. Morita[2], T. Miyata[2], T. Nakamura[2], J. Aketagawa[2], T. Muta[2], F. Tokunaga[2] and K. Ohashi[3]

[1]Department of Bacteriology, Osaka City University Medical School, Abeno-ku, Osaka 545, [2]Department of Biology, Faculty of Science, Kyushu University, Higashi-ku, Fukuoka 812 and [3]Hayashibara Institute for Biochemistry, Fujisaki, Okayama 702, Japan

Amoebocytes of horseshoe crabs (such as Limulus polyphemus and Tachypleus tridentatus) contain a coagulation system which is triggered by minute amounts of endotoxic lipopolysaccharide (LPS) and (1-3)-β-D-glucan and result in gelation of hemolymph. Limulus amoebocyte lysate (LAL) is now widely employed as a sensitive assay method for endotoxin. Iwanaga et al. (7), purified reaction components of the gelation cascade and clarified the mechanism of the gelation reaction. In the course of their extensive studies Tanaka et al., (15) discovered a potent anticoagulant, named Anti-LPS Factor (ALF), which specifically inhibits the activation of Factor C by LPS. ALF is a simple basic protein with a molecular weight of 11,600 Da and the unique chemical structure of this protein was described in detail by Iwanaga et al., in this volume and elsewhere (1, 8). In collaborative studies we have found interesting biological activities of ALF such as hemolysis of LPS sensitized erythrocytes (12) and growth inhibition of Gram negative bacteria (10).

In 1987 Iwanaga et al., (8) found another novel anticoagulant in LAL and purified it. This anticoagulant also inhibits the LPS-mediated activation of Factor C, and it was originally named LPS Binding Peptide (LBP). Although a more elegant name Tachyplesin I was coined for it, we use the name LPS Binding Peptide in this paper. LBP is a cyclic peptide composed of 17 basic and hydrophobic amino acids with two S-S bonds with a molecular weight of 2,300

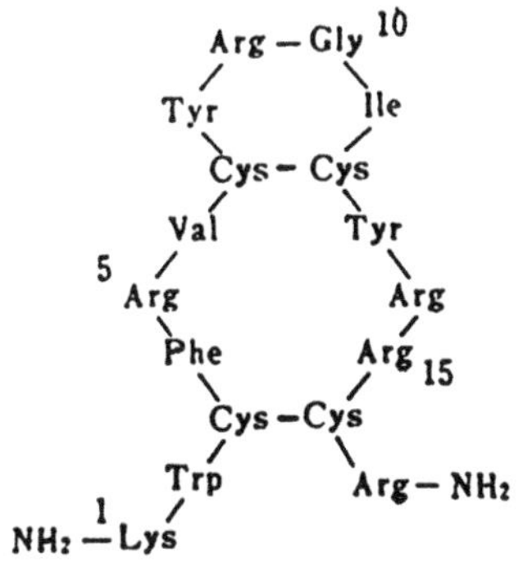

Fig 1. Structure of LPS binding peptide (Tachyplesin I)

Da (Fig 1). We investigated biological activities of LBP comparing with those of ALF and found that LBP also hemolyse LPS sensitized red blood cells (RBC). However important is a wide antimicrobial spectrum of LBP which effectively inhibit growth of Gram negative and Gram positive bacteria as well as some fungi. Furthermore, we demonstrate that both ALF and LBP combine to the lipid moiety of LPS and neutralize pyrogenicity of LPS. Biological significance of ALF and LBP in biological defense system of horseshoe crab is also discussed.

MATERIALS AND METHODS

ALF and LBP

ALF was isolated from the amoebocyte lysate of Tachypleus tridentatus (Japanese horseshoe crab) according to the method already reported by Morita et al., (10). Briefly, LAL was chromatographed on a Dextran sulfate Sepharose CL-6B column followed by gel filtration on a Sephadex G-50 column. LBP was purified from 0.1 N HCl extract of amoebocyte debris as described by Iwanaga et al. (8). Purity of ALF and LBP was confirmed by SDS-PAGE.

Lipopolysaccharides

Phenol extracted, purified LPSs from Escherichia coli 0113(S), Escherichia coli J5(Rc) and Salmonella minnesota 1114W(S) were used in this study. Re LPS from Salmonella minnesota R595(Re) was purified by phenol-chloroform-petroleum ether method (4). These LPS were dissolved in 0.15 M NaCl or in Tris buffered saline (Tris-HCl, pH 7.2, 50 mM + 0.15 M NaCl) by sonication for about 1 min.

LPS Sensitized Red Blood Cells (LPS=RBC)

Red blood cells were collected from human heparinized blood (O-type) and washed with Tris-saline three times. To 1 ml of 2.5% red blood cell suspension 0.5 ml of LPS solution (1 mg/ml) was gradually added and incubated at 37° for 30 to 60 min with gentle shaking. After the incubation the LPS sensitized RBC were washed several times with 10 ml of Tris-saline and the final concentration of LPS=RBC was adjusted to 0.5%. The LPS=RBC was checked by agglutination with antiserum to the bacterium from which the employed LPS was derived. The LPS=RBC was stored at 4° and used within a few days. For simplicity R595=RBC, for example, denotes the RBC sensitized with Salmonella minnesota R595 LPS.

Hemolysis of LPS=RBC

Fifty µl of the LPS-RBC was mixed with 50 µl of two-fold dilution series of ALF or LBP in each well of a U-bottom microplate, and mixed well by mechanical shaking. After incubation at 37° for 60 min, hemolysis was recorded by observing sedimented LPS=RBC or by measuring turbidities at 630 nm on a microplate reader (Corona MTP- 100P). Quantitative hemolysis was assayed as follows: In a microtube 50 µl of LPS=RBC and 50 µl of ALF or LBP solution with 100 µl of Tris-saline were incubated with a floating rack in a waterbath kept at 37° for 1 hr. After adding 2.3 ml of saline the tubes were centrifuged at 2,500 rpm for 10 min. Released hemoglobin concentrations in the supernatants were determined by measuring absorbances at 412 nm with a spectrophotometer (Hitachi 100-20).

Bacterial and Fungal Strains

The following strains of bacteria were used: Salmonella typhimurium strains LT2(S), SL134(SR), TV149(Ra), TV148(Rb), SL1069(Rc), SL1181 (Rd2) and SL1102(Re). These strains were given by courtesy of Dr. N. Kasai, Showa

University. Salmonella minnesota strains 1114W(S), R595(Re), Escherichia coli K12, Pseudomonas aeruginosa, Staphylococcus aureus strains 209P, ATCC25923, Staphylococcus epidermidis and Bacillus subtilis were stock strains of the Department of Bacteriology, Osaka City University Medical School. Candida albicans IMF 40002 and Cryptococcus neoformans IMF 40040 were kind gifts of Dr. T. Arai of Chiba University.

Culture Media

Heart infusion broth (Difco Laboratories, Detroit, Mich.) was used for subcultures of the bacteria. For growth inhibition tests of the bacteria a synthetic Jarvis's medium (9) supplemented with 2 mg/ml of yeast extract (Difco Laboratories, Detroit, Mich.) was employed. (Abbreviated as JY medium). The fungi were grown on Sabouraud broth supplemented with 1% myo-inositol.

Antimicrobial Activity

Bacteria grown on heart infusion broth at 37° overnight were diluted with JY medium to contain about 10^6 colony forming units (CFU)/ml according to calibrated tubidity-viable count relationships.

Typical incubation mixtures for growth inhibition experiments contained 20 μl of the bacterial suspension, 20 μl of serial dilutions of ALF or LBP and 160 μl of JY medium in each well of a flat bottom microplate for tissue culture (The Data Packing Corp., Cambridge, MA). After incubation at 37° for about 18 hr absorbances at 550 nm were measured on a microplate reader (Corona MTP-100P) taking the absorbance of a well filled with uninoculated JY medium as a reference.

For Candida albicans and Cryptococcus neoformans the Sabouraud-inositol medium was used and inocula were 20 μl of about 10^4 CFU/ml. Absorbance after two days growth at 30° was determined.

Minimal inhibitory concentrations of ALF or LBP against these bacteria and fungi were expressed as the lowest final concentrations (μg/ml) at which no growth was observed.

Bactericidal activity of ALF and LBP was determined by counting viable cells of ALF or LBP treated suspensions. Mixtures of 100 μl of bacterial (10^6 CFU/ml) or fungal (10^5 CFU/ml) suspension and 100 μl of ALF or LBP solution were kept at 37° for up to 60 min. Ten μl of 10-fold dilution of the treated suspensions was plated on nutrient agar for the bacteria and on Sabouraud agar for the fungi, and colonies were counted triplicately after overnight incubation at 37° for the bacteria and two days incubation at 30° for the fungi.

Pyrogen Test

Rabbit pyrogen test was kindly carried out by Dr. H. Kawasaki of National Institute of Hygiene Osaka Branch. Mixtures of equal volumes of various concentrations (10, 1 and 0.1 μg/ml) of LBP or ALF and Escherichia coli UKTB LPS (the Japanese Reference Endotoxin lot No. 1) (10 ng/ml) was kept at 22° for 30 min. Three to four rabbits weighing about 2 kg were intravenously injected with a 1 ml/kg dose of the mixture, and rectal temperatures of the rabbits were recorded for 4 hr. Fever indices were calculated from the temperature curves.

Double Diffusion in Gel

Formation of precipitation lines between ALF or LBP and various LPS was

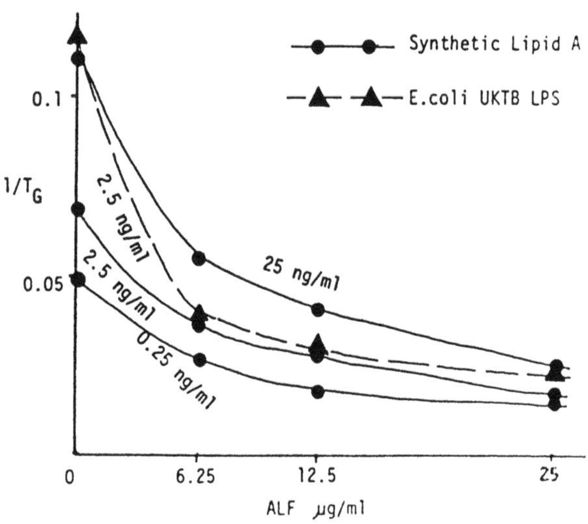

Fig 2. Inhibition of LAL gelation by ALF. The reaction mixtures were consisted of 100 µl of LAL 50 µl of various concentration of ALF and 50 µl of Escherichia coli UKTB LPS or synthetic lipid A (No. 506) dissolved in 0.025% triethylamine. TG means gelation time at 37°.

observed by double diffusion test in agarose gel dissolved in the Tris-saline (pH 7.2), 0.3 M acetate buffer (pH 4.6) and veronal buffer (pH 8.6). The precipitation lines formed were stained with amidoblack.

RESULTS

Inhibition of Limulus Gelation Reaction

Both ALF and LBP were discovered as potent anticoagulants which inhibit the activation of Factor C by LPS. It has already been demonstrated that an alternative pathway in the LAL cascade, the activation of Factor G by (1-3)-β-D-glucan, was not affected by ALF and LBP (7, 8). ALF inhibits the activation of Factor C by various LPS irrespective of their origins. As illustrated in Fig 2, gelation reactions of LAL by various LPS measured with a turbidimeter (Toxinometer ET201, Wako Pure Chemical Industry Co., Osaka) were effectively inhibited by ALF. The fact that chemically synthesized lipid A (6) was also inhibited by ALF suggests that ALF may interact with the lipid moiety of LPS.

Hemolysis of LPS Sensitized Red Blood Cells

At first we intended to test hemoagglutination of LPS sensitized RBC considering a possibility of polyvalent binding of ALF to LPS. When ALF was added to LPS=RBC, in our surprise, instantaneous hemolysis occurred even at room temperature.

LPS derived from S type (Salmonella minnesota 1114W and Escherichia coli 0113) as well as Re type (Salmonella minnesota R595) can effectively sensitize RBC for the hemolysis by ALF and human O or A or B type RBC, horse and chicken RBC sensitized with these LPS are all susceptible to the hemolysis. The minimal hemolytic concentration of ALF was dependent on the LPS concentration used for the sensitization of RBC, RBC sensitized with as low as 10 ng/ml of 1114W LPS were hemolysed by ALF at a higher concentration (50 µg/ml). In the optimal condition the minimal hemolytic concentration of ALF was 0.48 µg/ml, while LBP required 2 µg/ml or more for complete hemolysis. Human O RBC which was not treated with LPS was not completely hemolyzed at

Table 1. Hemolytic activity of anti-LPS factor on RBC sensitized with LPS

RBC sensitized with	Dilution of anti-LPS factor											
	2	4	8	16	32	64	128	256	512	1024	2048	Control
S. minnesota R595 LPS (Human RBC)	+	+	+	+	+	+	+	+	+	+	-	-
S. minnesota 1114W LPS (Human RBC)	+	+	+	+	+	+	+	+	+	+	+	-
S. minnesota 1114W LPS (Chicken RBC)	+	+	+	+	+	+	+	+	+	+	-	-
S. minnesota 1114W LPS (Horse RBC)	+	+	+	+	+	+	+	+	+	+	+	-
E. coli 0113 LPS (Human RBC)	+	+	+	+	+	+	+	+	+	-	-	-
None (Human RBC)	-	-	-	-	-	-	-	-	-	-	-	-
None (Chicken RBC)	-	-	-	-	-	-	-	-	-	-	-	-
None (Horse RBC)	-	-	-	-	-	-	-	-	-	-	-	-

Fifty μl of 0.5% RBC sensitized with LPS was mixed with 50 μl of a 2-fold serial dilution of anti-LPS factor in a microtiter U-plate and incubated at 37°C for 30 min. The concentration of original solution of anti-LPS factor was 2 mg/ml. +, hemolysis-positive; −, hemolysis-negative

the concentrations less than 250 μg/ml of ALF and 62.5 μg/ml of LBP. (Table 1 and Fig 3)

Neutralization of the Hemolysis by Free LPS

It was reasonably expected that free LPS added to the hemolytic system may bind to ALF and LBP and thus neutralize the hemolysis. When R595=RBC or 1114W=RBC were added to ALF or LBP preincubated with two-fold dilutions of free LPS the hemolysis was inhibited depending on the concentrations of free LPS irrespective of the origins of the LPS used for the sensitization (Fig 4). Escherichia coli 0113 native polysaccharide (the polysaccharide portion of the LPS) had no such inhibitory effect. These results provide an additional evidence for the binding capacity of ALF and LBP to the lipid moiety of LPS.

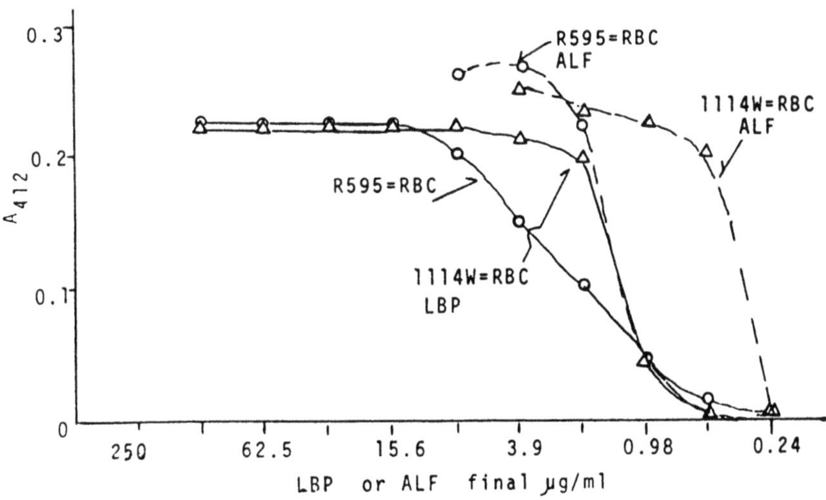

Fig 3. Hemolysis of LPS sensitized RBC by ALF and LBP. Released hemoglobin was measured by reading absorbance at 412 nm as described in Methods.

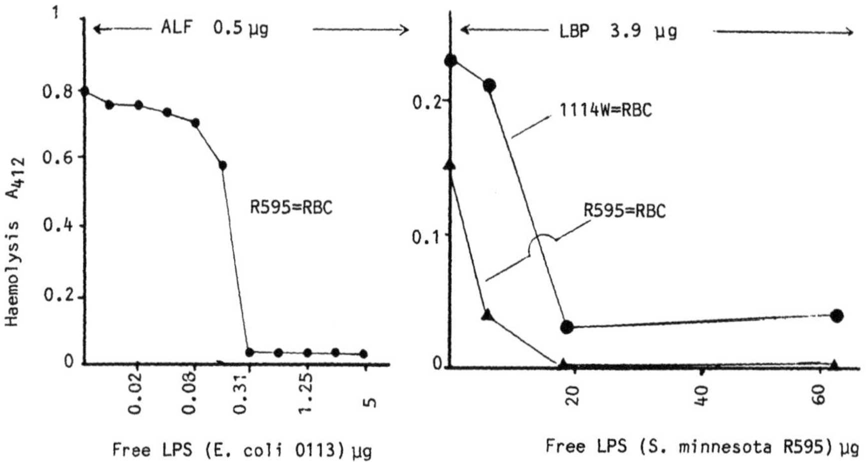

Fig 4. Neutralization of the hemolysis by free LPS. Fifty µl of various concentrations of Escherichia coli 0113 LPS or Salmonella minnesota R595 LPS was mixed with 50 µl of ALF or LBP solution, and then 100 µl of R595=RBC or 1114W=RBC was added. The doses of ALF and LBP were 0.5 µg and 3.8 µg respectively.

Kinetics of the Hemolytic Process

The hemolytic process of ALF and LBP was chased by measuring turbidity changes of R595=RBC treated with ALF and LBP as illustrated in Fig 5. The hemolysis by ALF completed within 1 min at 37°, while the process of LBP proceeded more slowly and it was incomplete at lower concentrations. The hemolysis by ALF proceeded rapidly at 37° and complete hemolysis occurred within 5 min even at 0° using higher concentrations (12). On the other hand, the hemolysis by LBP was not detectable at 0° after prolonged incubation for 80 min. (Fig 6)

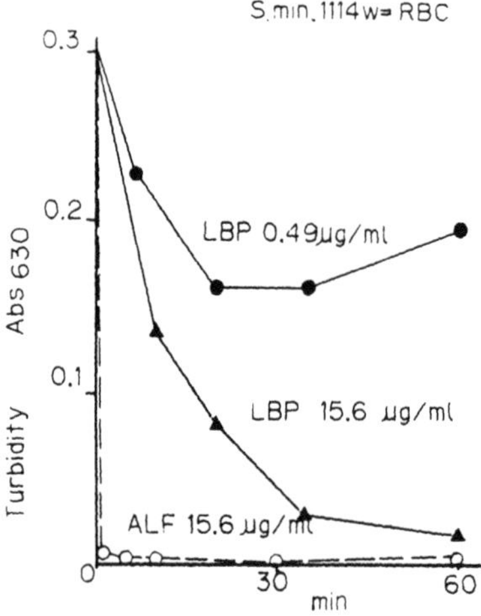

Fig 5. Time course of the hemolysis by ALF and LBP. ALF or LBP was mixed with 1114W=RBC at 37° and turbidities at 630 nm were read at the time indicated.

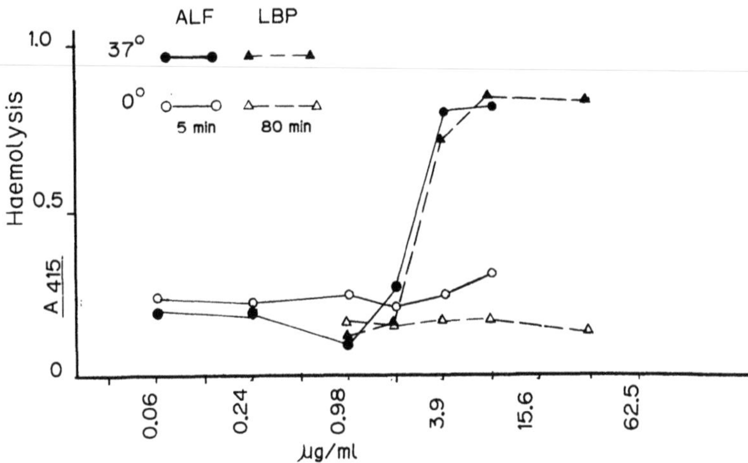

Fig 6. Effects of temperature on the hemolysis by ALF and LBP. Various concentrations of ALF or LBP were added to 1114W=RBC and incubated at 37° and 0°. Hemolysis was measured after 5 min for ALF and 80 min for LBP.

Effect of Human Serum on the Hemolysis

Another difference in the hemolysis by ALF and LBP is an inhibitory effect of human serum. Human homologous serum heated at 60° for 5 min tend to suppress the hemolysis by LBP, whereas hemolysis by ALF is not affected by the serum. (Fig 7)

Effect of ALF on Human Cells other than RBC

Human polymorphonuclear cells and mononuclear cells were separated from

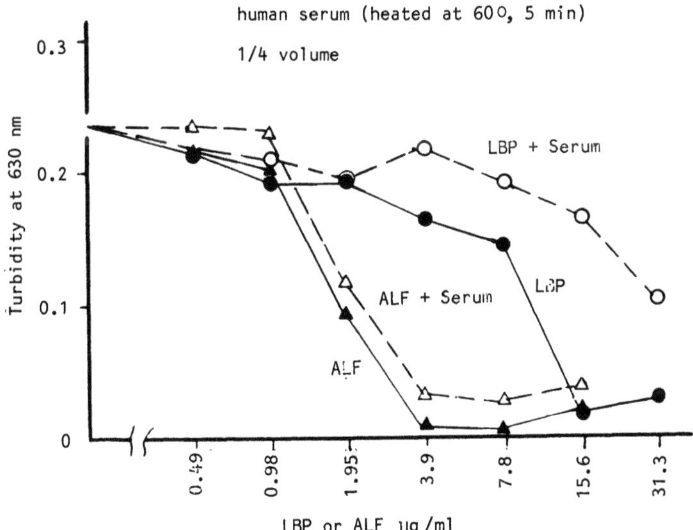

Fig 7. Effects of heated human serum on the hemolysis by ALF and LBP. Reaction mixtures contained 25 µl of ALF or LBP, 25 µl of human serum heated at 60° for 5 min, and 50 µl of R595=RBC. Turbidities at 630 nm were read after 60 min at 37°.

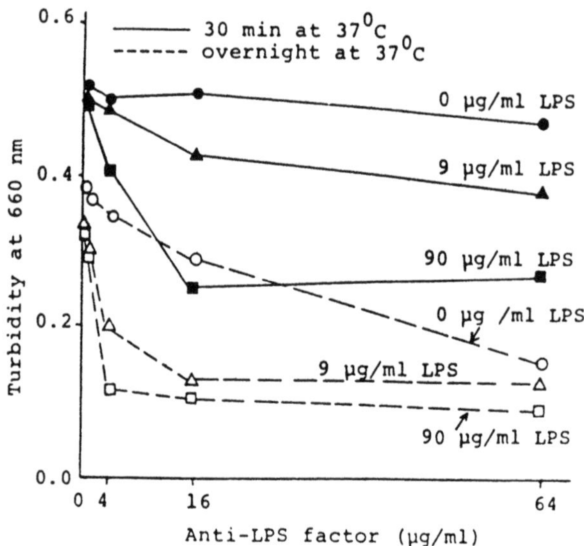

Fig 8. Cytolysis of LPS sensitized human leukemia cell K562 by ALF. One ml of K562 cell suspensions in PBS(6×10^6/ml) were sensitized with 9 and 90 μg/ml of Salmonella minnesota 1114W LPS at 37° for 30 min. The final concentration of the sensitized K562 cell was 2.5×10^6/ml. Turbidities at 37° after 30 min and overnight were measured.

heparinized blood by differential centrifugation in Mono Poly Resolving Medium (Flow Laboratories). Washed cells were sensitized with 1114W LPS in a similar way as LPS=RBC, and ALF was added to the cell suspensions. After incubation at 37° for 1 hr massive cytolysis was observed and Giemsa stain showed only disrupted cell debris. Unsensitized leukocytes treated with ALF seemed to be unaffected (data not shown).

Human leukemia cells K562 cultured in RPMI 1640 medium (Gibco, penicillin G 100 μg/ml, streptomycin 100 μg/ml, fetal calf serum 10%) under 5% CO_2 atmosphere for 5 days were sensitized with 1114W LPS. Fig 8 illustrates turbidity changes of the LPS sensitized leukemia cells in various concentrations of ALF. Marked decreases in the turbidities of the LPS sensitized cells depending on the concentrations of ALF as well as of LPS were observed. Massive cytolysis was microscopically observed in these cases too.

Antibacterial Activity of ALF

We have already reported that ALF exhibited growth inhibition against some, not all, strains of Gram negative bacteria (10). Among the strains tested Re type strains, Salmonella minnesota R595 and Salmonella typhimurium 1102, were most susceptible to the antibacterial action of ALF, and S strains such as Salmonella minnesota 1114W and Salmonella typhimurium LT2 were rather resistant to ALF. The sensitivity of the rough strains is most clearly illustrated in Fig 9. The susceptibility of these strains to ALF inversely related to the polysaccharide chain length of their LPS from the S strain through the Re strain. Viable cell counts demonstrated that ALF act as a bactericidal substance against the sensitive strains. On the other hand, the growth of Gram positive bacteria such as Staphylococcus aureus and Staphylococcus epidermidis was not affected by ALF (10). No lysozyme activity was detected with a large amount (33 μg) of ALF using Micrococcus lysodeikticus as an indicator (Fig 10). It was also demonstrated that the antibacterial activity of ALF was effectively adsorbed by free LPS and heat killed cells of Salmonella minnesota R595 (10).

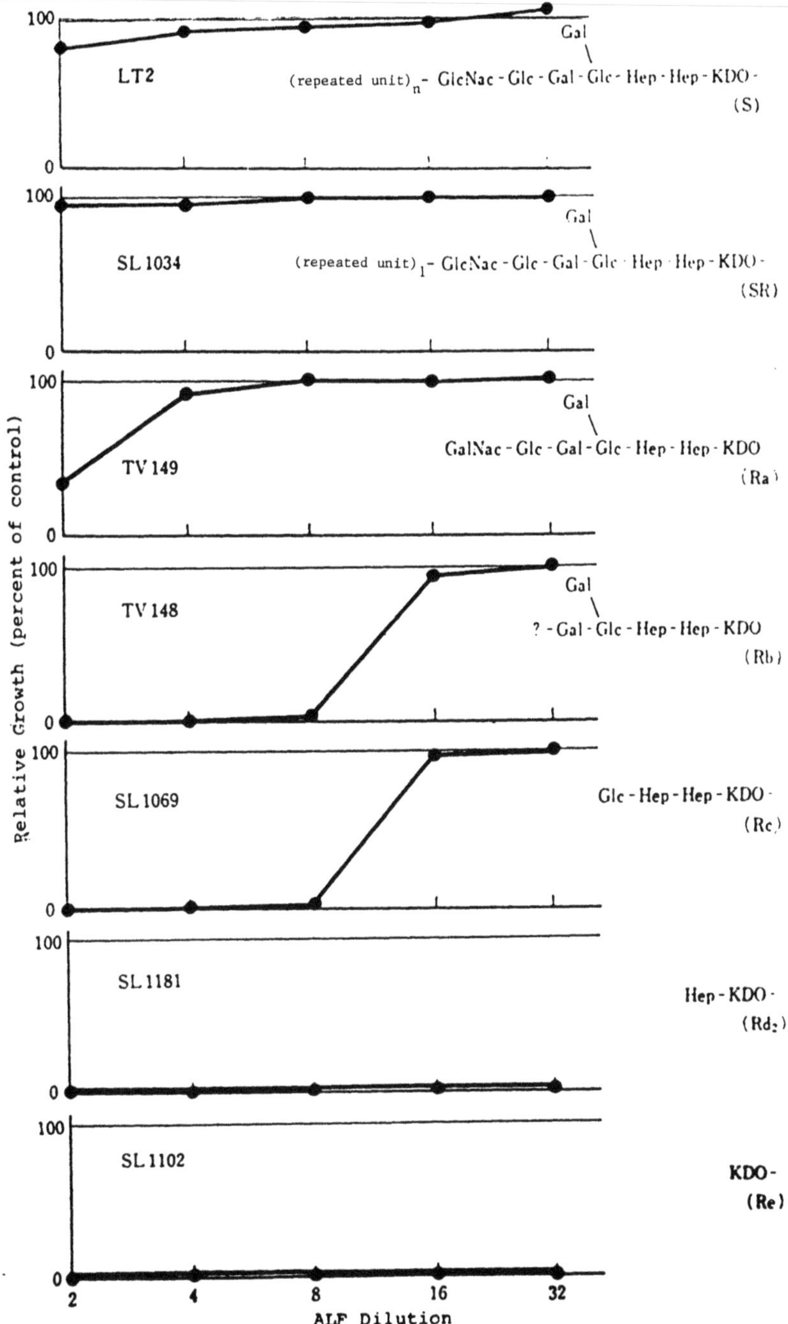

Fig 9. Sensitivity of various Salmonella typhimurium strains to ALF. The name of strains and their core and backbone saccharide structures are indicated. The treated bacteria were grown in Penassay medium at 37° for 18 hr. Relative growth was expressed as percent turbidities at 550 nm of controls without ALF. ALF dilutions 2, 4.....correspond to the final concentration of 3.31, 1.66....μg/ml.

Antimicrobial Activity of LBP

In the previous study of ALF Penassay medium which contain macromolecular components was used. In order to avoid possible interaction of the components with ALF and LBP, we reinvestigated antimicrobial activities of ALF and LBP employing a more simple JY medium.

In a preliminary experiment LBP and ALF applied on bacterial lawn plates produced distinct inhibition zones against several Gram negative as well as positive bacteria. The diameters of the inhibition zones approximately paralleled to the dose of LBP and ALF applied.

Minimal inhibitory concentrations (MIC) of LBP and ALF against several bacterial and fungal strains were determined by the microplate culture technique as described in the Methods. As summarized in Table 2, LBP displayed potent antimicrobial activity against a wide range of microorganisms. It was effective not only to Gram negative bacteria but to several smooth strains of Gram negative and Gram positive ones such as Staphylococcus species. Furthermore LBP inhibited growth of Candida albicans and Cryptococcus neoformans. ALF was found to be effective to both rough and smooth strains of Salmonella, but it was practically not effective to Staphylococcus, Candida and Cryptococcus.

Microbicidal Action of LBP

We are now investigating the mechanism of the antimicrobial action of ALF and LBP. Whatever the mechanism may be, ALF and LBP were found to be microbicidal towards the sensitive strains. As shown in Fig 11, viable cell counts of the susceptible strains decreased with time, and the D values which represent the time required for killing 90% of the original number of viable cells were 7 min for Salmonella typhimurium LT2 and 10 min for Escherichia

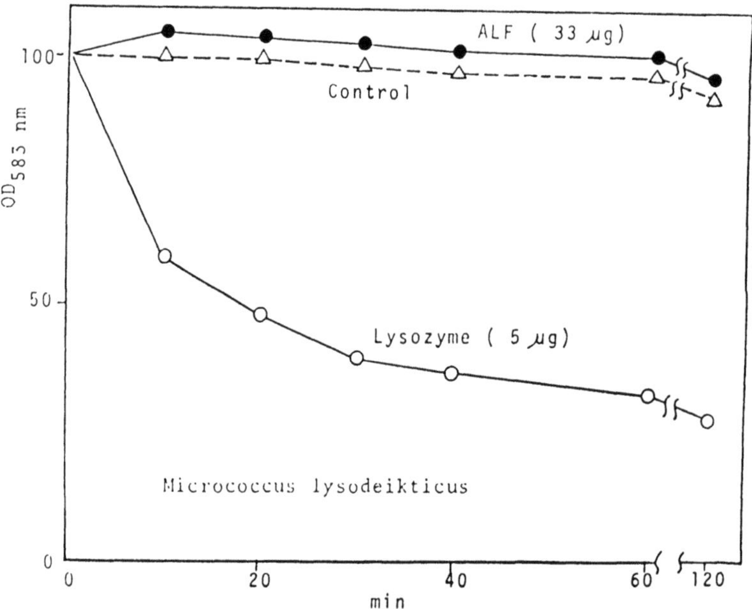

Fig 10. Test for lysozyme activity. Reaction mixtures contain 2.5 ml of Micrococcus leisodeikticus suspension and 0.5 ml of egg white lysozyme (10 µg/ml) or ALF (66 µg/ml) in 0.066 M phosphate buffer, pH 6.2.

Table 2. Antimicrobial activity of LBP and ALF

	Strains	MIC(μg/ml)	
		LBP	ALF
Gram(-)	Salmonella typhimurium LT2 (S)	3.13-6.25	6.25-12.5
	Salmonella typhimurium 1102 (Re)	0.78-1.56	6.25-12.5
	Salmonella minnesota 1114W (S)	12.5	
	Salmonella minnesota R595 (Re)	12.5	
	Escherichia coli K12	12.5	
	Pseudomonas aeruginosa	12.5	
Gram(+)	Staphylococcus aureus 209P	1.56-6.25	
	Staphylococcus aureus ATCC 25923	6.25	12.5<
	Staphylococcus epidermidis	6.25	
	Bacillus subtilis	3.13	
Fungi	Candida albicans IMF 40002	3.13	25<
	Cryptococcus neoformans IMF 40040	1.56	25<

coli K12. Killing of more larger fungal cells (Candida albicans) proceeded more slowly although the MIC values towards the Candida strain was as low as that for the sensitive bacteria.

Neutralization of Pyrogenicity of LPS by ALF and LBP

Because ALF and LBP interact with LPS and inhibit the activation of Factor C by LPS, it should be tested whether they neutralize biological activities of LPS in vivo or not. Results of neutralization of the pyrogenicity of LPS are given in Table 3. The fever indices of the mixture of LBP or ALF and Escherichia coli UKTB LPS decreased with the increasing doses of LBP and ALF. LBP seemed to be more potent in the neutralization in weight basis, but it should be considered that the molecular weight of LBP is about one fifth that of ALF. No toxic symptom other than the temperature rise was observed in these rabbits.

Precipitation Reaction in Gel

More direct evidence for binding capacities of ALF and LBP is provided by the fact that both produce sharp precipitation lines towards LPS in double diffusion test in agarose gel. The precipitation lines between ALF or LBP and various LPS fused each other irrespective of the origins of the LPS used, and the precipitation lines of ALF and LBP against one kind of LPS also fused (Fig 12). Single radial diffusion assays of ALF and LBP in LPS containing gel were also possible (data not shown).

DISCUSSION

Our previous and present studies on ALF and LBP isolated from horseshoe crab amoebocytes demonstrated that ALF and LBP have several interesting biological activities: 1) inhibition of the activation of Factor C by LPS in LAL system, 2) hemolysis of LPS sensitized RBC and leukocytes, 3) antimicrobial activities, 4) neutralization of pyrogenicity of LPS, and 5) precipitation reaction with LPS in gel. As a corollary of these results we can inevi-

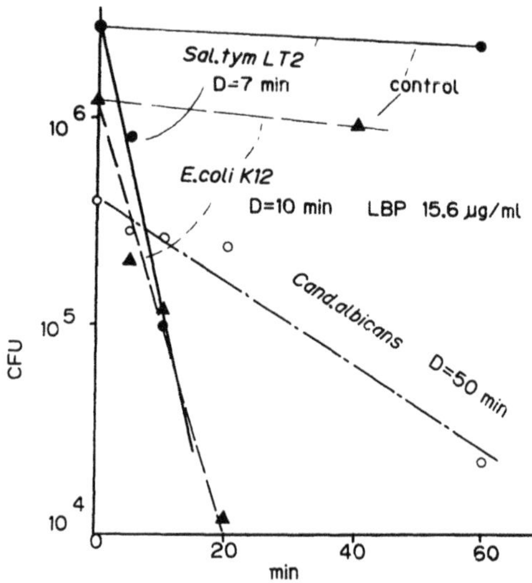

Fig 11. Microbicidal action of LBP. Mixtures of microbial suspensions and LBP were incubated at 37°, and 10 µl aliquotes were taken at the time indicated. Colony counts were made as described in Methods.

tably conclude that both ALF and LBP bind to the lipid moiety of various LPS. Several LPS binding proteins are known in higher animals such as "LPS receptor" of RBC, high density lipoprotein, a cationic protein of leukocytes, etc. However the chemical structures and biological functions of these proteins still remained unclear. ALF and LBP are a couple of the first example of LPS binding substances of animal origins whose whole chemical structures have already been elucidated.

Localization of basic as well as hydrophobic residues in ALF molecules which provide it an amphipathic nature have been demonstrated by Iwanaga et al. (1, 7, 8). The clusters of the basic and hydrophobic groups in ALF molecule and the peculiar cyclic peptide structure of LBP may constitute

Table 3. Neutralization of pyrogenicity of LPS

Dose		Fever index (% of control)	
LPS*	LBP or ALF	LBP	ALF
5 ng/kg	0 µg/kg	23.6 (100)%	
	0.05	21.0 (92.8)	23.6 (100)
	0.5	5.53 (23.4)	10.3 (43.6)
	5	4.60 (19.5)	6.53 (27.7)

* : E. coli UKTB LPS mixed with LBP or ALF was injected intravenously into 2-4 rabbits.

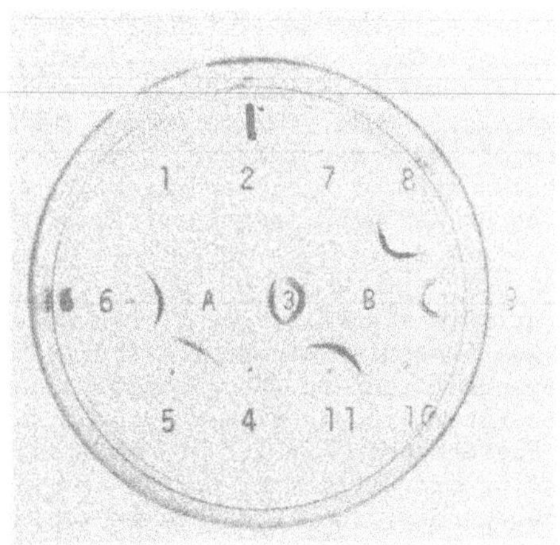

A=ALF B=LBP
1,4,7,10=E.coli J5
2,11 =S.min.1114W
3,6,9 =S.min.R595
5,8 =E.coli 0113

Fig 12. Precipitation reaction in gel of ALF and LBP towards various LPS. Each well contains 40 µl of 1,000 µg/ml of ALF or LBP, and 20 µl of 1,000 µg/ml of various LPS.

possible binding sites to acidic groups and fatty acyl chains of LPS. The basic and hydrophobic nature of the double cyclic peptide, LBP, recalls a cyclic peptide polymyxin B which is also known to bind LPS, but polymyxin B does not inhibit growth of Gram positive bacteria and fungi. Elucidation of the structure-activity relationship in near future may provide us more profound understanding about interaction of LPS and these LPS binding substances.

The most interesting finding in this study may be the antimicrobal activities of ALF and LBP. ALF inhibits the growth of rough strains of Gram negative bacteria, but it is not active towards Gram positive and fungal strains tested. On the other hand, LBP exhibited a broad spectrum of the antimicrobial activity. It is effective to Gram negative and Gram positive bacteria as well as to some fungal strains.

Deep rough strains of Enterobacteriaceae are generally more susceptible to many detergents and antibiotics than the smooth strains. In this study the most sensitive to ALF and LBP were the Re strains of Salmonella. It is possible that lack of long polysaccharide chains in their LPS may facilitate the access of ALF (11,600 Da) to the lipid moiety of LPS which is embedded in the lipid layer of the outer membrane of bacterial cells. Weiss et al., (16) purified bactericidal, membrane active and LPS binding proteins from human and rabbit leukocytes. They indicated that sensitivity of Salmonella typhimurium strains decreased in the order of Rd1>Rc>Rb>Ra>S depending on their saccharide chain lengths of LPS. Similar relationships were also found with ALF, but it is plausible that ALF and LBP may have affinities not only to LPS but to acidic membrane lipids as polymyxin B bind to both LPS and phospholipids such as phosphatidylethanolamine. Interpretation of the broad spectrum of LBP should be considered in this line.

Nachum et al., (11) reported presence of broad spectrum antibacterial substance(s) in LAL of Limulus polyphemus, but their chemical entities have not yet been described. In other invertebrates a number of antimicrobial isopeptides are known; for example, cecropins from silk worms (2, 3), sarcotoxins from flesh flies (13) and mellitins of bee venom (3). In addition, a broad spectrum antimicrobial peptide was recently isolated from Xenopus frog skin (17). In mammals antimicrobial peptides, defencins, were purified from polymorphonuclear leukocytes of human, rabbits and guinea pigs (5, 14). Common features of these peptides are their antimicrobial activities and relatively rich contents of basic and hydrophobic amino acids. However, no information about LPS binding capacities of these peptides is available as yet.

Biological and evolutional significances of ALF and LBP have not yet been fully elucidated. One feasible role of ALF and LBP seems to be the regulation which avoid overreactions of the gelation cascade as several regulatory components are integrated in other blood coagulation systems and the complement system. Furthermore, ALF and LBP may possibly play important roles in killing of invading microorganisms in the body of horseshoe crabs which are devoid of antibody formation, and they may constitute the defence corp along with other innate immunity systems such as phagocytic cells, agglutinins and the gelation cascade. However, we have less knowledge about cell physiology of horseshoe crab amoebocytes comparing with that of mammalian cells. We should be aware that nature might provide living creatures many purposeful mechanisms for their survival beyond our present imagination.

> "So many the outward shows be least themselves.
> The world is still deceived with ornament"
> W. Shakespeare, The Merchant of Venice, Act III, Sc. 2

ACKNOWLEDGEMENT

We wish to thank Dr. H. Kawasaki of National Institute of Hygiene for the pyrogen test.

REFERENCES

1. Aketagawa, J., Miyata, T., Ohtsubo, S., Nakamura, T., Morita, T., Hayashita, H., Miyata, T., Iwanaga, S, Tkao, T. and Shimonouchi, S., 1986, Primary structure of limulus anticoagulant anti-lipopolysaccharide factor. J. Biol. Chem. 261: 7357.

2. Boman, H. G., 1982, Humoral immunity in insects and the counter defence of some pathogen. Fortsch. Zool., 27, Zbl. Bakt. Suppl. 12, 211.

3. Boman, H. G. and Hultmark, D., 1987, Cell-free immunity in insects. Ann. Rev. Microbiol. 41: 103.

4. Galanos, C., Luderitz, O. and Westphal, O., 1969, A new method for the extraction of R lipopolysaccharide. Eur. J. Biochem. 9: 245.

5. Ganz, T., Selsted, M. E., Szklarek, D., Harwig, S. S. L., Daher, K., Bainton, D. F. and Lehrer, R. I., 1987, Defencins, natural peptide antibiotics of human neutrophil. J. Clin. Invest. 76: 1427.

6. Imoto, M., Yoshimura, H., Sakaguchi, N., Kusumoto, S. and Shiba, T., 1985, Total synthesis of Escherichia coli lipid A. Tetrahedron Lett. 26: 1545.

7. Iwanaga, S., Morita, T., Miyata, T., Nakamura, T. and Aketagawa, J., 1986, The hemolymph coagulation system in invertebrate animals. J. Protein Chem. 5: 255.

8. Iwanaga, S. et al., in this symposium, and Nakamura, T., Furunaka, H., Miyata, T., Tokunaga, F., Muta, T., Iwanaga, S., Niwa, M., Takao, T. and Shimonishi, Y., 1988, Tachyplesin, a class of antimicrobial peptide from the hemocytes of the horseshoe crab (Tachypleus tridentatus). Isolation and chemical structure. J. Biol. Chem. 263: 16709.

9. Jarvis, F. G., Mesenko, M. and Tibbs, K. E., 1960, Production of Vi antigen on a chemically defined medium by a coliform bacterium. J. Bacteriol. 80: 673.

10. Morita, T., Ohtsubo, S., Nakamura, T., Tanaka, S., Iwanaga, S., Ohashi, K. and Niwa, M., 1985, Isolation and biological activities of Limulus anticoagulant (anti LPS factor) which interact with lipopolysaccharide (LPS). J. Biochem. 97: 1611.

11. Nachum, R., 1979, Antimicrobial defense mechanisms in Limulus polyphemus, in: "Biomedical Applications of the Horseshoe Crab (Limulidae), E. Cohen ed., Alan R. Liss Publishing, N. Y., p. 513.

12. Ohashi, K., Niwa, M., Nakamura, T., Morita, T. and Iwanaga, S., 1984, Anti LPS factor in the horseshoe crab, Tachypleus tridentatus. Its hemolytic activity to the red blood cell sensitized with lipopolysaccharide. FEBS Lett. 176: 207.

13. Okada, M. and Natori, S., 1984, Mode of action of a bactericidal protein in the hemolymph of Sarcophaga peregrina (flesh fly) larvae. Biochem. J. 222: 119.

14. Selsted, M. E. and Harwig, S. S., 1987, Purification, primary structure, and antimicrobial activities of a guinea pig neutrophil defencin. Infect. Immun. 55: 2281.

15. Tanaka, S., Nakamura, T., Morita, T. and Iwanaga, S., 1980, Limulus anti-LPS factor, an anticoagulant which inhibits the endotoxin mediated activation of Limulus coagulation system. Biochem. Biophys. Res. Commun. 105: 717.

16. Weiss, J., Beckerdite-Quagliata, S. and Elsbach, P., 1980, Resistance of Gram-negative bacteria to purified bactericidal leukocyte proteins. J. Clin. Invest. 65: 619.

17. Zasloff, M., 1987, Magainins, a class of antimicrobial peptide from Xenopus frog skin: Isolation, characterization of two active forms, and partial cDNA sequence of a precursor. Proc. Natl. Acad. Sci., U.S.A., 84: 5449.

PRIMARY STRUCTURES AND FUNCTIONS OF ANTI-LIPOPOLYSACCHARIDE FACTOR AND TACHYPLESIN PEPTIDE FOUND IN HORSESHOE CRAB HEMOCYTES

T. Muta[1], T. Nakamura[2], H. Furunaka[2], F. Tokunaga[1], T. Miyata[1,2], M. Niwa[3] and S. Iwanaga[1,2]

[1]Department of Molecular Biology, Graduate School of Medical Science, [2]Department of Biology, Faculty of Science, Kyushu University 33, Fukuoka 812, and [3]Department of Bacteriology Osaka City University Medical School, Osaka 565, Japan

INTRODUCTION

The component of lipopolysaccharide (LPS) located in the cell surface of Gram-negative bacteria, has various biological activities, such as pyrogenicity, adjuvant activity, activation of macrophage and B lymphocyte antitumor activity, and so on (19). It is also known that LPS induces the activation and degranulation of horseshoe crab hemocytes and results in the hemolymph coagulation (2, 7). This cellular event is thought to be one of the self-defense mechanisms of horseshoe crab (12, 18, 23). The recent studies on the limulus coagulation system indicate that it consists of the sequential activations of at least three serine protease zymogens and subsequent conversion of coagulogen, an invertebrate fibrinogen-like substance, to coagulin gel (9, 10, 14-16, 21).

In 1982, a protein component that inhibits the coagulation cascade was found in the hemocyte lysate from Japanese (**Tachypleus tridentatus**) and American horseshoe crabs (**Limulus polyphemus**), and named anti-LPS factor (20). The purified protein specifically inhibits the LPS-mediated activation of limulus factor C (11) and has a strong antibacterial effect, especially on the growth of Gram-negative R-type bacteria (11). Moreover, it has hemolytic activity on the red blood cells sensitized with LPS (17) and cytolytic activity on LPS-sensitized polymorphonuclear leukocytes, mononuclear cells, and human leukemia cells (17). The whole amino acid sequence of anti-LPS factor isolated from **T. tridentatus** was determined in 1986. In our continued study of the limulus clotting system, we found here a new cationic peptide, named tachyplesin, in the hemocyte debris, which binds with LPS and displays antimicrobial activity against Gram-negative bacteria.

The present paper will describe the isolations and chemical structures of American **Limulus polyphemus** anti-LPS factor (13) and Tachyplesin peptide.

MATERIALS AND METHODS

Horseshoe crab (**Tachypleus tridentatus** and **Limulus polyphemus**) hemocytes were collected by the previous method (11). Factor C (14) and anti-LPS factor (11) were purified, respectively, from the hemocytes (**T. tridentatus**) as previously reported. Sephadex G-50 (fine) and CM Sepharose CL-6B were products of Pharmacia Fine Chemicals, Uppsala. LPS purified from **Escherichia**

coli 0111:B4 was purchased from List Biological Laboratories, Inc., CA. Boc-Val-Pro-Arg-pNA was a kind gift from Mr. S. Tanaka (Seikagaku Kogyo Co., Ltd., Tokyo). Trypsin treated with N-tosyl-L-phenylalanyl chloromethyl ketone was obtained from Worthington Biochemical Co., Freehold, NJ. Lysyl endopeptidase from **Achromobacter lyticus** M479-1 was obtained from Wako Pure Chemical Industries Ltd., Tokyo. Ethyleneimine was kindly supplied by Dr. S. Tsunasawa (Institute for Protein Research, Osaka University). Arginine α-amide was a generous gift from Dr. M. Hirata (Tokyo Research Laboratories, Kowa Co., Ltd., Tokyo). Cosmosil 5C18-P column was obtained from Nakarai Chemicals Ltd., Kyoto. All other chemicals were of analytical reagent grade.

Purification from L. polyphemus Anti-LPS Factor and its S-Pyridylethylation

The purification procedures of anti-LPS factor were essentially the same as those described previously (11), and its reduction and **S**-pyridylethylation were previously described (1).

Purification of Tachyplesin from Acid-Extract of Horseshoe Crab Hemocytes

About 50 g (wet weight) hemocytes were suspended in 200 ml of 20mM Tris-HCl buffer (pH 8.0) containing 50 mM NaCl, homogenized by the Physcotron (Nihon-Seimitsu Kogyo, Ltd.), and centrifuged at 8,000 rpm for 30 min in a Hitachi 20 PR-52 centrifuge. The hemocyte lysate in the supernatant was removed, and the precipitate was washed twice with 200 ml of the same buffer. The washed precipitate was then suspended in 100 ml of 20 mM HCL, homogenized, and centrifuged at 8,000 rpm for 30 min. The pellet was reextracted twice with 100 ml of 20 mM HCl. Finally, the combined acid-extracts were lyophilized. The lyophilized acid-extract was dissolved in 50 ml of 20 mM HCl and applied to a Sephadex G-50 column (3 x 90 cm). The gel filtration was carried out in 20 mM HCl at a flow rate of 40 ml/hr. The fractions containing tachyplesin were collected and the pH of the pooled fractions was adjusted to 6.0 with 1 M NaOH. The pooled fraction thus prepared was applied to a CM-Sepharose CL-6B column (2 x 15 cm), equilibrated with 20 mM sodium acetate buffer (pH 6.0). After washing the column with the same buffer, the elution was performed by a linear salt gradient from 500 ml each of the buffer with and without 1.5 M NaCl at a flow rate of 80 ml/hr. Finally, the column was washed with the buffer containing 1.5 M NaCl. All procedures for the purification of tachyplesin were performed under sterile conditions reported previously (14).

Tachyplesin Assay

The tachyplesin was assayed with the inhibitory activity towards the LPS-mediated activation of factor C. A mixture of LPS (0.2 μg/ml) and the sample in 100 μl of 50 mM Tris-HCl buffer (pH 8.0) containing human serum albumin (0.5 mg/ml) was preincubated for 5 min at 37°C, and 100 μl of factor C (0.3 μg/ml) in 50 mM Tris-HCl buffer (pH 8.0) containing human serum albumin (0.5 mg/ml) was added and further incubated for 15 min. Then, the factor C activity generated was measured by using Boc-Val-Pro-Arg-pNA as a specific chromogenic substrate for activated factor C, according to the method described previously (14). One unit of the tachyplesin activity was defined as the amount that inhibits 50% of the factor C activation under above condition.

Electrophoresis

Sodium dodecylsulfate-polyacrylamide gel electrophoresis (SDS-PAGE) was performed by the method of Weber and Osborn in the presence of 8 M urea. The gels were stained with Coomassie brilliant blue R250. The marker proteins for estimation of the molecular weight were myoglobin (Mr = 16,949), myoglobin I + II (14,404), myoglobin I (8,159), myoglobin II (6,214) and myoglobin III (2,512) from Seikagaku Kogyo Co., Ltd., Tokyo.

Determination of Protein Concentrations

The concentrations of purified tachyplesin, anti-LPS factor and factor C were determined by amino acid analysis.

Double Diffusion Test

The complexes between tachyplesin, anti-LPS factor or factor C and LPS were analyzed on a double diffusion method using 1% agarose gel plate as described previously (16).

Amino Acid Analysis, Sequence Determination and Fast Atom Bombardment (FAB) Mass Spectrometry

These methodologies and strategies used for determination of the primary structures have been described in detail previously (1, 9, 21).

RESULTS

Primary Structure of Limulus Polyphemus Anti-LPS Factor

The whole amino acid sequence of anti-LPS factor was determined by sequencing the S-alkylated protein and the peptides obtained by enzymatic cleavages of the protein with lysyl endopeptidase, clostripain, and SV-8, as shown in Fig 1.

Automated Edman degradation of the intact protein resulted in the identification of 20 amino acid residues from the NH_2-terminal end, except for position 19. Both PTH-Asn and PTH-Lys were detected at position 13. The S-alkylated protein (2.2 nmol) was digested with lysyl endopeptidase and the resulting peptide mixture was separated by reversed-phase HPLC. When the peptide K-6 was applied to the sequence analysis, two PTH-amino acids at every cycle were detected, indicating that the peptide contained two different peptides. Thus, the peptide K-6 was rechromatographed by the neutral pH buffer system, and the peptides K-6-1 and K-6-2 were separated. Finally, six major and two minor peptides were obtained in pure form. Through these procedures, all the peptides derived from the whole protein, except for a dipeptide corresponding Gly-48-Lys-49, were purified. The sum of the total residues of six major peptides and one additional glycine plus one additional lysine was in good agreement with that of the whole protein. The sequence analysis of eight peptides yielded 94% of the total sequence (95 out of 101 residues).

To obtain overlaps and confirm the sequences of lysyl endopeptidase peptides, the S-alkylated protein (2.2 nmol) was digested with clostripain. The resulting peptide mixture was separated by reversed-phase HPLC and five pure peptides were obtained. The peptide Cl-5 overlapped the peptides K-5 and K-6-1. However, the other clostripain peptides did not overlap the lysyl bonds. To obtain further overlaps, the S-alkylated protein was digested with SV-8 and the digest was subjected to reversed-phase HPLC. Because the S-alkylated material was not dissolved in 2 M urea, the digestion did not occur completely. Thus, the digest was a mixture consisting of more than 10 peptides with various lengths. Among them, the peptides, V8-2, V8-3, V8-5, and V8-7 were sequenced. The sequence of the peptide V8-7 was determined by Edman degradation up to 50 cycles, except for 19th, 44th, and 49th. This sequence corresponded to the NH_2-terminal portion of the whole protein and overlapped the peptides K-9, K-4, K-2, K-1, and K-6-2. The peptide V8-3

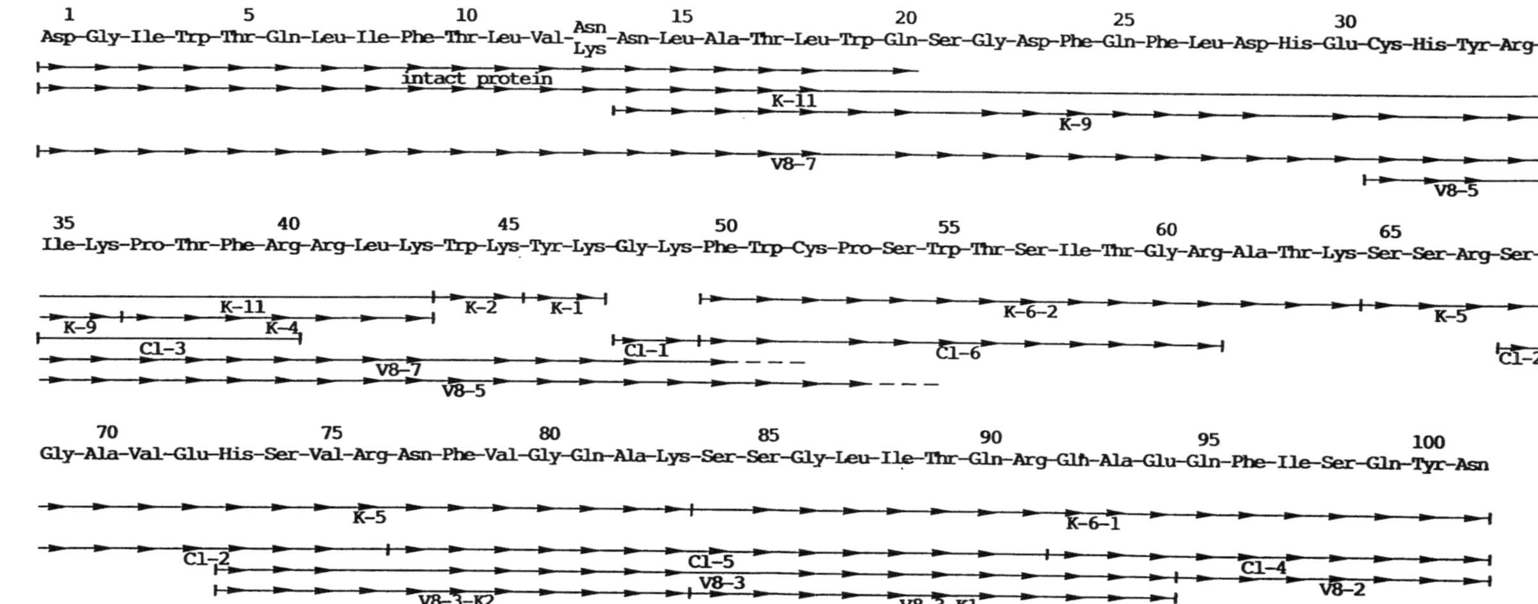

Fig 1. Amino acid sequence of anti-LPS factor from **L. polyphemus**. The residues marked with arrows are those identified by Edman degradation. Vertical lines represent the begining and the end of the lysyl endopeptidase (K), clostripain (Cl), and SV-8 (V8) peptides, respectively. The peptides, for which the actual lengths are not known, give a dashed line and they do not have a vertical line at the COOH-terminal end.

overlapped the peptides K-5 and K-6-1. V8-7 was further digested with lysyl endopeptidase and V8-7-K1 and V8-7-K2 were obtained.

Even with the overlaps mentioned above, we still failed to obtain a complete overlap at the Lys-Ser (residues 64 and 65) bond. However, the whole amino acid composition determined by acid hydrolysis of this protein coincided well with that derived from the sequence data, and the amino acid sequence of this region was fairly well conserved in both proteins from **T. tridentatus** and **L. polyphemus**, indicating that no other amino acid could be inserted between the Lys and Ser residues (residues 64 and 65).

The results described above permitted alignment of all the lysyl endopeptidase peptides and the whole amino acid sequence of S-alkylated anti-LPS factor, as shown in Fig 1. In this molecule two cysteine residues existed at the identical position with those of **T. tridentatus** anti-LPS factor. Since free sulfhydryl groups were not detected (1), these two cysteine residues must be linked with an intramolecular disulfide bridge as those of **T. tridentatus** anti-LPS factor.

A NEW CATIONIC PEPTIDE, TACHYPLESIN, FROM **TACHYPLEUS TRIDENTATUS** HEMOCYTES

Isolation of Tachyplesin

The acid extract prepared from the hemocyte debris was first fractionated on a Sephadex G-50 column. Tachyplesin appeared in a low molecular weight fraction and the tachyplesin activity was associated with a major peak of absorbance at 280 nm. The further purification was performed by using a CM-Sepharose CL-6B column, and tachyplesin was eluted at a higher concentration of NaCl (1.0 M) in the buffer. This indicated that tachyplesin is a highly basic substance. Through these procedures, about 26 mg of tachyplesin from 50 g of the wet hemocytes was obtained and the yield was about 42%. The purity of the preparation was examined by SDS-PAGE in the presence and absence of 2-mercaptoethanol, and it gave a single band with an apparent Mr of approximately 2,000.

Inhibitory Activity of Tachyplesin toward the LPS-Mediated Activation of Factor C

Fig 2 shows the inhibitory activity of tachyplesin towards the LPS-mediated activation of factor C, which is compared with that of anti-LPS factor previously isolated from the hemocytes. The potency of this inhibitory activity was evaluated from the dose-response curves of tachyplesin and anti-LPS factor on the LPS-mediated activation of the zymogen factor C. The effective dose for 50% inhibition was calculated to be 0.05 μg/ml for tachyplesin and 0.11 μg/ml for anti-LPS factor. Thus, the inhibitory activity of tachyplesin was two times higher than that of anti-LPS factor at the weight ratio. Moreover, this peptide as well as anti-LPS factor (11) had no effect on the amidase activity of activated factor C (factor $\overline{C}$), suggesting that tachyplesin is bound with LPS and neutralizes the LPS activity, resulting in the inhibition on the zymogen factor C activation.

Complex Formation between Tachyplesin and LPS

To demonstrate the interaction between tachyplesin and LPS, a double diffusion test was performed by using an agarose gel plate, as shown in Fig 3. The complex formation between tachyplesin and LPS was compared with those of other LPS-binding components, factor C and anti-LPS factor, isolated from the hemocytes (13, 14). The results indicated that tachyplesin binds with LPS, resulting in the formation of a precipitin line and forms a high molecular mass complex similarly as factor C and anti-LPS factor. Moreover,

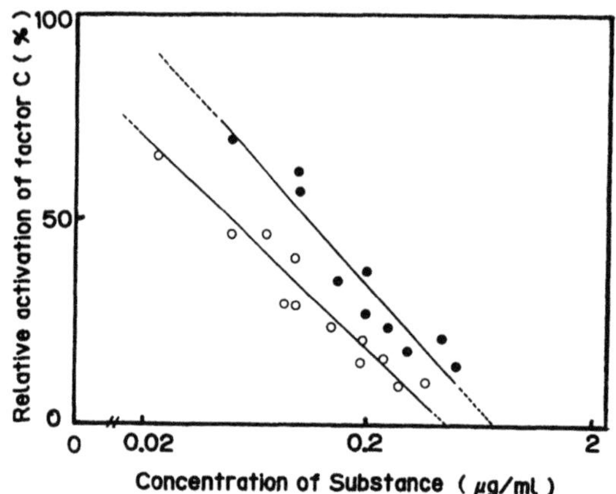

Fig 2. Inhibitory activity of tachyplesin on the LPS-mediated activation of factor C. LPS (0.2 μg/ml) was preincubated with various concentrations (0.05-1 μg/ml) of tachyplesin (O) or anti-LPS factor (●), in a total volume of 100 μl of 0.05 M Tris-HCl buffer (pH 8.0) containing human serum albumin (0.5 mg/ml) and then 100 μl of factor C (0.3 μg/ml) was added and the factor C activation was assayed as described in "MATERIALS AND METHODS". The relative activation of factor C was expressed, taking the amidase activity of factor $\overline{C}$ generated in the absence of tachyplesin as 100%.

tachyplesin was found to have an ability to bind acidic phospholipid such as phosphatidylglycerol and to form a complex with it (data not shown).

Amino Acid Sequence of Tachyplesin

The isolated tachyplesin consisted of 17 amino acid residues containing five Arg but no acidic amino acids and hexosamines. The amino acid sequence of tachyplesin was analyzed by automated Edman degradation using intact (10 nmoles) and S-pyridylethylated (15 nmoles) samples (Fig 4). The COOH-terminal residue was supposed to be arginine or its derivative by subtraction of the sequenced amino acid residues from total amino acids of the molecule. To identify the COOH-terminal residue, carboxypeptidases Y and B digestions were performed on intact and S-pyridylethylated samples. However, the quantity of free arginine liberated was only less than 3% of the original materials, suggesting that α-COOH group of the COOH-terminal arginine must have been masked. To confirm this result, intact tachyplesin was heated at 110°C for 10 hr with 30 mM HCl in an evacuated and sealed tube, and the resulting acid-treated material was digested again with carboxypeptidase B. By this treatment, 0.5 moles of free arginine per molecule of tachyplesin was estimated on amino acid analysis. These data made it possible to presume that the COOH-terminal arginine has been modified by α-amidation.

Identification of the COOH-terminal End of Tachyplesin

Since lysyl endopeptidase from **Achromobacter lyticus** specifically hydrolyzes the peptide bonds of the carboxyl sides of lysine and S-aminoethylcysteine residues, the S-aminoethylated tachyplesin was first digested with this enzyme to release the COOH-terminal residue from the molecule. The resulting COOH-terminal residue was coupled with phenylisothiocyanate and the phenylthiocarbamoyl derivative was analyzed by reversed-phase HPLC. In addition to a free lysine (actually its phenylthiocarbamoyl derivative) released from the NH_2-terminal end of tachyplesin, an unknown peak with the same retention time as that of authentic arginine α-amino was found. When this unknown peak was collected, hydrolyzed with 5.7 M HCl at 110°C for 12 hr, and phenyl-

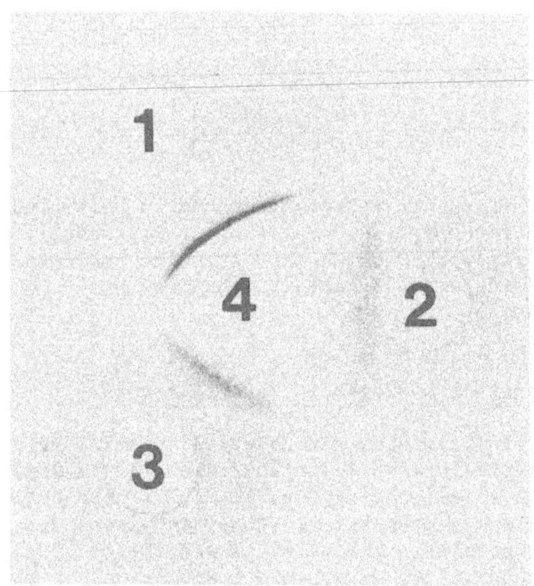

Fig 3. Analysis on the interaction of tachyplesin with LPS. The complex formations between tachyplesin, factor C or anti-LPS factor and LPS were analyzed in 1% agarose gel containing 50 mM Tris-HCL buffer (pH 8.0). The double diffusion was performed in a moist chamber at room temperature for 2 days. The precipitin lines formed between samples and LPS were stained with Coomassie brilliant blue R-250 after drying the gel plate using filter paper.
1. tachyplesin; 2. factor C; 3. anti-LPS factor; 4. LPS.

thiocarbamoylated again, the resulting material showed the same retention time as that of free phenylthiocarbamoyl-arginine. These results indicated that the COOH-terminal residue of tachyplesin is not arginine but arginine α-amide. The arginine α-amide residue at the COOH-terminal end was further confirmed by FAB mass spectrometric analysis using intact and acid-treated tachyplesin. The observed mass value of the intact peptide at $m/z = 2263.0$ (protonated form) corresponded to the theoretical value ($m/z = 2263.1$) calculated from the amino acid sequence of tachyplesin containing α-amide at the COOH-terminal end. The acid-treated tachyplesin provided the signals both at $m/z = 2263.0$ and 2264.0, although their ratio was unclear. Thereby, a part of the COOH-terminal arginine α-amide of tachyplesin had to be deamidated after its acid-treatment at 110°C for 10 h.

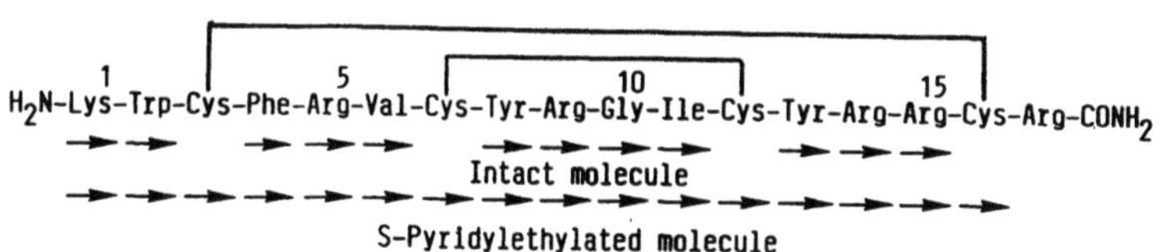

Fig 4. Amino acid sequence of tachyplesin. Residues identified by automatic Edman degradation are indicated by arrows. The position of disulfide bridges was identified by trypsin digestion of intact sample.

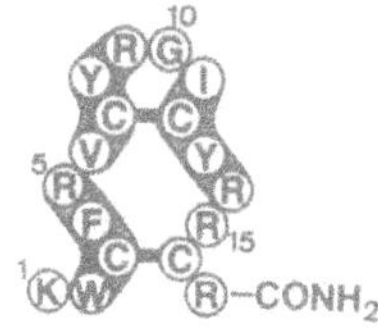

Fig 5. Repeated tetrapeptide sequence found in tachyplesin. Three tandem repeat of tetrapeptide consisting of hydrophobic amino acid-half-cystine-hydrophobic amino acid-arginine residues from the NH_2-terminal side are indicated by shadows.

Assignment of Disulfide Linkages in Tachyplesin

No **S**-pyridylethylcysteine was observed on amino acid analysis after treatment of tachyplesin with 4-vinylpyridine in the absence of dithiothreitol, although 4 residues of **S**-pyridylethylcysteine per molecule were quantitated after the **S**-alkylation. Thus, two intra-disulfide linkages must be found in the tachyplesin molecule. The position of the disulfide bridges was identified based on the amino acid compositions of the tryptic peptides derived from intact tachyplesin. Two major peptides were separated on a Cosmosil 5C18 column. The peptide T-1 consisted of a pentapeptide (Lys-1 to Arg-5) and a dipeptide (Cys-16 to Arg α-amide-17). The peptide T-2 contained both a tetrapeptide (Val-6 to Arg-9) and a pentapeptide (Gly-10 to Arg-14). These results indicated the presence of two disulfide linkages between Cys-3 and Cys-16 and between Cys-7 and Cys-12 in tachyplesin.

From all the results described above, the primary structure of tachyplesin was established as shown in Fig 5. This polypeptide consisted of a total of 17 amino acids with the molecular weight of 2,263.

DISCUSSION

Three genera including four species of horseshoe crabs are living in the world. Out of four species, American horseshoe crab, **L. polyphemus**, is known to be evolutionarily distant from the other three Asian species, based on the immunochemical and structural studies of four coagulogens (10). The sequence of **L. polyphemus** anti-LPS factor obtained here shows 83% sequence identity with that of Japanese horseshoe crab, **T. tridentatus** (1) (Fig 6). This value is even high comparing with that shown in their coagulogens (69%). As reported previously (9), coagulogen molecule has the lower homologous region consisting of the 28 amino acid residues long (named peptide C), which is cleaved off by a limulus clotting enzyme in its transformation to coagulin gel. If this region is ignored, the sequence homology of the remaining

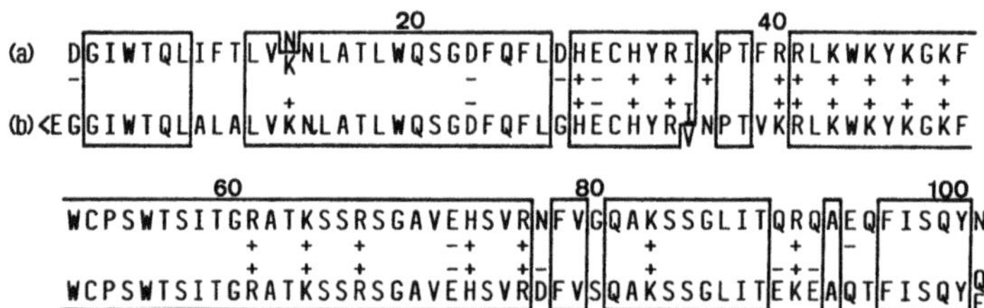

Fig 6. Alignment of the sequences of anti-LPS factors from **L. polyphemus** (a) and **T. tridentatus** (b). Identical residues are boxed and charged residues are indicated by + or - between the two sequences.

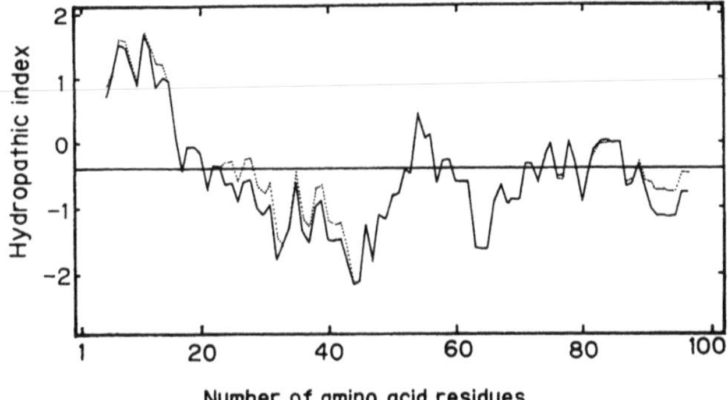

Fig 7. Hydropathy profiles of anti-LPS factors from **L. polyphemus** (——) and **T. tridentatus**(-----). Each hydropathic index is a mean hydropathy index value of 9 successive residues (6).

portion increases up to 73%, which become more comparable to the value obtained in this study. Nevertheless, the homology between two species of anti-LPS factors is high, which suggests that the entire molecule is closely related with the biological function.

Hydropathic characters (6) of anti-LPS factors derived from **L. polyphemus** and **T. tridentatus** are given in Fig 7. They show a typical amphipathic character, i.e., the NH_2-terminal region consisting of about 20 residues is highly hydrophobic and the remaining region contains positively charged residues and has relatively high content of serine. The region from Arg-41 to Lys-49 has basic amino acids at every second residues, and the region from Arg-61 to Arg-76 has them almost at every third residues. If these regions from Arg-41 to Lys-49 and from Arg-61 to Arg-76 make it possible to form β-sheet structure and α-helix, respectively, the positive charges would form a cluster at the same sides of the protein molecule. These two positive charge clusters may have an interaction with phosphate groups in the lipid A portion of LPS, and this character may be important to express the activity of this molecule for LPS-binding. Thus, it seems likely that anti-LPS factor interacts with LPS at the positively charged regions and perturbs a cell membrane structure at the NH_2-terminal hydrophobic region including up to approximately 27th residue. The region may have a sufficient length to go across a lipid bilayer like transmembrane α-helices of bacteriorhodopsin molecule, as shown in Fig 8.

It has been reported that the amino acid sequence of **T. tridentatus** anti-LPS factor shows the homology with α-lactalbumin/lysozyme family (1). **L. polyphemus** anti-LPS factor also shows almost equivalent homology. Since α-lactalbumin has a high affinity of Ca^{2+} binding site (3), we searched the potential Ca^{2+} binding site along the polypeptide chain of anti-LPS factor and found the existence of the sequence similar to that observed in the EF-hand structure (5), as shown in Fig 9. Since the regions from Glu-72 to Tyr-100 and from Gln-90 to Asn-101 gave the EF-hand alignment score, 9 and 6, respectively, the regions from Gln-81 to Gln-92 and from Gln-90 to Asn-101 are thought to be a Ca^{2+}-binding loop (22). The latter loop, however, gave lower alignment score, because the poly-peptide chain is terminated at Asn-101 so that there is no tail to form α-helix. In general, the scores of the region of other proteins which are known to actually bind Ca^{2+} are between 12 and 16. Our preliminary test on the Ca^{2+} binding ability of anti-LPS factor according to the method of Maruyama et al., (8) indicated that the dot blotted protein on a nitro-cellulose membrane is not able to bind $^{45}Ca^{2+}$, although bovine -lactalbumin used for the control can bind Ca^{2+}. Since anti-LPS factor contains lysine at the position Y (5), where is known to have

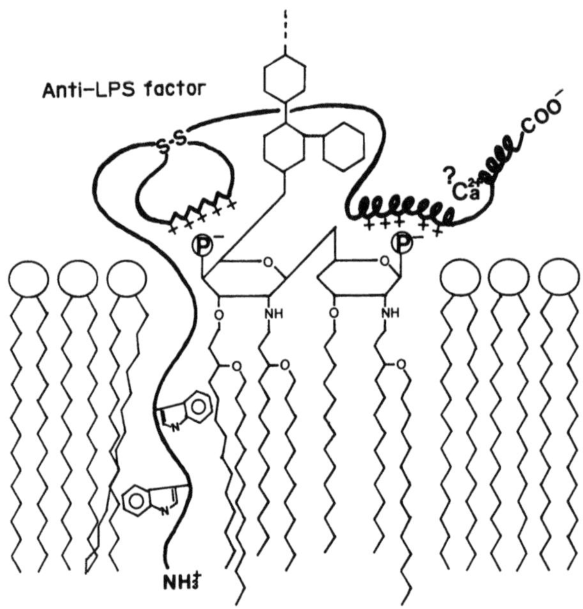

Fig 8. A speculative scheme of anti-LPS factor which interacts with LPS at the positively charged regions and perturbs a cell membrane structure at the NH_2-terminal hydrophobic region.

an oxygen atom as a Ca^{2+} ligand in other Ca^{2+} binding proteins, it might lose the high affinity Ca^{2+} binding site. There is a possibility, however, that the anti-LPS factor is an ancestral protein before duplications of EF-hand structure with Ca^{2+} binding, such as calmodulin and troponin C, which have four EF-hand structures. Recently, Stuart et al., have reported that the high affinity Ca^{2+} binding site in α-lactalbumin exists in the region from Lys-79 to Asp-88, which indicates a novel form of the Ca^{2+} binding site. The amino acid sequence of the Ca^{2+} binding site found in α-lactalbumin is not homologous to the corresponding sequence of anti-LPS factor. Thus, it might be reasonable that anti-LPS factor does not bind Ca^{2+}.

	-----α-helix----- ---Ca^{2+} binding loop--- ----α-helix----	Score
TEST	E L - - L L - - L O - O - O G - L O - - O L - - L L - - L	
(a)	Ⓔ H S V R N F V G Ⓠ A K S Ⓢ Ⓖ L Ⓘ Ⓣ Q R Ⓠ A E Q Ⓕ Ⓘ S Q Y	9
(b)	Ⓔ H S V R D F V S Ⓠ A K S Ⓢ Ⓖ L Ⓘ Ⓣ E K Ⓔ A Q T Ⓕ Ⓘ S Q Y	9
(c)	Q A K S S G L I T Ⓠ R Ⓠ A Ⓔ Q F Ⓘ Ⓢ Q Y Ⓝ	6
(d)	Q A K S S G L I T Ⓔ K Ⓔ A Ⓠ T F Ⓘ Ⓢ Q Y Ⓠ/Ⓔ	6

Fig 9. EF-hand like structure found in anti-LPS factors. The sequences of anti-LPS factors from **L. polyphemus**, (a) residues 72-100 and (c) residues 81-101, and from **T. tridentatus**, (b) residues 73-101 and (d) residues 82-102 are aligned by their correspondence to the test sequence (TEST) (22) to search EF-hand structures. Residues corresponding to the test sequence are circled and scored one point. The sum of scores are shown in the right. The abbreviations used for the test sequence are as follows: O. oxygen containing amino acids (D, N, E, Q, S, T); L, hydrophobic amino acids (L, I, V, F, M); G, glycine; E, glutamic acid.

In the course of these studies, we recently found a cationic peptide, tachyplesin, which inhibits the LPS-mediated activation of the zymogen factor C. Tachyplesin appears to exist very abundantly in the hemocyte debris, suggesting that it is one of the major cationic components of the hemocyte membrane. This cationic peptide is also able to bind tightly with **Escherichia coli**-type LPS (19) and to neutralize the factor C-activating activity of LPS similar to that of anti-LPS factor. In fact, the inhibitory activity of tachyplesin on the activation of the zymogen factor C mediated with LPS is comparable with that of anti-LPS factor (Fig 2). Although other biological significance of tachyplesin in the hemocytes is under investigation, the preliminary experiments indicate that the peptide displays antimicrobial activity against Gram-negative bacteria (**Salmonella typhimurium** and **Salmonella minnesota** R595). In the presence of tachyplesin at 2 μg/ml, **Salmonella** strains lost viability irreversibly (described in the accompanying paper by Niwa et al.). Therefore, tachyplesin seems very likely to act as antimicrobial peptide for the defense of horseshoe crab against microbial infections.

Tachyplesin is highly stable under a low pH and a high temperature, since the LPS-binding ability of tachyplesin was not affected even in 0.1% trifluoroacetic acid used for HPLC and by heat treatment in neutral pH buffer at 100°C for 30 min. This stability seems to be due to the rigid structure with two disulfide linkages. It is also of interest that tachyplesin shows a characteristic structure with three tandem repeats of tetrapeptide, namely, hydrophobic amino acid-Cys-hydrophobic amino acid-Arg, indicating its amphipathic nature closely associated with the biological activity (Fig 5). The COOH-terminal residue of tachyplesin contains an arginine α-amide, as identified by the chemical and FAB mass spectrometric analysis. The naturally occurring peptides containing arginine α-amide at the COOH-terminal have been reported in a scorpion polypeptide toxin and sarcotoxins from **Sarcophaga peregrina**.

The amino acid of sequence of tachyplesin was subjected to a computer-assisted search for homology with known sequences, using a data base "PRF/SEQDB" (Protein Research Foundation, Osaka, Japan). Despite the sequence similarities with any other cationic polypeptides could not be found, a partial sequence homology with some of proteins such as protease inhibitors and cytotoxic proteins has been noted. However, this homology seems insignificant to be discussed here.

ACKNOWLEDGEMENTS

This work was supported by a Grant-in-Aid for Scientific Research from the Ministry of Education, Science and Culture of Japan. We wish to express our thanks to Chizuko Takabayashi-Sueyoshi and Satsuki Kajiyama for amino acid and sequence analyses. We also thank Mizumo Akiyoshi and Nobuko Ueno for their expert secretarial assistances.

REFERENCES

1. Aketagawa, J., Miyata, T., Ohtsubo, S., Nakamura, T., Morita, T., Hayashida, H., Miyata, T., Iwanaga, S., Takao, T., and Shimonishi, Y., 1986, Primary structure of limulus anticoagulant, anti-lipopolysaccharide factor. J. Biol. Chem. 261: 7357.

2. Dumont, J. N., Anderson, E., Winner, G, 1986, Some cytologic characteristics of the hemocytes of limulus during clotting. J. Morphol. 119: 181.

3. Hiraoka, Y., Segawa, T., Kuwajima, K., Sugai, S., and Murai, N., 1980, α-Lactalbumin: A calcium metalloprotein. Biochem. Biophys. Res. Commun. 95: 1098.

4. Imoto, M., Kusumoto, S., Shiba, T., Naoki, T., Iwashita, H., Rietschel, E. T., Wollenweber H.-W., Galanos, C., and Lüderitz, T., 1983, Chemical structure of E. coli lipid A: Linkage site of acyl groups in the disaccharide backborn. Tetrahdr. Lett. 24: 4017.

5. Kretsinger, R. H. and Nockolds, C. E., 1973, Carp muscle calcium-binding protein II. Structure determination and general description. J. Biol. Chem. 218: 3313.

6. Kyte, J. and Doolittle, R. F., 1982, A simple method for displaying the hydropathic character of a protein. J. Mol. Biol. 157: 105.

7. Levin, J. and Bang, F. B., 1964, The role of endotoxin in the extracellular coagulation of limulus blood. Bull. Johns Hopkins Hosp. 115: 265.

8. Maruyama, K., Mikawa, T., and Ebashi, S., 1984, Detection of calcium binding proteins by ^{45}Ca autoradiography on nitrocellulose membrane after sodium dodecylsulfate gel electrophoresis. J. Biochem. 95: 511.

9. Miyata, T., Hiranaga, M., Umezu, M., and Iwanaga, S., 1984, Amino acid sequence of the coagulogen from **Limulus polyphemus** hemocytes. J. Biol. Chem. 259: 8924.

10. Miyata, T., Matsumoto, H., Hattori, M., Sakaki, Y., and Iwanaga, S., 1986, Two types of coagulogen mRNAs found in the horseshoe crab (**Tachypleus tridentatus**) hemocytes: Its molecular cloning and nucleotide sequence. J. Biochem. 100: 213.

11. Morita, T., Ohtsubo, S., Nakamura, T., Tanaka, S., Iwanaga, S., Ohashi, K., and Niwa, M., 1985, Isolation and biological activities of limulus anticoagulant (anti-LPS factor) which interacts with lipopolysaccharide (LPS). J. Biochem. 97: 1611.

12. Mürer, E. H., Levin, J., and Holme, R., 1975, Isolation and studies of the granules of the amebocytes of **Limulus polyphemus**, the horseshoe crab. J. Cell. Physiol. 86: 533.

13. Muta, T., Miyata, T., Tokunaga, F., Nakamura, T., and Iwanaga, S., 1987, Primary structure of anti-lipopolysaccharide factor from American horseshoe crab, **Limulus polyphemus**. J. Biochem. 101: 1321.

14. Nakamura, T., Morita, T., and Iwanaga, S., 1986, Lipopolysaccharide-sensitive serine protease zymogen (factor C) found in limulus hemocytes: Isolation and characterization. Eur. J. Biochem. 154: 511.

15. Nakamura, T., Horiuchi, T., Morita, T., and Iwanaga, S., 1986, Purification and properties of intracellular clotting factor, factor B, from horseshoe crab (**Tachypleus tridentatus**) hemocytes. J. Biochem. 99: 847.

16. Nakamura, T., Tokunaga, F., Morita, T., and Iwanaga, S., 1988, Interaction between lipopolysaccharide and intracellular serine protease zymogen, factor C, from horseshoe crab (**Tachypleus tridentatus**) hemocytes. J. Biochem. 103: 370.

17. Ohashi, K., Niwa, M., Nakamura, T., Morita, T., and Iwanaga, S., 1984, Anti-LPS factor in the horseshoe crab, **Tachypleus tridentatus**: Its hemolytic activity on red blood cell sensitized with lipopolysaccharide. FEBS Letters 176: 207.

18. Ornberg, R. L. and Reese, T. S., 1979, Secretion in limulus amebocytes is by exocytosis. Prog. Clin. Biol. Res. 29: 125.

19. Rietschel, E. T., Zähringer, U., Wollenweber, H.-W., Miragliotta, G., Musehold, J., Luderitz, T., and Schade, U., 1984, Bacterial endotoxins: Chemical structure and biological activity. Amer. J. Emergency Med. 2: 60.

20. Tanaka, S., Nakamura, T., Morita, T., and Iwanaga, S., 1982, Limulus anti-LPS factor: An anticoagulant which inhibits the endotoxin-mediated activation of limulus coagulation system. Biochem. Biophys. Res. Commun. 105: 717.

21. Tokunaga, F., Miyata, T., Nakamura, T., Morita, T., Kuma, K., Miyata, T., and Iwanaga, S., 1987, Lipopolysaccharide-sensitive serine protease zymogen (factor C) of horseshoe crab hemocytes: Identification and alignment of proteolytic fragments produced during the activation show that it is a novel type of serine-protease. Eur. J. Biochem. 167: 405.

22. Tufty, R. M. and Kretsinger, R. H., 1975, Troponin and parvalbumin calcium binding regions predicted in myosin light chain and T4 lysozyme. Science 187: 167.

23. Young, N. S., Levin, J., and Prendergast, R. A., 1972, An invertebrate coagulation system activated by endotoxin: Evidence for enzymatic mediation. J. Clin. Invest. 51: 1790.

INVESTIGATION OF ENDOTOXIN BINDING CATIONIC PROTEINS FROM GRANULOCYTES;

AGGLUTINATION OF ERYTHROCYTES SENSITIZED WITH RE-LPS

M. Hirata, M. Yoshida, K. Inada and T. Kirikae

Department of Bacteriology, School of Medicine
Iwate Medical University, Mirioka, 020 Iwate, Japan

Endotoxin has been found to cause cytotoxic damages of mouse bone marrow cells, especially granulocytes and macrophages, migration of marrow cells into circulation (3, 18-20), and increase in the tissue factor (tissue thromboplastin) activity in these cells (4-6). Tissue factor activity is found on the membrane surface of intact cells (i.e., cell suspension), and homogenization or sonic disruption of the cells weakened the tissue factor activity. This phenomenon is due to anticoagulant activity of cationic proteins (CAP) released from these cells (5, 7, 15). CAP from mouse bone marrow or rabbit granulocytes are the endotoxin (LPS)-binding proteins since (a) the mixture of LPS and CAP solution increased turbidity, and (b) preincubation of LPS with CAP inhibited some LPS activities (activation of blood coagulation factor XII, and lethality to mouse and tissue factor generation in mouse spleen cells) (5). Recently CAP was found to cause agglutination of erythrocytes sensitized with LPS, especially Re-LPS and lipid A.

In this study, binding mechanism of CAP to Re-LPS was investigated using two parameters, i.e., CAP-induced agglutination of erythrocytes sensitized with LPS and increase in turbidity of the CAP-LPS mixture.

MATERIALS AND METHODS

Endotoxin Preparations

The endotoxins of Salmonella typhimurium LT2(S) and TV160(Rb) were prepared according to the method of Westphal et al. Endotoxin preparations of S. minnesota (Ra ~ Re and lipid A), E. coli 08:K42 (S and Re) were kindly supplied through the courtesy of Dr. O. Lüderitz, Dr. C. Galanos and Dr. K. Jann (Max-Planck-Institut für Immunbiologie, Freiburg, Germany). All glassware and buffer solutions were heated at 250°C for 2 hr or autoclaved. A teflon homogenizer was soaked overnight in 95% ethanol containing 0.2 M NaOH and used for the extraction of cationic proteins from granulocytes.

Granulocytes

Peritoneal granulocytes were obtained from rabbits (weighing 2 ~ 3 Kg) that had received 500 ml of saline containing 0.25% sodium caseinate intraperitoneally 16 to 17 hr earlier (16).

Extraction of Cationic Proteins (CAP)

Granulocytes were washed two times with saline and homogenized in 0.1 M citric acid (15). After centrifugation at 40,000 x g for 30 min, cold ethanol was added to the supernatant (80% v/v) and crude CAP was precipitated.

Purification of CAP

Crude CAP was dissolved in 0.02 M HCl containing 0.3 M NaCl (pH 1.7) and subjected to purification by Fast Protein Liquid Chromatography (FPLC) on a Superose 12 column (1.0 x 30 cm, Pharmacia), equilibrated with the same solvent. The fractions containing LPS-binding activity (CAP-HA, as described later) were pooled and dialyzed against 0.1% acetic acid and lyophilized. This lyophilized sample was further applied to a column (1.0 x 5.0 cm of Heparin-Sepharose CL-6B (Pharmacia) equilibrated with 0.05 M Tris-HCl, pH 7.0, containing 0.1 M NaCl. Stepwise elution was performed with the same buffer containing 0.5 M and 2.0 M NaCl. Extraction and purification of CAP were performed under sterile conditions.

Sensitization of Erythrocytes with LPS

One ml of 1% erythrocyte suspension (human O type, C3H/HeN mouse or sheep) was mixed with 0.2 ml of LPS solution and incubated at 37°C for 30 min, followed by washing with phosphate buffered saline (PBS), and then the concentration of suspension was adjusted to 1.0%. In the case of S-LPS, the solution was heated at 100°C for 1 hr before sensitization of erythrocytes.

CAP-Mediated Hemagglutination

Fifty μl of 1.0% erythrocyte suspension sensitized with LPS was mixed with 50 μl of a 2-fold serial dilution of CAP in a microtiter U-plate and incubated at 37°C for 1 hr. Activity of CAP was expressed as a minimum agglutinating concentration (MAC) of CAP.

Passive Hemagglutination

Antibody titers (anti-S and anti-Re) of the immunized sera were assayed by passive hemagglutination in which sheep erythrocytes were sensitized with respective LPS preparations (21).

LPS-Induced Direct Hemagglutination

According to the method of Kirikae (8), 50 μl of 2-fold serial dilution of Re-LPS was added to 50 μl of 1.0% rabbit erythrocyte suspension, and incubated at 37°C for 3 hr. Minimum agglutinating concentration of Re-LPS was expressed as 1 HA unit.

Coagulation Study

Anticoagulant activity of CAP was expressed as prolongation of clotting time of human plasma (7). Briefly, 0.1 ml of CAP solution or FPLC fraction was preincubated with 0.1 ml of human plasma at 37°C for 3 min. Then, 0.1 ml of standard tissue thromboplastin (Simplastin, 250 ~ 500 μg/ml in 25 mM-$CaCl_2$) was added to the mixture and clotting time was measured.

Determination of Turbidity of the Mixture of CAP and LPS

The mixture of CAP and LPS was incubated at room temperature (23-24°C) and turbidity of the mixture was recorded at 340 nm.

RESULTS

CAP-Mediated Hemagglutination (CAP-HA)

Table 1 shows CAP-induced hemagglutination, designated as CAP-mediated hemagglutination or CAP-HA; Crude CAP agglutinated sheep, human and mouse erythrocytes which are sensitized with Re-LPS; Minimum agglutinating concentration (MAC) of CAP to sheep erythrocytes sensitized with Re-LPS (100 μg/ml) was 1.6 - 7.8 μg/ml.

MAC of CAP was inversely related to the amounts of LPS used for sensitization, i.e., a small amount of CAP agglutinated the erythrocytes sensitized with a large amount of Re-LPS. Human erythrocytes sensitized wth 10 μg/ml of Re-LPS were agglutinated by 50 μg/ml of CAP, however, those sensitized with 1 μg/ml of Re-LPS were not agglutinated by more than 100 μg/ml of CAP. In the case of mouse erythrocytes, a small amount of Re-LPS ($\leq$1 ug/ml) was adequate for sensitization to cause CAP-HA.

CAP-HA Activities of Several LPS Preparations

The activities of crude CAP and FPLC fraction to sheep erythrocytes sensitized with 100 μg/ml of several LPS preparations were compared (Table 2). Crude CAP could also agglutinate erythrocytes sensitized with lipid A, however, at least a 16-32 times larger amount of CAP was required as compared to the erythrocytes sensitized with Re-LPS (MAC; 25-50 vs 1.6 μg/ml). CAP did not agglutinate the erythrocytes sensitized with S ~ Rb-LPS. Re-LPS was more active than lipid A as to CAP-HA. A low concentration such as 4 ng/ml of FPLC fraction (fraction No. 14 of Fig 5, molecular weight was 50K to 70K) agglutinated the erythrocytes sensitized with Re-LPS. This fraction was 400 times more active than crude CAP. In Table 3, large amounts of LPS were used for sensitization of erythrocytes, i.e., 500 μg/ml of LPS preparations except for Re-LPS and lipid A, were used. CAP activities to erythrocytes sensitized with R-LPSs were higher than those with S-LPS since small amounts of CAP agglutinated erythrocytes sensitized with R-LPSs. CAP activities were thought to depend upon the structure of LPS used for sensitization. KDO component seemed to play an important role in the CAP-HA.

Table 1. Cationic Protein (CAP)-mediated Hemagglutination

Re-LPS used for sensitization (μg/ml)	Minimum agglutinating concentration of CAP(MAC, μg/ml)		
	Sheep RBC	Human RBC	Mouse RBC
100	1.6 ~ 7.8	12.5	-
10	-	50	-
1	-	> 100	25
0.1	-	-	50
0.01	-	-	100
0	500	> 100	> 100

Re-LPS.. S. minnesota R595 RBC ..Red blood cells
CAP .. Crude CAP(ethanol precipitate) - ..Not tested

Table 2. CAP-mediated Hemagglutination

Preparations used for sensitization (100 μg/ml)		MAC of CAP (μg/ml) Crude CAP*	FPLC-Fraction**
S. typhimurium	S	>100	>1.45
	Rb	>100	>1.45
S. minnesota	Ra	>100	>1.45
	Rb	>100	>1.45
	Rc	50 ~ 100	>1.45
	Re	1.6	0.004
	Lipid A	25-50	0.36 ~ 0.72

*Ethanol precipitate **Active fraction of FPLC

Inhibition of CAP-HA by LPS

CAP (pooled fraction of FPLC) solution was preincubated with each LPS preparation at 37°C for 30 min, and each reaction mixture was added to sheep erythrocytes sensitized with 100 μg/ml of Re-LPS. As indicated in Table 4, all LPS preparations, including lipid A, inhibited CAP-HA, and minimum inhibitory concentration of LPS preparations were 0.4 ~ 6.25 μg/ml. Therefore, it seemed that the binding of CAP to lipid A portion of Re-LPS attached on the membrane surface causes hemagglutination.

Table 3. CAP-mediated Hemagglutination

Preparations used for sensitization		μg/ml	MAC of CAP μg/ml
S. typhimurium	S	500	200
	Rb	500	50
E. coli 08:K42⁻	S	500	100
	Re	500	25
S. minnesota	Ra	500	200
	Rb	500	200
	Rc	500	100
	Rd1P+	500	100
	Rd1P-	500	50
	Rd2	500	50
	Re	100	12.5
	Lipid A*	100	50

*SRBC sensitized with 200-400 μg/ml of lipid A agglutinated spontaneously in PBS but did not in veronal-buffered saline.

Table 4. Inhibition of CAP-mediated HA by LPS Preparations or Lipid A

Preparations		Minimum inhibitory concentration μg/ml
S. typhimurium	S	3.13
	Rb	0.40
S. minnesota	Ra	1.56
	Rb	0.78
	Rc	6.25
	Rd1P+	1.56
	Rd1P-	0.40
	Rd2	3.13
	Re	6.25
	Lipid A	6.25

CAP (FPLC fraction, 97.5 μg/ml: MAC=12.2 μg/ml) solution was preincubated with each preparation at 37°C for 30 min, and each reaction mixture was added to SRBC sensitized with 100 μg/ml of Re-LPS.

Table 5. CAP-HA and PHA

Effects of Sensitization of SRBC with Re- and/or S-LPS

Sensitized with		CAP-HA	PHA titer	
Re-LPS*	S-LPS**	MAC (μg/ml)	Anti-S	Anti-Re
200	-	25	< 40	1280
100	-	50	< 40	1280
50	-	100	< 40	640
25	-	200	< 40	160
-	100	> 200	2560	< 40
200	100	25	2560	1280
100	100	50	2560	1280
50	100	200	2560	320
25	100	200	2560	160
-	-	> 200	< 40	< 40

*S. minnesota R595 **S. typhimurium LT2 SRBC suspension was sensitized with Re-LPS (200 ~ 25 μg/ml) for 40 min, then washed with PBS and resensitized with 100 μg/ml of S-LPS.

Table 6. Inhibitory Effects of CAP on the Binding of Re-LPS to SRBC

Sensitized with S-LPS + CAP		PHA titer Anti-S	Sensitized with Re-LPS + CAP		PHA titer Anti-Re
100	0	2560	100	0	1280
100	200	2560	100	200	40
50	0	2560	50	0	320
50	200	2560	50	200	20
25	0	640	25	0	160
25	200	640	25	200	< 20

S-LPS .. S. typhimurium LT2 Re-LPS .. S. minnesota R595
Mixture of LPS (μg/ml) and CAP (μg/ml) was preincubated at 37°C for 1 hr.

CAP-HA and Passive HA

Erythrocytes were sensitized with different amounts of Re-LPS, and effects of these sensitizations on CAP-mediated HA and antibody-mediated HA (passive HA using anti-S and anti-Re sera) were compared. As indicated in Table 5, anti-Re titer depended upon the amounts of Re-LPS, and CAP-mediated HA was inversely related to the amounts of Re-LPS used for sensitization. Erythrocytes sensitized with S-LPS reacted to anti-S serum but did not react to anti-Re serum. CAP did not agglutinate the erythrocytes sensitized with S-LPS, as already indicated in Table 2 and 3.

Erythrocyte suspension was sensitized with Re-LPS for 40 min, then washed with PBS and resensitized with S-LPS. Shown in PHA titer, these erythrocytes reacted to both sera, i.e., to anti-S and anti-Re sera. CAP-mediated HA was not affected by the resensitization.

Since the PHA titers using erythrocytes sensitized with 100 μg and 200 μg of Re-LPS were the same, the sensitization seemed to be adequate. These results indicate that CAP activity depended on amounts of Re-LPS attached on the erythrocyte membranes. Additional sensitization with S-LPS did not affect CAP-HA. Therefore, the binding site of Re-LPS on erythrocyte membranes must be different from that of S-LPS.

Inhibition of the Binding of Re-LPS to Erythrocytes by CAP

In this experiment, erythrocytes were sensitized with LPS alone or with the mixture of LPS and CAP preincubated for 1 hr, and binding capacity of S-LPS or Re-LPS to erythrocytes was determined by passive HA. As shown in Table 6, PHA titer of anti-Re decreased when Re-LPS was preincubated with CAP, however, anti-S titer did not change. This indicates that binding capacity of Re-LPS on erythrocyte membranes was abolished by preincubation of Re-LPS with CAP, but that of S-LPS was not. Therefore, the structure of Re-LPS binding site of erythrocyte membranes and that of CAP appeared to be very similar in nature. The possibility is further supported from the next finding.

Table 7. Inhibition of LPS-Induced Direct Hemagglutination by CAP or Polymyxin B

Re-LPS[a)] μg/ml (HA units)	Minimum inhibitory concentration μg/ml CAP	PxB
0.1(4HA)	10	-
0.2(8HA)	20	-
1.0(40HA)	50	25

a) Minimum agglutinating concentration of Re-LPS to rabbit erythrocytes was 0.024 μg/ml.

Re-LPS solution was preincubated with CAP or Polymyxin B (PxB) at 37°C for 50 ~ 60 min, then, the mixture was added to 1% rabbit erythrocyte suspension.

Inhibition of LPS-Induced Direct Hemagglutination by CAP

As shown in Table 7, Re-LPS (0.024 μg/ml) directly agglutinated rabbit erythrocytes, and this dose was expressed as 1 HA unit. Re-LPS (4 ~ 40HA) was preincubated with CAP or polymyxin B for 1 hr, and the mixture was added to rabbit erythrocyte suspension. Ten to 50 μg/ml of CAP inhibited LPS-induced direct HA. Fifty μg of CAP was equivalent to 25 μg of polymyxin B as to the inhibition of direct HA.

Binding of CAP to Re-LPS

Fig 1 shows the binding of CAP to Re-LPS. Re-LPS was incubated with CAP at 23°C for 30 min and turbidity of the mixture was determined. Addition of CAP solution to Re-LPS caused an increase of turbidity in proportion to the amounts of CAP. Binding of CAP to Re-LPS was shown to form an insoluble complex.

Effect of Ionic Strength on the Binding of CAP to LPS

Fig 2 shows the effect of ionic strength on the binding of CAP to Re-LPS. Re-LPS was incubated with CAP in 10 mM phosphate buffer, supplemented with several concentrations of NaCl. About 50% of the binding was inhibited by 200 mM NaCl. Inhibitory effects of NaCl on the binding was incomplete. The binding of CAP to Re-LPS was optimal under the condition of low ionic strength.

Effect of pH on the Binding of CAP to LPS

The data illustrated in Fig 3 indicates the effect of pH on the binding of CAP to Re-LPS or to lipid A. Re-LPS or lipid A was incubated with CAP at 23°C for 30 min under the condition of low ionic strength (10 mM buffer, pH 4.0 to 9.0) and turbidity was measured. The binding of CAP to LPS or lipid A was best expressed at pH 6.0 or from 6.0 to 7.0. In alkaline solution, the binding of CAP to LPS was very weak. On the contrary, binding of CAP to lipid A in acidic solution was not so affected. These results indicate that CAP binds to Re-LPS or to lipid A through ionic and hydrophobic bonds.

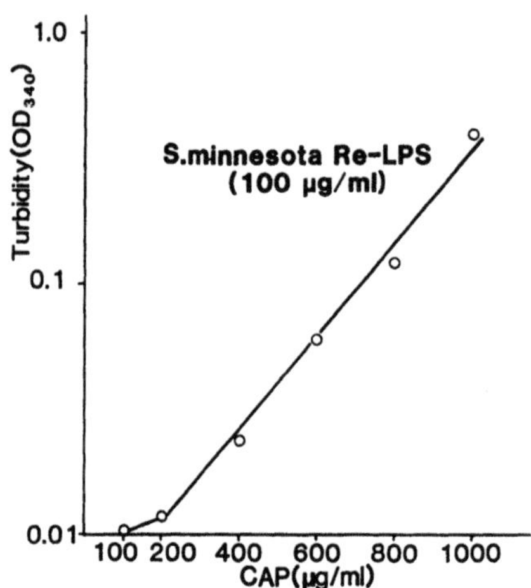

Fig 1. Re-LPS was incubated with equal volume of CAP in 10 mM phosphate buffer (pH 7.0) at 23°C for 30 min.

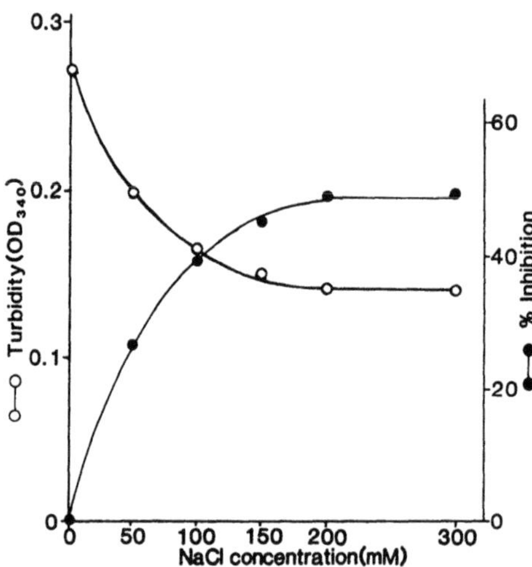

Fig 2. Re-LPS (100 μg/ml) was incubated with equal volume of CAP (500 μg/ml) for 10 min at 24°C in 10 mM phosphate buffer, pH 7.0, supplemented with the indicated concentrations of NaCl.

Binding Activities of CAP to LPS Preparations

CAP was incubated with each LPS preparation under the best condition for binding (pH 6.0 and low ionic strength) and the turbidity was recorded over a period of 30 min (Fig 4). Rapid increase of turbidity was marked in the mixture of CAP and Re-LPS or lipid A. The binding of CAP to S-LPS (E. coli 08 or S. typhimurium) was weak.

Reversible Binding of CAP to Re-LPS

Re-LPS was incubated with CAP solution at 23°C for 40 min, and the

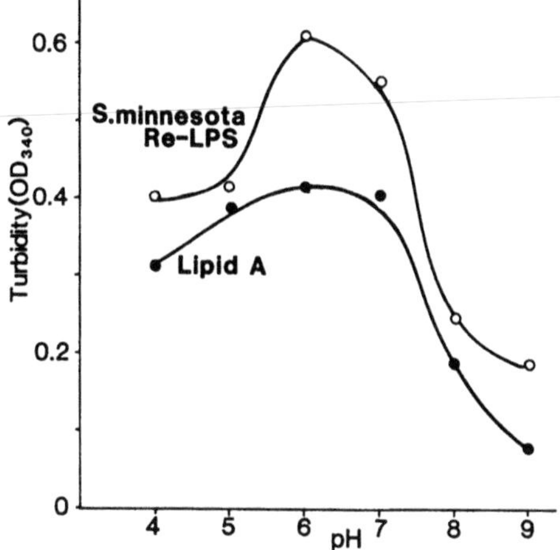

Fig 3. Re-LPS or lipid A (100 μg/ml) was incubated with CAP (500 μg/ml) for 30 min at 23°C in 10 mM sodium veronal-sodium citrate-HCl buffer.

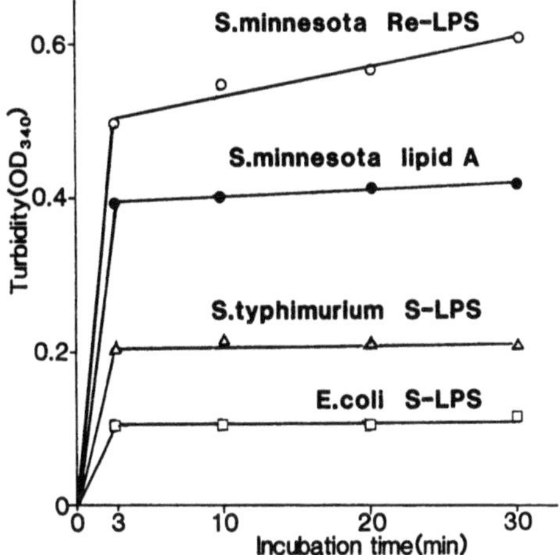

Fig 4. LPS or lipid A (100 μg/ml) was incubated with equal volume of CAP (500 μg/ml) at 23°C in 10 mM sodium veronal-sodium citrate-HCl buffer, pH 6.0.

mixture was divided into two portions. One was added to an equal volume of 10 mM buffer as control, and the other was added to 10 mM buffer containing 0.3 M or 0.6 M NaCl, and changes of turbidity were continuously recorded. Turbidity of the solution immediately decreased after the addition of 0.6 M NaCl. Decrease in the turbidity of the solution depended on the concentration of NaCl added to the buffer. Addition of a low concentration of NaCl caused temporary decrease in turbidity, followed by an increase in turbidity.

Gel Filtration of CAP

Fig 5 shows the gel filtration pattern of crude CAP on a Superose 12 column. Dash line indicates optical density at 280 nm, a solid line indi-

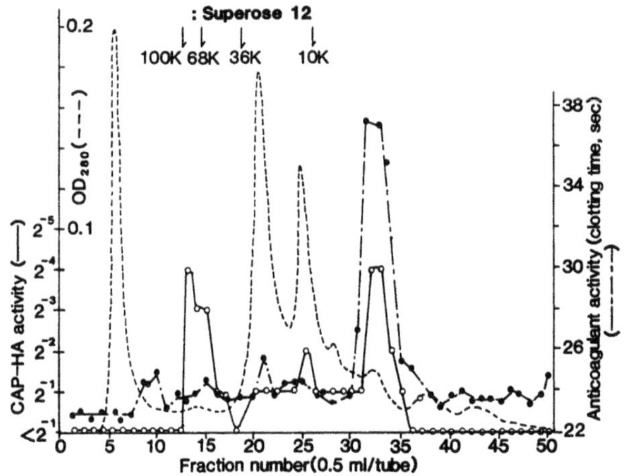

Fig 5.

cates CAP-HA activity, and chain line indicates the anticoagulant activity. Two fractions had CAP-HA activity and their molecular weights were around 68 K Dalton and less than 10 K Dalton. The first peak of the high molecular weight group had no anticoagulant activity, whereas the low molecular weight group had anticoagulant activity. As to anticoagulant activity, the dissociation of properties of crude CAP was found. In Fig 6, CAP was extracted from granulocytes by citrate-buffer, pH 5.0, containing 0.3 M-NaCl, and directly applied to gel filtration on a Superose 12 column. CAP-HA activity was also found in the two fractions. The shaded fraction with high molecular weight was then subjected to Affinity chromatography.

Affinity Chromatography

Fig 7 shows the elution profile of CAP on a Heparin-Sepharose CL-6B column. The CAP-HA activity was found in the fraction eluted with 2.0 M NaCl. Concerning the second peak with low molecular weight, anticoagulant activity of CAP was also eluted with 2.0 M NaCl (data is not shown here).

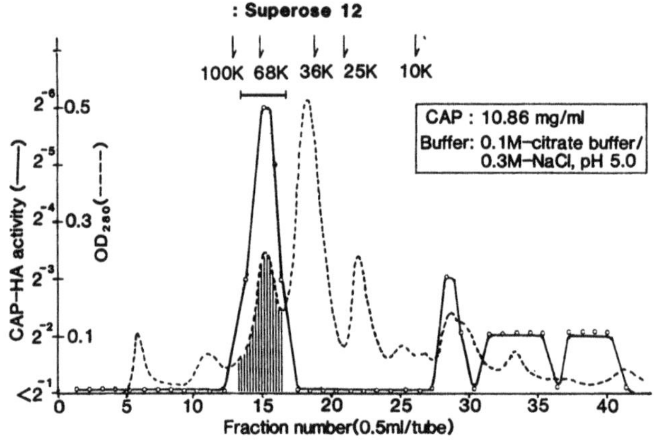

Fig 6.

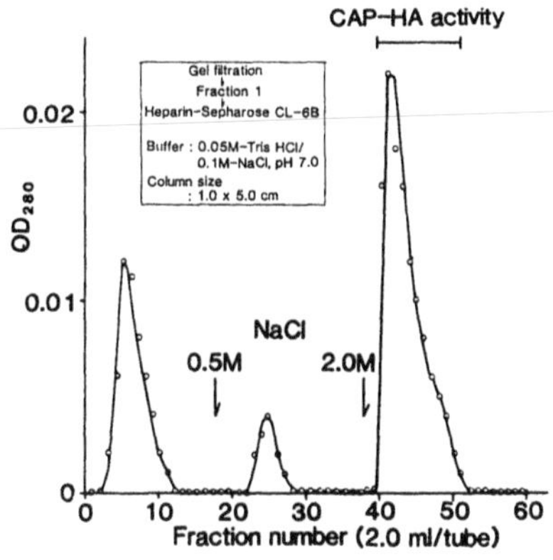

Fig 7.

DISCUSSION

Cationic proteins (CAP) isolated from liver and spleen of several animal species have been known to show anti-endotoxin activity (14). It has also been reported that CAP from granulocytes and macrophages have antibacterial activity (2, 9, 13, 16, 17) and anticoagulant activity (15).

Niwa and his coworkers have shown that anti-LPS factor, cationic protein, from limulus lysate also has anti-endotoxin and antibacterial activities, and this factor causes lysis of erythrocytes sensitized with LPS (11, 12).

Carr and Morrison have demonstrated that cationic antibiotic, polymyxin B, causes lysis of erythrocytes sensitized with Re-LPS (1). Kirikae has found that LPS, especially Re-LPS and lipid A, directly agglutinated erythrocytes from several animal species, such as mouse and rabbit, but did not agglutinate those from sheep and human (8). Contrarily, CAP agglutinated all of these erythrocytes sensitized with R-LPS. As to the CAP-mediated hemagglutination, activity of the CAP to erythrocytes sensitized with Re-LPS was higher than those sensitized with lipid A.

CAP-HA was inhibited by S-LPS, Re-LPS or lipid A after incubation of CAP with each LPS preparation. Therefore, the binding of CAP to lipid A portion of Re-LPS attached on the membrane surface is thought to cause hemagglutination. KDO component also seems to play an important role in the CAP-mediated hemagglutination.

CAP activity depended on the amount of Re-LPS attached to the erythrocyte membranes, however, CAP could not agglutinate erythrocytes sensitized with S-LPS.

The erythrocyte-sensitizing capacity of Re-LPS was inhibited by CAP, so far examined. Direct hemagglutination which shows attachment of LPS on erythrocyte surface was also inhibited by CAP. From these results, it seems that the binding site of Re-LPS to erythrocytes surface is similar to that of CAP. In other words, the acidical-charged and hydrophobic structure of Re-LPS micelle binds to both erythrocytes surface and CAP molecule.

Binding of CAP-to Re-LPS increased turbidity, as already observed in the mixture of polymyxin B and Re-LPS (10). The binding activity of CAP to Re-LPS was higher than that to lipid A or to S-LPS, and this phenomenon correlated well with the CAP-mediated hemagglutination. The binding of CAP to Re-LPS or to lipid A was optimal under the condition of low ionic strength, at pH 6 to 7. These findings indicate that the ionic and hydrophobic bonds of CAP to KDO-lipid A portions of Re-LPS, attached on the erythrocyte membranes, are involved in the induction of hemagglutination.

Antibacterial activity of CAP is well-known, and the same binding as CAP-HA may exhibit in the outer membrane of gram-negative bacteria, resulting in bacteriolysis.

By these investigations, the functional mechanism of LPS on cell surface, e.g., macrophages and B-lymphocytes could be analyzed. Furthermore, the defensive activities of CAP, such as antibacterial, anti-endotoxin and anticoagulant properties of CAP must participate in the host defense system.

ACKNOWLEDGMENTS

We would like to thank Dr. M. Niwa (Osaka City University) for his helpful discussion. We also wish to thank Drs. O. Lüderitz, C. Galanos and K. Jann (Max-Planck-Institute für Immunbiologie) for supplies of their preparations. We express our sincere gratitude to Dr. S. Tanaka (Seikagaku Kogyo Co. Ltd.) and Dr. S. Nakamura (Primate Research Institute, Kyoto University) for suggesting the method of extraction and purification of cationic proteins, and to Ms. V. L. Braymer for preparing the manuscript.

This work was supported by Grant-in-Aid for Scientific Research from the Ministry of Education of Japan (No. 60480167 and No. 61570214).

REFERENCES

1. Carr, C. and Morrison, D. C., 1984, Lipopolysaccharide interaction with rabbit erythrocyte membranes. Infect. Immun. 43: 600-606.

2. Ganz, T., Selsted, M. E., Szklarek, D., Harwig, S. S. L., Daher, K., Baiton, D. F. and Lehrer, R. I., 1985, Defensins: Natural peptide antibiotics of human neutrophils. J. Clin. Invest. 76: 1427-1435.

3. Hirata, M., 1975, Inhibitory effects of antihistamines and antiserotonins on the bone marrow reactions produced by Escherichia coli endotoxin in mice. J. Inf. Dis. 132: 611-616.

4. Hirata, M., Inada, K., Tsunoda, N. and Yoshida, M., 1980, Relationship between cells in bone marrow and intravascular coagulation in endotoxicosis, in: "Bacterial Endotoxins and Host Response", M. K. Argarwal, ed., Elsevier/North-Holland Biomedical Press, p. 255-272.

5. Hirata, M., Tsunoda, N., Suzuki, Y., Inada, K. and Yoshida, M., 1982, Endotoxemia and blood coagulation. 2. Anticoagulant activities of mouse bone marrow and spleen cells. Blood and Vessel. 13: 237-240.

6. Hirata, M., Yoshida, M., Tsunoda, N. and Inada, K., 1984, Endotoxemia and blood coagulation; Procoagulant activity of mouse bone marrow cells, in: "Bacterial Endotoxin: Chemical, Biological and Clinical Aspects", J. Y. Homma, S. Kanegasaki, O. Lüderitz, T. Shiba and O. Westphal, eds., Verlag Chemie, p. 351-362.

7. Hirata, M., Tsunoda, N. and Yoshida, M., 1987, Anticoagulant, cationic protein (CAP) isolated from granulocytes: Endotoxin-binding property of CAP, Blood and Vessel. 18: 592-594.

8. Kirikae, T., Inada, K., Hirata, M., Yoshida, M., Galanos, C. and

Lüderitz, O., 1986, Hemagglutination induced by lipopolysaccharides and lipid A. Microbiol. Immunol. 30: 269-274.

9. Lehrer, R. I., Selsted, M. E., Szklarek, D. and Fleischmann, J., 1983, Antibacterial activity of microbicidal cationic proteins 1 and 2, Natural peptide antibiotics of rabbit lung macrophages. Infect. Immun. 42: 10-14.

10. Morrison, D. C. and Jacob, D. M., 1976, Binding of polymyxin B to the lipid A portion of bacterial lipopolysaccharides. Immunochemistry. 13: 813-818.

11. Morita, T., Ohtsubo, S., Nakamura, T., Tanaka, S., Iwanaga, S., Ohashi, K. and Niwa, M., 1985, Isolation and biological activities of limulus anticoagulant (anti-LPS factor) which interact with lipopolysaccharide (LPS). J. Biochem. 97: 1611-1620.

12. Ohashi, K., Niwa, M., Nakamura, T., Morita, T. and Iwanaga, S., 1984, Anti-LPS factor in the horseshoe crab, Tachypleus tridentatus: Its hemolytic activity on the red blood cell sensitized with lipopolysaccharide. FEBS Letters. 176: 207-210.

13. Oderberg, H. and Olsson, I., 1975, Antibacterial activity of cationic proteins from human granulocytes. J. Clin. Invest. 56: 1118-1124.

14. Oroszlan, S. I., Mora, R. T. and Shear, M. J., 1963, Reversible inactivation of an endotoxin by intracellular protein. Biochem. Pharmacol. 12: 1131-1146.

15. Saba, H. I., Roberts, H. R. and Herion, J. C., 1967, The anticoagulant activity of lysosomal cationic proteins from polymorphonuclear leukocytes. J. Clin. Invest. 46: 580-589.

16. Selsted, M. E., Szklarek, D. and Lehrer, R. I., 1984, Purification and antibacterial activity of antimicrobial peptides of rabbit granulocytes. Infect. Immun. 45: 150-154.

17. Shafer, W. M., Martin, L. E. and Spitznagel, J. K., 1984, Cationic antimicrobial proteins isolated from human neutrophil granulocytes in the presence of diisopropyl fluorophosphate. Infect. Immun. 45: 29-35.

18. Yoshida, M., Hirata, M., Hatano, Y. and Inada, K., 1968, Hemorrhagic necrosis in mouse bone marrow induced by a single injection of endotoxin, and its application to the bioassay of endotoxin and to the study on biological activity of K-antigen. Japan J. Exp. Med. 38: 335-346.

19. Yoshida, M., Hirata, M. and Agarwal, M. K., 1976, Study on in vivo cytotoxicity caused by endotoxin injection, in: "Animal, Plant, and Microbial Toxins", A. Osaka, K. Hayashi and Y. Sawai, eds., Plenum Publishing Co., New York, p. 509-520.

20. Yoshida, M., Hirata, M. and Inada, K., 1973, Hemorrhage and necrosis in mouse bone marrow induced by endotoxin: A method assaying quantitative changes of the cellularities. Japan J. Exp. Med. 43: 393-402.

21. Yoshida, M., Kudoh, K., Hirata, M., Inada, K. and Ogasawara, M., 1984, Neutralizing effects of anti-Salmonella Re-antibody on endotoxic bone marrow reactions and induction of procoagulant activity, in: "Immunopharmacology of Endotoxicosis", M. K. Agarwal and M. Yoshida, eds., Walter de Gruyter, Berlin, p. 77-92.

INTERACTION OF BACTERIAL ENDOTOXIN (LPS) WITH FLUID PHASE AND MACROPHAGE MEMBRANE ASSOCIATED C1Q, THE FC-RECOGNIZING COMPONENT OF THE COMPLEMENT SYSTEM

M. Loos, B. Euteneuer and F. Clas

Institute of Medical Microbiology
Johannes Gutenberg-University, 6500 Mainz, FRG

INTRODUCTION

The bactericidal activity of normal serum was first described by Buchner in 1889 (10). This effect is abolished when serum has been incubated for 30 min at 56°C. Gram positives are less sensitive than Gram negative bacteria to direct killing, although gram positive cocci are opsonized by the action of serum mediated by antibodies and complement (22). It was found that most of the smooth strains of gram negative bacteria are serum resistant; whereas, the corresponding rough forms are extremely serum sensitive (32, 37). Thus evidence was provided that the composition of the bacterial surface may influence the reaction of the bacteria with the lytic system. The bacteriolytic properties of serum are mediated by the so called MAC (Membrane Attack Complex). This hydrophobic complex is inserted into cell membranes as a dimer and produces lysis (24). The antibody-dependent activation of the classical complement pathway as well as the activation of the alternative complement pathway by bacteria has been extensively studied. However, several bacterial strains are rapidly killed in non-immune sera. Furthermore, it was reported that C1 is absorbed to Mycoplasma pneumoniae in the absence of antibodies. The direct interaction with C1 and the activation of the classical complement cascade had even more biological consequences for these bacteria than activation of the alternative pathway (8).

Beside these humoral mechanisms of bacterial killing the phagocytic system plays an important role in host defense. Macrophages (MØ), which represent a central cell population cooperate with the cellular and humoral defense. Pathogenic bacteria can be divided into two groups (a) extracellular bacteria which are promptly killed after phagocytosis and (b) facultative intracellular bacteria which are resistant to intracellular killing unless MØ are activated. The phagocytic process involves contact between bacteria and cell receptors of the phagocytic system. This requires recognition and adhesion of the microbes. As studied extensively on polymorphonuclear leukocytes following ingestion, intracellular killing involves two major mechanisms, phagolysosome formation (20, 42) and generation of highly toxic oxygen products during the so called metabolic burst (5, 21).

There seems to be a connection between cellular defence and the bactericidal activity of serum. Synthesis in functionally active form of all components of the alternative and classical pathway up to and including C5 was found in mouse, guinea pig, and human MØ and monocytes (9, 12). Peritoneal MØ of NMRI-mice and of guinea pigs are able to synthesize active Clq and endogenous Clq is detectable in their membranes (26, 30, 31). There is striking evidence that MØ membrane-associated Clq has receptor functions for such molecules and structures which also interact with serum-Clq.

This report shows that serum Clq as well as MØ membrane-associated Clq interact directly with isolated LPS as well as LPS of intact Salmonella strains. Antibody-independent binding of serum-Clq to R-forms of S. minnesota and S. typhimurium initiates activation of the complement system leading to killing of these bacteria. MØ membrane-associated Clq and LPS are involved in attachment and endocytosis of the R-forms of these Salmonella strains. Adherence and ingestion of the bacteria is followed by the generation of oxygen radicals, lysosomal enzymes, IL-1 and prostaglandins (PGE_2). Adhesion is diminished by preincubation of the bacteria with purified Clq or by preincubation of MØ with monoclonal anti-Clq F(ab')2.

MATERIALS AND METHODS

Bacteria

The LPS-mutants (S, Ra, Rb, Rc, Rd, Re) of S. minnesota and S. typhimurium were kindly provided by G. Schmidt, Forschungsinstitut Borstel, FRG.

Cultivation

Salmonella were cultured in nutrient broth (Oxoid Ltd, Wesel, FRG) for ca. 16 hr or 4 to 5 hr until exponential growth was reacted. After being washed twice with 0.01 M phosphate buffered saline (PBS, pH 7.5) the suspensions were adjusted to the desired cell number.

Hemolytic Complement Assays

The methods for preparing sheep erythrocytes (E) sensitized with rabbit immunoglobulin G antibody (A) and coated with complement components to form the cellular intermediates (EA and EAC4) and VBS-S or VBS-ethylenediaminetetraacetate (VBS-EDTA) have been described by Rapp and Borsos (35).

Direct Cl and Clq Binding Assays

Samples containing 2×10^8 bacteria per ml and 1.3×10^{11} effective molecules of purified $C\bar{1}$ were incubated at 30°C and 4°C and samples were removed at selected times from 0 - 60 min. The control was the same amount of $C\bar{1}$ incubated with Veronal-buffered saline with low conductivity (VBS-S u = 0.065). After the samples were removed the $C\bar{1}$ bound bacteria were centrifuged and the remaining $C\bar{1}$ activity was assayed in each supernatant fluid. Data with the microbes were compared with those of the buffer-treated controls and the percentage of effective $C\bar{1}$ molecules consumed was plotted against time of incubation.

The monoclonal anti-Clq antibody which recognizes the globular portions of Clq has been described by Heinz et al. (19).

MØ

Ten-week-old female mice (strain NMRI; Ivanovas, Kisslegg, FRG) were injected intraperitoneally with 1 ml of thioglycolate broth (Oxoid, Ltd.). Four days later, exudative cells were harvested by washing the peritoneal cavity of each mouse with 5 ml of cooled PBS (4°C), collected by centrifugation (15 min; 250 x g), and suspended in culture medium to the desired cell concentration.

Phagocytosis Experiments

Assays for phagocytosis were done in Leighton tissue culture tubes. A total of 10^6 MØ per ml were suspended in M-199 with Earle salts (M199; Flow Laboratories Ltd., Bonn, FRG) without any antibiotics and serum components. One milliliter of each cell suspension was added to Leighton tubes and incubated for 60 min at 37°C in the presence of 5% CO_2 to allow the MØ to settle. Nonadhering cells were eliminated by washing twice with PBS. The MØ were then cultured for 24 hr in M-199 and washed twice with PBS prior to phagocytosis experiments. As detected by trypan blue exclusion, more than 95% of the cells were typical, well-spread viable MØ.

One portion of 3×10^8 bacteria/ml (Re-mutant or wild type) was added to the monolayers, and the monolayers were washed at intervals varying between 0 and 90 min. The MØ were rinsed six times with PBS to remove extracellular nonadherent bacteria. The MØ were lysed under hypotonic conditions by adding 1 ml of ice-cold sterile water for 30 min and mixing vigorously to suspend the ingested or cell-associated microorganisms. Lysis of MØ was observed directly by phase-contrast microscopy. The viability of bacteria was not affected by these procedures. The number of surviving bacteria was measured by colony counting from appropriate dilutions of cell lysate after growth overnight on blood agar plates.

Electron Microscopy

MØ cultivated for 24 hr were infected with S. minnesota Re-mutant in a ratio of 1:100. After an incubation period of 45 min and washing with PBS, MØ were fixed for ultrathin-section preparations with 2.5% glutaraldehyde in PBS for 20 min. The cultures were postfixed with 1% OsO_4 in PBS for 30 min. Samples were dehydrated in a graded ethanol series with uranyl acetate solution and lead citrate and then examined in a Philips electron microscope, model 301.

IL-1 Murine Thymocyte Assay (17)

PHA induced proliferation of thymocytes from 5 to 8 week old C3H/HeJ mice were used to determine IL-1 activity in the supernatants of NMRI mouse MØ. Single cell suspensions of thymocytes were prepared by gently pressing the thymus through a gauge wire mesh No. 60 into cold PBS. Aggregates were removed by a 10 min gravity sedimentation. The cells were washed twice with PBS and resuspended to a density of 1.5×10^7 cells/ml in RPMI containing 10% FCS and Penicillin-Streptomycin. Thymocytes were cultured for 72 hr at 1.5×10^6 cells/well in flat bottom 96/well microtest tissue culture plates (Intermed, Wiesbaden) in the presence or absence of 1.5 μg/ml PHA (Sigma) and various dilutions of the samples to be assayed for IL-1 activity. Cultures were pulsed with 0.2 μCi per well (Amersham Buchler, Braunschweig). For the final 24 hr of incubation cells were collected on filter paper with an automatic harvester. Because IL-1 is both directly mitogenic and synergistic with PHA in the induction of thymocyte proliferation, experimental results are usually presented for both types of activities. The results are expressed as the arithmetic mean Δcpm ^{3}H-thymidine incorporated = (cpm thymocytes + supernatant + PHA) - cpm of thymocytes + PHA).

PGE_2 Production and Measurements

MØ culture supernatants were collected after different times. The aliquots were frozen at -70°C and later assayed for PGE_2 using a specific RIA (Fa. Dupont, Dreieich).

β-glucuronidase

β-glucuronidase was assayed in culture supernatants and Triton-X 100 lysates of MØ using a method based on that of Fishman et al. (14). Reagents and samples used in the assay were as described in Sigma Technical Bulletin No. 325.

CL

The chemiluminescence (CL) response (electron emission) was assayed in a Bioluminat apparatus (Fa. Berthold, Wildbad, FRG) at 37°C by the method described by Euteneuer et al. (13). The CL intensity from each sample was measured as counts per minute for a 30 min period.

RESULTS

Interaction of Bacterial Endotoxin (LPS) with Fluid Phase C1q

Earlier reports have shown that bacterial LPS as well as intact gram negative bacteria are able to activate the complement system via the alternative pathway leading to a consumption of the five terminal components (7, 18, 36). Loos et al., (28) reported for the first time an antibody-independent binding of purified $C\bar{1}$ as well as native serum C1 to serum-sensitive strains of E. coli and K. pneumoniae. For further characterization of the interaction between bacteria and C1 it was of advantage to have bacterial strains with a defined surface composition. Serum-resistant smooth and serum-sensitive rough strains of S. minnesota and S. typhimurium were chosen: the serum-resistant wild type (S-form) and the serum-sensitive mutants with varying lipopolysaccharide (LPS) chain length (Ra, Rb, Rc, Rd, Re mutants (16)).

In a first set of experiments, we compared the binding of $C\bar{1}$ to the S-form and the Re-mutant. At an ionic strength of $u = 0.065$ the binding capacity of the S-form was saturated with 500 effective $C\bar{1}$ molecules per bacterium for the Re-form. However, similar binding studies performed at physiological ionic strength ($u = 0.15$) revealed that only the Re-form but not the S-form is able to bind C1 antibody-independently (data not shown). Fixation and transfer studies revealed that C1 was more tightly bound to the Re-form than to sensitized erythrocytes (EA) (25). First hints for direct binding of C1q to the bacterial surface came from experiments using fluoresceinated anti-C1q antibody: Under physiological conditions C1q was detectable only on the surface of the Re-form but not on the S-form (11).

According to these results it was obvious that certain bacterial-derived lipopolysaccharide (LPS) preparations bind directly to isolated C1 via C1q. To prove this assumption the binding capacity of isolated LPS preparations of the S- and the different R-mutants as well as of Lipid A for fluid phase C1 and C1q was tested in dose response curves. C1 and C1q bind directly to LPS and Lipid A. Binding of C1 to LPS occurs via C1q since the C1q- and C1-consuming capacity, expressed as 50% inhibition of C1 or C1q activity, is almost identical (Table 1). The C1q-LPS interaction appears to be influenced by the core and the O-specific sugar portion of LPS because the lipid A portion, which is identical in all LPS and extremely exposed in Re-mutants, has a strong C1q-binding capacity. As shown in Table 1 the LPS of the smooth form (wild type) of S. minnesota is substantially weaker than LPS of the rough form in its C1q- and C1-consuming capacity. Compared to S-form LPS, LPS of the Rb- and Rc-forms have a 10-fold and LPS of the Ra-, Rd-, and Re-forms have a 100-fold greater ability to consume C1q and C1. Therefore, it seems to be evident that the O-antigenic sugar chains prevent binding of C1q and C1 to the bacterial surface of the wild type.

Table 1. Binding of C1 and C1q to LPS and Lipid A of Salmonella minnesota mutants

LPS of S. minnesota strains	C1q	C1	ratio C1q/C1
	µg/ml necessary for 50% consumption		
S	380	350	1.1
Ra	15	6	2.5
Rb	50	35	1.4
Rc	40	35	1.1
Rd	1.3	1.6	0.8
Re	4	2.5	1.6
Lipid A	n.d.	24	-
			m.w. 1.4
LPS of E. coli 075	n.d.	0.77	-

Since erythrocytes (E) have a receptor for LPS and E-LPS can be formed, LPS-coated erythrocytes were used for further characterization of the interaction of LPS with the classical pathway. If C1 is bound to LPS via C1q, then binding of C1 should be prevented by purified C1q in a competitive fashion. The experiment shown in Fig 1 confirms this assumption. Incubation of E-LPS with different concentrations of purified C1q led to a C1q-dependent reduction of C1 uptake from 95 to 30%. Binding of $C\bar{1}$ to E-LPS resulted in the formation of an E-LPS-$C\bar{1}$ intermediate which was able to consume C4. The number of $C\bar{1}$ molecules taken up by E-LPS depends on the amount of LPS present on the erythrocytes. Therefore, the rate of C4 consumption also depends on the number of LPS molecules per cell. Similar to the direct interaction of E-LPS with C1, an interaction of gram negative bacteria with C1 and the classical pathway was found.

In further experiments the participation of the classical pathway in the bactericidal effect of normal human serum (NHS) was examined, using human selective complete C1q-deficient serum (6). About 1000 bacteria were incubated in each serum sample for 2 hr at 37°C; all sera were diluted 1:10 in 4 mM thioglycolate. As shown in Fig 2.2 Re-mutants of S. minnesota are serum sensitive while the wild type showed no sensibility to the bactericidal effect of normal serum. Furthermore, the serum-sensitive Re-mutant survived in the C1q deficient patient serum. The killing capacity could be restored by addition of purified C1q (6.5×10^{10} effective molecules per ml, i.e., 500 times less than the amount of C1q in NHS). The higher resistance of the S-form to NHS may reflect the weakness or inability of S-form LPS to bind C1q or C1. These findings were validated using electron microscopy and a ferritin-labeled antibody. Fig 2.1 shows the ultrathin sections of the S-form and the Re-mutant of S. minnesota. A conspicuous ferritin layer surrounds the Re-mutant indicating that a lot of cell-bound C1q could be detected by the antibodies on the bacterial surface (Fig 2.1 left). The S-form did not bind C1q since no ferritin grains were detectable on the outer membrane of the S-form (Fig 2.1a). The presented electron microscopic photographs confirm the observations of the hemolytic assays that C1q is bound only by the Re-mutant and not by the serum-resistant S-form of S. minnesota.

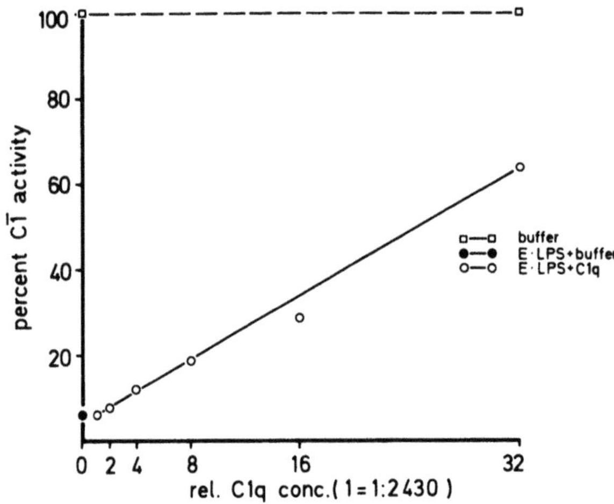

Fig 1. Purified C1q prevents binding of C1 to E-LPS. E-LPS (LPS of S. minnesota R-595) was preincubated with increasing amounts of purified C1q or with buffer as control. After washing, the cells were incubated with purified $C\bar{1}$. The consumption of $C\bar{1}$ was measured in the supernatants.

Interaction of Bacterial Endotoxin (LPS) with Macrophage Membrane-Associated C1q

Recently it was shown that macrophages synthesize C1q (26). Furthermore, C1q, the Fc-recognizing subcomponent of C1, is expressed in the membrane of macrophages (27, 30). The experiments presented so far have shown that C1q binds directly to the serum-sensitive Re-mutant but not to the S-form of S. minnesota. Therefore, the question arose whether MØ are able to differentiate between the C1q binding Re-mutant and the non-C1q binding S-form of Salmonella strains.

The ability of the MØ to adhere to bacterial pathogens is a prerequisite for phagocytosis. Uptake of bacteria (S- and R-forms) was performed in Lab-Tek tissue culture chamber/slides (Miles Laboratories, Napperville, IL) with 300 µl MØ at a cell number of 1×10^6 MØ/ml. MØ were incubated with bacteria for various periods of time. After washing, fixation and gram staining, adherent bacteria were examined by phase-contrast microscopy. The attachment of the Re-mutant was much greater than that of the wild type (data not shown). Fig 3 demonstrates the ingestion of the Re-mutant which followed the adherence. During the first 15 min of incubation of MØ with 3×10^8 cells of the Re-mutant, 1.4×10^5 bacteria were taken up. After 60 min, ingested bacteria were reduced to 7.4×10^4 cells. The observed increase in number of colonies after this time can probably be explained by an increase in number of organisms which were not killed. The adherence of the Re-mutant was dependent on MØ age, culture media and concentration of bacteria.

The attachment of the Re-mutant to the macrophage surface was demonstrated by ultrathin section preparations (Fig 4). Mitochondria are concentrated at the locus of ingestion (A) MØ membrane structures engulf the bacteria (B, C) and afterwards Salmonella are completely ingested. Lysosomes are detectable (C, D) and intracellular division of the Re-mutant is possible.

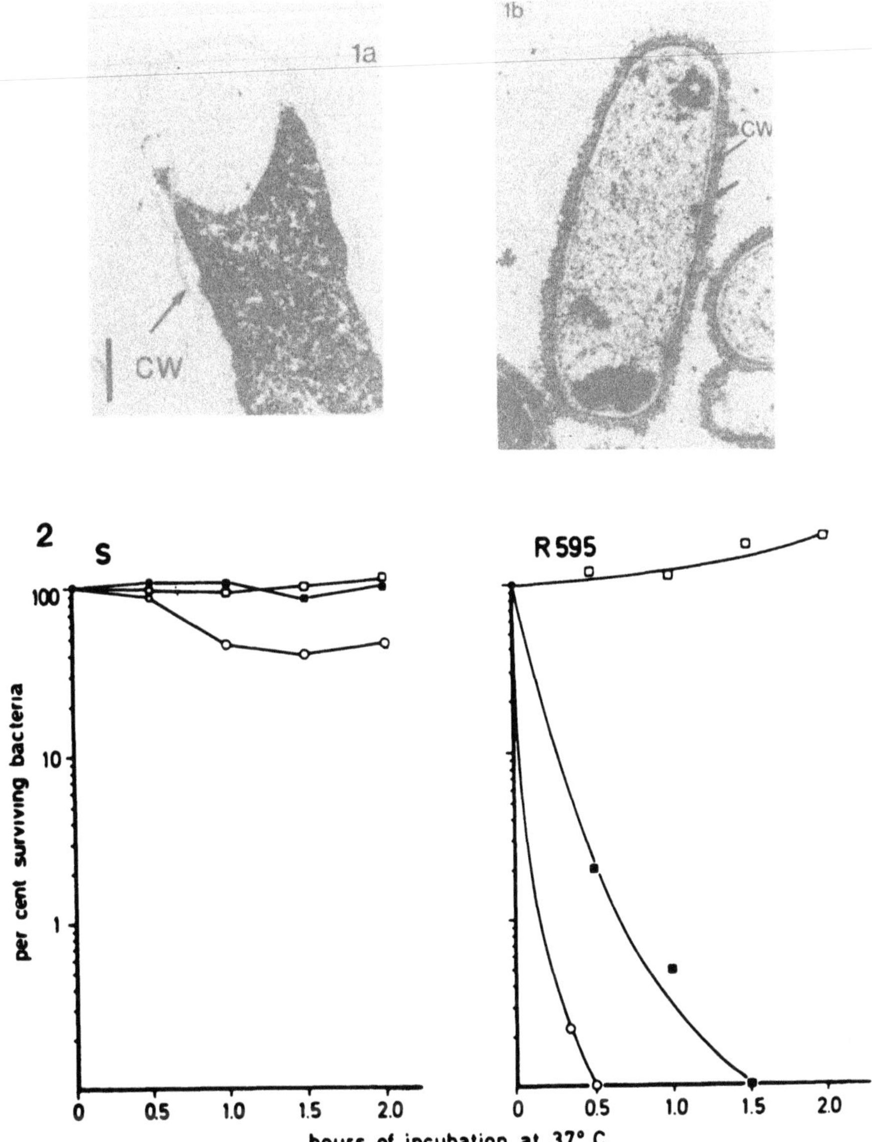

Fig 2.

1. Ultrathin sections of the S- and Re-forms of S. minnesota. The bacteria were treated with purified C1q, anti-C1q IgG, and anti-IgG labeled with ferritin. The S-form (1a) presents no ferritin outside the cell wall (CW); whereas the cell wall of the Re-form (1b) is surrounded by an intensive layer of ferritin (←), indicating the presence of C1q antigen. The bar represents 200 nm.
2. Bactericidal activity of a selective complete C1q-deficient human serum (10%) before (□) and after (■) the addition of highly purified C1q (6.5×10^{10} effective molecules per ml) on the S-form (left) and the Re-form (right) of S. minnesota. Buffer-treated bacteria were used as 100% controls. The open circles represent the data obtained with 10% NHS on the same number of bacteria (10^{3} per ml).

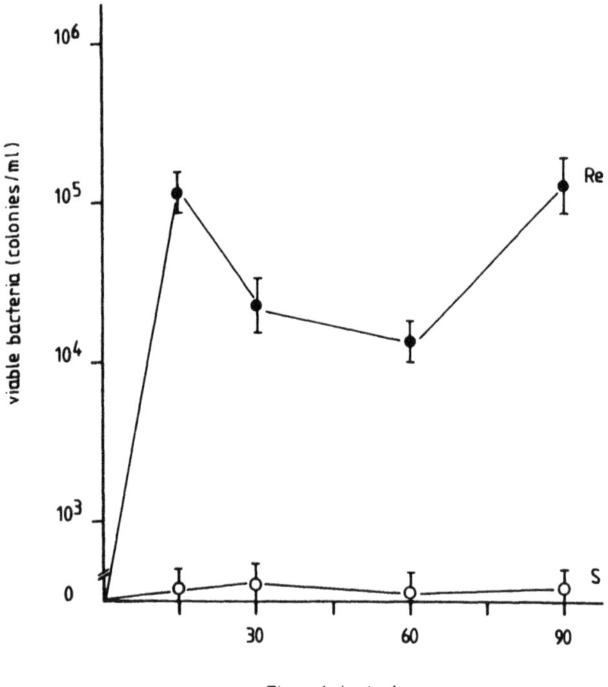

Fig 3. Time-dependent uptake of S. minnesota by macrophages. 1 x 10^6 macrophages were incubated with 3 x 10^8 bacteria for different lengths of time. After washing six times with PBS, macrophages were lysed with cold water and viable intracellular bacteria were determined by the amount of cell forming units (CFU).

Phagocytosis is accompanied in PMN and MØ by the triggering of an oxidative burst (41). This oxidative burst is accompanied by production of superoxide anions (O_2^-), hydrogen peroxide (H_2O_2) and hydroxyl radicals (•OH). Beside PMN, MØ need a further stimulation by thioglycolate (23) or BCG (Bacillus Calmette-Guerin) (4, 33).

Because of the strong binding affinity of the Re-mutant in contrast to the wild types, the Re-mutants of S. minnesota and S. typhimurium induced an increased chemiluminescent (CL) signal in guinea pig MØ as well as in mouse MØ. Binding was inhibited by purified Re-form LPS and the CL-signal was dose dependently blocked by preincubation of MØ with native LPS (13).

The MØ response to bacterial stimulus was measured by release of IL-1, PGE2 and lysosomal enzymes like β-glucuronidase. For the determination of extracellular β-glucuronidase supernatants were collected every 24 hr for a period of 7 days and stored in aliquots at -80°C until assayed. Intracellular β-glucuronidase activity was assayed after lysis of the monolayers with 0.1% Triton-X and subsequent freezing and thawing. Exposure of MØ to the Re-mutant for only 30 min stimulates release of lysosomal enzymes from the cells. At day 2 β-glucuronidase activity in the (Fig 5) culture supernatant showed a rapid and linear increase. After 5 days a maximal activity

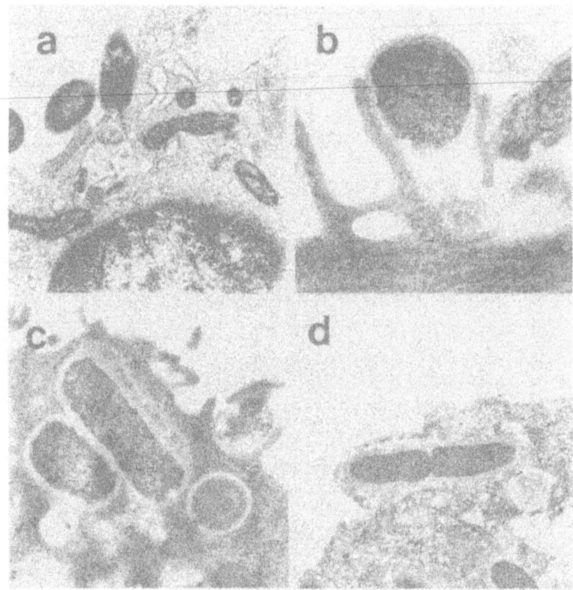

Fig 4. Ultrathin sections of macrophages after incubation of MØ with the Re-mutant of S. minnesota.
a: Concentration of mitochondria at the locus of ingestion (x 19990)
b: Ingestion through filamentous structures (x 56316)
c: Intracellular bacteria lying beside a lysosome (x 37620)
d: Intracellular division of bacteria (x 21660)

of $26U/10^7$ cells was obtained. Incubation of MØ with the Re-mutant caused a nearly five-fold increase of activity compared to the untreated control. The wild type induced a maximal activity of $7.8\ U/10^7$ MØ at day 5, i.e., a 0.4-fold increase of β-glucuronidase activity over control values. The intracellular content of β-glucuronidase was reduced by the Re-mutant from 4U to $2.3U/10^7$ MØ at day 5. The wild type induced a decrease to $1U/10^7$ MØ. Determination of the intracellular and extracellular protein content as well as the release of LDH from the cells as a cytoplasmatic marker led to the conclusion that the observed extracellular increase of β-glucuronidase activity is due to an increased enzyme synthesis. This is in agreement with the results of Allison and Davies (3) who showed that MØ synthesize during phagocytosis an increased amount of lysosomal hydrolases. Phagocytosis is also associated with an increase in hexosemonophosphate (HMP)-activity to trigger secretion of lysosomal enzymes (38). These observations are in agreement with our own results: The Re-mutant which induced an increase in β-glucuronidase also triggered an oxidative burst in the MØ which is associated with a rise of HMP-activity.

In the next experiment stimulation of IL-1 synthesis by Salmonella was investigated. IL-1 activity in the culture supernatants was assayed in the comitogenic assay on C3H/HeJ thymocytes in the presence of suboptimal doses of phytohemagglutinin (17). The low proliferative effect of lectins like PHA was markedly enhanced by IL-1 (40). The results (Fig 6) represent the values obtained in 1:4 dilution of cell supernatants. The levels of IL-1 activity in supernatants were expressed as cpm values of ^{3}H-thymidine incorporated by thymocytes. Exposure of MØ to the Re-mutant stimulated incorporation of ^{3}H-thymidine. Therefore, contact of macrophages with the Re-mutant led to a significant increase of IL-1 production with a maximum on day 4. In contrast, MØ infected with the wildtype induce a constant rise in IL-1 produc-

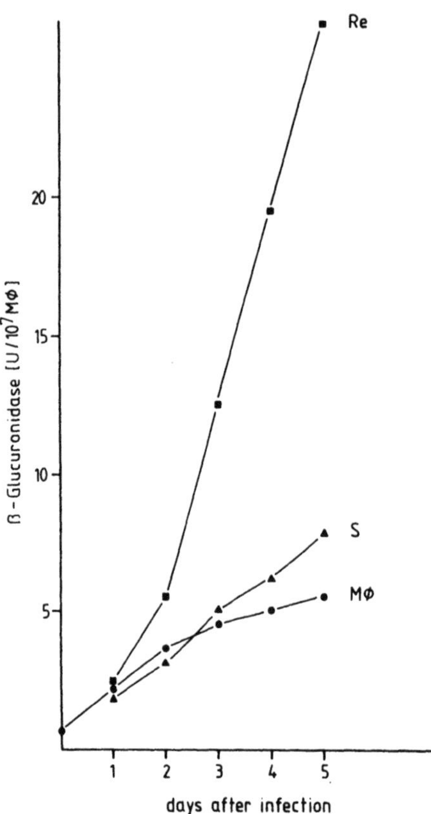

Fig 5. β-glucuronidase activity in macrophage supernatants after incubation with the wild type and the Re-mutant of S. minnesota. Comparison to a medium-treated control culture of MØ. 5 x 10^6 MØ/ml were cultivated for 24 hr in M199 without antibiotics. After washing the cell cultures two times, MØ were incubated with bacteria in a ratio of 1:10. After 30 min any bacteria not ingested were removed by six washing steps and MØ were further cultivated in M199 medium containing Penicillin and Streptomycin.

tion comparable with the amount of IL-1 produced on day 1 by MØ infected with the Re-mutant. This constant level induced by the S-form may be due to membrane fractures or free LPS in the exponential growth culture of the bacteria.

It has been amply documented that macrophages are the major producers of prostaglandins, thromboxanes, and other arachidonic acid metabolites among leukocytes. Stimulation of arachidonic acid conversion may occur in response to a number of stimuli, including the Fc fragment of immunoglobulins, immune complexes, lymphokines, endotoxin and others (1).

1 x 10^6 MØ/ml which had been cultivated for one day were incubated with the Re-mutant or the wild type for 30 min. After several washing steps MØ were further incubated in new culture medium with Penicillin and Streptomycin. PGE-content of the culture supernatants was detected after different times (Fig 7). The Re-mutant induced a release of PGE_2. After 30 min a concentration of 24 ng PGE_2/ml was measured compared to 1-2 ng PGE_2/ml by MØ without bacteria. Maximal release of PGE_2 (>25 ng/ml) from MØ was observed 60-90 min after incubation with the Re-mutant. An enhanced PGE_2-production could also be observed for the wild type. The highest levels (11 ng PGE_2/ml)

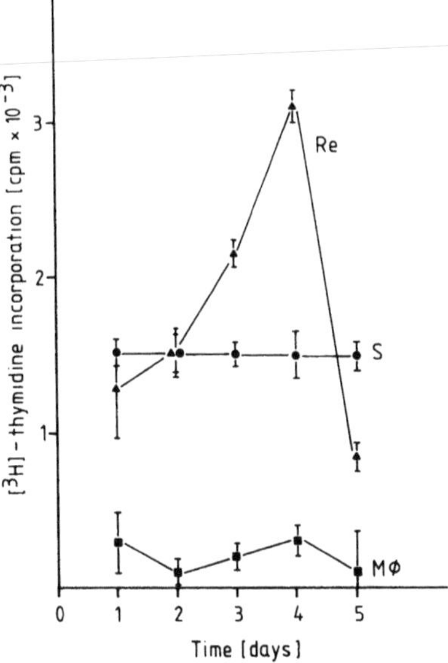

Fig 6. IL-1 production by MØ after incubation with the Re-mutant or the wild type of S. minnesota, normally without any contact to bacteria. IL-1 activity was expressed as incorporation of ^{3}H-thymidine. Cell supernatants were diluted 1:4.

being reached between 80-90 min. After 90 min PGE_2 levels decreased in cell samples to below the starting level.

These experiments provide evidence that indeed MØ are able to differentiate between the serum sensitive, C1q-binding Re-form and the serum resistant, non-C1q-binding S-form of Salmonella strains. Adhesion and uptake of the Re-form is accompanied by a series of biological events which have also been described to occur through interaction of MØ with LPS. Since LPS binds directly to C1q and endogenous C1q is incorporated into the membrane of MØ, it was of interest to test whether membrane-associated C1q is involved in the binding of the Re-form to MØ. To answer this question two sets of experiments were performed. In one experiment the Re-form was preincubated with purified C1q before the bacteria were incubated with MØ. It turned out that the adhesion of the bacteria to MØ and the generation of oxygen radicals in MØ were markedly reduced by the C1q coated Re-form (Fig 8). In the second experiment MØ were treated with different concentrations of a monoclonal anti-C1q $F(ab')_2$ antibody before incubation with the Re-form. The anti-C1q $F(ab')_2$ monoclonal antibody reduced dose dependently the generation of oxygen radicals in MØ (Fig 8). Both experiments support the assumption that MØ membrane-associated C1q is involved in the uptake of the C1q-binding Re-form.

DISCUSSION

Today, direct cooperation between humoral (complement system and antibodies) and cellular immune systems (macrophages and lymphocytes) has been very well documented. MØ and the complement system as antigen unspecific compartments of the immune system have a main function in the early stage of host defense against microorganisms, i.e., bacteria and viruses. In this report we investigated the interaction of the complement system and MØ with different Salmonella strains, especially the interaction between fluid phase C1q, the Fc-recognizing subcomponent of the first component of complement, and of MØ-membrane-associated C1q which is synthesized by MØ. Our results

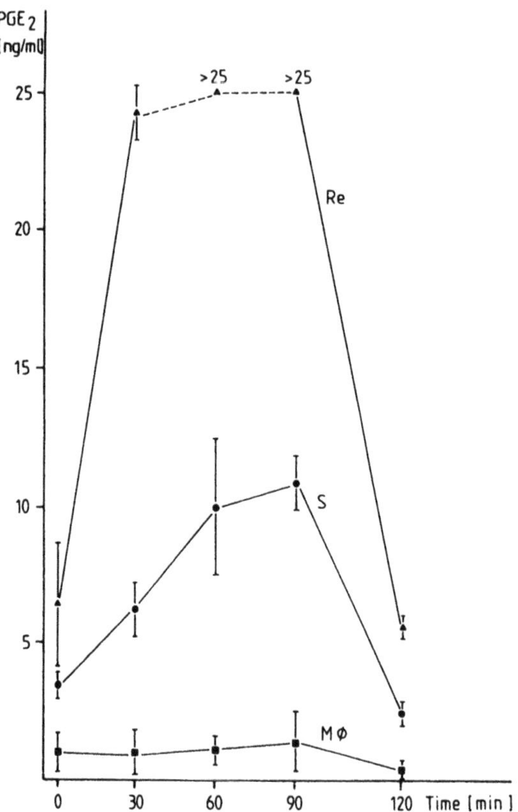

Fig 7. PGE_2-synthesis after contact with the Re-mutant and the S-form of S. minnesota, compared to untreated control.

demonstrate a low-binding affinity of Clq to Salmonella wild types (S-forms) and a strong affinity to the Re-mutants (Fig 2). These experiments show the importance of bacterial cell wall structures in binding to fluid phase as well as to MØ membrane-associated Clq.

Using mutant bacteria which differ in their LPS composition, we found that LPS is one important reactant for Clq in the bacterial membrane (Fig 1). The lipid A portion of LPS binds Clq directly. This binding seems to be amplified by a portion of the KDO, the core polysaccharide (Table 1). However, the O-antigenic sugar chain of LPS abrogates the Clq binding capacity of LPS (Table 1). This may explain why S-form of Salmonella strains are relatively serum-resistant. The Re-mutants which contain mainly lipid A and portions of KDO showed the strongest Clq binding capacity and were rapidly killed in NHS. Since the killing of the Re-mutant was abrogated in a complete selective Clq deficient serum and was restored upon addition of purified Clq, the Cl subcomponent Clq initiates the activation of the complement sytem leading to killing of these bacteria (Fig 2). This takes place even in the absence of antibodies (Fig 1). Therefore, direct binding of Clq to these bacteria may represent the biological function which is ascribed to so called "natural antibodies".

MØ have been shown to synthesize Clq and endogenous Clq is incorporated into the membrane of MØ (26, 30). Therefore, we also tested the hypothesis

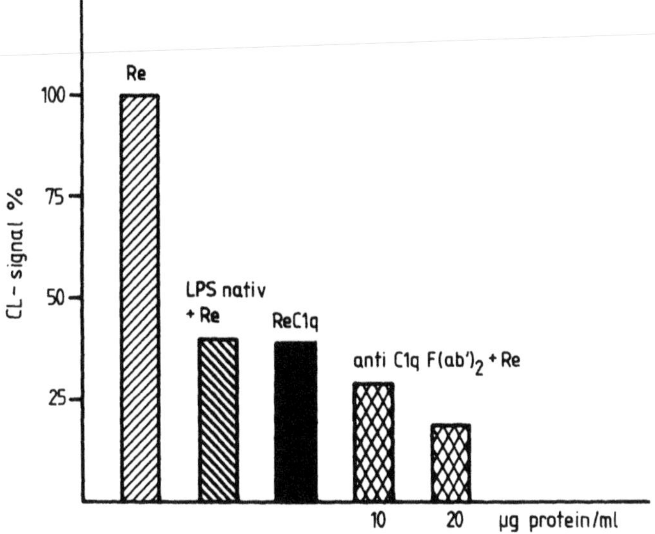

Fig 8. Influence of native LPS, C1q and anti-C1q $F(ab')_2$ on the Re-form-induced CL-Signal of macrophages. (i) Re-mutants were preincubated with purified C1q before exposure to MØ. (ii) MØ were preincubated with LPS or different amounts of an anti-C1q $F(ab')_2$ antibody.

that MØ can differentiate between the C1q binding Re-mutant and the non-binding wild type. Similar to Friedberg and Shilo (15), who used a test system containing fetal calf serum, we found a different uptake of S. minnesota strains under serum free conditions. In agreement with these authors we also found a quick decrease in cell number after uptake of the Re-mutant while the wild type which possesses a complete core and the O-antigenic sugar chains could evade ingestion. The process of ingestion is an active one, because mitochondria concentrate at the point of ingestion. Bacteria lie in a phagosome and, as seen in Fig 4, an intracellular division of bacteria is detectable. Intracellular replication of S. typhimurium was also found in 1979 by Lowrie et al. (29). Contact of the Re-mutant of S. minnesota and S. typhimurium strains with MØ surface triggers an oxidative burst (13). The importance of reactive oxygen products in defence of infections was described some years ago. Patients with chronic granulomatous disease which had a lack of activated MØ suffered chronic diseases which disappeared when an outer source of H_2O_2 was given. Beside this process on the MØ surface a further reaction of the MØ to bacterial stimuli was detected as lysosomal enzyme release (Fig 5). To trigger enzymatic activity specific receptors were needed. As mentioned by Schnyder and Baggiolini (39) enzyme activation is induced through an oxidative burst or through biochemical reactions connected with hexosemonophosphate (HMP)-shunt activity. Regulation of enzyme activation through IL-1 was described by Pantalone and Page (34). IL-1 content in MØ culture supernatants was also increased after stimulation with the Re-mutant (Fig 6). Furthermore, a rise in production of PGE_2 was also detected after incubation of MØ with Re-bacteria (Fig 7). Aderem and colleagues (2) stated that the ester-linked 3-OH myristic acid of the lipid A portion of LPS is necessary for triggering secretion. Former investigations demonstrated a dose dependent blockade of Fc-receptor activity on MØ. LPS of the Re-mutant showed the best reactivity (13). It was concluded that the Re-mutant binds to Fc-recognizing membrane structures and other membrane constituents. Yagawa et al. (43), found that expression of Fc-receptors on the plasma membrane of guinea pig peritoneal MØ was suppressed by long term exposure to lipopolysaccharide (LFS) or muramyl dipeptide. IgG 2 as well as IgG I receptors to be involved.

Our recent findings (26, 27) identified C1q as an Fc-recognizing subcomponent. Binding of FPLC purified C1q to the Re-mutant led to a reduction of 50-60% in binding tests as well as in CL-studies. MØ membrane-associated C1q (30) seems to be involved in binding of gram negative bacteria to MØ. Our investigations led to the hypothesis that endogenous C1q participates as a membrane associated molecule in the attachment of the Re-mutant. Furthermore, C1q seems to have receptor function which leads to further cellular events. However, these experiments do not rule out that besides LPS and C1q other bacterial and MØ membrane constituents and structures participate in the interaction between bacteria and MØ as well as with the complement system. But there is no doubt that these components are involved in the natural defence against gram negative bacteria (Fig 9).

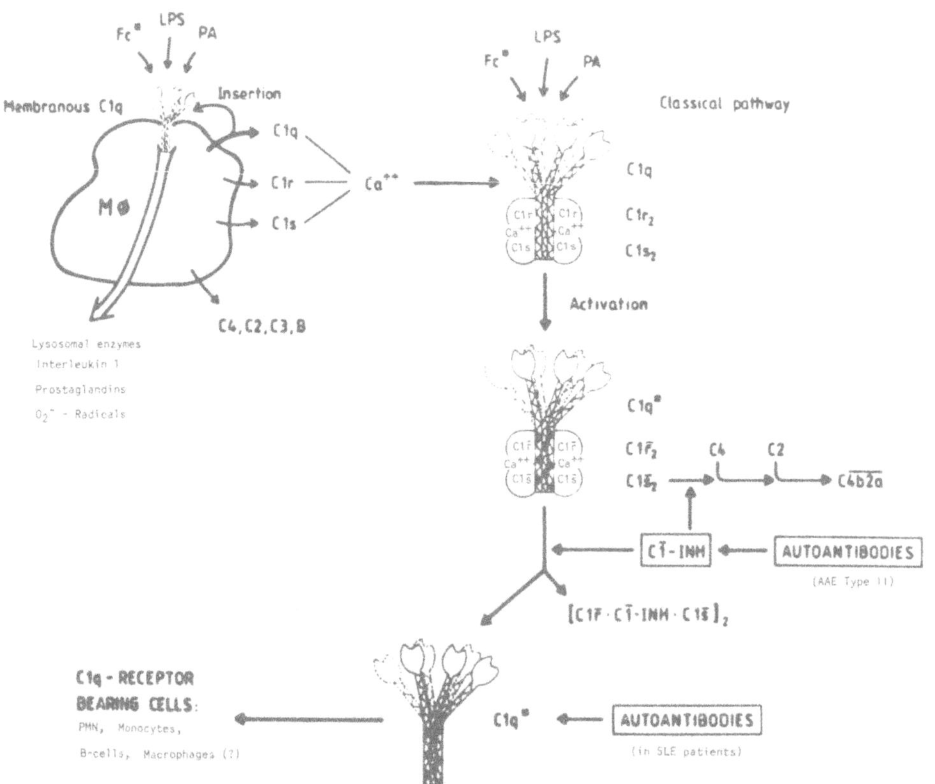

Fig 9. Schematic diagram of the biological role of C1q in the fluid phase as part of the classical complement pathway and of endogenous macrophage membrane-associated C1q. Both C1q forms interact directly with Fc of immunoglobulins, LPS of gram negative bacteria and polyanionic molecules (PA). All three C1q binding structures induce activation of the classical complement cascade as well as activation of macrophages.

REFERENCES

1. Aaskov, J. G. and Halliday, W. J., 1971, Requirement for lymphocyte-macrophage interaction in the response of mouse spleen cultures to pneumococcae polysaccharide. Cell Immunol. 2: 335.

2. Aderem, A. A., Cohen, D. S., Wright, S. D. and Cohn, Z. A., 1986, Bacterial lipopolysaccharides prime macrophages for enhanced release of arachidonic acid metabolites. J. Exp. Med. 164: 165.

3. Allison, A. C. and Davis, P., 1975, Increased biochemical and biological activities of mononuclear phagocytes exposed to various stimuli, with special reference to secretion of lysosomal enzymes, in: "Mononuclear phagocytes in immunity, infection and pathology", R. van Furth, ed., Blackwell Scientific Publications, Oxford, p. 487.

4. Ando, M., Suga, M., Sugimoto, M. and Tokuomi, H., 1979, Superoxide production in pulmonary alveolar macrophages and killing of BCG by the super-oxide-generating system with or without catalase. Infect. Immunol. 24: 404.

5. Babior, B. M., 1978, Oxygen-dependent microbial killing by phagocytes. N. Engl. J. Med. 298: 659-668.

6. Berkel, I. A., Loos, M., Sanal, O., Mauff, G., Gungen, Y., Ors, V., Ersoy, F. and Yegin, O., 1979, Clinical and immunological studies in a case of selective complement Clq deficiency. Clin. Exp. Immunol. 38: 52-63.

7. Bjornson, A. B. and Bjornson, H. W., 1977, Activation of complement by opportunist pathogens and chemotypes of Salmonella minnesota. Infect. Immun. 16: 748-753.

8. Bredt, W., Wellek, B., Brunner, H. and Loos, M., 1977, Studies on the interaction between myoplasma pneumoniae and the first component of complement. Infect. Immun. 15: 7-12.

9. Buchner, H., 1889, Uber die bakterientötende Wirkung des zellfreien Blutserums. Zentralbl. Bakteriol. 5: 817-823.

10. Burger, R., 1988, Complement biosynthesis: Factors of the alterna- tive pathway, in: "The Complement System," K. Rother and G. O. Till, eds., Springer Verlag, Heidelberg, p. 70-80.

11. Clas, F. and Loos, M., 1981, Antibody-independent binding of the first component of complement (C1) and its subcomponent Clq to the S- and R-forms of Salmonella minnesota. Infect. Immun. 31: 1138-1144.

12. Cole, F. S. and Colten, H. R., 1988, Complement biosynthesis: Factors of the classical pathway, in: "The Complement System," K. Rother and G. O. Till, eds., Springer Verlag, Heidelberg, p. 44-70.

13. Euteneuer, B., Störkel, S. and Loos, M., 1986, Contributions of Clq, bacterial lipopolysaccharide and porins during attachment and ingestion phases of phagocytosis by murine macrophages. Infect. Immun. 51: 807-815.

14. Fishman, W. H., Kato, K., Antiss, C. L. and Green, S., 1967, Human serum β-glucuronidase; its measurement and some of its properties. Clin. Chim. Acta. 15: 435.

15. Friedberg, D. and Shilo, M., 1970, Role of cell wall structure of Salmonella in the interaction with phagocytes. Infect. Immun. 2: 279.

16. Galanos, C., Lüderitz, O., Rietschel, E. T. and Westphal, O., 1977, Newer aspects of the chemistry and the biology of bacterial lipopolysaccharides with special reference to their lipid A component, in: "Biochemistry of lipids II", T. W. Goodwin, ed., University Park Press, Baltimore, 14: 239-335.

17. Gery, I., Gershon, R. K. and Waksman, B. H., 1972, Potentiation of the T-lymphocyte response to mitogens. 1. The responding cell. J. Exp. Med. 136: 128.

18. Gewurz, H., Shin, H. S. and Mergenhagen, S. E., 1968, Interactions of the complement sytem with endotoxic lipopolysaccharide: consumption of each of six terminal complement components. J. Exp. Med. 128: 1049-1057.

19. Heinz, H.-P., Dlugonska, H., Rüde, E. and Loos, M., 1984, Monoclonal anti-mouse macrophage antibodies recognize the globular portions of Clq, a subcomponent of the first component of complement. J. Immunol. 133: 400-404.

20. Hirsch, J. G. and Cohn, Z. A., 1960, Degranulation of polymorphonuclear phagocytes following phagocytosis of microorganisms. J. Exp. Med. 112: 1005-1014.

21. Johnston, R. B., 1978, Oxygen metabolism and the microbicidal activity of macrophages. Fed. Prod. 37: 2759-2764.

22. Johnston, R. B., Klemperer, M., Alper, C. A. and Rosen, R. S., 1969, The enhancement of bacterial phagocytosis by serum. The role of complement components and two cofactors. J. Exp. Med. 129: 1275-1290.

23. Johnston, R. B., Godzik, C. A. and Cohn, Z. A., 1978, Increased superoxide anion production by immunologically activated and chemically elicited macrophages. J. Exp. Med. 148: 115.

24. Kolb, W. B. and Müller-Eberhard, H. J., 1975, The membrane attack mechanism of complement isolation and subunit composition of the C5b-9 complex. J. Exp. Med. 141: 724-735.

25. Loos, M., 1982, Antibody-independent activation of Cl, the first component of complement. Ann. Immunol. (Inst. Pasteur) 133C: 165-179.

26. Loos, M., 1983, Biosynthesis of the collagen-like Clq molecule and its receptor functions for Fc and polyanionic molecules on macrophages. Curr. Top. Microbiol. Immunol. 102: 1-56.

27. Loos, M., Müller, W., Boltz-Nitulescu, G. and Förster, O., 1980, Evidence that Clq, a subcomponent of the first component of complement is an Fc-receptor of peritoneal and alveolar macrophages. Immunobiol. 157: 54.

28. Loos, M., Wellek, B., Thesen, R. and Opferkuch, W., 1978, Antibody-independent interaction of the first component of complement with gram-negative bacteria. Infect. Immun. 22: 5-9.

29. Lowrie, D. B., Aber, V. R. and Carrol, M. E. W., 1979, Division and

death rates of Salmonella typhimurium inside macrophages. Use of penicillin as a probe. J. Gen. Microbiol. 110: 409.

30. Martin, H., Heinz, H.-P., Reske, K. and Loos, M., 1987, Macrophage C1q: Characterization of a membrane form of C1q and of multimers of C1q subunits. J. Immunol. 138: 3863.

31. Müller, W., Hanauske-Abel, H. and Loos, M., 1978, Biosynthesis of the first component of complement by human and guinea pig peritoneal macrophages. Evidence for an independent production of the C1 subunits. J. Immunol. 121: 1578.

32. Muschel, L.-H. and Larsen, L. L., 1970, The sensitivity of smooth and rough gram-negative bacteria to the immune bactericidal reaction. Proc. Soc. Exp. Biol. Med. 133: 345-348.

33. Nathan, C. F. and Root, R. K., 1977, Hydrogen peroxide release from mouse peritoneal macrophages: Dependence on sequential activation and triggering. J. Exp. Med. 146: 1648.

34. Pantalone, R. and Page, R. L., 1977, Enzyme production and secretion by lymphokine activated macrophages. J. Reticuloendothel. Soc. 21: 343.

35. Rapp, H. J. and Borsos, T., 1970, Molecular basis of complement action. Appleton-Century-Crofts, New York.

36. Root, R. K., Ellman, L. and Frank, M. M., 1972, Bactericidal and opsonic properties of C4-deficient guinea pig serum. J. Immunol. 109: 477-486.

37. Rowley, D., 1968, Sensitivity of rough gram-negative bacteria to the bactericidal action of serum. J. Bacteriol. 95: 1647-1650.

38. Schnyder, J. and Baggiolini, M., 1978, Secretion of lysosomal hydrolases by stimulated and non-stimulated macrophages. J. Exp. Med. 148: 435.

39. Schnyder, J. and Baggiolini, M., 1978, Role of phagocytosis in the activation of macrophages. J. Exp. Med. 148: 1449.

40. Smith, K. A., Lachman, L. B. and Oppenheim, J. J., 1980, The functional relationship of the interleukins. J. Exp. Med. 151: 1551.

41. Stahelin, H., Suter, E. and Karnovsky, M. L., 1956, Studies on the interaction between phagocytes and tubercle bacilli I. Observations on the metabolism of guinea pig leukocytes and the influence of phagocytosis. J. Exp. Med. 104: 121.

42. Stossel. T. P., 1975, Phagocytosis: recognition and ingestion. Semin. Hematol. 12: 83-116.

43. Yagawa, K., Kaku, M., Ichinose, Y., Nagao, S., Tanaka, A., Aida, Y. and Tomoda, A., 1985, Down-regulation of Fc-receptor expression in guinea pig peritoneal exudate macrophages by muramyl dipeptide or lipopolysaccharide. J. Immunol. 134: 3705.

FURTHER CHARACTERIZATION OF MONOCLONAL ANTIBODIES TO LIPOPOLYSACCHARIDE OF SALMONELLA MINNESOTA STRAIN R595

B. J. Appelmelk[1], J. Cohen[3], A. Silva[3], A. M. J. J. Verweij-van Vught[1], H. Brade[4], J. J. Maaskant[1], W. F. Schouten[1], O. Mol[1], A. Honing[1], L. G. Thijs[2], and D. M. MacLaren[1]

[1]Department of Medical Microbiology and [2]Medical Intensive Care Unit, Vrije Universiteit, Amsterdam, The Netherlands
[3]Infectious Diseases Unit, Royal Postgraduate Medical School, Hammersmith Hospital, London, U.K.
[4]Forschungsinstitut Borstel, Borstel, FRG

INTRODUCTION

It is well recognized that neutralization of endotoxin (lipopolysaccharide, LPS) by means of antibodies, could be of value in reducing the high mortality due to Gram-negative sepsis and septic shock. Of particular interest would be the availability of a single antiserum (or: monoclonal antibody), effective against the three bacterial species which are most often implicated, i.e., **Escherichia coli, Klebsiella pneumoniae,** and **Pseudomonas aeruginosa.** A polyclonal antiserum, raised against a rough bacterial mutant of **E. coli** (strain J5) was found to have such cross-protective abilities, and to significantly reduce mortality in human septic shock (21). An intrinsic problem in the use of polyclonal antisera is the difficulty in knowing to which epitope(s) cross-protective antibodies is (are) directed. To answer this question monoclonal antibodies (mAbs) to the (LPS) core (and: lipid A) region have been prepared and tested for protection. The philosophy is that, since the LPS core region and the toxic lipid A part of the major Gram-negative species contain common structural elements, this core-lipid A part would be the ideal candidate for evoking cross-reactive monoclonal antibodies with LPS-neutralizing abilities. Indeed, the preparation of such cross-protective mAbs has been reported by at least two research groups (8, 19).

We have prepared monoclonal antibodies directed at LPS from **S. minnesota** R595 (3). The structure of R595 LPS has been determined recently (17): this very simple LPS consists of an α-2.4-linked KDO-KDO disaccharide (KDO: 3-deoxy-D-**manno**-octulosonic acid), which in turn is α-ketosidically linked to the 6' OH of the non-reducing glucosamine of lipid A. In addition to these structural data, KDO-containing synthetic substructures of R595 LPS have been prepared (10, 14). Consequently, the tools are available to determine the exact epitope specificities of anti-R595 LPS mAbs, which is important for understanding the biological effects of such Mabs. The anti-R595 LPS Mabs mentioned above have been tested for their aiblity to neutralize homologous endotoxin (4): ascites was mixed with R595 LPS and injected into actinomycin D-treated mice. Some mAbs were found to be protective (up to a 90 fold increase in LD_{50} was observed), while others were without effect. No correlation was found between ability to neutralize and (sub)class and approximate

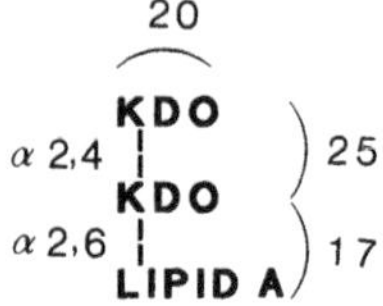

Fig 1. Epitope-specificities of three monoclonal antibodies directed at lipopolysaccharide of **Salmonella minnesota** strain R595.

affinity; moreover, some protective Mabs were very low titered, while some non-protective ones were highly titered. In other words protective clones did not seem to possess a single, common property. As noted above, it is very likely that the epitope specificity is important with regard to the biological effect of anti-core Mabs. For some of the clones, the exact binding site has been determined (Fig 1): the binding site of clone 17 (protective) involves parts of KDO and lipid A (manuscript in preparation); clone 20 (protective) binds to an epitope involving the lipid A-distal KDO monosaccharide; clone 25 (non-protective) is specific for α -2.4-linked KDO-KDO disaccharide (5), i.e., an epitope localized between that of clone 17 and that of clone 20. It is beyond dispute that the protective clones 17 and 20 do not have the common property of binding to the same epitope. Even more, 17 and 20 recognize epitopes which do not even seem to be adjacent, i.e., the epitopes of these Mabs are localized very near to (clone 17) or very far from (clone 20) the lipid A part. In fact, these epitopes seem to be interspersed by the non-protective one recognized by clone 25. However, these observations are based on a two-dimensional structural formula of R595 LPS (17), and thus the three dimensional conformation of this LPS is not taken into account. It could be that the binding sites of clones 17 and 20 are spatially close, due to the three-dimensional conformation of R595 LPS. This question is addressed in this paper by the use of the cyclic peptide antibiotic polymyxin B (PMB) as an independent probe for the three-dimensional structure of R595 LPS. The background of our experimental set-up was: a) that PMB binds to the lipid A-KDO region (12, 13) and b) that PMB has LPS neutralizing abilities in a variety of animal models (16), including the acinomycin D model which we have used (see Results).

In this paper we test the hypothesis that, due to conformational effects, the epitopes of the protective clones 17 and 20 are spatially close to the PMB binding site. In addition we investigate the ability of the anti-R595 LPS clones to cross-react with heat-killed cells and isolated LPS of **E. coli, K. pneumoniae** and **P. aeruginosa**. Finally, the ability of one of the Mabs (clone 20) to protect against lethal sepsis is investigated.

MATERIALS AND METHODS

Monoclonal Antibodies

Monoclonal antibodies to R595 LPS have been described before (3-5). They were coded as nos. 14-29. They were obtained by immunization of Balb/c mice with a variety of R595 vaccines: heat- and acetone-killed cells; live bacteria; boiled cells treated with alkali. Long as well as short duration vaccination protocols were followed. Selection of clones after fusion (using conventional procedures) was based on isotype and on reactivity in ELISA (1) with LPS from various rough strains of **S. minnesota** (strains R595, R7, R5, R345 and R60, i.e., chemotypes Re to Ra). Bovine serum albumin (BSA)-complexed LPS were used as coating antigens; horseradish peroxidase (HRP) labeled conjugates were used throughout.

Effect of Polymyxin B on R595 LPS Lethality

R595 LPS (List, Campbell, CA, USA), in doses of 1 and 10 ng/mouse) was mixed with 100 μg PMB (Pfizer, Brussels) and with 20 μg actinomycin D (Merck, Sharp and Dohme, Rahway, N.J. USA) and injected intravenously (i.v.) into 2 groups of 6 mice. In the control groups of mice, LPS plus actinomycin D only, was injected. LD_{50} figures were based on one-week-survival data.

Inhibition Studies with PMB

Culture supernatants from clones 17, 20, and 25 were diluted such, that the specific optical density (OD 492), measured by ELISA, using R595 LPS-BSA coated wells, amounted to 1.5. BSA-coated wells served as controls for non-specific binding. The various individually diluted antibodies were then mixed with PMB in the concentration range of 3.1 μg/ml to 102.4 mg/ml PMB (in two-fold steps); mixing was followed by the usual ELISA procedure. The amount of competing PMB which resulted in 50% reduction of specific OD (i.e., OD 492 = 0.75 after subtraction of control value) was calculated from the inhibition curves obtained. This parameter was called the PMB inhibition index.

Cross-Reaction Studies

The ability of the clones to cross-react with heterologous LPS and bacteria was investigated in ELISA. The bacteria used were smooth strains of **E. coli** (serotype 0111:B4) and **P. aeruginosa** (both strains were kindly provided by Dr. E. J. Ziegler, San Diego, CA, USA) as well as a clinical isolate of **K. pneumoniae** (kindly supplied by Dr. N. T. Rapson, Wellcome Research Laboratories, Beckenham, U.K.). Approximately 5 x 10^7 cells per well of heat-killed (1 hr at 100^oC) bacteria in phosphate-buffered saline, pH 7.5, (PBS) were used for coating. Smooth form LPS of **E. coli, P. aeruginosa** and **K. pneumoniae** were obtained from List Biological Laboratories (Campbell, USA) and 0.1 μg LPS, dissolved in 100 μl 0.01 M carbonate buffer, pH 9.6, was applied per well. Appropriately coated wells without Mab, but with conjugate, served as background controls. Clone 20 was further investigated for binding to 3 rough bacterial strains: **S. minnesota** R595; **P. aeruginosa** strain 18S (provided by Dr. T. L. Pitt, Central Public Health Laboratory Service, London, U.K.). This strain has been described before (15); **K. pneumoniae** strain LEN-113 (obtained from Dr. Kato, Nagoya University, Nagoya, Japan). LPS of this strain has a structure very similar to LPS of the already described strain LEN-111 03^-K1^- (9). Lastly, the reactivity of clone 20 to bi-phosphoryl lipid A of **E. coli** F515 was determined, and compared with reactivity to LPS from strain R595.

Cross-protection Experiments

The ability of clone 20 to protect against lethal sepsis was investigated in a variety of animal models:

1) The mucin-hemoglobin (Mu/Hb) model (2, 11). The strains of **E. coli** 0111:B4, **K. pneumoniae** and **P. aeruginosa** described above were used for challenge. In the Mu/Hb model, the LD_{50} obtained with a particular strain depends on the actual amount of Mu/Hb which is intraperitoneally (i.p.) co-injected with the bacteria; thus, the LD_{50} can be manipulated at will, from as high as 10^7 colony forming units (CFU), to as low as a single bacterial cell. Mucin from procine stomach (type II) was purchased from Sigma (St. Louis, MO, USA); dried bovine hemoglobin was obtained from BBL (Cockeysville, MD, USA). For **E. coli** 0111:B4, 70 mg Mu and 15 mg Hb was injected into each mouse; for **K. pneumoniae:** 70 mg Mu and 25 mg Hb; for **P. aeruginosa:** 70 mg Mu and 10 mg Hb. Challenge doses of approximately 0.1, 1.0, 10 and 100 CFU were injected into 4 groups of 6 Swiss-albino mice. In all cases, 1 ml containing

the appropriate amounts of Mu/Hb and bacteria was injected. In this model most of the deaths occur within 36 hr after challenge and no more occur after one week, which was taken as the end-point. For immunoprotection experiments, 0.3 ml ascites of clone 20 was given i.v. 3 hr before challenge. The control mice received 0.3 ml pyrogen-free PBS.

2) Prevention of lethal sepsis by treatment of mice with a combination of antibody and gentamicin (18). This model, by including therapy with antibiotics, may mimic more closely than the Mu/Hb model, in the situation of human sepsis. In addition, a potential advantage with regard to demonstrating protection, is the extra chance given to the antibody to neutralize the endotoxin, liberated by antibiotic activity. Two different forms of this model were used:

a) For **E. coli** and **P. aeruginosa** the protection experiments were as follows: 0.2 ml of hybridoma culture supernatant of clone 20 (= 10 μg Mab) was injected i.v., 1.5 hr before challenge. Control mice received 0.2 ml of pyrogen-free saline or culture medium lacking Mab. No antibiotics were present in medium or supernatant. The endotoxin content of the supernatant was < 50 pg/ml as determined by a chromogenous LAL assay described previously (7). The bacterial inocula were 3×10^8 for **E. coli** and 0.7×10^8 for **P. aeruginosa.** The bacteria were injected i.v. Gentamicin was given in a dose of 2 mg/kg/day in two daily i.v. injections of 0.2 ml, starting 2 hr after challenge.

b) For protection experiments with **K. pneumoniae**, mice were made neutropenic by injecting 300 mg/kg cyclophosphamide, i.v., 48 and 24 hr before challenge with 0.3×10^9 CFU. Otherwise the model was the same as described above. It was essential to use cyclophosphamide, since in non-neutropenic mice irreproducible lethality figures were obtained when **K. pneumoniae** was used for challenge.

RESULTS

Effect of Polymyxin B on R595 LPS Induced Endotoxic Lethality

Incubation of R595 LPS with 100 μg PMB had a profound effect on the number of endotoxic deaths. When the mixture was injected into actinomycin D-sensitized mice, the LD_{50} for R595 LPS incubated with saline was 1 ng; for the PMB-treated R595 LPS an LD_{50} of > 21.6 ng was obtained. In the PMB treated groups, 11/12 mice survived, in the control group only 3/12 ($p < 0.005$).

In Vitro Inhibition Studies with Polymyxin B

The ability of PMB to compete **in vitro** with monoclonal antibodies (clones 17, 20 and 25) for binding to R595 LPS is shown in Table 1 and is expressed as the PMB index. In this Table, the ability of Mabs to protect mice in vivo against R595 LPS (data taken ref. 4) is expressed as the protection factor (the increase in LD_{50} in mice given Mab compared to mice which had received saline). Table 1 shows that the three clones tested were all sensitive to inhibition by PMB, although the extent to which this occurred varied substantially; while binding of clone 17 was diminished to 50% by 3.1 μg/ml PMB clone 20 required > 3.2 mg/ml, i.e., a 1000-fold difference; clone 25 required an intermediate amount. Clearly, no correlation is present between the ability to protect and the PMB index.

Cross-reactivity Studies

The ability of anti-R595 to cross-react with heterologous bacteria and

Table 1. Comparison between the ability of monoclonal antibodies directed at LPS of **Salmonella minnesota** strain R595 to protect against LPS (protection factor) and their competitive inhibition by polymyxin B (PMB index).

Clone number	Protection factor	PMB index
17	91#	3.1 μg/ml
20	46#	> 3.2 mg/ml
25	4.7**	100 μg/ml

#Clones 17 and 20 are protective ($p < 0.001$).
**Clone 25 is not protective ($p < 0.05$).

LPS is shown in Table 2. Clones 17 and 22 did not cross react at all; clones 15, 16, 21, 25, 26, 27 and 29 exhibited a very limited degree of cross-reactivity: while some binding could be demonstrated with selected antigens, no binding was observed with others. Clone 19 exhibited a low binding to all antigens tested. Clones 14, 20 and 28 were the "best" cross-reactive clones. Clone 20 is of particular interest, as it is the only cross-reactive clone which was also protective in the actinomycin D model (4).

When tested by ELISA for reactivity with R595 LPS and biphosphoryl lipid A, the results shown in Table 3 were obtained. It is evident that the responses to these two antigens were virtually identical.

Table 2. Cross-reactivity* of anti-R595 LPS monoclonal antibodies

Clone no.	LPS			Bacteria		
	E. coli	**Klebsiella**	**Pseudomonas**	**E. coli**	**Klebsiella**	**Pseudomonas**
14	0.2	1.2	0.2	0.7	0.9	0.8
15	0.1	0	0	0	0	0.2
16	0.1	0.1	0.1	0	0	0.1
17	0	0	0	0	0	0
19	0.2	0.1	0.2	0.1	0.2	0.1
20	0.1	0.9	0.1	0.3	0.8	0.6
21	0	0.1	0	0	0	0
22	0	0	0	0	0	0
25	0.1	0.1	0	0	0	0.1
26	0.1	0	0.1	0	0	0.2
27	0.2	0.1	0	0	0	0
28	0.2	0.1	0.2	0.3	0.2	0.3
29	0.1	0	0.3	0	0	0.2

*Cross-reactivity is expressed as optical density at 492 nm.

Table 3. Ability of clone 20 to react* with heat-killed rough bacterial cells, R595 LPS and lipid A

Dilution of antibody	Antigen tested: LPS		Heat-killed bacterial cells**		
	lipid A	R595 LPS	R595	LEN-113	18S
1/10	2	2	1.5	2.0	1.9
1/20	1.9	1.9	1.0	1.7	1.5
1/40	1.1	1.3	0.7	1.0	1.1
1/80	0.7	0.7	0.5	0.5	0.7
1/160	0.5	0.5	0.3	0.4	0.4
1/1280	0.1	0.2	0.2	0.2	0.2

*The results are expressed as optical densities, measured at 492 nm.
R595 = **Salmonella minnesota rough strain R595 (Re-chemotype); LEN-113 and 18S are rough strains of **Klebsiella pneumoniae** and **Pseudomonas aeruginosa**, respectively.

The reaction of clone 20 to three rough bacterial strains is also indicated in Table 3. The results obtained with the three strains were very much alike.

Cross-protection Experiments

Based on the results obtained above, clone 20 was selected for protection studies with live bacteria as a challenge. The results obtained in the mucin-hemoglobin model are shown in Table 4. No protective effect could be demonstrated.

Table 4. Cross-protection experiments with anti-core Mab clone 20 in the mucin-hemoglobin lethal sepsis model.

Challenge organism		Approximate challenge dose (CFU): 0.1	1	10	100
		No. deaths/no. mice challenged			
Escherichia coli					
	Saline	0/12	7/12	10/12	11/12
	Clone 20	0/12	5/12	6/12	12/12
Klebsiella pneumoniae					
	Saline	1/6	2/6	5/6	6/6
	Clone 20	0/6	3/6	4/6	6/6
Pseudomonas aeruginosa					
	Saline	1/6	1/6	6/6	6/6
	Clone 20	0/6	4/6	6/6	6/6

Table 5. Effect of clone 20 on lethal sepsis due to **Escherichia coli** in gentamicin treated mice.

No. of Experiments	Total no. of mice	Mortality (%)	
		24 hr	48 hr*
Mab group: 6	36	0	0
Controls : 6	36	42	72

*No deaths occurred after 48 hr.

Additionally, clone 20 was tested in combination with gentamicin treatment of mice. The results obtained in this model are shown in Tables 5-7. It is clear that clone 20 was effective against challenge with **E. coli** 0111:B4 (Table 5). Furthermore, it seemed to delay death following challenge with **P. aeruginosa** (Table 6). Clone 20 had no effect in the neutropenic mouse model following challenge with **K. pneumoniae** (Table 7).

DISCUSSION

Firstly, in this paper it is clearly shown that PMB when mixed with R595 LPS leads to a decreased number of endotoxic deaths in actinomycin-D sensitized mice. This model was used by us before (4), when we demonstrated neutralization of R595 LPS by specific Mabs.

This positive outcome led us to suggest that a common mechanism could underlie protection mediated by PMB and Mabs: i.e., that the protective clones 17 and 20 possessed the common property of binding at, or close to the PMB binding site, while clone 25 would bind further away. When the epitopes recognized by these three clones are drawn into the (schematic) structural formula of R595 LPS (Fig 1), this hypothesis seems unlikely. However, this takes no account of possible conformational effects, which could bring the binding sites of clones 17 and 20 close to each other, as well as close to the PMB binding site. This was tested by means of **in vitro** inhibition studies in which increasing amounts of PMB were allowed to compete with Mab for binding to R595 LPS coated on ELISA plates. Our results (Table 1) show that only micrograms of PMB were required to compete effectively with clone 17, while milligrams were required in the case of clone 20. Intermediate amounts were required in the case of clone 25. This is exactly the same

Table 6. Effect of clone 20 on lethal sepsis due to **Pseudomonas aeruginosa** in gentamicin treated mice.

No. of Experiments	Total no. of mice	Mortality (%)				
		Day 1	Day 2	Day 3	Day 4	Day 5*
Mab group: 5	30	3	33	47	47	47
Controls : 5	30	23	47	60	63	63

*No deaths occurred after 5 days

Table 7. Effect of clone 20 on lethal sepsis due to **Klebsiella pneumoniae** in gentamicin treated, neutropenic mice.

No. of Experiments		Total no. of mice	Mortality (%)				
			Day 1	Day 2	Day 3	Day 4	Day 5*
Mab group:	2	12	0	50	50	83	92
Controls :	2	12	0	33	50	92	92

*No deaths occurred after day 5.

order as predicted from two-dimensional data (Fig 1). It is clear that no correlation exists between protection factor and PMB inhibition index.

Our results suggest:

a) That the two-dimensional structure of the R595 LPS molecule is closely mimicking its conformation in space.

b) that we have no evidence in favor of our hypothesis that protective epitopes have the common property of being spatially close. And thus, despite our detailed knowledge of several epitope-specificities, at present we are unable to understand the effect - or lack of effect - of anti-R595 LPS Mabs on LPS endotoxicity.

c) that the PMB inhibition index may be used to determine the approximate epitope localization of anti-core antibodies. A low index means binding close to the lipid A-core junction, a high one means binding further away. This assumption has been validated now by use of four other monoclonal antibodies with defined binding sites (not shown).

From the data shown in Table 2, it is clear that very little cross-reactivity of Mabs with heterologous smooth LPS or bacteria was observed. Only clones 14, 19, 20 and 28 bound to all antigens tested. Clones 14 and 20 bound somewhat better to heat-killed cells of smooth **E. coli** and **P. aeruginosa**, than to purified smooth LPS. However, the optical densities obtained were lower than when rough strain bacteria or rough LPS were used as coating antigen (not shown). Reactivity of clones 14 and 20 with **K. pneumoniae** was peculiar; firstly, LPS reacted better than bacteria, and secondly, the responses obtained were of the same order as reaction with rough bacteria/LPS (not shown). However, the reactions to other strains of **K. pneumoniae** were lower (not shown), which indicates that the particular **Klebsiella** described here, is unusual with regard to cross-reactivity. It could even be that strong reactivity to the **Klebsiella** tested here is not due to interaction with the core, but to cross-reaction with other, antigenically related structures.

The binding data shown in Table 2 can be interpreted in several ways: do they mean that, generally speaking, core structures in purified LPS are more concealed than in the case of heat-killed cells? Or, alternatively is the binding observed a result of nonspecific sticking of the clones to surfaces which are partly charged, and partly hydrophobic. In this regard, it is of interest that those clones which gave the highest optical densities in these experiments (i.e., clones 14, 20 and 28) were the only ones within this panel possessing the IgM isotype. It is known that IgM antibodies in particular, can bind "promiscuously" to a broad diversity of non-related antigens, including the plastic surface of ELISA plates. Such promiscuous binding is more likely to be explained by nonspecific interactions (stickiness) than by specific antigen/antibody interaction. What clearly is missing are procedures capable of discriminating between nonspecific binding to smooth LPS/bacteria and specific antigen/antibody interaction.

The following example shows how results based on ELISA data alone can be misleading. When clone 20 was allowed to react with R595 LPS and lipid A coated on ELISA plates the results presented in Table 3 were obtained. These results indicate that clone 20 is specific for an epitope present in free lipid A, as well as in covalently linked lipid A, i.e., R595 LPS. However, detailed studies using synthetic core and lipid A structures, in combination with passive hemolysis have demonstrated (5) unequivocally that clone 20 is specific for KDO, and not for lipid A. Binding in ELISA of clone 20 to lipid A, however strong it may be, is most likely due to nonspecific interaction and not to specific recognition of antigen. Consequently, the binding of clone 20 with cells of the three rough bacterial strains tested (Table 3), with smooth strains and LPS (Table 2) may be at least partly due to nonspecific interaction.

Despite our uncertainty with regard to interpreting our cross-reactivity data, we decided to test anti-R595 LPS Mabs in lethal sepsis models. The obvious choice for this purpose was clone 20. This clone was the only one within our panel which had been shown before to neutralize R595 LPS in the actinomycin D model (4), and which also demonstrated binding to heterologous bacteria. The decision to use the Mu/Hb model was based on earlier experiments (2) in which we had shown that a polyclonal antiserum, raised against the **Escherichia coli** rough strain J5, was protective in this model, and not in non-compromised mice. Our explanation was that, by immunocompromizing the mice, which resulted in very low LD_{50}s, the ratio of antibody to challenge is much higher than in the case of non-compromised animals, where only very high doses of bacteria have lethal effects.

Despite the extremely low LD_{50} (approximately 1 CFU/animal), and despite the injection of a considerable amount of Mab 20 (0.3 ml ascites) no improved survival was observed (Table 4). We can only speculate about these negative outcomes; the obvious two questions are: is this the "wrong" clone, i.e., is it ineffective at neutralizing LPS during sepsis, or is this the "wrong" animal model. With regard to the Mu/Hb model, it could be that by compromising the mice to such a severe degree, defense systems like phagocytosis or complement action are completely blocked, thus nullifying the protective effects of an antibody. We therefore decided to set-up an additional animal model, in which non- or less severely compromised animals were subjected to bacterial challenge. The chosen model, i.e., treatment with Mab plus gentamicin has the additional advantage of demonstrating potentially synergistic effects; killing is then mediated by the antibiotic, while the LPS thus liberated, could be neutralized by the Mab. According to this reasoning, the opsonic/bactericidal properties are less crucial in this model. Table 5 shows clearly the effectiveness of clone 20 following challenge with **E. coli**. Although hybridoma culture supernatant instead of fully purified antibody was used, it is very likely that the antibody itself was responsible for the protective effect: a) neither pyrogen-free saline, nor hybridoma growth medium without clone (not shown) had any protective effect, and b) the endotoxin levels in the preparation injected were very low, i.e., less than 10 pg of endotoxin was present in the injected antibody sample. The (virtual) absence of endotoxin antibody preparations is of utmost importance when **in vivo** immunoprotection experiments are done. Recently, it has been shown that the presence in antibody preparations of nanogram amounts of endotoxin could lead to a nonspecific increase in resistance to sepsis, thus giving the false impression that the antibody itself possessed protective properties (6, 20). The results obtained with the other two challenge strains illustrate the difficulty of extrapolating **in vitro** to **in vivo** results; some delay of death was observed when **P. aeruginosa** was injected while the Mab appeared ineffective in the **Klebsiella** model. From the binding data (Table 2), just the opposite would have been expected.

It would be of interest to increase the dose of Mab to see whether or not a decrease in final mortality can be obtained for **P. aeruginosa.** The total lack of effect on mortality due to **K. pneumoniae** might have several explanations: is the capsule hindering binding of the Mab to its target, i.e., the core, despite use of antibiotics? Is neutrophil function indispensable? Or alternatively, is the core structure so different that no recognition takes place?

SUMMARY

We have shown here that despite the use of monoclonal antibodies with well-defined epitope-specificities, and despite testing them in the most simple animal model available (i.e., mixing of homologous LPS with Mab prior to injection), we are not yet able to explain why some of the antibodies were effective and others not. For some of the clones (e.g., clone 20), an even better definition of binding sites is currently taking place in an attempt to obtain this understanding. We also do not yet understand why clone 20 was not effective in the mucin model, while using much lower amounts of injected antibody, and much higher challenge doses, this Mab was effective against **E. coli** in the gentamicin-treated mouse model. Very clear is, however, that in order to be protective in the latter model, Mabs are not required to be specific for lipid A.

In the future it will be essential to develop procedures which measure specific interaction between smooth LPS/bacteria and antibodies to the LPS core region. In addition, it will be of great help when the chemical structure of non-substituted, rough-form LPS, as occurring in smooth LPS preparations, would be defined. This applies also to O-substituted core molecules.

ACKNOWLEDGEMENTS

Part of the work was supported by the Praeventiefonds, The Hague, The Netherlands (J. J. M.), and the Wellcome Trust, London, U. K. (J. C.). We gratefully acknowledge the material support to J. C. and A. F. by Celltech Ltd., Slough, U. K. E. J. Ziegler and N. T. Rapson were so kind to provide bacterial strains.

REFERENCES

1. Appelmelk, B. J., Verweij-van Vught, A. M. J. J., MacLaren, D. M., and Thijs, L. G., 1985, An enzyme-linked immunosorbent assay (ELISA) for the measurement of antibodies to different parts of the Gram-negative lipopolysaccharede core region. J. Immunol. Meth. 82: 199.

2. Appelmelk, B. J., Verweij-van Vught, A. M. J. J., Maaskant, J. J., Schouten, W. F., Thijs, L. G., and MacLaren, D. M., 1986, Use of mucin and hemoglobin in experimental murine Gram-negative bacteremia enhances the immunoprotective action of antibodies reactive with the lipopolysaccharide core region. Antonie van Leeuwenhoek 52: 537.

3. Appelmelk, B. J., Verweij-van Vught, A. M. J. J., Maaskant, J. J., Schouten, W. F., Thijs, L. G., and MacLaren, D. M., 1987, Monoclonal antibodies detecting novel structures in the core region of **Salmonella minnesota** lipopolysaccharide. FEMS Microbiol. Lett. 40: 71.

4. Appelmelk, B. J., Verweij-van Vught, A. M. J. J., Brade, H., Maaskant, J. J., Schouten, W. F., Thijs, L. G., and MacLaren, D. M., 1988, Production, characterization and biological effects of monoclonal antibodies to different parts of the Gram-negative lipopolysaccharide core region, in: "Bacterial endotoxins: pathophysiological effects, clinical significance and pharmaceutical control," J. ten Cate, H. Buller, A. Sturk, and J. Levin, eds., Alan R. Liss, Inc., New York (in press).

5. Brade, L., Kosma, P., Appelmelk, B. J., Paulsen, H., and Brade, H., 1987, Use of synthetic antigens to determine the epitope specificities of monoclonal antibodies against the 3-deoxy-D-**manno**-octulosonate region of bacterial lipopolysaccharide. Infect. Immun. 55: 462.

6. Chong, K-T., and Huston, M., 1987, Implications of endotoxin contamination in the evaluation of antibodies to lipopolysaccharides in a murine model of gram-negative sepsis. J. Infect. Dis. 156: 713.

7. Cohen, J., and McConnell, J. S., 1984, Observations on the measurement and evaluation of endotoxemia by a quantitative **Limulus** lysate microassay. J. Infect. Dis. 150: 916.

8. Dunn, D. L., Ewald, D. C., Chandan, N., and Cerra, F. B., 1986, Immunotherapy of Gram-negative sepsis, A single murine monoclonal antibody provides cross-general protection. Arch. Surg. 121: 58.

9. Kato, N., Ohta, M., Kido, N., Ito, H., Naito, S., and Kuno, T., 1986, Stability of the nexagonal lattice structure formed by an R-form lipopolysaccharide of **Klebsiella**: decrease in the stability by electrodialysis and recovery by addition of the magnesium. Microbiol. Immunol. 30: 13.

10. Kosma, P., Gass, J., Schulz, G., Christian, R., and Unger, F. M., 1987, Artifical antigens: synthesis of polyacrylamide copolymers containing 3-deoxy-D-**manno**-2-octulopyranosylono (KDO) residues. Carbohydr. Res. 167: 39.

11. Marks, M. I., Ziegler, E. J., Douglas, H., Corbeil, L. B., and Braude, A. I., 1982, Induction of immunity against lethal **Haemophilus influenzae** type b infection by **Escherichia coli** core lipopolysaccharide. J. Clin. Invest. 69: 742.

12. Moore, R. W., Bates, N. C., Hancock, R. E. W., 1986, Interaction of polycationic antibiotics with **Pseudomonas aeruginosa** lipopolysaccharide and lipid A studied by using dansylpolymyxin. Antimicrob. Agents Chemother. 29: 496.

13. Morrison, D. C., Jacobs, D. M., 1976, Binding of Polymyxin B to the lipid A portion of bacterial lipopolysaccharides. Immunochemistry 813: 13.

14. Paulsen, H., and Schuller, M., 1987, Synthesis of KDO-containing lipid A analogues. Liebigs Ann. Chem. 1987: 247.

15. Pitt. T. L., MacDougal, J., Penketh, A. R. L., and Cooke, E. M., 1986, Polyagglutinating and non-typable strains of **Pseudomonas aeruginosa** in cystic fibrosis. J. Med. Microbiol. 21: 179.

16. Rifkind, D., 1967, Prevention by polymyxin B of endotoxin lethality in mice. J. Bacteriol. 93: 1463.

17. Tacken, A., Rietschel, E. T., and Brade, H., 1986, Methylation analysis of the heptose/3-deoxy-D-**manno**-2-octulosonic acid region (inner core) of lipopolysaccharide from **Salmonella minnesota** rough mutants. Carbonhydr. Res. 149: 279.

18. Trautmann, M., Muller-Leutloff, Y., Hofstaetter, T., Seiler, F. R., and Hahn, H., 1985, Experimental **Klebsiella** septicemia in mice: treatment with specific antibodies from the rabbit alone and in combination with the gentamicin. Infection 13: 37.

19. Teng, N. H., Kaplan, H. S., Hebert, J. M., Moore, C., Douglas, H., Wunderlich, A., and Braude, A. I., 1985, Protection against Gram-negative bacteremia and endotoxemia with human monoclonal IgM antibodies. Proc. Natl. Acad. Sci. USA 82: 1790.

20. Woods, J. P., Black, J. R., Barritt, D. S., Connell, T. D., and Cannon, J. G., 1987, Resistance to meningococcemia apparently conferred by anti-H8 monoclonal antibody is due to contaminating endotoxin and not to specific immunoprotection. Infect. Immun. 55: 1927.

21. Ziegler, E. J., McCuthan, J. A., Fierer, J., Glauser, M. P., Sadoff, J. C., Douglas, H., Braude, A. I., 1982, Treatment of Gram-negative bacteremia and shock with human antiserum to a mutant **Escherichia coli**. N. Engl. J. Med. 307: 1225.

SPECIFICITY AND FUNCTION OF MONOCLONAL ANTIBODIES REACTIVE WITH DISCRETE STRUCTURAL ELEMENTS OF BACTERIAL LIPOPOLYSACCHARIDE

M. Pollack, K. Oishi, J. Chia, M. Evans, G. Guelde and N. Koles

Department of Medicine, Uniformed Services University
F. Edward Hébert School of Medicine
Bethesda, Maryland, U.S.A.

ABSTRACT

We examined the binding and functional activities of monoclonal antibodies (mAbs) reactive with different structural elements of **Escherichia coli** and **Salmonella minnesota** LPS. O-side chain-reactive mAbs were highly specific for homologous, smooth LPS, bound avidly to intact bacteria, mediated complement-dependent bactericidal and/or opsonic activity, and protected against live, homologous IP challenges in mice. Core- and lipid A-specific mAbs, on the other hand, were more cross-reactive, although this cross-reactivity was severely restricted by the relative inaccessability of epitopes in the core/lipid A region. This was reflected in the general inability of these mAbs to react with isolated smooth LPS or wild type bacteria, or to mediate bactericidal or opsonic functions. No LPS-reactive mAbs, regardless of molecular specificity, was able to block LPS- or lipid A-induced TNF production by RAW 264.7 macrophages, thus raising doubts concerning the putative endotoxin-neutralizing properties of mAbs reactive with the core/lipid A complex.

Bacterial lipopolysaccharides (LPS) exhibit a complex identity. They represent an essential structural element of the outer membrane of all Gram-negative bacteria (7); they are toxins (5); they mediate a variety of immunomodulatory activities; and they are important bacterial surface antigens (2). In general, LPS macromolecules consist of three genetically, biochemically, and antigenetically distinct regions or domains: the O-side chain, core oligosaccharide, and lipid A moiety (15). Of these three regions, the O-side chain is the most phylogenetically diverse. It also represents the most antigenetically exposed element on isolated or cell-associated, native LPS. The core and lipid A structures, in contrast, are relatively conserved among different bacteria and are less accessible to antibody attack by virtue of overlying sugars contained in the O-side chain or outer core (8).

In this study, we investigated selected functional activities of monoclonal antibodies (mAbs) specific for different epitopes within the three major structural domains of **Escherichia coli** and **Salmonella minnesota** LPS. The possible endotoxin-neutralizing and antibacterial properties of these mAbs were our particular focus.

MATERIALS AND METHODS

LPS and lipid A preparations are described elsewhere (10). Murine mAbs were prepared as previously described (9). Binding of mAbs to isolated LPS or lipid A was evaluated by enzyme-linked immunosorbent assay (ELISA) and by passive hemolysis assay (PHA) (9). Protection experiments were performed in 6 week old, outbred Swiss-Webster mice. Groups of 40 mice were injected i.v. with 1 mg of mAb contained in 0.2 ml of clarified ascites fluid appropriately diluted with normal saline. Within one hour, the mice were challenged i.p. with approximately 5 LD_{50}'s of bacteria suspended in normal saline containing 5% hog gastric mucin. Cumulative mortality was recorded after 5 days and compared by Chi square test with that obtained in mice that received a "nonsense" mAb (#13-17) employed as a negative control. Homologous rabbit antiserum raised against the LPS produced by each challenge strain was administered in conjunction with each live challenge.

Monoclonal antibody binding to intact bacteria was assessed by flow cytometry. Washed, log phase bacteria were incubated at $4^{o}C$ for 30 min with approximately 100 µg/ml of mAb, washed, reincubated under the same conditions with fluorescein isothiocyanate-conjugated monoclonal rat anti-mouse kappa light chain antibody, washed again, and fixed with 1% paraformaldehyde. The bacteria were analyzed using a FACS II flow cytometer (Becton-Dickinson) with an argon ion laser set at 500 mW of power.

Murine RAW 264.7 macrophages were maintained as a monolayer in DMEM (Hazleton Research Products, Inc., St. Leneka, KS) supplemented with 5% fetal calf serum, glutamine, penicillin and streptomycin. Eighteen hours prior to assay, the macrophages were harvested by scraping, washed, counted, and seeded onto 96-well microculture plates at a density of 1 x 10^{6} cells per well. After overnight incubation, the monolayers were washed with medium and incubated at $37^{o}C$ for 4 hr with a mixture of LPS (or lipid A) and mAb, which had been preincubated together at $37^{o}C$ for 30 min. Tumor necrosis factor (TNF) bioactivity was determined in a cytotoxicity assay employing actinomycin D-sensitized murine L-929 fibroblasts (12). Forty thousand L cells, suspended in 100 ul of medium, were seeded into the wells of a 96-well microculture plate and incubated overnight. Serially diluted TNF-containing macrophage supernatants, recombinant murine TNF standard, and media controls were added in 50 ul aliquots to L cell monolayers in the presence of 2 µg/ml of actinomycin D. After 18 hr incubation at $37^{o}C$, the plates were washed, stained with 0.2% crystal violet, and optical density measured spectrophotometrically at 550 nM. One unit of TNF bioactivity was defined as the reciprocal supernatant titer producing 50% cytolysis, and corresponded to approximately 1-10 pg of recombinant murine TNF.

Complement-mediated bactericidal activity of mAbs was determined by incubating appropriate dilutions of mAb, at $37^{o}C$ for 30 min, with 2 x 10^{7} bacteria in 1 ml of veronal-buffered saline containing 0.1% gelatin, 0.3 mM $CaCl_2$, and 2.0 mM $MgCl_2$. The presensitized bacteria were then washed and incubated at $37^{o}C$ for 60 min in the presence of 10% normal human serum previously absorbed with heat-killed bacteria (10% AbsNHS). Samples were removed for quantitative culture and bacterial killing expressed as log 10 cfu/ml in samples containing heat-inactivated AbsNHS - log 10 cfu/ml in fresh AbsNHS.

The opsonic activity of mAbs was evaluated by determining the uptake of radiolabeled bacteria by human PMNs in the presence of complement. **E. coli** 0111:B4 bacteria were labeled by overnight growth in the presence of ^{3}H-N-acetyl-glucosamine (specific activity = 34.2 Ci/mmol) in MOPS medium containing 0.4% glucose and 0.1 mM galactose. Assay mixtures contained 0.1 ml of ^{3}H-labeled bacteria (2 x 10^{8} cfu/ml) presensitized with appropriate dilutions of mAb, 0.2 ml of 2.5% fresh (or heat-inactivated) AbsNHS, and 0.2 ml of

Ficoll-Hypaque separated human PMN's (5×10^6 cells per ml). Following incubation of reaction mixtures at 37°C for 60 min, with constant mixing, 200 µl aliquots were removed to two silicon-coated glass tubes and centrifuged for 10 min at 160 x g and 2,000 x g, respectively. Counts per minute determined on the pellet obtained at the higher centrifuge setting was considered as total radioactivity, and cpm of the pellet formed at the lower centrifuge setting was taken as cell-associated radioactivity. Opsonic activity was expressed as percent uptake = PMN-associated cpm - total cpm.

RESULTS AND DISCUSSION

Monoclonal antibodies were generated against epitopes on the O-side chain, core oligosaccharide, and lipid A of **E. coli** and **Salmonella** LPS. Representative binding data, obtained by PHA, are shown in Table 1. This and similar analyses indicated that O-side chain-specific mAbs reacted exclusively with homologous smooth LPS (e.g., see mAb 04-4C4 in Table 1). Core-specific mAbs, on the other hand, generally reacted only with those rough mutant LPS's on which the relevant core epitope was adequately exposed (Table 1). Thus, for example, mAbs specific for epitopes in the hexose, heptose, and KDO regions of the core oligosaccharide were restricted in their reactivity to rough mutant chemotype LPS bearing their respective epitopes at or near the nonreducing terminus of the core oligosaccharide. Moreover, lipid A-specific mAbs were either totally incapable of recognizing their respective epitopes on smooth or rough LPS (e.g., J23-4E12 in Table 1), or able to react only with rough LPS having the most rudimentary (i.e., Re chemotype) core component (data not shown). The mAb designated J18-8D2 (Table 1) demonstrated an interesting specificity pattern in so far as it reacted with both Rc chemotype LPS and with lipid A. This was interpreted as representing mAb multispecificity, i.e., the ability to recognize two or more similar but

Table 1. Binding activity in the passive hemolysis assay of O-side chain-, core, and lipid A-reactive monoclonal antibodies (mAbs)

	MAb (specificity)							
LPS/lipid A	04-4C4 (O)	S1-3A5 (C)	J7-3G7 (C)	J7-4D2 (C)	J7-5C10 (C)	J18-8D2 (C,L)	Y1-4A6 (C)	J23-4E12 (L)
Smooth LPS								
E. coli 026:B6	-	-	-	-	-	-	-	-
E. coli 055:B5	-	-	-	-	-	-	-	-
E. coli 0111:B4	10,240	-	-	-	-	-	-	-
E. coli 0127:B8	-	-	-	-	-	-	-	-
E. coli K235	-	-	-	-	-	-	-	-
S. minnesota	-	160	-	-	-	-	-	-
S. typhimurium	-	160	-	-	-	-	-	-
Rough LPS								
E. coli K12, mm294 (Ra)	-	160	10	-	-	-	40	-
S. minnesota R60 (Ra)	-	10,240	40	-	-	-	-	-
S. minneosta R345 (Rb)	-	160	40	-	-	-	-	-
E. coli J5 (Rc)	-	-	40,960	40,960	163,840	10,240	160	-
S. minnesota R5 (Rc)	-	-	-	-	40,960	2,560	160	-
S. minnesota R7 (Rd)	-	-	-	-	-	-	160	-
S. minnesota R595 (Re)	-	-	-	-	-	-	2,560	-
E. coli K12, D31m4 (Re)	-	-	-	-	-	-	2,560	-
Lipid A								
E. coli K12, D31m4	-	-	-	-	-	640	-	40,960
E. coli J5	-	-	-	-	-	640	-	-
S. minnesota R595	-	-	-	-	-	640	-	40,960
Synthetic lipid A								
LA-15-PP (506)	-	-	-	-	-	640	-	40,960

Note: Data represent reciprocal titers of monoclonal antibody-containing mouse ascites fluid. Minus signs indicate a titer < 1:10. O = O-side chain; C = core oligosaccharide; L = lipid A.

distinct epitopes on the same antigen. In this case, the epitopes may have involved one or both of the L-glycerol-D-mannoheptose-4'-phosphate groups present on Rcp+ LPS (4, 7) and the structurally similar glucosamine-4'-phosphate at the nonreducing end of the lipid A backbone (11).

Shown in Fig 1 are 17 mAbs that reacted with **S. minnesota** wild type (smooth) or rough mutant chemotype LPS. Each mAb, indicated by clone number, appears beneath that part of the **Salmonella** LPS macromolecular structure recognized by the mAb in question, as inferred from binding data obtained with various rough mutant and smooth LPS antigens. This figure emphasizes our identification of mAbs which recognize epitopes in all three major structural domains of native **Salmonella** LPS.

We next evaluated the binding of mAbs reactive with different structural elements of LPS to intact bacteria. Typically, O-side chain-specific mAbs such as S1-3H5 (see Table 2) reacted with the homologous, smooth, wild type strain, while demonstrating little or no reactivity against rough mutant chemotypes lacking the O-side chain. In this case, interestingly, the S1-3H5 mAb did show some binding activity against **S. minnesota** Ra and Rc chemotype bacteria, suggesting that these rough mutants may synthesize small amounts of complete core with attached O-side chains. Core-specific mAbs generally reacted with rough mutant chemotypes corresponding to the isolated LPS against which reactivity had been previously demonstrated (Table 2). There were, however, a number of exceptions to this correlation between mAb reactivity with isolated and bacterium-associated LPS. Examples were the failure of mAb S1-3A5 to react with **S. minnesota** Ra chemotype bacteria despite its reactivity with purified Ra chemotype LPS, and the ability of J7-5C10 and J8-5G4 to recognize an epitope on Re mutant bacteria in the absence of reactivity with isolated Re chemotype LPS (Table 2). Similarly, lipid A-specific mAbs reacted with some rough mutant bacteria, although their reactivity was more restricted against purified core glycolipids. The reactivity of J23-4E12 with Rc and Re chemotype bacteria (Table 2), in contrast with its inability to react with isolated Rc and Re LPS (Table 1), illustrates this point. Despite the ability of some core- and lipid A-specific mAbs to react with certain rough mutant chemotype bacteria whose core structure was more complete than that of the homologous strain, these mAbs rarely reacted with smooth LPS (Table 2).

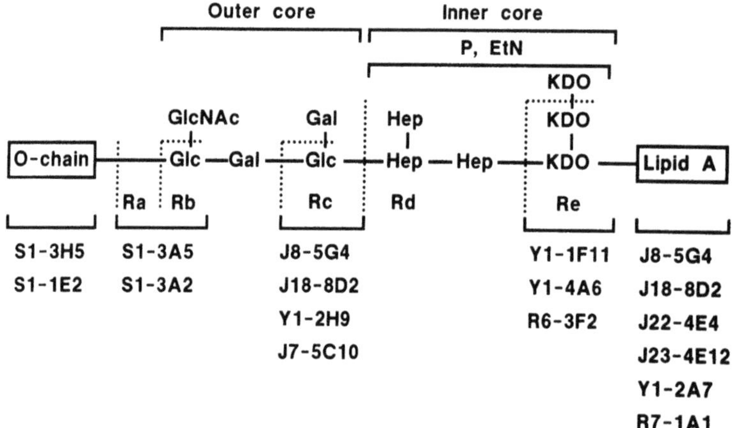

Fig 1. Monoclonal antibodies (mAbs) reactive with discrete structural elements of **Salmonella minnesota** LPS. Hybridoma clone designations are indicated under those parts of the LPS structure recognized by the mAbs produced by the clones.

Table 2. Binding of LPS-specific monoclonal antibodies (mAbs) to wild type and rough mutant **Salmonella minnesota** bacteria determined by flow cytometry

MAb	Specificity[1]	LPS chemotype			
		Wild type	Ra	Rc	Re
S1-3H5	O-side chain	99.2[2]	18.9	4.0	0.3
S1-3A5	Ra/Rb	0.3	0.7	0.9	0.3
J7-5C10	Rc	0.1	0.4	80.8	94.5
J8-5G4	Re/lipid A	0.2	0.6	93.2	88.8
Y1-1F11	Re	0.0	0.5	1.8	94.0
J23-4E12	lipid A	0.1	3.0	92.7	91.1

[1]Determined by ELISA, PHA with purified LPS, lipid A.
[2]Percent of bacteria exhibiting fluorescence after subtraction of negative control value.

Antibodies that react with LPS may, theoretically, express functionality through endotoxin-neutralizing or antibacterial properties. We examined selected examples of each.

Endotoxin-neutralizing activity was evaluated in an **in vitro** assay of LPS- or lipid A-induced tumor necrosis factor (TNF) secretion by murine RAW 264.7 macrophages. MAbs specific for epitopes on the O-side chain, core oligosaccharide, or lipid A moiety were preincubated with rough or smooth LPS, or lipid A, before adding the mixture to macrophage cultures. Subsequently harvested culture supernatants contained high levels of TNF, as measured in a cytotoxicity assay employing actinomycin D-sensitized L-929 fibroblasts. None of the mAbs examined caused a significant reduction in LPS- or lipid A-induced TNF production (Table 3). Likewise, high-titered lipid A-specific antisera had no discernible blocking effect on TNF induction by synthetic **E. coli** lipid A (6) (data not shown). Polymyxin B, on the other hand, caused $\geq 90\%$ inhibition of LPS- and lipid A-induced TNF production when preincubated with either molecular species. To the extent that a) TNF represents an important mediator of **in vivo** endotoxicity (1), and b) the **in vitro** assay described above accurately reflects **in vivo** events, the failure of LPS-specific mAbs to block LPS-induced TNF production suggests a lack of endotoxin-neutralizing activity in physiologically meaningful terms. Moreover, preliminary **in vivo** data indicate that O-side chain-, core-, and lipid A-specific mAbs also fail to block LPS- or lipid A-induced lethality in D-galactosamine-sensitized mice (Pollack, M., Koles, N., unpublished data). These **in vivo** data appear to corroborate the apparent inability of LPS-specific mAbs to block **in vitro** endotoxicity.

Since LPS represents an important surface antigen of Gram-negative bacteria, and the antibacterial properties of certain LPS-specific antisera have been well documented (16), we examined the complement-dependent bactericidal and opsonic activities of LPS-reactive mAbs as a function of epitope specificity, whole cell binding, and isotype. Murine mAbs representing all IgG subclasses, and IgM, were produced against determinants on the O-side chain of **E. coli** 0111:B4 LPS. All of these mAbs mediated complement-dependent bactericidal activity (Fig 2). The extent of this activity, however, varied markedly among antibodies of different isotypes. The IgM mAbs were most active in bactericidal assays, an IgG2a mAb was intermediate in activity, and the remaining IgG isotypes were least active. Differences

Table 3. Effect of O-side chain-, core-, and lipid A-reactive monoclonal antibodies (mAbs) on LPS- and lipid-A induced tumor necrosis factor (TNF) production by RAW 264.7 macrophages

MAb	Isotype	Specificity	Inhibition of TNF induced by **E. coli** 0111 LPS	**E. coli** J5 LPS	**E. coli** D31m4 LPS	**E. coli** lipid A
04-2H7	IgM	**E. coli** 0111:B4 O-side chain	-			
J7-5C10	IgM	**E. coli** J5 (Rc) core		-		
J8-1C2	IgM	**E. coli** J5 (Rc) core; **E. coli** D31m4 (Re) core		-	-	
J18-8D2	IgG2a	**E. coli** J5 (Rc) core; **E. coli** lipid A		-		-
Y1-4A6	IgG3	**E. coli** D31m4 (Re) core			-	
J23-4E12	IgM	**E. coli** lipid A				-
50-9	IgM	negative control	-	-	-	-
PMB		--	+	+	+	+

NOTE: LPS or lipid A (0.05 ug) was incubated with mAb (0.1-1,000 ug) at $37^{o}C$ for 30 min before adding the mixture to 1×10^6 RAW 264.7 macrophages. Macrophage supernatants were collected 4 hr later for TNF assay. Inhibition < 5%, minus sign; >50%, plus sign; not done, blank. PMB = polymyxin B.

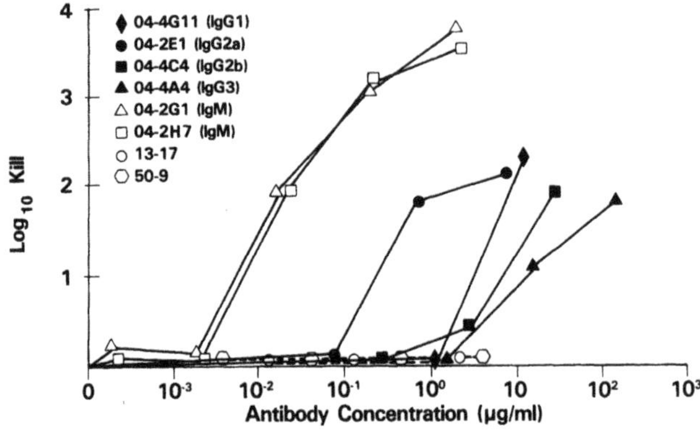

Fig 2. Complement-mediated bactericidal activity of O-side chain-specific monoclonal antibodies (mAbs) against **E. coli** 0111:B4. The mAbs designated 13-17 and 50-9 react with irrelevant antigens and are included as negative controls. Assays were performed in the presence of 1% absorbed, fresh normal human serum.

in the avidity of the various mAbs, estimated by RIA employing radiolabeled mAbs (Guelde, G., Pollack, M., unpublished data), did not appear to account for observed differences in bactericidal activity. What did seem to correlate best with this functional activity was relative C_3-binding activity (13) which corresponded closely to complement-dependent bacterial killing (data not shown). The bactericidal activity of O-side chain-specific mAbs demonstrated in the case of **E. coli** 0111:B4 was not a universal finding. MAbs generated against O-side chains of **S. minnesota** LPS, for example, mediated very little killing, and immunotype-specific mAbs produced against **Pseudomonas aeruginosa** LPS demonstrated no complement-dependent killing.

Core- and lipid A-reactive mAbs demonstrated no complement-dependent killing of **E. coli** 0111:B4 or **S. minnesota** wild type bacteria. This result was anticipated by the inability of such mAbs to bind smooth strains. An attempt was made to evaluate the possible bactericidal activity of core- and lipid A-reactive mAbs against rough mutant bacteria with which they reacted. However, the extreme susceptibility of these strains to the lytic action of complement alone (3), precluded any meaningful analysis of the possible contribution of mAbs to this process, even under low complement conditions.

We next evaluated the opsonic activity of mAbs directed against different elements of the LPS macromolecule. As expected, O-side chain-specific mAbs exhibited marked complement-dependent enhancement of bacterial uptake by human PMNs (Fig 3), and this was matched by activity in an opsonophagocytic bacterial killing assay (data not shown). The relative opsonic activity of mAbs reactive with the O-side chain of **E. coli** 0111:B4 LPS conformed to the same hierarchy as complement-dependent bactericidal activity (data not shown). Because both activities correlated with the complement-fixing efficiency of the various mAbs, it was assumed that this was the basis for observed differences in respect to both mAb functions. Unlike complement-dependent bactericidal activity, opsonic activity was expressed by all O-side chain-reactive mAbs examined, irrespective of specificity. This applied to mAbs that reacted with **S. minnesota** and **P. aeruginosa** as well as **E. coli** 0111:B4 LPS. In contrast, mAbs specific for determinants on the core oligosaccharide or lipid A exhibited little or no opsonic activity against smooth bacteria (Fig 3). Some of these same mAbs did, however, enhance the complement-mediated uptake of rough mutant strains at sub-bactericidal complement concentrations. Limited observations, employing **E. coli** J5 as the test strain, suggested that the relative opsonic activity of various core- and lipid A-reactive mAbs mays have been influenced both by epitope specificity and by isotype (Oishi, K., Pollack, M., unpublished data).

Protection experiments employing selected O-side chain-, core-, and lipid A-reactive mAbs were performed in mice challenged i.p. with both rough and smooth strains. Representative data (Table 4) indicate that O-side chain-specific mAbs were highly protective against infections produced with homologous, wild type bacteria. Core- and lipid A-specific mAbs, on the other hand, elicited no significant protection against either wild type or rough mutant bacteria. It appeared, in fact, from these and other protection data that neither antisera nor mAbs directed against epitopes in the core/lipid A complex protected against live challenge with rough bacteria in this murine model. It is unclear whether this observation reflected an artifact of the model, such as the large inoculum of rough bacteria required to produce a lethal infection, or some implicit features(s) of the interaction between core and lipid A-specific antibodies and their respective determinants on rough strain LPS or intact bacteria.

It would appear from these data that mAbs which recognize epitopes on different structural elements of LPS exhibit very different specificity and function. On the one hand, O-side chain-reactive mAbs are highly specific for homologous, smooth LPS, bind avidly to intact bacteria, mediate

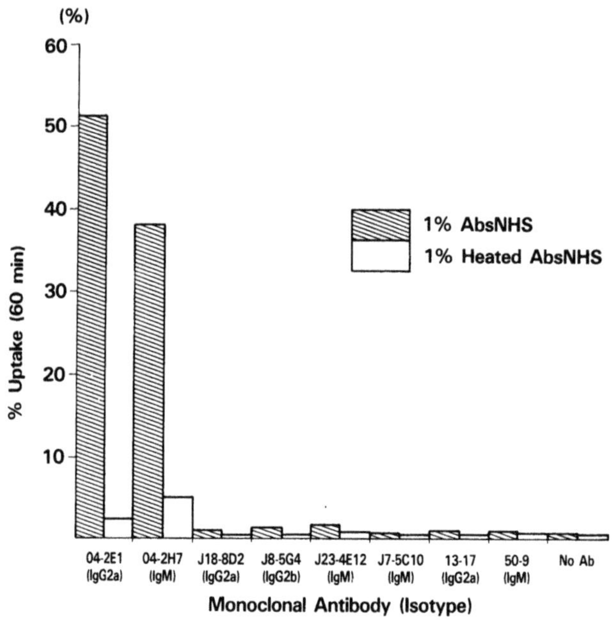

Fig 3. Complement-mediated opsonic activity of LPS-reactive monoclonal antibodies (mAbs) against **E. coli** 0111:B4 bacteria. MAb specificities were as follows: 04-2E1 and 04-2H7, wild type (O-side chain); J7-5C10, Rc mutant (core); J8-5G4, Rc mutant (core) and lipid A; J23-4E12, lipid A; 13-17 and 50-9, irrelevant antigens. AbsNHS = absorbed (fresh) normal human serum.

complement-dependent bactericidal and/or opsonic activity, and protect against live challenge. Core- or lipid A-specific mAbs, on the other hand, tend to be more cross-reactive, although this cross reactivity is severely restricted by the relative inaccessibility of particular epitopes in the core/lipid A complex. This is reflected in the general inability of these mAbs to react with either isolated smooth LPS or wild type bacteria. Epitope

Table 4. Protective activity of O-side chain-, core-, and lipid A-reactive monoclonal antibodies against i.p. challenges with wild type **Salmonella minnesota** and rough mutant strains in mice

		Percent survival for each challenge strain			
Antibody	Specificity	Wild type	Ra	Rc	Re
antiserum	homologous LPS	100*	100*	38	3
S1-1E2	wild type LPS	100*	-	-	-
S1-3A5	Ra, Rb LPS	10	23	-	-
J7-5C10	Rc LPS	0	-	58	-
J18-8D2	Rc LPS, lipid A	18	-	48	18
Y1-4A6	Re LPS	8	-	-	8
J23-4E12	lipid A	8	28	30	13
13-17	negative contro	5	5	40	3

Groups of 40 outbred Swiss-Webster mice received 1 mg of mAb i.v. 1 hr prior to i.p. challenge with 2-5 LD50's of bacteria in 5% hog gastric mucin.
*p < 0.05.

inaccessibility may be the major factor responsible for the limited antibacterial and protective capacity of core- and lipid A-specific mAbs. Other as yet poorly defined immunochemical factors may contribute to the low functional activities of these mAbs. One obvious difference, for example, between core- (or lipid A-) related epitopes and those determined by the repeating oligosaccharide subunit structure of the O-side chain, is the relatively small number of "copies" of the former per LPS molecule (and per bacterium) compared with the latter. This difference in epitope density no doubt influences the comparative functional activities of mAbs specific for different regions of the LPS macromolecule.

Whereas our data substantiate the antibacterial activities of O-side chain-specific antibodies, they do not support the putative antiendotoxic properties of antibodies directed against determinants in the core/lipid A region of LPS (14). It should be noted, however, that these data are quite limited, having been generated in highly artificial **in vitro** and **in vivo** murine models, and their general applicability is unclear. Particularly relevant, in this regard, are substantial interspecies differences in respect to LPS responsiveness. Also critical are the particular physiochemical forms assumed by LPS **in vivo** during the course of an actual infection, either cell-associated or free, intact or fragmented; the pathogenic role played by each form of LPS; and the ability of mAbs specific for particular elements of the LPS macromolecule to recognize these forms under **in vivo** conditions and to express a functional activity as a consequence of this recognition process.

REFERENCES

1. Beutler, B. and Cerami, A., 1987, Cachectin: more than a tumor necrosis factor. N. Eng. J. Med. 716: 379.

2. Brade, H., Brade, L., Schade, U., Zahringer, U., Holst, O., Kuhn, H.-M., Rozalski, A., Rohrscheidt, E. and Rietschel, E. Th., 1988, Structure, endotoxicity, and antigenicity of bacterial lipopolysaccharides (endotoxins, O-antigens), in: "Bacterial endotoxins: pathophysiological effects, clinical significance and pharmacological control", J. Levin, H. R. Buller, S. W. TenCate, S. J. H. VanDeventer, A. Sturk, eds., Alan R. Liss Publishing, New York.

3. Clas, F. and Loos, M., 1980, Killing of S and Re forms of **Salmonella minnesota** via the classical pathway of complement activation in guinea pig and human sera. Immunology 40: 547.

4. Fuller, N. A., Wu, M. C., Wilkinson, R. G. and Heath, E. C., 1973, The biosynthesis of cell wall lipopolysaccharide in **Escherichia coli** VII. Characterization of heterogenous "core" oligosaccharide structure. J. Biol. Chem. 248: 7938.

5. Galanos, C., Luderitz, O., Rietschel, E. Th. and Westphal, O., 1977, Newer aspects of the chemistry and biology of bacterial lipopolysaccharides, with special reference to the lipid A component, in: "Biochemistry of lipids.II", T. W. Goodwin, ed., University Park Press, Baltimore.

6. Imoto, M., Yoshimura, H., Kusumoto, S. and Shiba, T., 1984, Total synthesis of lipid A, active principle of bacterial endotoxin. Proc. Jpn. Acad. Ser. B. Phys. Biol. Sci. 60: 285.

7. Luderitz, O., Freudenberg, M. A., Galanos, C., Lehmann, V., Rietschel, E. Th. and Shaw, D. H., 1982, Lipopolysaccharides of gram-negative bacteria. Current Topics in Membranes and Transport 17: 79.

8. Luderitz, O., Staub, A. M. and Westphal, O., 1966, Immunochemistry of O and R antigens of **Salmonella** and related **Enterobacteriaceae**. Bacterial Rev. 30: 192.

9. Pollack, M., Chia, J. K. S., Koles, N. L., Miller, M. and Guelde, G., 1988, Monoclonal antibodies that recognize epitopes in the core and lipid A region of lipopolysaccharides, in: "Bacterial endotoxins: pathophysiological effects, clinical significance, and pharmacological control", J. Levin, H. R. Buller, J. W. TenCate, S. J. H. VanDeventer and A. Sturk, eds., Alan R. Liss Publishing, New York.

10. Pollack, M., Raubitschek, A. A. and Larrick, J. W., 1987, Human monoclonal antibodies that recognize conserved epitopes in the core-lipid A region of lipopolysaccharides. J. Clin. Invest. 79: 1421.

11. Rietschel, E. Th., Wollenweber, H. W., Brade, H., Zahringer, U., Linder, B., Seydel, V., Bradaczek, H., Barnickel, G., Labischinski, H. and Giesbrecht, P., 1984, Structure and conformation of the lipid A component of lipopolysaccharides, in: "Handbook of endotoxin. Vol 1: chemistry of endotoxin", E. Th. Rietschel, ed., Elsevier Science Publishers, Amsterdam.

12. Ruff, M. and Gifford, G., 1980, Purification and physio-chemical characterization of rabbit tumor necrosis factor. J. Immunol. 125: 1671.

13. Spiegelberg, H. L., 1974, Biological activities of immunoglobulins of different classes and subclasses. Adv. Immunol. 19: 259.

14. Teng, N. N. H., Kaplan, H. S., Hebert, J. M., Moore, C., Douglas, H., Wunderlich, A. and Braude, A. I., 1985, Protection against Gram-negative bacteremia and endotoxemia with human monoclonal IgM antibodies. Proc. Natl. Acad. Sci. U.S.A. 82: 1790.

15. Wilkinson, S. G., 1977, Composition and structure of bacterial lipopolysaccharides, in: "Surface carbohydrates of the prokaryotic cell", I. W. Sutherland, ed., Academic Press, New York.

16. Young, L. S., 1972, Human immunity to **Pseudomonas aeruginosa**. II. Relationship between heat-stable opsonins and type-specific lipopolysaccharides. J. Infect. Dis. 126: 277.

MECHANISMS OF NEUTRALIZATION OF ENDOTOXIN BY MONOCLONAL ANTIBODIES TO O AND R DETERMINANTS OF LIPOPOLYSACCHARIDE

T. Sagawa, *Y. Hitsumoto, *M. Kanoh, *S. Utsumi and S. Kimura

Second Department of Surgery, *Department of Microbiology
Ehime University, School of Medicine, Shigenobu-cho
Onsengun, Japan (791-02)

INTRODUCTION

The protective potentials of antibodies to O and R core regions of lipopolysaccharide (LPS) have been amply substantiated (2, 7). However, the efficacy of antibodies to the toxic lipid A moiety itself is still ambiguous, and how antibodies to regions distal from lipid A can neutralize the toxicity remains to be clarified. We have compared the effects of mouse monoclonal antibodies (mAbs) of IgG class to these three regions of LPS on the biological activities as well as micellic structure of LPS, in order to shed light on the mechanism of neutralization of endotoxin by these antibodies.

MATERIALS AND METHODS

Monoclonal Antibodies

LPS from **S. minnesota**, an O-defective J5 (Rc) strain of E. coli and a synthetic lipid A of the **E. coli** type (Dai-ichi Chemical Corp.) coupled to Keyhole Limpet hemocyanin (3) were used as immunogens. Balb/c mice were primed with each immunogen in Freund's complete adjuvant (100 μg, i.p.) then boosted weekly without adjuvant (50-250 μg, i.v.). Hybridoma with Sp2/O-Ag14 cells were prepared according to (5) and cell lines producing antibodies specific for S. minnesota LPS alone (anti-O, IgG3), J5 but also crossreactive with LPS of S. minnesota (anti-R, IgG1) and for lipid A (anti-A, IgG3) were established by repeating cloning. Monoclonal antibodies were purified from culture or peritoneal fluids by using Protein A-Cellulofine columns (Seikagaku Kogyo LTD).

Effects of mAbs on LPS Activities

LPS from **S. minnesota** (Boivin) was used throughout this study, since this, after being treated at pH 9.6, could bind nearly equal amounts of anti-O, anti-R and anti-A mAbs in ELISA. For the protectivity to endotoxin shock, C57Bl/6 mice (5-7 wks) given a prophylactic dose (100 μg, i.v.) of each mAb or saline were challenged 2 hr later with D-galactosamine (2.6 mmoles/kg, i.p.) and 20 LD_{50} of LPS (10 ng, i.v.) and mortality within 24 hr was scored. For the anti-pyrogenic effect, rabbits were given mAbs (500 μg, i.v.) 2 hr prior to LPS (0.8 μg/kg, i.v.) and change in the rectal temp. was followed. Unimmunized rabbits gave a biphasic fever response with peaks at 60 and 180 min, respectively. TNF production by BCG-activated macrophages in response to various concentrations of LPS in the presence or absence of mAbs (10 μg/ml) was assayed at intervals by the lytic activity to actinomycin D-treated L929 cells by the Crystal violet method (1). Effects of mAbs on LPS-induced IL-1 and PGE_2 productions were tested in the similar manner, but resident unactivated peritoneal macrophages were used. IL-1 was assayed by the thymocyte proliferation method (4) and PGE_2 by RIA.

Analysis of Immune Complexes

The size distribution of LPS-antibody complexes was analyzed by the sedimentation in a 9-41% sucrose density gradient at 30000 rpm for 16 hr with ^{125}I-labeled mAbs.

RESULTS

Results are summarized in Table 1. Both anti-O and anti-R mAbs reduced mortality of mouse endotoxin shock and abrogated the second fever onset in rabbits, in agreement with the previous report (6). The anti-A mAb used here was practically without effect in these systems. Parallel to the protective potentials of these mAbs were their effects on the TNF-producing activity of LPS in vitro. Thus 10 μg of anti-O or anti-R reduced the activity of 10 μg of LPS to that of 0.1 μg or less, whereas the same amount of anti-A could hardly reduce the activity of LPS. To the contrary, both anti-O and anti-R mAbs enhanced the IL-1 production in 2 hr culture at least 2-fold. However, the effects of these mAbs on the PGE_2 production was quite singular. The anti-R greatly enhanced the PGE_2 production during the first 30 min period of incubation when no detectable PGE_2 was produced otherwise, whereas the anti-O mAb suppressed the production during entire incubation period of 2 hr. Again, the effect of anti-A mAb was obscure.

Table 1. Summary of the Effects of Anti-O, Anti-R and Anti-Lipid A mAbs to the Biological Activities of LPS and Analysis of Immune Complexes

mAbs	Protectivity	Fever suppression	in vitro			Complex Formation with LPS
			TNF production	IL-1 production	PGE_2 production	
Anti-O	+	+	↓	↑	↓	restricted to homologous LPS +++ large(> 19S)
Anti-R	+	+	↓	↑	↑	crossreactive +++ small(9S)
Anti-Lipid A	—	—	→	→	→	crossreactive poor midium(~ 14S)

Fig 1 shows the sedimentation patterns of these mAbs with or without LPS. The bulk of anti-O mAb was associated with complexes larger than 19S, leaving only a small amount of unbound antibody in the 7S region (Fig 1a). The anti-R mAb, in contrast, formed small and much homogeneous complexes of approximately 9S with LPS (Fig 1b). Although self-aggregation of the IgG3 anti-A mAb obscured the sedimentation pattern of its complexes, it was still obvious that only a small portion of this antibody was associated with LPS and the size of complexes was on average smaller than those with anti-O but definitely larger than complexes formed with anti-R (Fig 1c).

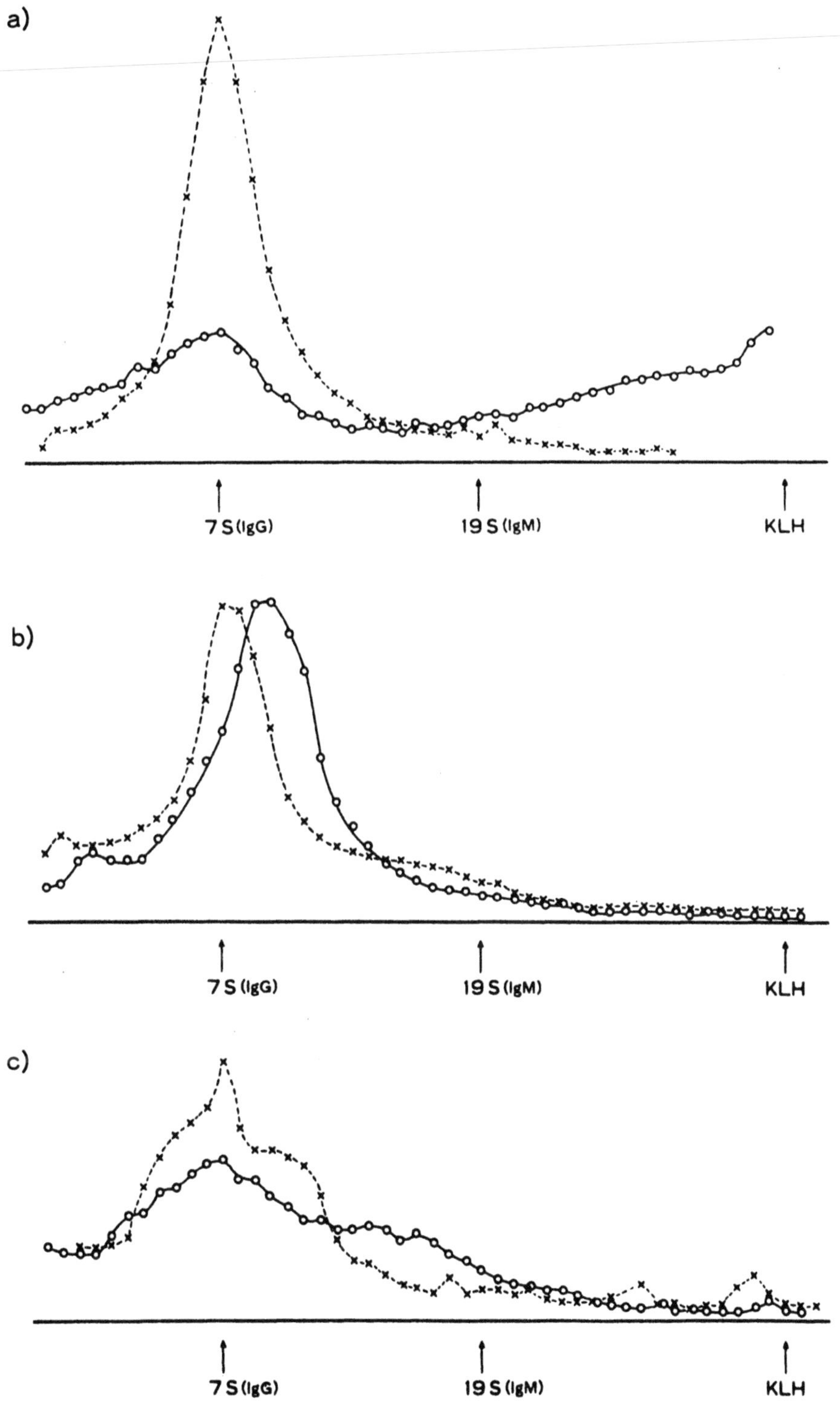

Fig 1. Sucrose density gradient sedimentation patterns of ^{125}I labeled a) anti-O, b) anti-R and c) anti-lipid A mAbs with (o——o) or without x----x) LPS.

DISCUSSION

LPS is believed to be in slow transitions among polydisperse lamellar micelles but, unlike more stable vesicular micelles of phospholipids, a rapid equilibrium may also exist between these open micelles of LPS and its monomeric or oligomeric forms. In order to interpret the present results, we postulate that the TNF- and PGE_2-inducing activities of LPS are largely exerted by the large micellic and small oligomeric forms, respectively. The binding of anti-O antibody molecules to the outermost surface of a micelles will not disrupt the micellic structure but sterically block the interaction of LPS with cells, while such large immune complex will be readily cleared by the Fc receptor-mediated phagocytosis. On the other hand, antibody binding to a region more close to lipid A would interfere with the hydrophobic association between LPS molecules and therefore disrupt the micellic structure, resulting in the reduction in the TNF-inducing activity but enhancing the PGE_2-inducing activity of LPS. Antibody to lipid A, though reactive with exposed areas of small LPS micelles, would not be able to access the core region of large micelles nor disrupt micellic structure.

REFERENCES

1. Aggarwall, B. B., Kohr, W. J., and Harkins, R. N., 1985, Human tumor necrosis factor. Production, purification and characterization. J. Biol. Chem. 260: 2345.

2. Braude, A. I., Douglas, H., and Ziegler, E. J., 1977, Antibody to cell wall glycolipid of gram-negative bacteria: Induction of immunityto bacteremia and endotoxemia. J. Infect. Dis. S136: S167.

3. Galanos, C., Luderitz, O., and Westphal, O., 1971, Preparation and properties of antisera against the lipid A component of bacterial lipopolysaccharides. Eur. J. Biochem. 24: 110.

4. Mizel, S. B., Oppenheim, J. J., and Rosenstreich, D. L., 1978, Characterization of lymphocyte activating factor (LAF) produced by a macrophage cell line. P 388D1. J. Immunol. 120: 1497.

5. Oi, V. T., and Herzenberg, L. A., 19o80, Immunoglobulin-producing hybrid cell lines. in: "Selected methods in cellular immunology". B. B. Mishell, ed., W. H. Freeman Co., San Francisco.

6. Radvany, R., Neale, N. L., and Nowotny, A., 1966, Relation of structure to function in bacterial O-antigens. VI. Neutralization of endotoxic O antigens by homologous O-antibody. Ann. N.Y. Acad. Sci. 133: 763.

7. Ziegler, E. J., Douglas, H., and Braude, A. I., 1982, Treatment of gram-negative bacteremia and shock with human antiserum to a mutant Escherichia coli. N. Egl. J. Med. 307: 1225.

SECTION IV.

CELLULAR INTERACTIONS

POSSIBLE REFRACTORY SITE ON LPS-INDUCED INTERLEUKIN 1 PRODUCTION IN C3H/HEJ PERITONEAL MACROPHAGES

M. Nakano, Y. Terada, H. Matsumura and H. Shinomiya

Department of Microbiology, Jichi Medical School
Tochigi 329-04, Japan

INTRODUCTION

The C3H/HeJ strain of mice is known to be unresponsive to LPS (20), and this peculiar characteristic of these mice has greatly contributed to the analysis of the complex processes involved in the cell activation by LPS as a negative control. The unresponsiveness of these mice is believed to be attributed to a mutation of a single gene locus on chromosome 4 that has been designated as the LPS-gene with normal (n) and defective (d), alleles, respectively (26). Because C3H/HeJ mice carry the LPS-defective gene (Lps^d), their macrophages cannot secrete interleukin 1 (IL-1) in response to LPS (21). Determining the location of where the blocking sites are phenotypically expressed by the defective gene may provide us with a useful approach for elucidating the triggering by LPS, because it must be one of the important sites of this pathway. In a previous paper (22), we demonstrated that the C3H/HeJ macrophages are unresponsive to the calcium ionophore A23187 as well as LPS, and we suggested that the blocking sites expressed phenotypically by the Lps^d are shared by LPS- and A23187-stimulated processes. In the present study, we intend to elucidate the difference of intracellular signal transmission on the LPS-induced IL-1 production in macrophages between LPS-responsive C3H/He mice and LPS-unresponsive C3H/HeJ mice.

MATERIALS AND METHODS

Mice

C3H/He and C3H/HeJ mice were bred and maintained in our animal colony under standard care. Male and female mice were used between 7 to 20 wk of age. In individual experiments, sex and age-matched were used.

Culture Media

RPMI 1640 medium was prepared from powdered stock (Flow Laboratories Co., Ltd., Rockville, MD) and supplemented with 0.2% $NaHCO_3$, 10 mM HEPES, 1 mM pyruvate, 2 mM L-glutamine, 5 x 10^{-5} M 2-mercaptoethanol, 100U/ml of penicillin, 100 μg/ml of streptomycin, and 1 or 9% heat-inactivated fetal calf serum (FCS; Lot 100379, HyClone Laboratories, Logan, UT) (FCS-RPMI medium). FCS was selected according to the content of LPS (less than 0.1 ng/ml by the Toxicolor Test, a type of Limulus amebocyte lysate assay; Seikagaku Kogyo Co., Ltd., Tokyo).

Reagents

LPS was prepared from Salmonella typhimurium LT2 by phenol-water extraction as described (27) and further purified by repeated centrifugation at 100,000 x g for 60 min. A23187, PMA and Quin 2 acetoxymethyl ester were obtained from Sigma Chemical Co., St. Louis, MO. Ionomycin was purchased from Calbiochem, La Jolla, CA. A23187 and ionomycin were initially dissolved in dimethyl sulfoxide (DMSO). LPS and PMA were dissolved in phosphate-buffered saline and ethanol, respectively. The calmodulin antagonists W-5 and W-7 and the protein kinase C antagonist H-7 were obtained from Seikagaku-Kogyo Co., Ltd., Tokyo, and they dissolved in distilled water. Recombinant human IL-1β was given to us by Ohtsuka Pharmaceutical Co., Tokushima, Japan. The stocked solutions of these reagents were diluted with culture medium when used.

Preparation of Macrophages

Peritoneal exudate cells (PEC) were obtained from the peritoneal cavities of mice according to the procedures described in the previous paper (22). The PEC were dispensed onto 24-well flat-bottomed tissue culture plates (1 x 10^6 cells/1 ml of 1% FCS-RPMI medium/well) and incubated for 2 hr at 37°C in a humidified atmosphere of 5% CO_2 and 95% air. The nonadherent cells were washed off by two vigorous rinses with warm medium. The remaining adherent cells were >95% macrophages, as determined by morphologic criteria, phagocytosis, and nonspecific esterase staining. Regardless of the preparation from C3H/He or C3H/HeJ mice, similar numbers of adherent cells were obtained in the wells.

Production of IL-1 by Macrophages

After the final washing, macrophage monolayers were overlaid with 1 ml of 1% FCS-RPMI medium. Various concentrations of LPS, A23187, ionomycin or PMA were added when the cultures were initiated. W-5, W-7 or H-7 was added to the cultures just before adding the stimulants mentioned above. The cultures were incubated at 37°C in a humidified atmosphere of 5% CO_2 and 95% air. At various time intervals, the supernatants of the cultures were collected for the determination of extracellular IL-1. The residual adherent macrophages were disrupted by freeze-thawing and sonication in order to determine intracellular IL-1.

IL-1 Assay

IL-1 was assayed by the slightly modified method of Mizel et al. (15). The detailed procedures have been described in our previous paper (22). The activity was expressed by the [^{3}H]thymidine incorporation (counts per min) into the C3H/HeJ thymocytes in cultures or by the units that were calculated from the incorporation in comparison with those of human recombinant IL-1β as the standard IL-1.

Extraction of Cytoplasmic RNA and the Hybridization

Total cellular RNA was extracted from the macrophages by the guanidinium isothiocyanate-cesium chloride method (3). Then, northern blot and dot blot hybridization were performed according to the instructions of Maniatis et al. (11). In brief, the RNA was electrophoresed in a 1.2% agarose-formaldehyde gel containing ethidium bromide (0.2 ng/ml) and transferred onto a nitrocellulose membrane filter. The filter was hybridized with our synthetic ^{32}P-end-labeled murine IL-1β oligonucleotide probe (42 mer) in 4-fold-diluted SSPE-solution (0.15 M NaCl, 10 mM sodium phosphate, pH 7.0 and 1 mM EDTA dissodium) containing 50% formaldehyde, 50-fold-diluted Denhardt's solution and 10% sodium dodecyl sulfate (SDS) at 45°C for 20 hr. After washing, the filter was exposed to a film (Fuji Rx, Tokyo, Japan) with an intensifying screen at -70°C for 48 hr.

Assay of Protein Kinase C (PKC)

The macrophages were disrupted by sonication in Tris-HCl-buffered solution (20 mM, pH 7.5) supplemented with 2 mM EDTA, 5 mM EGTA, 2 mM phenylmethlsulfonyl fluoride (PMSF), 10 mM 2-mercaptoethanol, 0.25 M sucrose and 0.1% Triton X-100, and then centrifuged at 100,000 x g for 60 min. PKC activity in the supernatant was determined by the incorporation of [gamma-^{32}P]ATP into histone type III-s according to the measuring method described by Castagna et al. (1).

Assay for Calmodulin (CaM)

The soluble form of CaM was extracted from the homogenate of macrophages with EGTA-solution according to the method of Kakiuchi et al. (7, 23). Its activity as a modulator and the Ca^{2+}-sensitivity of CaM were determined by its ability to activate phosphodiesterase (PDE) (7). Pig brain CaM (Boehringer Mannheim, Mannheim, West Germany) was used as the standard.

Assay for Calmodulin-Binding Proteins (CaMBP)

Macrophages were disrupted by freeze-thawing and sonication in the 20 mM Tris-HCl buffered solution (pH 7.5) containing 1 mM EGTA, 1 mM $MgSO_2$, 0.2 mM dithiothreitol, 0.34 M sucrose, 1 mM PMSF, leupeptin (2 μg/ml) and pepstatin (10 μg/ml) (1 x 10^9 macrophages/100 ml solution), and then centrifuged at 50,000 x g for 1 hr. CaMBP in the supernatants were assessed autoradiographically by modifications (10, 24) of the method of LaPorte and Strom (9).

Quantitation of Protein

Contents of protein in the samples were determined by the method of Lowry (10).

RESULTS

Effect of LPS or A23187 on IL-1 Production by C3H/He and C3H/HeJ Macrophages

The capabilities of C3H/He and C3H/HeJ macrophages to produce IL-1 were examined. As shown in Fig 1, the samples that were mixed of the dialyzed supernatants and disrupted cells from the cultures of C3H/He macrophages stimulated with either LPS or A23187 for 48 hr contained IL-1 activities, while those with C3H/HeJ macrophages did not. Although C3H/HeJ macrophages were refractory to LPS and A23187, this does not mean that C3H/HeJ macrophages lack the capability to produce IL-1. When C3H/HeJ macrophages as well as C3H/He macrophages were stimulated with PMA, these macrophages produced IL-1 (22).

Kinetics of Extracellular and Intracellular IL-1 Production by C3H/He and C3H/HeJ Macrophages

IL-1 produced by macrophages in vitro is released into the culture medium. However, large amounts of IL-1 still remain in the intracellular cytosol and cell membrane. The kinetics of the production of extracellular and intracellular IL-1 from these C3H/He and HeJ macrophages by the stimulation with LPS or A23187 were examined (Fig 2). Significant amounts of extracellular and intracellular IL-1 were produced by C3H/He macrophages after the induction by these stimulants (Figs 2A and 2B). The kinetics of intracellular IL-1 production in C3H/He macrophages are different from those of the extracellular production. The intracellular IL-1 levels increased

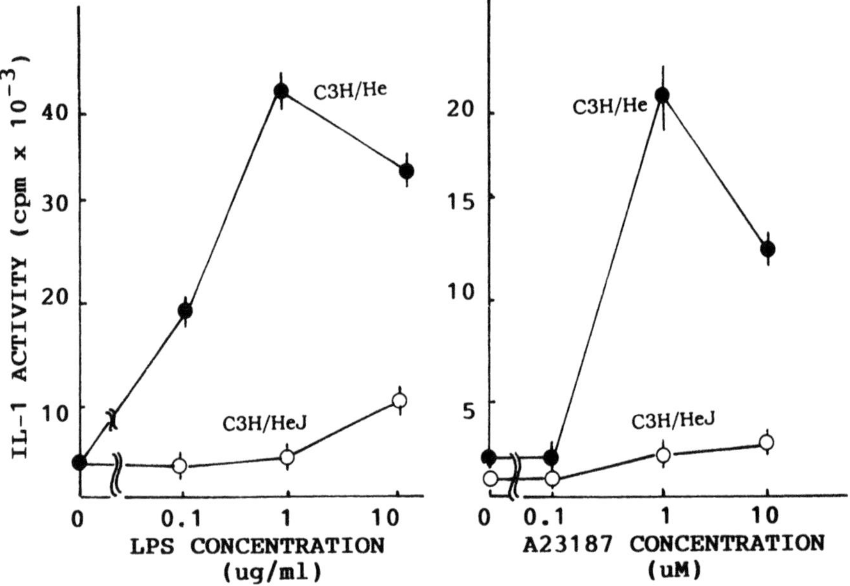

Fig 1. IL-1 production by C3H/He and C3H/HeJ macrophages stimulated with LPS (left panel) or A23187 (right panel). Adherent macrophages prepared from the PEC (1 x 10^6/ml/culture) of C3H/He (closed circles) or C3H/HeJ (open circles) mice were cultured for 48 hr in the presence of LPS (0.1 to 10 μg/ml) or A23187 (0.1 to 10μM). Then, IL-1 activity of the sample that was mixed of the culture supernatant and the disrupted cells was assayed. Each point represents the mean cpm of triplicate cultures ± SD.

more quickly after the stimulations by these activators, reached maximum at 24 hr, and then dropped (Fig 2B). The ability of LPS to induce extracellular or intracellular IL-1 was greater than that of A23187. On the other hand, C3H/HeJ macrophages did not produce any extra- or intracellular IL-1 after the stimulation by A23187 (Figs 2C and 2D). C3H/HeJ macrophages stimulated by LPS showed low levels of intracellular IL-1 activity (Fig 2D).

Expression of IL-1β mRNA in the Macrophages

In order to examine whether the blocking site(s) on IL-1 production by C3H/HeJ macrophages is pre- or post-translational, the expression of mRNA for IL-1 in the macrophages was examined by northern blot analysis. When the cultured C3H/He macrophages were stimulated either by LPS or A23187, IL-1β mRNA was detected in the macrophages at 2 hr after the stimulation and reached the plateau after 12 hr. However, no detectable IL-1β mRNA was seen in C3H/HeJ macrophages after the induction by these stimulants. These results indicate that the defective point in the IL-1 production of C3H/HeJ macrophages must be located on the intracellular signaling pathway before the expression of IL-1 mRNA.

Influx of Free Ca^{2+} to the Cytoplasm

Intracellular calcium ions ($[Ca^{2+}]i$) are known to play some important role in intracellular signal transmission. In order to elucidate whether the increase of $[Ca^{2+}]i$ is related to the difference in the abilities between C3H/He and C3H/HeJ macrophages to produce IL-1 in the response to A23187 induction, the amounts of $[Ca^{2+}]i$ in the macrophages were quantified by measuring fluorescence intensity in macrophages which were preloaded with

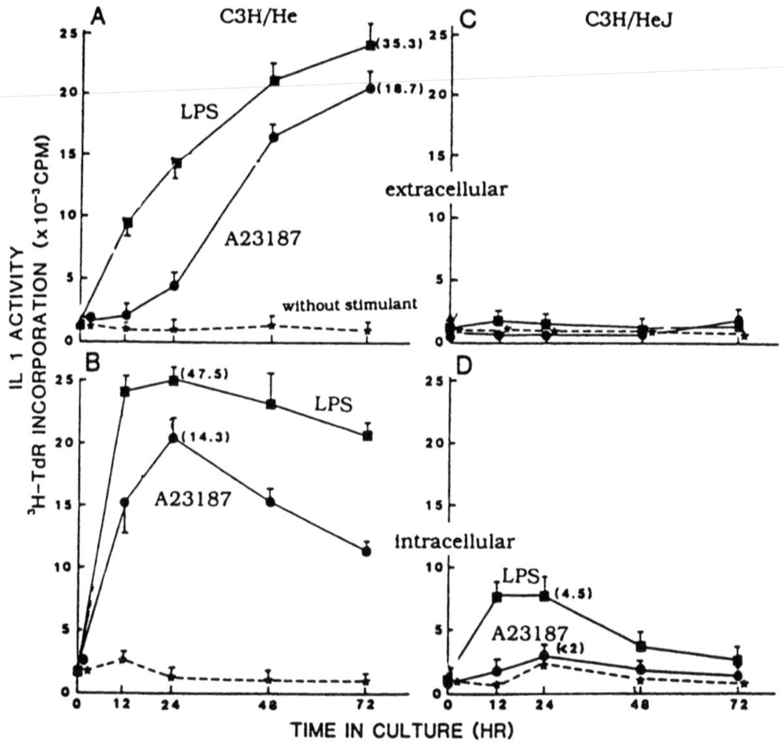

Fig 2. Kinetics of extracellular and intracellular IL-1 production by C3H/He and C3H/HeJ macrophages stimulated with LPS or A23187. Adherent macrophages prepared from the PEC (1 x 10^6/ml/culture) of C3H/He (A and B) or C3H/HeJ (C and D) mice were cultured in the presence or absence of LPS (10 µg/ml) or A23187 (10^{-6}M) for the time indicated on the abscissa. Then, the supernatants and the cultured cells were collected separately. The cells were sonicated. After the dialyzation, the IL-1 activity in the supernatants (extracellular IL-1: A and C) or in the macrophages (intracellular IL-1: B and D) were assessed. Each point represents the mean cpm of triplicate cultures ± SD. The values in parenthesis indicate the units/ml of the maximum IL-1 activity in the related samples.
■——■, LPS; ●——●, A23187; *------*, without stimulant.

Quin 2 and then stimulated. As shown in Figure 3, the fluorescence intensity of the C3H/HeJ macrophages stimulated by A23187 was almost equal to that of the C3H/He macrophages. Addition of LPS to the cultures did produce an increase in $[Ca^{2+}]i$. These results suggest that the site refractory to A23187 on the pathway for the production of IL-1 in C3H/HeJ macrophages exists after the process of $[Ca^{2+}]i$ increase.

Effect of H-7, a PKC Inhibitor, on IL-1 Production by C3H/He Macrophages

PMA is capable of activating PKC (1) and inducing IL-1 production by both C3H/He and C3H/HeJ macrophages (22). In order to examine the relation between A23187-induced IL-1 production and the activity of PKC, the effect of H-7 (5), a PKC inhibitor, was examined on the C3H/He macrophage cultures in the presence of A23187 as the inducer of IL-1. However, the production was not blocked by 3.1 to 50 µM of this inhibitor.

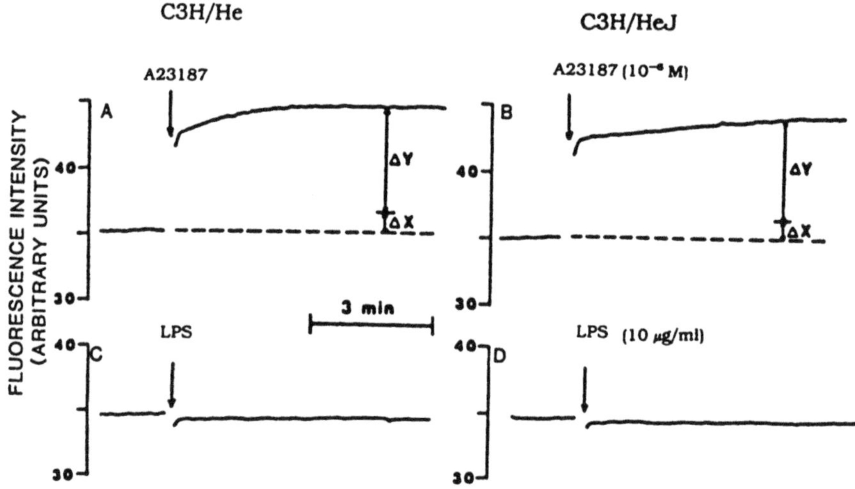

Fig 3. Effects of A23187 and LPS on the macrophage $[Ca^{2+}]i$. C3H/He (A and C) or C3H/HeJ (B and D) macrophages were preloaded with Quin 2 and then stimulated (arrow) with A23187 (10^{-6}M) (A and B) or LPS (10 μg/ml) (C and D). ΔX, augmentation of fluorescence when macrophages not loaded with Quin 2 were stimulated with A23187. ΔY, the increase of $[Ca^{2+}]i$-specific fluorescence.

Activities of PKC in C3H/He and C3H/HeJ Macrophages

In order to clarify whether or not the activity of PKC in the C3H/HeJ macrophages is affected, the activities in the supernatant obtained from the disrupted C3H/He or C3H/HeJ macrophages was assessed as described in "Materials and Methods". As shown in Figure 4, the PKC activity of C3H/HeJ macrophages was not different from that of C3H/He macrophages.

Effect of CaM Antagonists on IL-1 Production by C3H/He Macrophages

The CaM-system is another calcium-dependent intracellular signaling pathway (16). Therefore, we examined whether calmodulin participates in the production of IL-1 by using the CaM antagonists W-5 and W-7 (6, 17). W-5 interacts more weakly with CaM than W-7 (17). As shown in Figure 5, A23187-induced extracellular IL-1 production by C3H/He macrophages was almost completely blocked by W-7 (25 μM or 100 μM) and it was partially (25 μM) or almost completely (100 μM) blocked by W-5. At these concentrations, A23187-induced intracellular IL-1 production was also inhibited (data not shown). In contrast, LPS-induced IL-1 production was inhibited only by high doses of W-7. No suppressive effects of these antagonists were observed on PMA-induced IL-1 production even at high concentrations. These results suggest that calmodulin is important in A23187-stimulated IL-1 production, and that the actions of A23187 and LPS seem to be different, although both of them were unable to stimulate C3H/HeJ macrophages to produce IL-1.

The inhibitory effects of W-7 and W-5 on A23187-induced IL-1 production were confirmed by monitoring the mRNA levels by northern blot analysis. The C3H/HeJ peritoneal macrophages were stimulated with A23187 (10^{-6}M) in the presence or absence of W-7 or W-5 (5 to 100 μM), and the expression of IL-1β mRNA was determined by dot hybridization. When 20 μM or more W-7 was added to the cultures, the expression of IL-1β mRNA was completely blocked. The effect of W-5 is weaker than that of W-7, and 100 μM W-5 partially inhibited the expression.

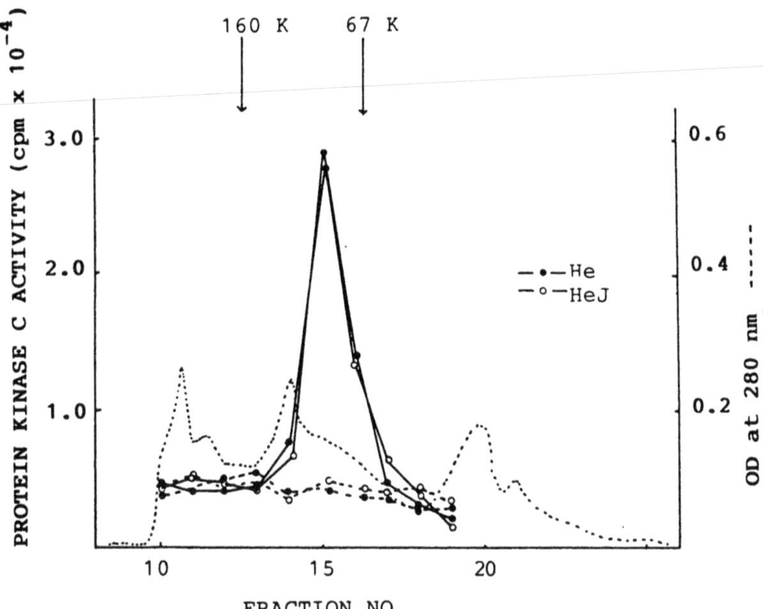

Fig 4. PKC activity in the extracts from C3H/He or C3H/HeJ macrophages. The extracts containing PKC were obtained from the PEC of C3H/He (closed circles) or C3H/HeJ (open circles) mice and fractioned by G3000SW gel filtration as described in "Materials and Methods". Then, the PKC activity in each fraction was determined. ——, PKC activity in the presence of Ca^{2+}; -----, PKC activity in the presence of EGTA; ......, absorbance at 280 nm.

CaM Activity in C3H/He and C3H/HeJ Macrophages

The results that we have described so far strongly suggest that the calcium-dependent CaM system is one of the major pathways for the production of IL-1 after the stimulation with calcium ionophore, and the defective point of C3H/HeJ is located on a process in this pathway. Therefore, we next examined whether the CaM of C3H/HeJ macrophages itself has some functional defect. C3H/He or C3H/HeJ macrophages were homogenized, and the CaM was extracted from the homogenates by EGTA. The activity in the extract was determined by examining the ability to activate phosphodiesterase (PDE) in the diluted solutions and the requirement for Ca^{2+} in the activation of PDE. As shown in Figure 6, the activities in the solution obtained from C3H/HeJ macrophages were almost the same as those from C3H/He macrophages. These results indicate that the function of calmodulin itself in C3H/HeJ macrophages is not different from that in C3H/He macrophages.

Deficiency of CaMBP in C3H/HeJ Macrophages

In order for CaM to function, CaMBP is necessary (2). Among the many types of CaMBP, Speaker et al. (25), recently reported macrophage- specific CaMBP. Therefore, we examined if there are any differences in this protein between C3H/He and C3H/HeJ macrophages at 24 hr after the stimulation by LPS. The CaMBP extracted from the macrophages was detected by electrophoresis on polyacrylamide gel, and autoradiograms of the proteins were made (Fig 7). When the C3H/He macrophages were stimulated with LPS, some of the proteins capable of binding to CaM were very markedly increased. In contrast, a trace amount of the protein was seen in the C3H/HeJ macrophages after the stimula-

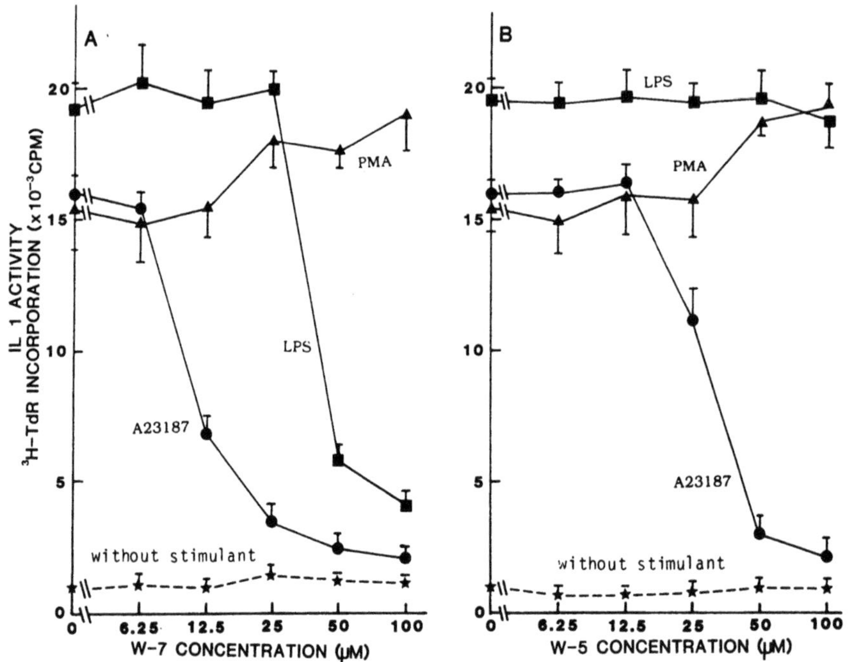

Fig 5. Effect of CaM antagonists, W-7 or W-5, on IL-1 production in C3H/He macrophages stimulated by LPS, A23187 or PMA. C3H/He macrophages (1 x 10^6/ml/culture) were cultured in the presence of A23187 (10^{-6}M), LPS (1 μg/ml) or PMA (10^{-5}M) with or without W-7 or W-5 for 48 hr. Then, IL-1 activities in the supernatants were assayed as described for Figure 1.

tion by LPS. These results indicate that the generation and/or recruitment of some of the CaMBP by LPS in C3H/HeJ macrophages were genetically hampered.

DISCUSSION

IL-1 is one of the cytokines, hormone-like factors with divergent biological effects including the augmentation of mitogenesis by immature thymocytes, the differentiation of peripheral T lymphocytes to express cell surface markers and produce lymphokines, the promotion of antibody production by B lymphocytes, the stimulation of the hypothalamic fever center, and the productions of acute phase protein, collagenese and prostaglandin (17). Although LPS is a powerful inducer for IL-1-producing cells, and the macrophages of C3H/He mice respond to LPS and produce IL-1, the macrophages of C3H/HeJ mice are refractory to LPS stimulation of IL-1 production (21, 22); (Figs 1 & 2). In the present study, we demonstrated that calcium ionophores, A23187 and ionomycin, have phenomenologically similar attributes to LPS in the stimulation of IL-1 production by the macrophages of these LPS responder and nonresponder strains of mice, although, on the other hand, PMA can induce IL-1 production from both types of macrophages.

The IL-1 mRNA was hardly detectable in the unstimulated macrophages, but when stimulated by LPS, they can express it quickly (4, 13). There are two types of IL-1 mRNA, α and β types. The amount of IL-1β mRNA is at least 10-fold greater than that of IL-1α mRNA in human peritoneal blood monocytes stimulated with LPS (12). In our results, C3H/He macrophages could express IL-1β mRNA after the stimulation with either LPS or A23187, while C3H/HeJ macrophages could not. We have not examined the expression of IL-1α mRNA,

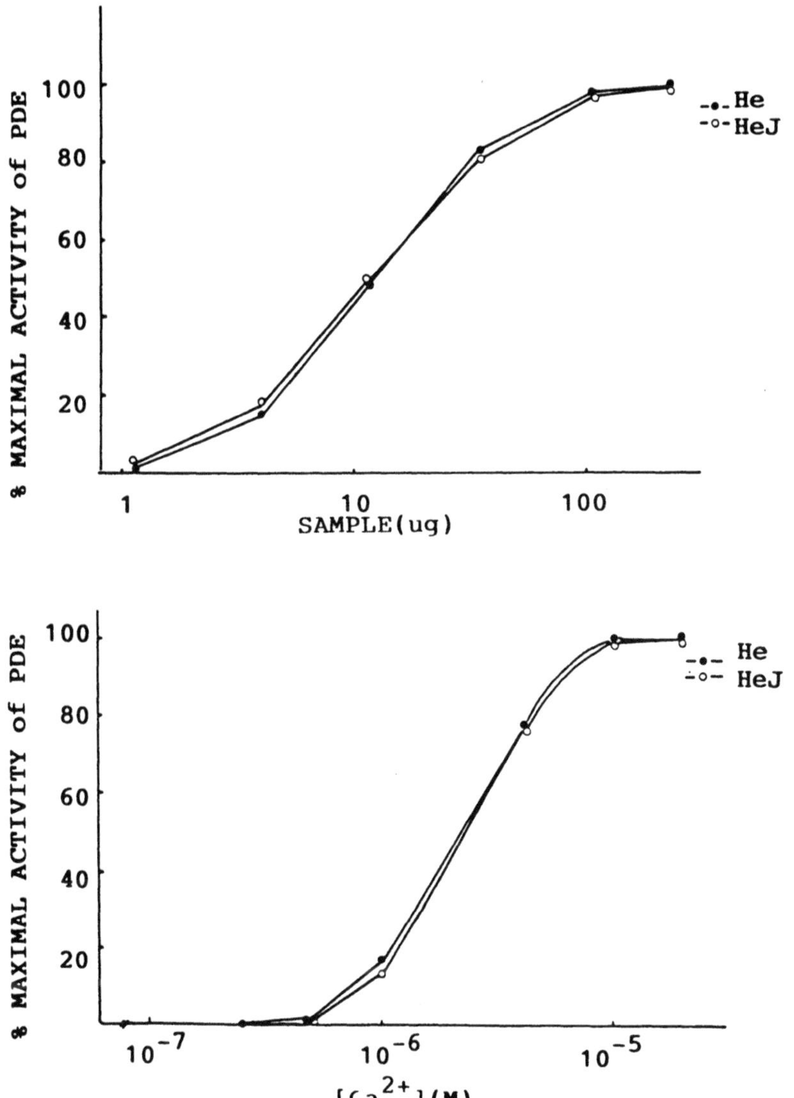

Fig 6. Activity of CaM in the samples extracted from C3H/He or C3H/HeJ macrophages and its dependency on Ca^{2+}. Upper panel shows the CaM activities in the samples, which are estimated by the ability to activate PDE. The content of protein (i.e., crude CaM) in the samples is indicated on the abscissa. The lower panel shows the Ca^{2+} dependency of the sample (100 μg protein) in the activation of PDE.

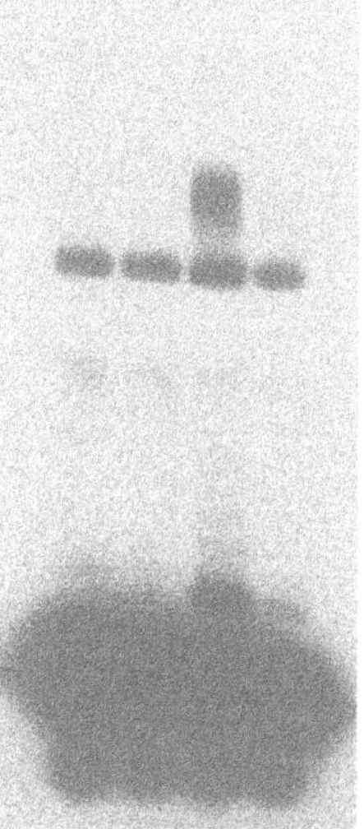

Fig 7. Autoradiogram of CaMBP in the extracts from C3H/He or C3H/HeJ macrophages. The macrophages (10^6/ml/culture) were cultured in the presence or absence of LPS (2 μg/ml) for 24 hr. Then, CaMBP was extracted and detected by electrophoresis on a polyacrylamide gel. The location is determined by autoradiography.

but Koide and Steinman have reported that no IL-1α mRNA is detected in keratocytes of C3H/HeJ mice after stimulation by LPS (8).

A23187 was shown to Ca^{2+}-specifically induce IL-1 production in human peripheral blood monocytes (14) and mouse peritoneal macrophages (21). However, LPS-nonresponsive C3H/HeJ macrophages could not respond to A23187 or ionomycin as well as LPS. Therefore, it is likely that the intracellular pathways responding to the calcium ionophores may share some processes with those in the pathways for LPS response, and some point on these shared processes in C3H/HeJ macrophages may be affected. However, the mode of action of LPS is different from that of the calcium ionophores since LPS does not elevate $[Ca^{2+}]i$ at all, but the calcium ionophores do (Fig 3).

Prpic et al., demonstrated that LPS and lipid A cause increased breakdown of phosphatidylinositol 4,5-bisphosphate (PIP_2), which led to enhanced intracellular levels of calcium and also to enhanced protein phosphorylation, presumably mediated by PKC (19). They presumed that the LPS-mediated hydrolysis of PIP_2 is likely to be an important mediator of the biological activities of LPS. PMA is a powerful PKC activator (1), and it can induce IL-1 production in C3H/HeJ macrophages as well as in C3H/He macrophages (21). However, the activation of PKC seems to be unrelated to the pathway of LPS-induced IL-1 production, because we could not find any difference in the activities between C3H/He and C3H/HeJ macrophages (Fig 4). Furthermore, we could not find any inhibitive effects of H-7, a PKC inhibitor, on A23187-induced IL-1 production by C3H/He macrophages. These results suggest that PKC activation is not essential for the production of IL-1 by the macrophages stimulated with A23187 or LPS.

The CaM system is another calcium-dependent intracellular signaling pathway (2). CaM antagonists inhibited A23187-induced IL-1ß mRNA expression and the IL-1 production (Fig 5) by C3H/He macrophages at a reasonable concentration. W-7, one of the stronger antagonists, also inhibited the LPS-induced IL-1 production (Fig 5). These findings indicate that the CaM-system is intimately related to the intracellular pathways on LPS and A23187-induced IL-1 production. If this is so, the defective point in C3H/HeJ macrophages unresponsive to LPS or A23187 should have some relation to the CaM-system. However, the CaM itself in C3H/HeJ macrophages seems to be intact, because the extracted CaM from the C3H/HeJ macrophages was as functional as the CaM from C3H/He macrophages (Fig 6).

In order for CaM to function, CaMBP is necessary (2). Orlow et al., reported that the resident C3H/HeJ macrophages as well as the C3H/He macrophages acquire CaMBP if they are allowed to develop in culture in the presence of LPS for 3 days (18). However, we demonstrated that there is no up-regulation of the macrophage-specific CaMBP by LPS in the 24-hr cultured C3H/HeJ macrophages in comparison with the C3H/He macrophages (Fig 7). The CaMBP that appears in the early stage after LPS-stimulation should be related to IL-1 production, because the IL-1 production is initiated at an early time after the stimulation. The Lps^d mutation may be related with the failure of regulating CaMBP in the early stage. A mutation on CaMBP has already been described by Speaker et al. (25). They found a mutant cell line from the macrophage-like mouse cell line, which was resistant to trifluoperazine, an inhibitor of CaM function, and these cells possessed a decrease in CaM binding activity.

Considering these findings together, it seems to be possible that the Lps^d dysfunction directly or indirectly affects a certain common step situated in both the Ca^{2+}-CaM initiated process and the LPS-initiated one, and a defect in CaMBP might be one of the most important candidates for Lps^d.

ACKNOWLEDGMENTS

This work was partially supported by Grants from the Ministry of Culture, Education and Science in Japan.

REFERENCES

1. Castagna, M. Y., Takai, Y., Kaibuchi, K., Sano, K., Kikkawa, U. and Nishizuka, Y., 1982, Direct activation of calcium-activated, phospholipid-dependent protein kinase by tumor-promoting phorbol ester. J. Biol. Chem. 257: 7847.

2. Cheung, W. Y., 1980, Calmodulin plays a pivotal role in cellular regulation. Science 207: 19.

3. Chirgwin, J. M., Przybyla, A. E., Macdonald, R. J. and Rutter, W. J., 1979, Isolation of biologically active ribonucleic acid from sources enriched in ribonuclease. Biochemistry 18: 5294.

4. Fenton, M. J., Clark, B. D., Collins, K. L., Webb, A. C., Rich, A. and Auron, P. E., 1987, Transcriptional regulation of the human prointerleukin 1b gene. J. Immunol. 138: 3972.

5. Hidaka, H., Inagaki, M., Kawamoto, S. and Sasaki, Y., 1984, Isoqunolinesulfonamides, novel and potent inhibitors of cyclic nucleotide dependent protein kinase and protein kinase C. Biochemistry 23: 5036.

6. Hidaka, H., Sasaki, Y., Tanaka, T., Endo, T., Ohno, S., Fujii, Y. and Nagata, T., 1981, N-(6-aminopexyl)-5-chloro-1-naphthalenesulfonamide, a

calmodulin antagonist, inhibits cell proliferation. Proc. Natl. Acad. Sci. U.S.A. 78: 4354.

7. Kakiuchi, S., Yasuda, S., Yamazaki, R., Teshima, Y., Kanada, K. and Soube, K., 1982, Quantitative determinations of calmodulin in the supernatant and particulate fractions of mammalian tissues. J. Biochem. 92: 1041.

8. Koide, S. and Steinman, R. M., 1987, Induction of murine interleukin 1: stimuli and responsive primary cells. Proc. Natl. Acad. Sci. U.S.A. 84: 3802.

9. Laporte, D. C. and Strom, D. R., 1978, Detection of calcium-dependent regulatory protein binding components using ^{125}I-labeled calcium-dependent regulatory protein. J. Biol. Chem. 253: 3347.

10. Lowry, O. H., Rosebrough, N. J., Farr, A. L. and Randall, R. J., 1951, Protein measurement with the Folin phenol reagent. J. Biol. Chem. 193: 265.

11. Maniatis, T., Fritsch, E. F. and Sambrook, J., 1982, "Molecular Cloning," Cold Spring Harbor Laboratory, New York.

12. March, C. J., Mosley, B., Larsen, A., Cerretti, P., Braedt, G., Price, V., Gillis, S., Henney, C. S., Kronheim, S. R., Grabstein, K., Conlon, P. J., Hopp, T. P. and Cosman, D., 1985, Cloning, sequence and expression of two distinct human interleukin-1 complementary DNAs. Nature 315: 641.

13. Matsushima, K., Taguchi, M., Kovaks, E. J., Young, H. A. and Oppenheim, J. J., 1986, Intracellular localization of human monocytes associated interleukin 1 activity and release of biologically active IL-1 from monocytes by trypsin and plasmin. J. Immunol. 136: 2883.

14. Matsushima, K. and Oppenheim, J. J., 1985, Calcium ionophore (A23187) increases interleukin 1 (IL 1) production by human peripheral blood monocytes and interacts synergistically with IL 1 to augment concanavalin A-stimulated thymocyte proliferation. Cell. Immunol. 90: 226.

15. Mizel, S. B., Oppenheim, J. J. and Rosenstreich, D. L., 1978, Characterization of lymphocyte-activating factor (LAF) produced by the macrophage cell line, P388D1. I. Enhancement of LAF production by activated T lymphocytes. J. Immunol. 120: 1497.

16. Nishikawa, M., Tanaka, T. and Hidaka, H., 1980, Ca^{2+}-calmodulin-dependent phosphorylation and platelet secretion. Nature 287: 863.

17. Oppenheim, J. J., Stadler, B. M., Siraganian, R. P., Mage, M. and Mathieson, B., 1982, Lymphokines: Their role in lymphocyte responses. Properties of interleukin 1. Fed. Proc. 47: 257.

18. Orlow, S. J., Rosenstreich, D. L., Pifco-Hirst, S. and Rosen, O. M., 1985, Purification and distribution of a novel macrophage-specific calmodulin-binding glycoprotein. J. Immunol. 134: 449.

19. Prpic, V., Weiel, J. E., Somers, S. D., DiGuiseppi, J., Gonias, S. L., Pizzo, S. V., Hamilton, T. A., Herman, B. and Adams, D. O., 1987, Effects of bacterial lipopolysaccharide on the hydrolysis of phosphatidylinosotol-4,5-bisphosphate in murine peritoneal macrophages. J. Immunol. 139: 526.

20. Rosenstreich, D. L., 1985, Genetic control of endotoxin response: C3H/HeJ mice, in: "Handbook of Endotoxin," L. J. Berry, ed., Elsevier/North-Holland Biomedical Press, New York, 3: 82.

21. Rosenstreich, D. L., Vogel, S. N., Jacques, A. R., Wahl, L. M. and Oppenheim, J. J., 1978, Macrophage sensitivity to endotoxin: genetic control by a single codominant gene. J. Immunol. 121: 1664.

22. Shinomiya H. and Nakano, M., 1987, Calcium ionophore A23187 does not stimulate lipopolysaccharide nonresponsive C3H/HeJ peritoneal macrophages to produce interleukin 1. J. Immunol. 139: 2730.

23. Soube, K., Yamazaki, R., Yasuda, S. and Kakiuchi, S., 1981, Identity of the particulate form of calmodulin with soluble calmodulin. FEBS Lett. 129: 215.

24. Speaker, M. G., Sturgill, T. W., Orlow, S. J., Chia, G. H., Pifcko-Hirst, S. and Rosen, O. M., 1980, The effects of trifluoperazine on the macrophage-like cell line, J774. Ann. N. Y. Acad. Sci. 356: 162.

25. Speaker, M. G., Orlow, S. J., Sturgill, T. W. and Rosen, O. M., 1983, Characterization of a calmodulin-binding protein that is deficient in trifluoperazine-resistant variants of the macrophage-like cell line J774. Proc. Natl. Acad. Sci. U.S.A. 88: 329.

26. Watson, J., Kelly, K. Largen, M. and Taylor, B. A., 1978, The genetic mapping of a defective LPS response gene in C3H/HeJ mice. J. Immunol. 120: 422.

27. Westphal, O. and Lüderitz, O., 1954, Chemische erforschung von lipopolysacchariden gram-negative bakterien. Angew. Chem. 66: 407.

THE ROLE OF 13-HYDROXYLINOLEIC ACID IN THE ACTIVATION OF MACROPHAGES BY LIPOPOLYSACCHARIDE

U. F. Schade, I. Burmeister, R. Engel, H. Lode and I. Kozka

Forschungsinstitut Borstel, Institut fur Experimentelle Medizin und Biologie, D-2061 Borstel, FRG

INTRODUCTION

Bacterial lipopolysaccharides (LPS, endotoxin) are known to activate various functions and morphological properties of mononuclear phagocytes both in vivo and in vitro (11, 15). Recently, it has been reported that phagocytosis in bone marrow derived macrophage cultures was stimulated with LPS, indicating a direct interaction between endotoxin and the cells (4). The mechanism of the activation of monocytes is unknown. However, some LPS induced phenomena require the presence of arachidonic acid metabolites, e.g., the LPS-induced production of collagenase (1) and the release of interleukin 1 (5). In order to determine the possible role of cyclooxygenases and lipoxygenases in the activation of macrophages by LPS, the effects of several inhibitors of these enzymes on the binding and uptake of zymosan particles by macrophages primed with LPS was investigated and a lipoxygenase product, 13-hydroxyoctadecadienoic acid (13-HODD) was isolated from activated cells. Addition of exogenous 13-HODD led to increased association/uptake of zymosan with the cells. Therefore, our results suggest that 13-HODD is possibly involved in the activation process of macrophages by LPS.

MATERIALS AND METHODS

Lipopolysaccharide

LPS from S. abortus equi and free lipid A from E. coli which had been prepared according to (6) were kind gifts of Dr. H. Brade (Forschungsinstitut Borstel).

Macrophages

Resident mouse peritoneal macrophages (NMRI mice, 6-8 weeks) were used throughout the experiments described here (3).

Assay for Zymosan Association

Quantitative determination of the phagocytic capacity of macrophages was determined as described (16). Adherent macrophages (2×10^5 on glass coverslips) were incubated with LPS (10 - 100 ng/ml, 20 h), and fluorescent zymosan was added. The cells were allowed to take up particles (10 min) and the association index (AI) was determined using a fluorescent microscope, after washing the cultures and fixation with methanol. (AI = number of cells with bound particles x bound particles/ total number of cells counted x 100/total number of cells counted). Samples were prepared in triplicates and the stimulation was expressed as the multiple of the AI of untreated cell cultures which was set to 1 ± standard deviation (S.D.).

Determination of 13-Hydroxyoctadecadienoic Acid (13-HODD)

Macrophages (2 x 10^6) were incubated with LPS (100 ng/ml, 20 hr), the supernatants discarded and the remaining cells solubilized (2 ml 0.25% desoxycholate, containing 250 ng prostaglandin B1 as internal standard). After the addition of ethanol (2ml), the fluid phase was evaporated in a vacuum centrifuge and the residue hydrolyzed (1 N NaOH in methanol, 37°C, 1 hr). The hydrolysate was acidified (pH 3.5), extracted (3 x 1 ml $CHCl_3$), evaporated under nitrogen and analyzed by reverse phase HPLC (5um RP-18, acetonitril/H_2O, UV-detection at 280/235 nm). Chiralphase HPLC was carried out on a DNBPG-Chiral phase HPLC-column (Baker) according to (9). 13-HODD, eluting from the RP-HPLC was collected, converted to the methylester and chromatographed on the chiral column with hexane/isopropanol (99.4/0.6) as eluent (UV-detection at 235 nm). Soybean lipoxygenase (Sigma) was used to produce 13(S)-HODD as described in (8). Racemic 13-HODD was obtained by photooxidation of linoleic acid in the presence of methylene blue according to (2).

RESULTS

Stimulation of Zymosan Binding to Macrophages

Mouse peritoneal macrophages, after pretreatment with endotoxin in vitro were significantly stimulated in their capacity to bind zymosan particles. Optimal stimulation of the uptake was observed at doses between 50-150 ng/ml (Fig 1).

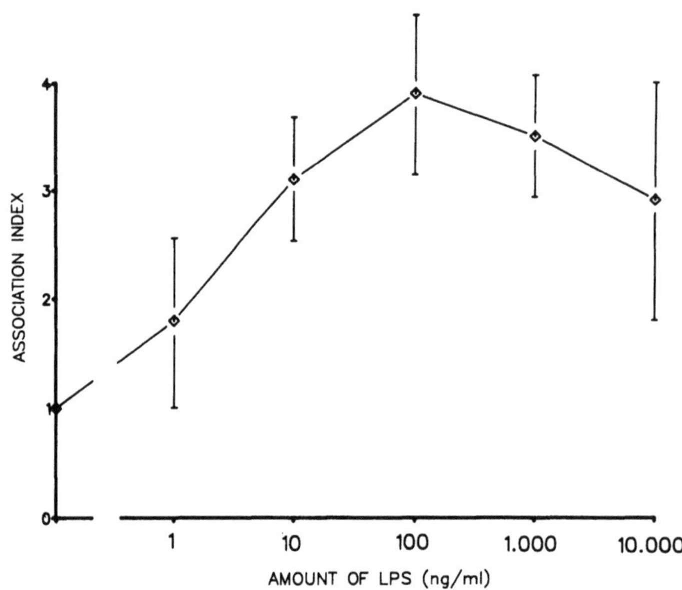

Fig 1. The effect of LPS on the phagocytic capacity of mouse peritoneal macrophages (uptake of zymosan particles).

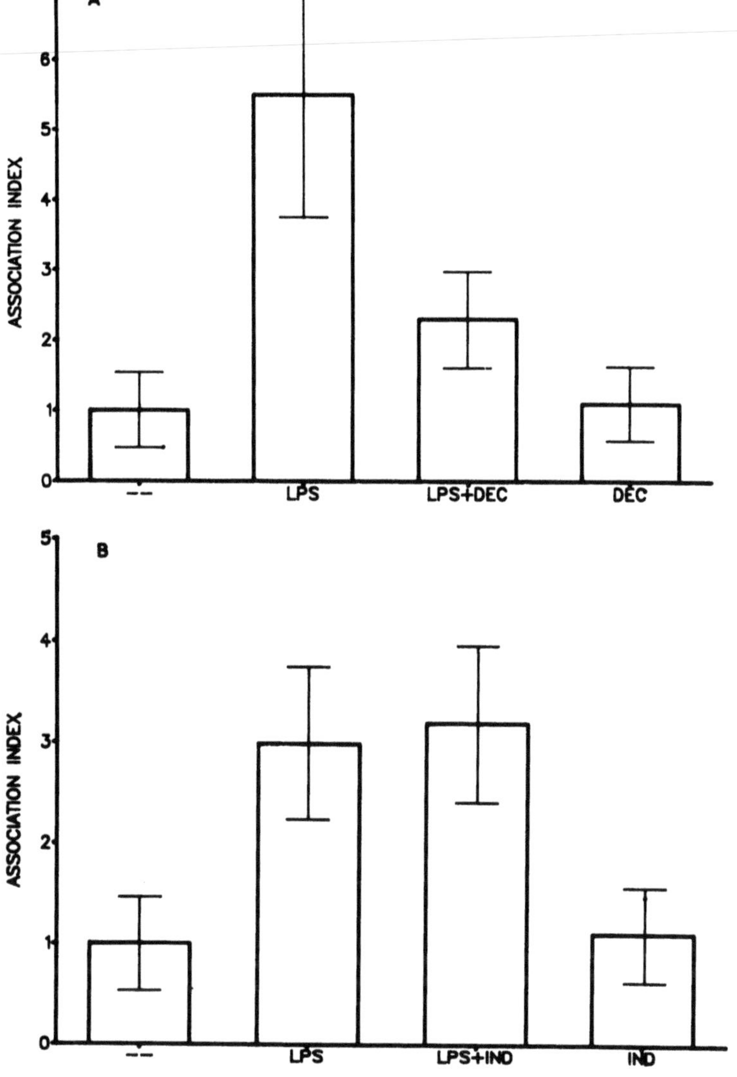

Fig 2. Association indices determined in the presence of LPS, DEC and indomethacin in macrophage cultures.

The activation of zymosan association was dose dependent (Fig 1) and could be achieved with bacterial and synthetic free lipid A (data not shown).

Involvement of Lipoxygenases in the Activation of Macrophages by Endotoxin

In order to test the possible involvement of lipoxygenases or cyclooxygenases in the activation of macrophages, LPS pretreatment of cell-cultures was carried out in the presence of a series of inhibitors of these enzymes. Examples of experiments with diethylcarbamazine (DEC, lipoxygenaseblocker, 7) and indomethacin (Indo, cyclooxygenaseblocker) are presented in Fig 2. The AI of cells treated with LPS was 5.6 ± 1.4. Treatment of macrophages with DEC in addition to LPS resulted in an AI of 3.3 ± 0.6 (2.6 uM) and 2.2 ± 0.3 (26 uM) respectively (Fig 2 A).

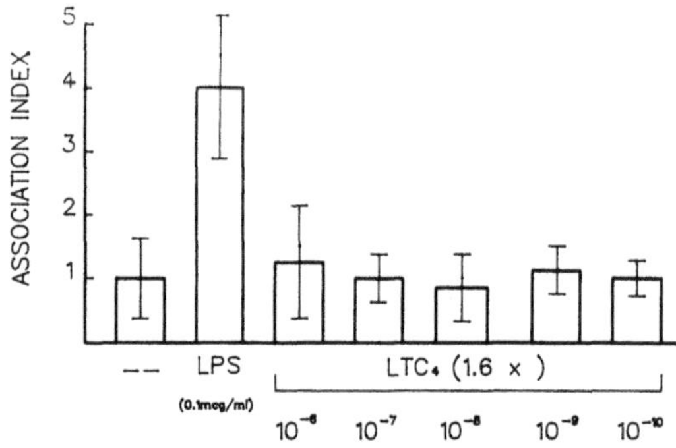

Fig 3. Association indices of macrophages pretreated with LPS or LTC4.

In contrast, the cyclooxygenase inhibitor indomethacin (0.3 uM) did not influence the LPS-induced activation of particle ingestion (Fig. 2 B). Neither DEC nor indomethacin influenced the basal zymosan phagocytosis of untreated macrophages.

The Influence of Lipoxygenase Products on Zymosan Association

Synthetic leukotrienes were tested for their ability to stimulate phagocytic properties of resident macrophages. Cell cultures were incubated with LTC4 and LTB4 (10^{-9} - 10^{-5} Mol, 20 hr) and binding of zymosan determined. As shown in Fig 3, pretreatment with LTC4 did not alter the uptake of particles by macrophages. Also, preincubation with LTB4 was uneffective (data not shown).

However, when peritoneal macrophages were preincubated with the lipoxygenase product 13-HODD (derived from incubation of linoleic acid with soybean lipoxygenase, see material and methods), the binding of zymosan compared to untreated controls was increased (Fig 4).

Incubation of the cells with 3.3 x 10^{-9} M 13-HODD led to an AI comparable to that achieved with 100 ng LPS/ml. In order to exclude possible LPS contamination of the 13-HODD sample, the macrophage pretreatment was carried out in the presence of polymyxine B (PMX) at a concentration which abolished the effect of 100 ng LPS/ml (Fig 4). 13-HODD stimulated the binding capacity of the cells for zymosan also in the presence of polymyxine B.

Determination of 13-HODD in LPS-Stimulated Macrophages

Mouse peritoneal macrophages (2 x 10^{7}) were incubated with LPS (100 ng/ml, 20 hr), the supernatants discarded, the remaining cells lysed and hydrolysates were prepared as described in the materials and methods section. After HPLC, a compound was isolated which eluted with the retention time of synthetic 13-HODD and had the same UV-spectrum. GC-MS analysis of the methylester, trimethylsilyl ether, confirmed the identity of the material isolated from macrophages as 13-HODD. In order to determine the configuration of the macrophage product, the methylester was applied to chiral phase HPLC. For comparison, a racemic mixture of 13-HODD and 9-HODD methylesters (prepared by photolysis of linoleic acid) and 13-HODD (prepared with the help of soybean lipoxygenase) were also analyzed by chiral phase HPLC. As shown in Fig 5, 13-HODD from macrophages eluted with the retention time of 13-HODD from soybean lipoxygenase and, therefore, possesses the (S)-configuration (8).

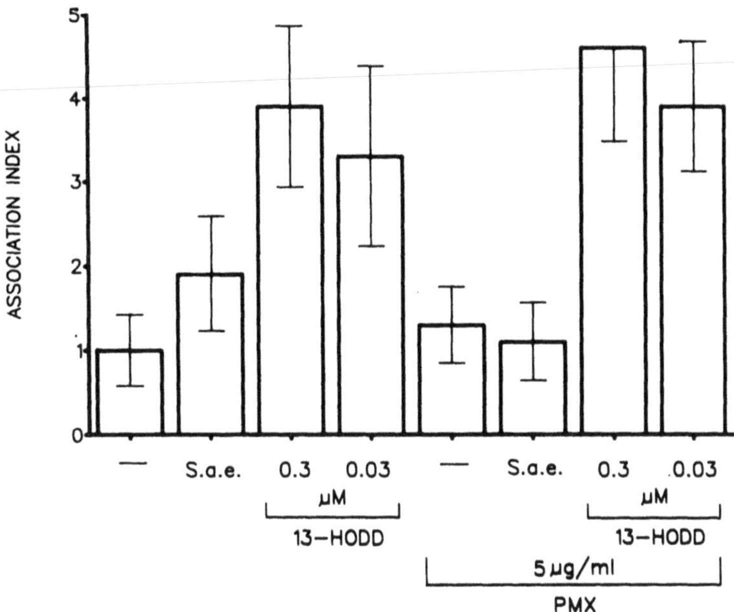

Fig 4. Association indices of macrophages pretreated with LPS or 13-HODD (PMX = Polymyxine B).

Quantitation of 13-HODD in LPS-Stimulated Macrophages

13-HODD from unstimulated and LPS-activated macrophages was isolated and quantitatively determined by HPLC. As shown in Table 1, LPS-treatment increased the content of 13-HODD in hydrolysates of macrophages significantly.

DISCUSSION

The activating potential of lipopolysaccharides for mononuclear phagocytes has been recognized for several experimental parameters like the tumoricidal action (15), release of superoxide anion (13) and the release of lysosomal enzymes (12). We have found that treatment of mouse peritoneal macrophages in vitro with endotoxin increases the association/uptake of zymosan particles by these cells. In order to define the possible involvement of eicosanoids in this LPS effect, inhibitors of the two pathways of arachidonic acid metabolism present in macrophages (lipoxygenase and cylooxygenase) were tested for their influence on the activation of the cells. When macrophages were incubated with DEC, the LPS-induced activation (enhanced zymosan association) was prevented. Indomethacin, however, did not interfere with increased zymosan association (16). DEC is an inhibitor of lipoxygenases while indomethacin blocks cyclooxygenase. Since DEC prevented LPS action, it is concluded that lipoxygenases are involved in the activation of macrophages with LPS.

It has been shown that LPS induces the synthesis of LTC4 in macrophages (10). In order to find out whether LTC4 is involved in the activation of macrophages by LPS, it was tested for its effects on phagocytic properties of macrophages. As shown in Fig 3, LTC4 has no influence on this cellular function. Pretreatment with 13-HODD, however, led to a stimulation of macrophages comparable to LPS (Fig 4).

Recently it was found that lipoxygenase products (mono-HETE's) are integrated into phospholipids of macrophages and polymorphonucleated neutro-

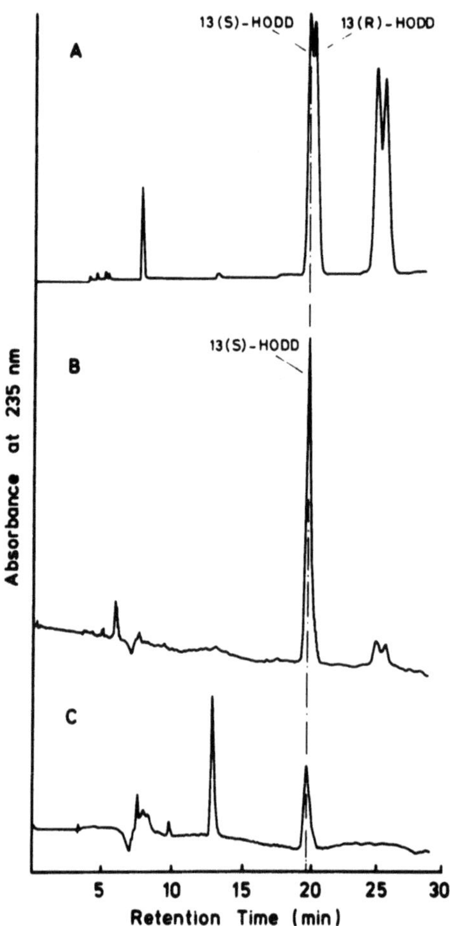

Fig 5. Chiral phase HPLC of a racemic mixture of 13- and 9-HODD (A), 13-HODD prepared by lipoxygenase (B), and 13-HODD from macrophage hydrolysates (C).

Table 1. Quantitative determination of 13-HODD in quiescent and LPS-stimulated macrophages

Pretreatment of macrophages	13-HODD formed
	(pg/μg protein)
[1]Pi/Nacl	32 ± 5
LPS (100 ng/ml, 20 h)	178 ± 14

[1]Pi/NaCl: phosphate buffered saline

phils (14, 18). Our findings show, that endogenously synthesized 13-HODD is present in macrophages in a bound form. Since mammalian lipoxygenases catalyze the oxygenation of unsaturated fatty acids with high regio- and stereoselectivity (8), the identification of the product from stimulated macrophages as 13 (S)-HODD (Fig 5) (17) indicates its enzymatic origin. LPS stimulated macrophages contained about 8 times more 13-HODD than unstimulated controls.

In summary, our results show that LPS-primed macrophages produce increased amounts of 13-HODD and can be stimulated by this compound. These findings suggest that this linoleic acid metabolite is involved in the activation of macrophages by LPS.

ACKNOWLEDGEMENTS

The skilled technical assistance of Ms. S. Fuchs and S. Cohrs is kindly appreciated. This study was supported by grant Scha 402/1-2 from the Deutsche Forschungsgemeinschaft. I. Burmeister is a recipient of a scholarship of the Kultusminister of Schleswig-Holstein (3156.45-7-2). LTC4 and LTB4 were generously donated by Dr. J. Rokach, Merck-Frosst, Canada.

REFERENCES

1. Bhatnagar, R., Schade, U., Rietschel, E. T. and Decker, K., 1982, Involvement of prostaglandin E and adenosine 3',5'-mono-phosphate in lipopolysaccharide stimulated collagenase release by rat Kuppfer cells. Eur. J. Biochem. 125: 125.

2. Camp, R. D. R., Mallet, A. I., Woollard, P. M., Brain, S. D., Black, A. K. and Greaves, M. W., 1983, The identification of hydroxy fatty acids in psoriatic skin. Prostaglandins 26: 431.

3. Conrad, R. E., 1981, Induction and collection of peritoneal exudate macrophages, in: "Manual of macrophage methodology," H. B. Herscowitz, H. T. Holden, J. A. Bellanti and A. Ghaffar, eds., Marcel Dekker, New York.

4. Cooper, P. H., Mayer, P. and Baggiolini, M., 1984, Stimulation of phagocytosis in bone marrow derived mouse macrophages, by bacterial lipopolysaccharide: correlation with biochemical and functional parameters. J. Immunol. 133: 913.

5. Dinarrelo, C. A., Bishai, J., Rosenwasser, L. J. and Coceani, F., 1984, The influence of lipoxygenase inhibitors on the in vitro production of human leukocytic pyrogen and lymphocyte activating factor (interleukin-1), Int. J. Immunopharmac. 6: 43.

6. Galanos, C. and Luderitz, O., 1984, O, Lipopolysaccharide: properties of an amphipathic molecule in: "Handbook of endotoxin, vol 1: chemistry of endotoxin," E. Th. Rietschel, ed., Elsevier Science Publishers, B. V. Amsterdam New York Oxford.

7. Hagmann, W. and Keppler, D., 1982, Leukotriene antagonists prevent endotoxin lethality. Naturwissenschaften 69: 594.

8. Hamberg, M. and Samuelsson, B., 1967, Oxygenation of unsaturated fatty acids by the vesicular gland of sheep. J. Biol. Chem. 242: 5344.

9. Kuhn, H., Wiesner, R., Lankin, V. Z., Nekrasov, A., Alder, L. and Schewe, T., 1987, Analysis of the stereochemistry of lipoxygenase-derived

hydroxypolyenoic fatty acids by means of chiral phase HPLC. Anal. Biochem. 160: 24.

10. Luderitz, T., Schade, U. F. and Rietschel, E. T., 1986, Formation and metabolism of leukotriene C4 in macrophages exposed to bacterial lipopolysaccharide. Eur. J. Biochem. 155: 377.

11. Morland, B. and Kaplan, G., 1977, Macrophage activation in vivo and in vitro. Exp. Cell Res. 108: 279.

12. Morland, B., 1979, Studies on selective induction of lysosomal enzyme activities of mouse peritoneal macrophages. J. Reticuloendothel. Soc. 26: 79.

13. Pabst, M. J. and Johnston, R. B., 1980, Increased production of superoxide anion by macrophages exposed in vitro to muramyl dipeptide or lipopolysaccharide. J. Exp. Med. 151: 101.

14. Pawlowski, N. A., Scott, W. A., Andreach, M. and Cohn, Z. A., 1982, Uptake and metabolism of monohydroxyeicosatetraenoic acids by macrophages. J. Exp. Med. 155: 1653.

15. Rosenstreich, D. L. and Vogel, S. N., 1980, Central role of macrophages in the host response to endotoxin, in: "Microbiology-1980", D. Schlessinger, ed., Am. Soc. Microbiol. Washington : 11.

16. Schade, U. F., 1986, Involvement of lipoxygenases in the activation of mouse macrophages by endotoxin. Biochem. Biophys. Res. Commun. 38: 842.

17. Schade, U. F., Burmeister, I. and Engel, R., 1987, Increased 13-hydroxyoctadecadienoic acid content in lipopolysaccharide stimulated macrophages. Biochem. Biophys. Res. Commun. 147:695.

18. Stenson, W. F. and Parker, C. W., 1979, 12-L-Hydroxy-5,8,10,14-eicosatetraenoic acid, a chemotactic fatty acid, is incorporated into neutrophil phospholipids and triglyceride. Prostaglandins 18: 285.

MODULATION OF INTERLEUKIN 1 PRODUCTION BY ENDOTOXIN, PERTUSSIS TOXIN, AND INDOMETHACIN

T. W. Klein, C. A. Newton, F. R. Vogel, H. Friedman, M. Lucas*, A. Rodloff* and H. Hahn*

University of South Florida, College of Medicine, Tampa, Florida USA, *Institute for Medical Microbiology, Free University of Berlin, Berlin, FRG

INTRODUCTION

Bordetella pertussis is the causative agent of whooping cough and little is known concerning the pathophysiology of the disease process. This is partially due to the fact that there is no suitable animal model for studying whooping cough. This microorganism produces a variety of toxins and biologically active extracellular products (10) including endotoxin (LPS) and the ADP-ribosylating toxin called pertussis toxin. **B. pertussis** endotoxin is typical in that it is composed of lipid A, a KDO residue and a polysaccharide portion (1, 4). This endotoxin has many of the biological properties of endotoxins from the family **Enterobacteriacea** including lethal toxicity, B lymphocyte mitogenicity, induction of the Shwartzman phenomenon, and pyrogenicity. In addition, crude LPS and the isolated polysaccharide group have been demonstrated to induce the formation of interleukin 1 in human monocyte preparations (1, 4). However, purified lipid A was unable to induce IL 1 in monocytes, but was pyrogenic (1).

The immunomodulating potential of endotoxins has led some authors to speculate that vertebrates have evolved cellular receptors capable of recognizing LPS and aiding lymphocytes and macrophages to make vigorous responses to pathogenic microorganisms (2). It is also likely, however, that the microorganisms under pressure to evolve, might have adapted by means of producing "virulence" components to counteract the LPS-induced augmented host defenses. One such evasive virulence factor which appears to down regulate LPS augmented responses is pertussis toxin (5, 16, TW Klein, FR Vogel, B Lozier, and WE Stewart, Abstr. Annu. Meet., Am. Soc. Microbiol., 1985, E20, p. 78). Pertussis toxin (PT) has been demonstrated to disrupt the control of the adenylate cyclase system in various cells by catalyzing the ADP-ribosylation of the Gi protein resulting in the "uncoupling" of Gi from the inhibitory receptor and thereby causing a loss of inhibitory receptor agonist action (12). However, studies in other cell systems suggest that PT might, in addition to affecting the activity of adenylate cyclase, also affect G proteins controlling the activity of the enzyme phospholipase C (13). Recently, we and others have observed (5; TW Klein, et al., Abstr. Ann. Meet., Am. Soc. Microbiol, 1985, E20, p. 78) that pertussis toxin can counteract the LPS augmenting capacity of interleukin 1 production. In the present series of studies we wished to further examine the potential interaction of multiple microbial toxins in regulating the production of IL 1 which is known to be involved in host resistance mechanisms.

MATERIALS AND METHODS

Animals

Female mice of strains BDF1 and C3H/HeJ were obtained from Jackson Laboratories, Bar Harbor, ME. The BDF1 mice were used as a source of macrophages while the C3H/HeJ mice were used as a source of thymocytes for the IL 1 assay. The mice were housed and cared for according to NIH guidelines and were used in experiments at either five to eight weeks of age (C3H/HeJ) or six to nine weeks of age (BDF1).

Drugs and Reagents

Pertussis toxin was kindly provided by Rino Rappuoli, Sclavo Research Center, Siena, Italy. The toxin was purified from the culture supernatant of a **B. pertussis** culture (strain BP165) by affinity chromatography as described (14). PT was diluted in phosphate buffered saline (PBS) and added to the cultures at the concentrations indicated. **Escherichia coli** (E. coli) strain 0127:B8, LPS was purchased from Calbiochem, San Diego, CA. The LPS was a phenol-water extracted material which was further purified by chromatography. The LPS was solubilized and sterilized for use by boiling in PBS for 30 min prior to use. Indomethacin was purchased from Sigma Chemical Co., St. Louis, MO and was initially dissolved in 0.1 M Na_2CO_3 prior to diluting in tissue culture medium for use. **Legionella pneumophila**, serogroup 1, bacteria were grown and killed with formalin as previously described (6). The killed bacteria were suspended in PBS and adjusted to the working concentration of approximately 3×10^9 bacteria/ml. The bacteria were added to the macrophage cultures to achieve a final concentration of 10^8/ml. The complete tissue culture medium used throughout these studies was RPMI 1640 medium (Gibco Laboratories, Madison, WI) supplemented with 10% fetal calf serum (Hyclone Laboratories, Logan, UT), penicillin (100 units/ml), streptomycin (100 ug/ml), L-glutamine, and 2-mercaptoethanol (5×10^{-5}M).

Peritoneal Cells

Resident peritoneal cells were obtained from BDF1 mice by peritoneal lavage with RPMI 1640 medium. Lavaged leukocytes were pooled, diluted in tissue culture medium and washed by centrifugation. The washed cells were adjusted to a final concentration of 5×10^5 cells/ml. The peritoneal cells (0.1 ml) were plated in 96 well flat-bottom tissue culture plates (Costar), incubated for 2 hr in 5% CO_2, rinsed vigorously several times with warm tissue culture medium to remove nonadherent cells, and subsequently treated with the various drugs and toxins.

IL 1 Production and Assay

Peritoneal macrophage cultures, in 96 well plates, were treated with either LPS or **L. pneumophila** bacteria and in some instances also treated simultaneously with either indomethacin or indomethacin plus pertussis toxin and incubated for 18 to 24 hr at 37°C in 5% CO_2. Following incubation, 0.1 ml of supernatant was removed from each culture and transferred to a fresh 96 well tissue culture plate. These supernatant samples were refrigerated and subsequently assayed for soluble IL 1 activity as previously described (6). The residual culture cells were washed and fixed with paraformaldehyde and analyzed for membrane associated interleukin 1 as previously described (9). Briefly, treated macrophages were washed two times with warm complete tissue culture medium and fixed in 1% paraformaldehyde in PBS for 15 min at room temperature. Following fixation, the paraformaldehyde was removed by several cycles of washing with complete tissue culture medium followed by 1 to 2 hr incubation in complete tissue culture medium at 37°C. To the paraformaldehyde fixed and rinsed cells were added thymocyte suspensions (1.5×10^6

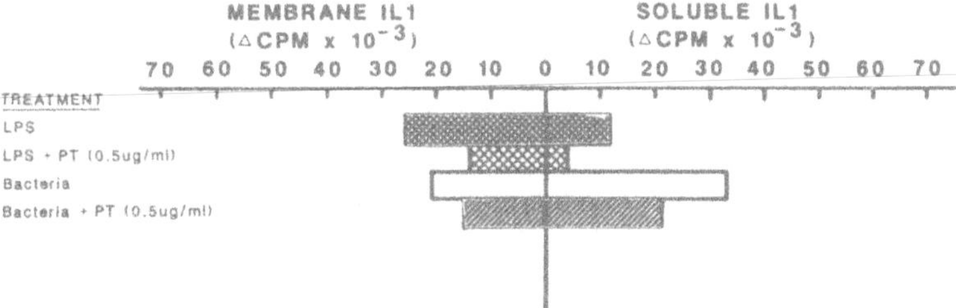

Fig 1. Inhibition of mIL1 and sIL1 activity by pertussis toxin. Macrophages were treated with either LPS (10 µg/ml) or **Legionella pneumophila** bacteria (10^8 bacteria/ml) in either the presence or absence of pertussis toxin (PT). See Materials and Methods for details.

cells/ well) prepared from C3H/HeJ endotoxin low responder mice. A submitogenic concentration of concanavalin A (0.2 µg/ml) was also added to each well. These cultures as well as thymocyte cultures containing test supernatants were incubated for 48 hours, pulsed with 0.5 uCi ^{3}H-thymidine (ICN) for 18 to 20 hr and the incorporated radioactivity determined following harvesting and counting in a scintillation counter.

RESULTS

The interactive effect of multiple virulence factors released from bacteria on the modulation of host resistance mechanisms has become an area of active investigation. Several years ago we reported (16) that pertussis toxin suppressed antibody formation possibly by inducing the formation of interferon gamma. Alternatively, the modulation of antibody production could have resulted from a pertussis toxin induced modulation of other cytokine formation and subsequently we (T.W. Klein et al., Abstr. Ann. Meet., Am. Soc. Microbiol., 1985, E20, p. 78) and others (5) demonstrated that the formation of both soluble IL 1 (sIL 1) and membrane IL 1 (mIL 1) were suppressed by the toxin. Figure 1 demonstrates the PT effect on the mIL 1 response and the sIL 1 response of mouse peritoneal macrophages stimulated by either a soluble stimulus such as LPS or stimulated by the interaction with the whole bacterial cell. The data show that pertussis toxin suppresses the formation of both forms of IL 1 induced in response to both forms of the stimulating agent. Also of interest was the finding that both bacterial cells and LPS produce equivalent amounts of mIL 1 but that the whole bacteria appeared to promote the release of sIL 1 from the macrophages to a greater extent than the LPS.

Prostaglandins formed in response to stimulation with LPS have been reported to negatively regulate the formation of IL 1 (7, 8). Treatment of cells, therefore, with a cyclooxygenase inhibitor such as indomethacin should augment interleukin 1 production. Figure 2 shows that stimulation of peritoneal macrophages with either LPS or Legionella bacteria in the presence of indomethacin substantially enhances the amounts of sIL 1 but appears to have little affect on the production or expression of mIL 1. Prostaglandins modulate IL 1 production at the molecular level possible by altering cAMP regulated systems (7). Because pertussis toxin has been reported to regulate cAMP production (12), it seemed possible that the simultaneous treatment of cells with both indomethacin and pertussis toxin may result in drug antagonism or interference effects. Figure 3 shows that PT can down-regulate the expression of both functional forms of IL 1 by mechanisms independent of cyclooxygenase activity. It is possible, therefore, that pathways other than the prostaglandin/cAMP pathway are involved in the PT induced down-regulation of IL 1 production.

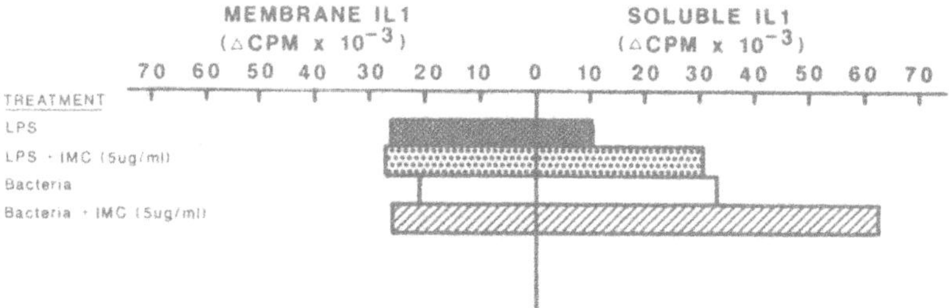

Fig 2. Enhancement of sIL1 activity by indomethacin. Macrophages were treated with either LPS (10 ug/ml) or **Legionella pneumophila** bacteria (10^8 bacteria/ml) in either the presence of absence of indomethacin (IMC). See Materials and Methods for details.

DISCUSSION

The observation that LPS induced cells to produce a lymphocyte activating factor (LAF; IL 1) and release this substance into the culture supernatant was reported 18 years ago (3). Until recently, however, the molecular events responsible for the production and release of this immunopotentiating factor were not understood. Presently we know that LPS binds to responding cells by an as of yet ill defined receptor moiety and that within hours following this binding the cell responds by producing prostaglandin E 1 (PGE_1) and IL 1 possible by mechanisms involving the phosphatidylinositol/ phospholipase C pathway coupled to the activation of protein kinase C (17). Evidence suggests that as the concentration of PGE increases it causes a transient increase in cAMP (7) through the protein kinase A pathway which may be responsible for the observed down-regulation of IL 1 production. Such a bidirectional control and antagonism between the protein kinase C (PKC) and the protein kinase A (PKA) pathways has been proposed (15).

The inhibitory effect of prostaglandin on IL 1 production appears to occur at a post-transcriptional stage of gene expression (7) and can be prevented by the simultaneous addition to macrophage cultures of drugs such as indomethacin which inhibit the cyclooxygenase enzyme activity thereby lowering the production of prostaglandins (7, 8). This augmention of IL 1 production in the presence of indomethacin is demonstrated in Fig 2. Jakway and DeFranco have reported (2, 5) that LPS modulates B cell and macrophage function by activating the receptor coupled Gi component thus inhibiting adenylate cyclase activity. To support this hypothesis, the authors reported that the pretreatment of cell membranes with LPS abolished the ADP-ribosylating activity of Gi by pertussis toxin and conversely the pretreat-

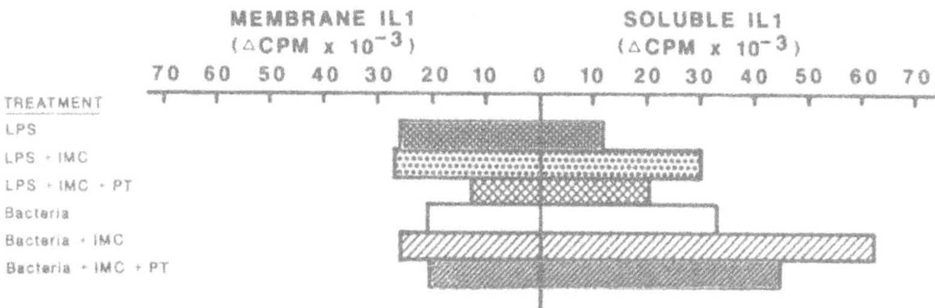

Fig 3. Inhibition by pertussis toxin of mIL1 and sIL1 activity in presence of indomethacin. Macrophages were treated as in Figure 2 and also treated with pertussis toxin (PT; 0.5 μg/ml). See Materials and Methods for details.

ment of cells with pertussis toxin diminished the IL 1 producing capacity of macrophages. In the latter case, the toxin was suggested to uncouple Gi from any inhibitory effect on adenylate cyclase and thus prolong the increase in cyclic AMP and further depress IL 1 production. Because of our interest in examining the interactive nature of the simultaneous addition of microbial toxins on immune responsiveness, we were studying the effect of PT on LPS induced IL 1 production. We observed as reported by Jakway (5) that the pretreatment of macrophages with pertussis toxin decreased a subsequent effect of LPS on IL 1 production. However, we also noticed that the simultaneous addition of both PT and LPS to the cultures also decreased IL 1 production (Fig 1). This result was somewhat unexpected because PT has been reported to inactivate Gi only when Gi is in the inactive form and not once it has been activated as would possibly be the case in the presence of LPS (5, 12). Our results suggested to us that in the case of simultaneous addition of LPS and PT, either the PT was inactivating Gi more rapidly than the LPS could activate it or the PT was suppressing IL 1 production by mechanisms other than adenylate cyclase/protein kinase A pathway. Nakamura and Ui (13) reported that PT can decrease phosphatidylinositol breakdown and other events involved in membrane signal transduction by an ADP-ribosylating reaction which does not result in the enhanced accumulation of cAMP. In addition, G proteins have been reported to regulate both adenylate cyclase (PKA pathways) and phosphoinositidase C (PKC pathway) (17). Because of this we felt it was possible that the PT could be inhibiting through both PKA and PKC and would therefore inhibit IL 1 production in the relative absence of prostaglandins and PKA activation as in the case of the indomethacin-treated cell. Figure 3 shows that the simultaneous addition of LPS, PT and indomethacin results in reduced mIL 1 and sIL 1 levels relative to the indomethacin only treated group. In the relative absence of prostaglandins production, pertussis toxin is still able to suppress IL 1 production by the macrophage suggesting that the toxin can inhibit by mechanisms other than prostaglandin/cAMP. Studies are currently in progress to determine the phosphoinositidase C and PKC activity of resident macrophage populations under the conditions of simultaneous stimulation with both LPS and PT. It is hoped from these studies to better understand the molecular changes in cells responding to multiple membrane perterbations caused by the encounter with multiple microbial toxins.

ACKNOWLEDGEMENTS

We thank Mrs. Sally Baker for the typing and preparation of this manuscript.

REFERENCES

1. Caroff, M., Cavaillon, J., Fitting, C. and Haeffner-Cavaillon, N., 1986, Inability of pyrogenic, purified Bordetella pertussis lipid A to induce interleukin-1 release by human monocytes. Infect. Immun. 54: 465.

2. DeFranco, A. L., Gold., M. R. and Jakway, J. P., 1987, B-lymphocyte signal transduction in response to anti-immunoglobulin and bacterial lipopolysaccharide. Immunol. Rev. 95: 161.

3. Gery, I., Gershon, R. K. and Waksman, B. H., 1972, Potentiation of the T-lymphocyte response to mitogens. J. Exper. Med. 136: 128.

4. Haeffner-Cavaillon, N., Cavaillon, J., Moreau, M. and Szabo, L., 1984, Interleukin 1 secretion by human monocytes stimulated by the isolated polysaccharide region of the Bordetella pertussis endotoxin. Mol. Immunol. 21: 389.

5. Jakway, J. P. and DeFranco, A. L., 1986, Pertussis toxin inhibition of B cell and macrophage responses to bacterial lipopolysaccharide. Science 234: 743.

6. Klein, T. W., Newton, C. A., Blanchard, D. K., Widen, R. and Friedman, H., 1987, Induction of interleukin 1 by Legionella pneumophila antigens in mouse macrophage and human mononuclear leukocyte cultures. Zbl. Bakt. Hyg. A 265: 462.

7. Knudsen, P. J., Dinarello, C. A. and Strom, T. B., 1986, Prostaglandins post transcriptionally inhibit monocyte expression of interleukin 1 activity by increasing intracellular cyclic adenosine monophosphate. J. Immunol. 137: 3189.

8. Kunkel, S. L., Chensue, S. W. and Phan, S. H., 1986, Prostaglandins as endogenous mediators of interleukin 1 production. J. Immunol. 136: 186.

9. Kurt-Jones, E. A., Beller, D. I., Mizel, S. B. and Unanue, E. R., 1985, Identification of a membrane-associated interleukin 1 in macrophages. Proc. Natl. Acad. Sci. USA 82: 1204.

10. Manclark, C. R. and Cowell, J. L., 1984, in: "Bacterial Vaccines", R. Germanier ed., Academic Press, Inc., Orlando, FL, p. 69-106.

11. Mitchell, B. and Kirk, C., 1986, G-protein control of inositol phosphate hydrolysis. Nature 323: 112.

12. Moss, J., Stanley, S. J., Watkins, P. A., Burns, D. L., Manclark, C. R., Kaslow, H. R. and Hewlett, E. L., 1986, Stimulation of the thiol-dependent ADP-ribosyltransferase and NAD glycohydrolase activity of Bordetella pertussis toxin by adenine nucleotides, phospholipids, and detergents. Biochem. 25: 2720.

13. Nakamura, T. and Ui, M., 1985, Simultaneous inhibitions of inositol phospholipid breakdown, arachidonic acid release, and histamine secretion in mass cells by islet-activating protein, pertussis toxin. J. Biol. Chem. 260: 3584.

14. Nicosia, A., Perugini, M., Franzini, C., Casagli, M. C., Borri, M. G., Antoni, G., Almoni, M., Neri, P., Ratti, G. and Rappuoli, R., 1986, Cloning and sequencing of the pertussis toxin genes: operon structure and gene duplication. Proc. Ntl. Acad. Sci. USA 83: 4631.

15. Nishizuka, Y., 1986, Studies and perspectives of protein kinase C. Science 233: 305.

16. Vogel, F. R., Klein, T. W., Stewart, W. E., Igarashi, T. and Friedman, H., 1985, Immune suppression and induction of gamma interferon by pertussis toxin. Infect. Immun. 49: 90.

17. Wightman, P. D. and Raetz, C. R. H., 1984, The activation of protein kinase C by biologically active lipid moieties of lipopolysaccharide. J. Biol. Chem. 259: 10048.

IMMUNOPHARMACOLOGIC ASPECTS OF LIPOPOLYSACCHARIDE ENDOTOXIN ACTION WITH SPECIAL REFERENCE TO CYCLIC NUCLEOTIDES

J. W. Hadden

Program of Immunopharmacology, Department of Internal Medicine, University of South Florida College of Medicine Tampa, Florida 33612

INTRODUCTION

Lipopolysaccharides (LPS) are responsible for the immunopharmacologic activities of the endotoxins of gram-negative bacteria. This chapter will discuss their immunopharmacologic actions and the evidence that their actions are mediated in part by cyclic nucleotides. The lipopolysaccharides are ubiquitous in nature and have many immunomodulatory activities. As a result, many immunologists consider them ever present nuisances perturbing their experiments. Clearly in the context of endotoxemia and sepsis the toxicities of endotoxins on the body's defense systems, including hyperpyrexia, intravascular coagulation, reticuloendothelial system (RES) blockade, etc., can be considered host destructive. On the other hand, in the absence of disease, low doses of endotoxins may be considered positive immunoregulators contributing to more effective host defense. It is possible to envision them as being part of the host defense mechanism. It may be that the nonpathogenic gastrointestinal flora provides a continuous low level of LPS acting as hormonal signals to promote the development and enhance the function of the entire immune system. Endotoxins regulate, either directly or indirectly, almost every phase of the development and function of the natural and specific immune defense systems of the body. They generally promote growth and function of the cell populations involved. They do so at low concentrations (ng/ml), i.e., at concentrations which may be periodically, even regularly, achieved locally and perhaps also systemically. Finally, they appear to act via the cyclic nucleotide pathways by which many of the body's hormones act and many of the molecules mediating immune function are also thought to act. They, therefore, qualify as messengers acting via receptors and hormonal pathways in physiologically constructive ways.

Immunopharmacologic Actions of Endotoxin

In Vivo Studies

Endotoxins by nature of their polysaccharide components are antigenic and through their diversity elicit antibodies capable of neutralizing their function and limiting their immunotoxic and dysregulatory actions on the system. The lipid A moiety is generally considered to provide the basis of the immunoregulatory functions although there is not unanimity on this point for all aspects of the nonspecific action of LPS on the immune system and evidence for a role of the polysaccharide moiety exists (see Nowotny in this text). The many actions of LPS on the immune system have been reviewed extensively in this book and elsewhere (see 48, 62). Endotoxins generally enhance host resistance to pathogen challenge, particularly when administered prior to challenge. They enhance resistance to transplantable tumors and are part of tumor destructive processes initiated by bacterial immunotherapies such as BCG, C. Parvum and mixed bacterial vaccines (9). They are potent adjuvants for antibody production when administered with or following antigen. They restore humoral immunity in aged mice, enhance responses to weak antigens, render tolerogenic doses of antigen immunogenic and prevent the induction of B cell but not T cell tolerance. They inhibit cellular immune responses under circumstances where they enhance humoral immunity yet they enhance cellular immunity to unrelated antigens including delayed-type hypersensitivity, graft-versus-host reaction, and allograft rejection. They expand the reticuloendothelial and hematopoietic systems and enhance nonspecific resistance mechanisms. LPS also promotes complement (C) activation via the alternate pathway which produces activated C_3. B cells and macrophages bear C_3 receptors and C_3 activation plays a role in stimulating these cells. LPS-induced production of chemotactic peptides C_3A and C_5A may also participate in granulocyte and macrophage chemotaxis and accumulation.

In Vitro Studies

The cellular targets and molecular mediators of these various LPS actions are summarized in Figure 1.

B Lymphocyte

LPS is a polyclonal B cell activator. In vitro studies (23, 43) have clearly demonstrated that LPS nonspecifically activates resting B cells to proliferate and to produce various classes of immunoglobulins. With antigen, LPS stimulates clonal expansion of antigen-reactive B cells and accelerates their differentiation into antibody secreting cells. LPS's effects on macrophages contribute to B cell differentiation and activation through the elaboration of interleukin I (IL1) and, B cell growth and stimulating factor (IL4, IL5, IL6) (36, 37, 74). Williamson and coworkers (72) suggested that the direct B cell effects of LPS are mediated by lipid A while those involving the macrophage are mediated by the polysaccharide moiety of LPS. In the

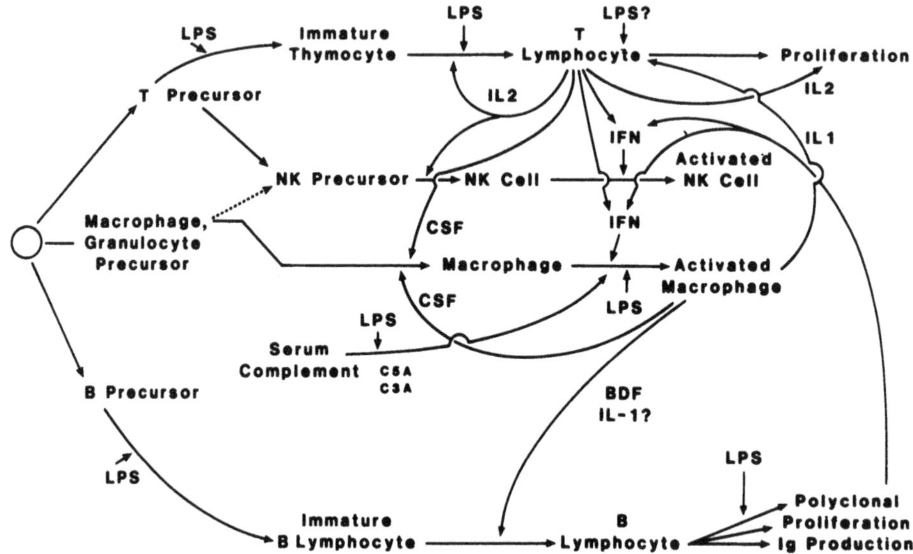

Fig 1. Cellular sites of the immunopharmacologic action of LPS.

context of a T-dependent antigen challenge, the effects of endotoxin on T helper cells contribute antigen specific T helper factors and/or B cell growth factor. Suppressor mechanisms for LPS-induced B cell responses have been described and are apparently mediated by macrophages and T and B cells (73). LPS also induces mature B cells to make colony stimulating factor (CSF-GM).

Besides the resting B cell, the immature B lymphocyte is a target of LPS-induced macrophage and T cell-produced growth and differentiation factors (IL4, IL5 & IL6). In addition, the precursor of the B cell (pre B cell) is a target of direct LPS action (34, 56, 57). LPS induces pre B cell differentiation in vitro as measured by induction of complement and other surface B cell receptors. Thus, LPS regulates directly or indirectly B cell differentiation from the earliest known precursor to the immunoglobulin producing plasma cell.

Macrophage

Extensive studies demonstrate that many macrophage functions are very sensitive to stimulation by LPS including phagocytosis, migration, lysosomal enzyme content, metabolism, secretion, microbicidal activity and cytotoxicity (1, 7, 14, 48, 54, 61). Macrophage microbicidal activity is stimulated directly by LPS alone and in conjunction with lymphokines like gamma interferon (γIFN). These macrophage activities are important in the enhancement of nonspecific resistance mechanism. LPS also induces macrophages to secrete a number of important mediators regulating other cell populations. LPS induces macrophage-derived: 1) IL1 which regulates T cells by inducing interleukin II (IL2); 2) colony stimulating factors (CSF) which induce clonal growth of macrophage and granulocyte precursors; 3) endogenous pyrogen which provides the mechanism for LPS-induced fever; 4) B cell growth and differentiation factors which regulate B cell maturation and function as discussed; 5) alpha interferon (αIFN) which induces antiviral resistance; 6) tumor necrosis factor (TNF); and 7) prostaglandins.

T Cell

LPS induces prothymocytes to differentiate in culture into cells bearing the markers of intrathymic lymphocytes (56, 57). We (10, 31, 32), showed that, in addition to IL2, LPS induces immature thymocytes to mature into mitogen-responsive T cells. Several studies (21, 51, 66, 67) have shown that, while LPS does not induce polyclonal activation of thymocytes, it does synergize with concanavalin A (Con A) to increase T cell proliferation. Whether this latter effect is mediated entirely by IL1 produced by thymic macrophages is not clear since mixed thymocyte populations were used in these studies. Phytohemagglutinin (PHA) and Con A responses of human peripheral blood lymphocytes, mainly T cells, are synergistically augmented by LPS (58) another action which may be mediated by monocyte-produced IL1. LPS stimulates growth of one T cell line and a small population (3%) of splenic T cells (65). These studies indicate that T cells at various stages of development are sensitive to LPS action. A major role of IL1 is the induction of IL2 by T cells; thus, LPS induces IL2 indirectly via its effect on macrophages. Whether LPS induces other T cell-produced lymphokines such as macrophage activating factor (MAF), migration inhibitory factor (MIF), colony stimulating factor (CSF) and gamma IFN remains to be determined.

Direct effects of endotoxin on other cells involved in immune expression such as granulocytes, natural killer cells, mast cells, etc., need to be clarified; however, LPS does activate granulocytes (69), platelets (16), and NK cells (17). In general, the effects of LPS on the immune system are positive ones to promote maturation and function of B and T lymphocytes, macrophages and NK cells.

Cyclic Nucleotides in Immunoregulation by LPS

Cyclic AMP and cyclic GMP represent intracellular messengers of hormone action. They are not the only messengers since different mechanisms are involved in the actions of steroid hormones, thyroid hormone, growth hormone, etc. A large number of studies have probed the roles played by these two cyclic nucleotide systems in the action of various agents on cells of the immune system (for further information in this area see 8, 12, 29). These agents include the heat stable bacterial enterotoxins (18, 20). Lewis Thomas and coworkers (5) were the first to implicate cyclic nucleotides in bacterial endotoxin action and subsequently a number of papers have suggested that cyclic nucleotides are important in LPS actions on various immune cell populations.

B Lymphocyte Proliferation

Watson (66-68) was the first to show that LPS induces early increases in cyclic GMP levels in mouse spleen lymphocytes without significant effects on cyclic AMP levels. He showed that exogenous cyclic GMP but not cyclic AMP can induce proliferation in these cells (69). Exogenous cyclic AMP inhibits the action of LPS to induce B cell proliferation, and the inhibition is reversed by cyclic GMP (67). He postulated that, cyclic GMP is part of the mitogenic signal in B lymphocytes.

The effect of LPS to increase cyclic GMP levels in B lymphocytes was confirmed by others (6, 59, 60). Freedman (22) extended the observation to show that, like T cell mitogens, LPS induces early calcium influx in murine splenocytes, cyclic AMP inhibited LPS-induced calcium influx, cyclic GMP enhanced the uptake, and cyclic AMP antagonized the effect of cyclic GMP. Using fluorescein-labeled antisera to the cyclic nucleotides and their protein kinases, Largen and Votta (40) found that LPS rapidly decreases the number of cells staining for cyclic AMP. LPS had no effect on the cells staining for Type I or II cyclic AMP-dependent protein kinase but markedly increased the number of cells staining for cyclic GMP-dependent protein kinase. Similarly, Ohara, et al. (49) showed that microinjection of antibodies to cyclic GMP suppressed and to cyclic AMP enhanced LPS-induced B lymphocyte proliferation. These collected observations parallel those made in T lymphocytes activated by PHA or Con A (29, 33) and support a role for cyclic GMP and calcium in B lymphocyte activation by LPS.

B and T Precursor Cell Differentiation

LPS induces prothymocyte maturation in the Komuro-Boyse assay and B cell maturation in a similar assay (34, 56, 57). In these studies cyclic AMP and agents which increase cyclic AMP induce both prothymocyte and pre B cell differentiation. The effect of LPS in both assays was enhanced by theophylline which inhibits cyclic AMP phosphodiesterase and antagonized by imidazole which promotes cyclic AMP catabolism. Theophylline potentiates induction by agents like poly A:U, choleratoxin, and prostaglandin PGE_1; and imidazole antagonizes their induction. We showed that in these circumstances LPS increases cyclic AMP but not cyclic GMP levels (30). Fairchild and Cohen (19) have also provided support for a parallelism of LPS- and cyclic AMP-induced B cell differentiation in mouse bone marrow cells. These observations suggest that, in contrast to that on mature B cell proliferation, LPS action to induce both T and B cell maturation is mediated by cyclic AMP.

Thymocyte and T Lymphocyte Proliferation

We observed that LPS induces peanut agglutinin positive (PNA+), immature cortical thymocytes to mature to a Con A-responsive state characteristic of the PNA-, mature thymocyte (30, 31). This action is shared by thymic epithelial cell supernatants and IL2 but not by thymosin. These results imply that LPS acts to differentiate the PNA+ cell to make it Con A responsive rather than an action to allow Con A to induce immature thymocyte proliferation by overcoming a deficiency in IL1 and, therefore, IL2 in the response. To clarify the point PNA+ cells were incubated for 24 hr with endotoxin and washed four times to remove all but trace endotoxin (<1 ng) before Con A was added. Under these circumstances a marked Con A response was induced by LPS, absent in the control. These experiments show that the action of LPS occurs prior to the action of Con A, and causes a Con A-unresponsive population to become responsive. They indicate that the action of LPS is not mediated by macrophage-produced IL1. That the effect is LPS and probably lipid A is specific was confirmed by the relative inability of C3H/HeJ mice to respond compared to C57Bl/6 or BALB/c mice and by the action of polymyxin B to prevent the response. Preliminary data indicate that LPS induces early two fold increases of cyclic GMP but no change of cyclic AMP levels in PNA+ thymocytes (30).

The addition of LPS on unfractionated thymocytes results in an augmentation of basal thymidine incorporation and Con A responses of mature thymocytes and this effect is comparable to the effect of exogenously added IL1 and is probably mediated by thymic macrophages. The effects of LPS on thymus cyclic nucleotide levels have previously been studied (46, 63). These groups showed that LPS increases cyclic AMP levels in unfractionated mouse thymocytes. The increases occurred with LPS concentrations above 1 µg/ml and ranged up to 12 fold. LPS induces PG production in blood leukocyte populations and results in the production of cyclic AMP (50). The cyclic AMP increases observed with LPS in thymocytes may well result from the induction of prostaglandin synthesis by thymic macrophages. Naylor (46) observed that thymocytes induce early increases in cyclic GMP levels of PNA-mature thymocytes. Our preliminary data indicate that LPS increases cyclic GMP levels of PNA-mature thymocytes. It is notable that the effect of LPS to promote mature thymocyte proliferation in response to Con A is mimicked by cyclic GMP but not cyclic AMP (66) and the effects of LPS to induce T suppressor cell function has been related to the cyclic AMP changes (73). Under these circumstances, it seems that the cyclic GMP changes induced by LPS in mature T cells are related to the enhancement of proliferation and the cyclic AMP changes are related to suppressor influences. However, more experiments are needed to clarify what the mechanisms are.

Macrophage

Macrophage modulation by LPS is a central phenomenon in the immunopharmacology of LPS. LPS at high concentrations induces macrophage prostaglandin synthesis (39) and, therefore, corresponding cyclic AMP increases in association with collagenase induction (4). We (28) previously examined the effects of LPS on macrophage microbicidal activity under circumstances in which macrophages show enhanced listericidal capacity following stimulation with LPS. We (30) observed that low concentrations of LPS induce early increases in macrophage cyclic GMP levels without significant effect on cyclic AMP levels. It is notable that CSF, PMA, MDP and tuftsin, all of which have similar effects as LPS on macrophages, i.e., activation for cytotoxicity and monokine production, also raise macrophage levels of cyclic GMP (11, 12, 27).

LPS is known to induce production of IL1, CSF, and alpha IFN by macrophages and alpha IFN, IL2 and CSF by lymphocytes. Many of these factors have apparent cyclic nucleotide mediation. IL1 has been reported to induce late changes but not early changes in cyclic GMP levels of lymphocytes (38). Alpha IFN has been reported to induce cyclic GMP increases in lymphoid cells (53). CSF1 has been reported by us to increase cyclic GMP levels in macrophages (27) and IL2 has been shown to increase cyclic GMP levels in PNA+ thymocytes as well as mitogen-primed blood lymphocytes (32). Thus each of the mediators induced by LPS has been implicated in inducing cyclic GMP in one or another cell or circumstance.

The foregoing, although incomplete, attests to important roles played by cyclic nucleotides in the direct action of LPS and in the indirect action of LPS-induced mediators on various cell populations. While interesting, these studies have intrinsic defects which limit conclusions about the relationship of LPS action to the cyclic nucleotide change and of these changes to the subsequent biological response. A wide variety of LPS preparations have been used; the roles of Lipid A and polysaccharide components and contaminating enterotoxins have not been assessed for some of the biological responses or any of the cyclic nucleotide responses. The cell populations employed, while generally enriched, were not purified. Thus LPS-induced direct versus indirect actions have not been assessed for some of the biological responses or any of the cyclic nucleotide responses. The levels of cyclic nucleotides have been measured without attention to the contribution of prostaglandin influence, often without purification of the cyclic nucleotide (in the case of cyclic GMP, an essential issue), and without phosphodiesterase inhibitors (to block cyclic nucleotide turnover and to show that the effect is on production and not catabolism). Importantly, with one exception (40), experiments are lacking to show the relation of cyclic nucleotide change to metabolic events which would link the cyclic nucleotide to the effector response. The possible importance of endotoxin mechanism in normal development and regulation of immune function make it important to correct these deficiencies.

Transmembrane Signals in LPS Action

Both the beneficial and the toxic actions of LPS must involve a great variety of both direct and indirect mechanisms. For the purposes of this discussion, it is relevant to discuss those mechanisms which relate to the cyclic nucleotide changes discussed. A large number of recent reports have elaborated the mechanisms by which surface ligands induce transmembrane signals which give rise to cyclic nucleotide second messengers and to other second messengers like protein kinase C and intracellular free calcium ion ([Ca++]i). These pathways are likely sites for endotoxin positive actions on cells of the immune system (see Fig 2).

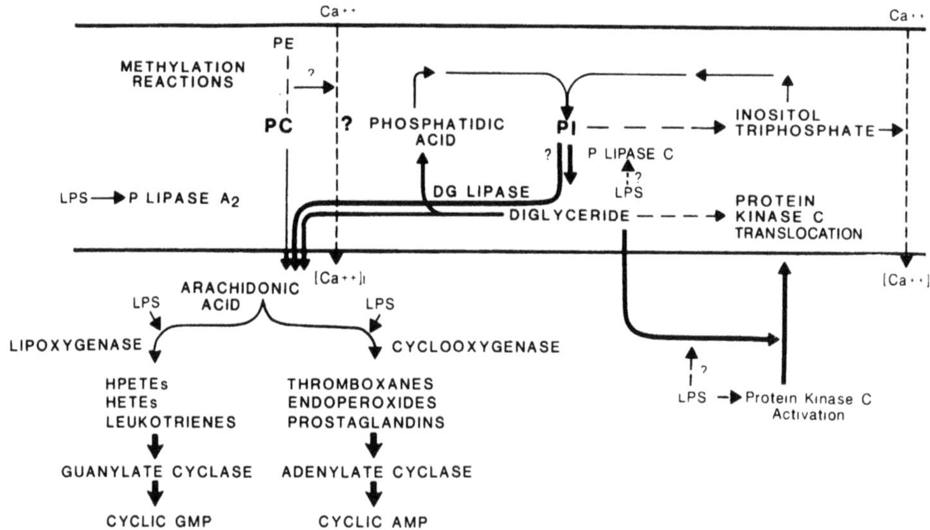

Fig 2. Transmembrane signaling mechanisms in the action of LPS.

With respect to LPS effect to modify cyclic AMP levels in cells of the immune system, two pathways are likely. LPS actions to induce macrophage production of arachidonic acid metabolites like thromboxane, prostacylin, and prostaglandins have been well documented (15, 39, 44, 46). Macrophage-derived prostaglandins through their action to directly stimulate adenylate cyclase are likely candidates for effects of LPS to increase cyclic AMP levels in cells of the immune system. Another action which may relate LPS to cyclic AMP may be, like bacterial enterotoxins (18, 20), through modification of "G" proteins regulatory for adenylate cyclase. Such actions remain to be demonstrated to account for "up regulation" of adenylate cyclase by LPS. The effects of "down regulation" of adenylate cyclase by LPS for beta adrenergic and prostaglandin induced activation have been observed in both lymphocytes and macrophages (35, 64). These effects may, on the one hand, involve inhibitory "G" proteins. On the other hand, protein kinase C-mediated phosphorylation of adenylate cyclase has been described as part of IL2 action (2) and since LPS has been described to activate protein kinase C in macrophages, (71), LPS could "down reglate" adenylate cyclase in this manner.

It seems more relevant to relate protein kinase C activation by LPS to activation events linked to cyclic GMP production in lymphocytes and macrophages. Lectin mitogens and phorbol myristage acetate (PMA) have been reported to activate protein kinase C and to stimulate cyclic GMP production in lymphocytes. The link here may involve phosphorylation and activation of guanylate cyclase (13, 33).

Other actions of LPS may also contribute to guanylate cyclase activation. Several investigators (41, 55) have implicated LPS in the activation of the lipoxygenase pathway in macrophages leading to production of leukotrienes and other eicosanoids. These products have been implicated in the direct activation of guanylate cyclase of leukocytes and lymphocytes (13, 25, 33). Thus, it seems likely that LPS induces guanylate cyclase activation of lymphocytes and macrophages by the activation of protein kinase C and/or metabolites of arachidonic acid.

The actions of LPS on both adenylate and guanylate cyclase are in significant part the result then of release of arachidonic acid from membrane phospholipids such as phosphotidyl inositol (PI) and choline (PC). These release mechanisms are thought to be regulated mainly by phosphol ilipase C in lymphocytes and both phospholipase C and A2 in macrophages. So far, only phospholipase A2 in macrophages has been explored as a target of LPS action. Liu, et al., (42) have observed that LPS, while not having lipase activity itself, activates endogenous phospholipase A2. This activation reduces membrane fluidity and results in the release of arachidonic acid. The free arachidonic acid may then be converted by macrophages into cyclooxygenase products like prostaglandins or by macrophages, and perhaps lymphocytes, to lipoxygenase products like hydroperoxy and hydroxy eicosatetranoic acids (HPETE's and HETE's) and leukotrienes (LTC4 and LTB4). These products in turn activate their appropriate cyclic nucleotide cyclases. The activation of these oxygenases are associated with the generation of hydrogen peroxide, superoxide anion and free oxygen radicals. These are well known products of LPS action and may relate both to enhanced bactericidal as well as to toxic effects (24, 52).

It seems likely that phospholipase C will also be a target of LPS activation. In addition to giving rise to the release of free arachidonic acid, phospholipase C action yields free diacylglycerol. Diacylglycerol is a central activator of protein kinase C (47) and its release would account for the activation of protein kinase C by LPS (42). Most activators of phospholipases A and C protein kinase C are associated with phosphatidyl inositol (PI) turnover and/or phospholipid methylation (PC formation). Studies on the effects of LPS on PI turnover have so far been negative (3, 26). These cycles are often linked to mechanisms of calcium influx and increases in [Ca++]i. Freedman (22) has shown that LPS increases calcium influx in B lymphocytes but the mechanism is not known. It remains to be determined what other transmembrane signaling mechanisms are involved in LPS action as a B cell mitogen.

The transmembrane signaling mechanisms which give rise to the cyclic nucleotide changes noted center on LPS action to release arachidonic acid from membrane lipids through the action of phospholipases. The conversion of arachidonic acid to prostaglandins via cyclooxygenases and to eicosanoids via lipoxygenases are pathways activating adenylate and guanylate cyclase, respectively. Additional actions of LPS on protein kinase C, perhaps via the diglyceride, diacylglycerol, would also contribute to cyclic nucleotide cyclase regulation as well as other activation processes. Modulations by LPS of other transmembrane signaling mechanisms remains to be explored. Further experimental development in this area using defined endotoxins and components and purified cell populations is warranted. The many positive effects of endotoxins indicate that, as the molecule can be detoxified without losing important biological activities powerful immunopharmacologic agents will emerge.

CONCLUSION

Endotoxins are likely candidates for positive regulators of the development and differentiation of T and B lymphocytes and macrophages and various granulocyte populations. The evidence indicating nontoxic physiological roles is more compelling than that supporting toxicity and suggests a reevaluation of the beneficial effects of endotoxins on immune function. The cyclic nucleotides are likely to be involved in many of the actions of endotoxin. The pharmacologic data are strong in indicating a role for cyclic AMP in actions of endotoxin to induce precursor cell differentiation and for cyclic GMP in actions of endotoxin to promote proliferative or secretory functions of mature lymphocytes and macrophages. In addition, endotoxin-induced mediators such as CSF, IFN, IL1 and IL2 appear to involve cyclic nucleotide mechanisms.

REFERENCES

1. Apte, R., Hertogs, C. and Pluznik, D., 1980, Regulation of lipopolysaccharide-induced granulopoiesis and macrophage formation by spleen cells. J. Immunol. 124: 1223.

2. Beckner, S. K. and Farrar, W. L., 1986, Interleukin 2 modulation of adenylate cyclase. J. Biol. Chem. 261: 3043.

3. Betel, I., Martijnse, J. and VandenBerg, K., 1974, Absence of an increase in phospholipid turnover in mitogen-stimulated B lymphocytes. Cell Immunol. 14: 2568.

4. Bhatnager, R., Schade, U., Rietschel, E. and Decker, K., 1982, Involvement of prostaglandin E and adenosine 3',5'-monophosphate in lipopolysaccharide-stimulated collagenase release by rat Kupffer cells. Eur. J. Biochem. 125: 125.

5. Bitensky, M. W., Gorman, R. E. and Thomas, L., 1971, Selective stimulation of epinephrine-responsive adenyl cyclase in mice by endotoxin. Proc. Soc. Biol. Med. 138: 773.

6. Bomboy, J. D., Jr. and Graber, S. E., 1980, Stimulation of cyclic 3',5'-guanosine monophosphate levels in rat spleen cells by lipopolysaccharide preparations. J. Lab. Clin. Med. 95: 654.

7. Bonney, R. J. and Humes, J. L., 1984, Physiological and pharmacological regulation of prostaglandin and leukotriene production by macrophages. J. Leuk. Biol. 35: 1.

8. Bourne, H. R., Lichtenstein, M., Melmon, K. L., Henney, C. S., Weinstein, Y. and Shearer, G. M., 1974, Modulation of inflammation and immunity by cyclic AMP. Science 184: 19.

9. Carswell, E. A., Old, L. J., Kassel, R. L., Green, S., Fiore, N. and Williamson, B., 1975, An endotoxin-induced serum factor that causes necrosis of tumors. Proc. Natl. Acad. Sci. 72: 3666.

10. Chen, S. S., Tung, J. S., Good, R. A. and Hadden, J. W., 1983, Changes in surface antigens of immature thymocytes under the influence of T cell growth factor and thymic factors. Proc. Natl. Acad. Sci. 80: 5980.

11. Coffey, R. G. and Hadden, J. W., 1982, Phorbol myristate acetate stimulation of lymphocyte guanylate cyclase and cyclic GMP phosphodiesterase and reduction of adenylate cyclase. Cancer Res. 43: 150.

12. Coffey, R. G. and Hadden, J. W., 1985, Neurotransmitters, hormones and cyclic nucleotides in lymphocyte regulation. Fed. Proc. 44: 112.

13. Coffey, R. G. and Hadden, J. W., 1985, Stimulation of lymphocyte guanylate cyclase by arachidonic acid and HETEs, in: "Prostaglandins, Leukotrienes, and Lipoxins," J. M. Bailey, ed., Plenum Press, New York.

14. Cohen, Z. A. and Morse, S., 1960, Functional and metabolic properties of polymorphonuclear Leukocytes. II. The influence of a lipopolysaccharide endotoxin. J. Exp. Med. 111: 689.

15. Cook, J. A., Wise, W. C. and Halushka, P. V., 1981, Thromboxane A2 and prostacyclin production by lipopolysaccharide-stimulated peritoneal macrophages. J. Reticul. Soc. 30: 445.

16. DesPrez, R. M., 1964, Effects of bacterial endotoxin on rabbit platelets. IV. The divalent ion requirements of endotoxin induced and immunologically induced platelet injury. J. Exp. Med. 124: 971.

17. Djeu, J., Heinbaugh, J., Holden, H. and Herberman, R., 1979, Augmentation of mouse natural killer cell activity by interferon and interferon inducers. J. Immunol. 122: 175.

18. Evans, D. J., Jr., Chen, C., Curlin, G. T. and Evans, D. G., 1972, Stimulation of adenyl cyclase by Escherichia coli enterotoxin. Nature New Biol. 236: 137.

19. Fairchild, S. and Cohen, J., 1978, B lymphocyte precursors, J. Immunol. 12: 1227.

20. Field, M., Graf, L. H., Jr., Laird, W. and Smith, P. L., 1978, Heat-stable enterotoxin of Escherichia coli: In vitro effects on guanylate cyclase activity, cyclic GMP concentration, and ion transport in small intestine. Proc. Natl. Acad. Sci. 75: 2800.

21. Forbes, J., Nakao, Y. and Smith, R., 1975, T mitogens trigger LPS responsiveness in mouse thymic cells. J. Immunol. 114: 1004.

22. Freedman, M. H., 1979, Early biochemical events in lymphocyte activation. Cell Immunol. 44: 290.

23. Gery, I., Kruger, J. and Spiegel, S., 1972, Stimulation of B lymphocytes by endotoxin: Reactions of thymus-deprived mice and karyotypic analysis of dividing cells in mice bearing T6-T6 thymus grafts. J. Immunol. 108: 1088.

24. Ghezzi, P., Saccardo, B. and Bianchi, M., 1986, Role of reactive oxygen intermediates in the hepatoxicity of endotoxin. Immunopharmacol. 12: 241.

25. Graff, G., Stephenson, J. H., Glass, D. B., Haddox, M. K. and Goldberg, N. D., 1978, Activation of soluble splenic cell guanylate cyclase by prostaglandin endoperoxides and fatty acid hydroperoxides. J. Biol. Chem. 253: 7662.

26. Grugg, S. A. and Harmony, J. A. K., 1985, Increased phosphatidylinositol metabolism is an important but not an obligatory early event in B lymphocyte activation. J. Immunol. 134: 4087.

27. Hadden, E. M., Sadlik, J. R., Coffey, R. G. and Hadden, J. W., 1982, Effects of phorbol myristate acetate (PMA) and lymphokine on cyclic GMP levels and proliferation of macrophages. Cancer Res. 42: 3064.

28. Hadden, J. W., Englard, A., Sadlik, J. R. and Hadden, E. M., 1979, The comparative effects of isoprinosine, levamisole, muramyl dipeptide and SM1213 on lymphocyte and macrophage proliferation and activation in vitro. Int. J. Immunopharmacol. 1: 17.

29. Hadden, J. W., and Coffey, R. G., 1982, Cyclic nucleotides in mitogen induced lymphocyte proliferation. Immunol. Today 3: 299.

30. Hadden, J. W., Galy, A., Hadden, E., Touraine, J-L. and Coffey, R., 1986, Cyclic nucleotides in the immunopharmacology of lipopolysaccharide endotoxins, in: "Immunobiology and Immunopharmacology of Bacterial Endotoxins," A. Szentivanyi, H. Friedman, and A. Nowotny, eds., Plenum Press, New York.

31. Hadden, J. W., Specter, S., Galy, A., Touraine, J-L. and Hadden, E., 1986, Thymic hormones, interleukins, endotoxin and thymomimetic drugs in T lymphocyte ontogeny, in: "Advances in Immunopharmacology III," L. Chedid, J. W. Hadden, F. Spreafico, P. Dukor and Willoughby, D., eds., Pergamon Press, Oxford.

32. Hadden, J. W., Hadden, E. M. and Coffey, R. G., 1987, Interleukin II increases cyclic GMP levels in immature thymocytes and mitogen-primed T lymphocytes. Int. J. Immunopharmacol. 9: 851.

33. Hadden, J. W., 1987, Transmembrane signals in the activation of T lymphocytes, in: "Mechanisms of Lymphocyte Activation and Immune Regulation," S. Gupta, W. E. Paul, and A. S. Fauci, eds., Plenum Press, New York.

34. Hammerling, U., Chin, A. and Scheid, M., 1975, The ontogeny of murine B lymphocytes. J. Immunol. 115: 1425.

35. Hazeki, K., Mori, Y., Ui, M., 1986, Induction of refractories of cyclic AMP responses to prostaglandin E1 and epinephrine by prior exposure of guinea pig macrophages to lipopolysaccharide. Arch. Biochem. Biophys. 246: 772.

36. Hoffman, M., Weiss, O., Koenig, S., Hirst, J. and Oettgen, H., 1975, Suppression and enhancement of the T cell dependent production of anti-

body to SRBC in vitro by bacterial lipopolysaccharide. J. Immunol. 114: 738.

37. Hoffman, M., Galanos, C., Koenig, S. and Oettgen, H., 1977, B cell activation by lipopolysaccharide. J. Exp. Med. 146: 1640.

38. Katz, S., Kierszenbaum, F. and Waksman, B., 1978, Mechanisms of action of lymphocyte-activating factor. J. Immunol. 121: 2386.

39. Kurland, J. and Bockman, R., 1978, Prostaglandin E production by human blood monocytes and mouse peritoneal macrophages. J. Exp. Med. 147: 952.

40. Largen, M. T. and Votta, B., 1983, Immunocytochemical evidence for 3',5'-cGMP and 3',5'-cGMP-dependent protein kinase involvement in lymphocyte proliferation. J. Cyclic Nucleo. Prot. Phosphoryl. Res. 9: 231.

41. Luderitz, O., Schade, U., Rietschel, E. Th., 1986, Formation and metabolism of leukotriene C4 in macrophages exposed to bacterial lipopolysaccharide. Eur. J. Biochem. 155: 377.

42. Lui, M-S., Ghosh, S. and Yang, Y., 1983, Change in membrane lipid fluidity induced by phospholipase A activation: A mechanism of endotoxin shock. Life Sci. 33: 1995.

43. Melchers, F. and Anderson, J., 1974, IgM in bone marrow-derived lymphocytes. Eur. J. Immunol. 4: 181.

44. Moore, R. N., Urbacek, R., Wahl, L. M. and Mergenhagen, S. E., 1979, Prostaglandin regulation of colony-stimulation factor production by lipopolysaccharide stimulated murine leukocyte. Infect. Immun. 26: 408.

45. Morris, D. D. and Moore, J. N., 1987, Endotoxin-induced production of thromboxane and prostacyclin by equine peritoneal macrophages. Circ. Shock 23: 295.

46. Naylor, P. Camp, C. Phillips, A., Thurman, G. and Goldstein, A., 1978, Effect of thymosin and lipopolysaccharide on murine lymphocyte cyclic AMP. J. Immunol. Meth. 20: 143.

47. Nishizuka, Y., 1984, The role of protein kinase C in cell surface signal transduction and tumor promotion. Nature 308: 693.

48. Nowotny, A., 1983, "Beneficial Effects of Endotoxin," Plenum Press, New York.

49. Ohara, J. and Watanabe, T., 1982, Microinjection of macromolecules into normal murine lymphocytes by cell fusion techniques. J. Immunol. 128: 1090.

50. Oppenheim, J., Koopman, W., Wahl, L. and Dougherty, S., 1980, Prostaglandin E2 rather than lymphocyte-activating factor produced by activated human mononuclear cells stimulates increases in murine thymocyte cAMP. Cell Immunol. 49: 64.

51. Ozato, K., Adler, W. and Ebert, J., 1975, Synergism of bacterial lipopolysaccharide and concanavalin A in the activation of thymic lymphocytes. Cell Immunol. 17: 532.

52. Peavy, D. L. and Fairchild, E. J., 1986, II, Evidence for lipid peroxidation in endotoxin-poisoned mice. Infect. Immun. 52: 613.

53. Rochette-Egly, C. and Tovey, M. G., 1982, Interferon enhances guanylate cyclase activity in human lymphoma cells. Biochem. Biophysica. Res. Commun. 107: 105.

54. Russell, S. W., 1986, Involvement of endotoxin in macrophage activation for antitumor immunity, in: "Immunobiology and Immunopharmacology of Bacterial Endotoxins," A. Szentivanyi, H. Friedman, and A. Nowotny, eds., Plenum Press, New York.

55. Schade, U. F., 1986, Involvement of lipoxygenases in the activation of mouse macrophages by endotoxin. Biochem. Biophys. Res. Commun. 138: 842.

56. Scheid, M., Hoffmann, M., Komuro, K., Hemmerlin, U., Abbott, J., Boyse, E., Cohen, G., Hooper, J., Schulof, R. and Goldstein, A., 1973, Differentiation of T cells induced by preparations from thymus and by nonthymic agents. J. Exp. Med. 138: 1027.

57. Scheid, M. P., Goldstein, G. and Boyse, E. A., 1978, The generation and regulation of lymphocyte populations. J. Exp. Med. 147: 1727.

58. Schmidtke, J. and Najarian, J., 1975, Synergistic effects on DNA synthesis of phytohemagglutinin or concanavalin A and lipopolysaccharide in human peripheral blood lymphocytes. J. Immunol. 114: 742.

59. Shenker, B. J. and Gray, I., 1979, Cyclic nucleotide metabolism during lymphocyte transformation. I. Cell. Immunol. 43: 11.

60. Shenker, B. J. and Gray, I., 1979, Cyclic nucleotide metabolism during lymphocyte transformation. II. Cell. Immunol. 43: 23.

61. Strauss, B. S. and Stetson, C. A., 1960, Studies on the effect of certain leukocytes of peripheral blood. J. Exp. Med. 112: 653.

62. Szentivanyi, A., Friedman, H. and Nowotny, A., "Immunobiology and Immunopharmacology of Bacterial Endotoxins," Plenum Press, New York.

63. Tsien, W-H., Sampson, M. and Sheppard, H., 1981, The elevation of mouse thymus cell cyclic adenosine monophosphate (cAMP) by lipopolysaccharide. Immunopharm. 3: 253.

64. VanOosterhout, A. J. M., TenHave, G. A. M. and Nijkamp, F. P., 1986, Endotoxin-induced reduction of β-adrenoceptor number in guinea pig splenic lymphocyte membranes. Agents Actions 19: 361.

65. Vogel, S., Hilfiker, M. and Caulfield, M., 1983, Endotoxin-induced T-lymphocyte proliferation. J. Immunol. 130: 1774.

66. Watson, J., 1975, The influence of intracellular levels of cyclic nucleotides on cell proliferation and the induction of antibody synthesis. J. Exp. Med. 141: 97.

67. Watson, J., 1976, The involvement of cyclic nucleotide metabolism in the initiation of lymphocyte proliferation induced by mitogens. J. Immunol. 117: 1656.

68. Watson, J., 1977, Involvement of cyclic nucleotides as intracellular mediators in the induction of antibody synthesis, in: "Comprehensive Immunology," R. A. Good and S. B. Day, eds., Plenum Press, New York.

69. Watson, J., Epstein, R. and Cohn, M., 1973, Cyclic nucleotides as intra-

cellular mediators of the expression of antigen-sensitive cells. Nature 246: 404.

70. Weissman, G. and Thomas, L., 1964, On a mechanism of tissue damage by bacterial endotoxins, in: "Bacterial Endotoxin," M. Landy and W. Braun, eds., Rutgers University Press, New Brunswick.

71. Wrightman, P. and Raetz, C., 1984, The activation of protein kinase C by biologically active lipid moieties of lipopolysaccharide. J. Biol. Chem. 259: 1048.

72. Williamson, S., Wannemuehler, M., Kirillo, E., Pritchard, D., Michalek, S. and McGhee, J., 1984, LPS regulation of the immune response: separate mechanisms for murine B cell activation by lipid A (direct) and polysaccharide (macrophage-dependent) derived from bacteroide LPS. J. Immunol. 133: 2294.

73. Winchurch, R. A., Hilberg, C., Birmingham, W. and Munster, A., 1982, Lipopolysaccharide-induced activation of suppressor cells: reversal by an agent which alters cyclic nucleotide metabolism. Immunol. 45: 147.

74. Wood, D. and Cameron, P., 1976, Stimulation of the rlease of a B cell activating factor from human monocytes. Cell. Immunol. 21: 133.

MECHANISMS OF ENDOTOXIN STIMULATION OF MONOCYTES IN WHOLE BLOOD

B. Osterud, J. O. Olsen and L. Wilsgard

Institute of Medical Biology, University of Tromso, Tromso, Norway

INTRODUCTION

Bacterial lipopolysaccharide endotoxins are potent inflammatory agents that have many physiologic and biochemical effects in vivo. Although a wide variety of biological responses to endotoxin have been well characterized, the molecular mechanism by which endotoxin influences cellular functions is still not established.

Many of the effects of endotoxin are mediated by monocyte/macrophages. Since most of the studies regarding endotoxin stimulation of these cells have been carried out in cell cultures, many diverging results have been reported. This has probably arisen from the variability in monocyte/macrophage functions dependent on how many days the cells have been cultured.

Gram negative organisms may cause severe pathological changes in the blood and blood vessels and frequently result in ultimate death (10). One of the systems that appear to be triggered is the coagulation system whereby disseminated intravascular coagulation (DIC) is induced.

In 1975 it was shown that monocytes in cell cultures could be stimulated by endotoxin to produce thromboplastin (tissue factor) (21). Thromboplastin is the most potent activator of the coagulation system (18), and its appearance on the surface of monocytes during gram negative septicemia is thought to account for the early induction of DIC (16). This has been quite obvious in mengococcal septicemia (17), probably due to the very high concentration of circulating endotoxin. In these patients it was found that a direct relationship between the level of thromboplastin activity in circulating monocytes and the clinical picture as judged by the fatal outcome. In order to find new ways to treat patients with meningococcal septicemia it became necessary to study the mechanism of activation of monocytes in blood as expressed by induced thromboplastin synthesis.

The role of complement in Gram negative septicemia has been challenged several times. Garner et al., (5) found that in complement depleted animals, shock and DIC could not be elicited by endotoxin infusion. Of special interest was the observation that the factor VII level increased after the injections of two doses endotoxin in the decomplemented dogs, where in dogs with intact complement, endotoxin induced rapid fall in factor VII level. The fall was probably associated with an exposure of thromboplastin on circulating monocytes, and subsequent binding of factor VII to exposed thromboplastin (1, 14). Some years ago we found indeed a mandatory role for complement in the endotoxin induced thromboplastin synthesis of monocytes (15).

The intracellular signals involved in blood cell activation have been studied extensively during the last years. Two systems seem to be essential for cell activation. These are the phospholipase C and the phospholipase A2 dependent pathways. The phospholipase A2 release and subsequent metabolization of the arachidonic acid has been documented to be mandatory for the oxygen burst in macrophages (19).

Platelets were found to play a role in the endotoxin induced thromboplastin synthesis of monocytes several years ago (12), and more recently it was suggested that the platelet generation of 12-HETE could account for this effect (9). The present study was undertaken to learn more about the endotoxin stimulation of monocytes in whole blood with special references to the intracellular signals involved in this cell activation.

MATERIALS AND METHODS

Cell Stimulation System

Blood was drawn into heparin anticoagulant (10 µg/ml) in plastic tubes. One ml aliquots were incubated with 2 ng endotoxin/ml (E. coli 026: B6, Difco Laboratories) for 2 hr in a rotating incubator (180 rpm) at 37°C. The reaction was stopped by adding 0.1 ml 2% EDTA to each test sample.

In the experiments where blood cells were recombined with plasma that had been treated in several ways, heparinized blood was centrifuged at 1500 x g for 10 min. Plasma was pipetted off, and the blood cells resuspended in 0.15 M NaCl, and once more centrifuged at 1500 x g for 10 min. The blood cells were then recombined with the treated plasma, added endotoxin and incubated as above.

Isolation of Monocytes

Heparinized blood was mixed with equal volume of 0.15 M NaCl and applied on top of 1.5 ml Lymphopaque (Nycomed, Oslo) in plastic tubes and centrifuged at 450 x g for 15 min as described (13). The isolated monocytes were counted and frozen at -70°C until testing of thromboplastin activity.

Measurement of Thromboplastin

The thromboplastin activity was measured by incubating the test samples with factor VII and factor X in the presence of Ca++ as previously described (13, 16), followed by the quantitation of generated factor Xa. The activity obtained in the factor Xa assay was related to the factor Xa obtained in the same system by testing dilutions of a crude thromboplastin preparation from human brain as reported (16).

INACTIVATION OF THE COMPLEMENT SYSTEM AND REMOVAL OF PLASMA COMPLEMENT FACTORS

Heparinized blood was centrifuged at 1500 x g for 10 min at room temperature. The plasma was pipetted off into plastic tubes, and either heated at 56°C for 30 min to inactivate the complement system, or subjected to Bio-Rex 70 (Bio-Rad, Labs, Richmond, CA) that had been equilibrated with buffer composed of 0.08 M NaCl, 2 mM EDTA and 0.05 M sodium phosphate (pH 7.3). After stirring for 30 min the Bio-Rex 70 was removed from the plasma by centrifugation at 12000 x g for 10 min. C1q and D were isolated from freshly prepared human plasma as reported (22).

Cobra Venom Factor

Cobra venom factor (CVF) was obtained from Crodis Labs (Miami, FL). The venom from Naja naja kaouthia was used.

Binding/Uptake of Endotoxin

Endotoxin (100 ng/ml blood) was added to heparinized blood and incubated at various time-intervals. Then the mononuclear cells were isolated as described above on Lymphopaque, and then washed once with 10 ml sterile 0.15 M NaCl. After centrifugation at 1500 x g for 10 min, the cell pellet was resuspended in 0.2 ml 0.15 M NaCl and frozen at -70°C until tested for endotoxin.

Measurement of Endotoxin

Endotoxin was measured by utilizing a combination of Limulus amebocyte lysate (LAL) and a chromogenic substrate. LAL (0.1 ml) was preincubated at 37°C for 5 min and added to 0.1 ml test sample, and then incubated for 30 min at 37°C. The test samples had been heated at 75°C for 5 min prior to incubation with the LAL. 0.2 ml of chromogenic substrate S-2423 (Kabi Vitrum, Sweden) was added to the LAL test sample, and the mixtures were incubated at 37°C for 3 min. To stop the reaction, 0.2 ml of 50% acetic acid was added plus 0.2 ml pyrogen free water. Released p-nitroaniline was read in a spectrophotometer at 405 nm. The method has been described in detail by Friberger et al. (4). The endotoxin standard was obtained from the kit of Coatest Endotoxin (E. coli 0111:B4, 2ng) Kabi Vitrum.

Preparation of Platelet Rich Plasma (PRP) and Granulocytes

Heparinized blood was centrifuged at 140 x g for 15 min at room temperature to obtain PRP.

Granulocytes were isolated by adding 0.6 ml Dextran T-500 (6 g/100 ml 0.15M NaCl) to 2.0 ml heparinized blood. This was allowed to sediment for 1 hr at room temperature. The upper part, consisting of white cells and platelets, was applied on top of 1.5 ml Lymphopaque, and then centrifuged at 450 x g for 20 min. The mononuclear cell band was pipetted off, whereas the granulocytes at the bottom part were resuspended and washed in 5 ml sterile 0.15 M NaCl and then centrifuged at 1500 x g for 10 min. The granulocytes were finally resuspended in either platelet poor plasma or platelet rich plasma, and immediately used for further experiments in recombination with mononuclear cells or buffer as controls.

RESULTS

The Binding/Uptake of Endotoxin to White Cells in Whole Blood

When endotoxin (100 ng/ml) was added to whole blood followed by the isolation of the various blood cells, a substantial amount of the endotoxin could be detected in the mononuclear cell fraction as shown in a typical experiment in Table 1. Neither isolated platelets nor granulocytes were found to possess endotoxin activity (data not shown).

Separation of blood cells and plasma followed by recombination and subsequent incubation with endotoxin resulted in a lower uptake/binding of the endotoxin (line 2 of Table 1). Similar reduction in endotoxin induced thromboplastin synthesis upon separation and recombination of the cells with the plasma has been observed (Osterud, unpublished data).

Table 1. The Binding/uptake of Endotoxin to Monocytes in Whole Blood

Incubation mixture	ENDOTOXIN CONC. (ng/ml) Incubation time (hrs) 0	1	2
Blood + endotoxin	0.5	22.4	17.9
Cells + plasma + endotoxin	0.2	9.1	4.8
Cells + heat inactivated plasma + endotoxin	0.1	0.4	1.2
Cells + Bio-Rex ads. plasma + endotoxin	0.1	2.0	2.1

Heat inactivation of the plasma at 56°C for 30 min prior to the recombination with the blood cells resulted in an abolished binding/uptake of endotoxin (line 3 of Table 1). Similar adsorption of plasma with Bio-Rex 70, which removes Clq and D, caused also near 80% reduction in binding/uptake of endotoxin.

<u>Endotoxin Induced Thromboplastin Synthesis in Monocytes Recombined with Plasma Treated in Various Ways to Inactivate the Complement System</u>

Complement factors removed from plasma by treatment with cobra venom factor (CVF) for 3 hr at 37°C prior to recombination of blood cells, followed by incubation with endotoxin, caused a dose dependent reduction in induced thromboplastin synthesis in monocytes, as shown in Table 2. Treatment with 1.0 U/ml of CVF reduced the endotoxin induced thromboplastin synthesis 80%.

Table 2. The Effect of Endotoxin on Monocytes in Plasma Depleted of Complement Factor by Cobra Venom Factor (CVF)

Concentration of CVF (U/ml)	Thromboplastin Act. x $10^{-3}/10^{6}$ cells $\pm$ S.D.
0	40.0 $\pm$ 5.3
1.0	8.1 $\pm$ 3.1
2.0	5.1 $\pm$ 2.3
4.0	3.1 $\pm$ 1.5

Table 3. The Effect of Complement on Endotoxin Stimulation of Monocytes in Whole Blood

Blood cells recombined with	Thromboplastin Act. x $10^{-3}/10^{6}$ cells $\pm$ S.D.
Plasma	0.6 $\pm$ 0.2
Plasma + Ex	26.4 $\pm$ 5.2
Heat-inactivated plasma + Ex	0.7 $\pm$ 0.3
Rio-Rex 70 ads. plasma + Ex	1.1 $\pm$ 0.4
Bio-Rex 70 ads. plasma + C1q + Ex	12.1 $\pm$ 2.9
Bio-Rex 70 ads. plasma + D + Ex	11.6 $\pm$ 2.2

As reported earlier (15) we found a striking effect by inactivation of plasma at 56°C on the endotoxin induced thromboplastin synthesis of blood monocytes. Table 3 illustrates that the heat inactivation completely abolished the stimulating effect of endotoxin on monocytes recombined with heat inactivated plasma. Furthermore, removing C1q and D in the complement system, caused also a total block of the endotoxin effect on the monocytes (line 4 of Table 3). However, about 50% of the abolishing effect could be reduced by either adding back isolated C1q (50 µg/ml) or D (0.4 µg/ml) to the Bio-Rex adsorbed plasma, demonstrating that both C1q in the classical pathway and D in the alternative pathway, support the effect of endotoxin in inducing thromboplastin synthesis in blood monocytes.

The Effect of A Phospholipase A2 Inhibitor on the Endotoxin Induced Synthesis of Thromboplastin in Blood Monocytes

In order to learn more about the intracellular signals involved in the endotoxin stimulation of monocytes as expressed by induced thromboplastin synthesis, heparinized blood was incubated with 2 ng endotoxin/ml blood in the presence of various concentrations of 2.4. dibromoacetophenone. As can be seen from Table 4, a dose dependent inhibition of the induced thromboplastin synthesis was obtained. Thus, the release of arachidonic acid (20:4) appeared to be mandatory for the endotoxin stimulation of monocytes in blood.

Inhibition of Endotoxin Induced Thromboplastin Synthesis in Monocytes by a Lipoxygenase Inhibitor

The phospholipase A2 inhibitor showed that the release of arachidonic acid is an essential feature in the endotoxin stimulation of monocytes. It was therefore of interest to see whether a lipoxygenase inhibitor also might influence the stimulatory effect of endotoxin. In contrast to the effect of the phospholipase A2 inhibitor, the lipoxygenase inhibitor, nordihydroguaiaretic acid (NDGA), appeared to have variable inhibitory effect on endotoxin stimulation of different individuals. Thus, in individuals with very sensitive monocytes (high responders), the inhibition was close to 80%, whereas in the low responders, no effect of the NDGA was observed on the endotoxin induced thromboplastin synthesis (Table 5).

Table 4. The Effect of Phospholipase A2 Inhibitor (2.4 Dibromoacetophenone) on Endotoxin Induced Thromboplastin Synthesis in Blood Monocytes

Inhibitor conc. (μM)	Thromboplastin Act. x $10^{-3}/10^{6}$ cells $\pm$ S.D.
0	32.0 $\pm$ 6.8
1	33.8 $\pm$ 8.5
5	25.4 $\pm$ 4.6
10	13.5 $\pm$ 4.3
20	0.8 $\pm$ 0.2
50	0.3 $\pm$ 0.2

Enhancement of Endotoxin Induced Thromboplastin Synthesis by Platelets

By separating the white and red cells from platelet rich plasma (PRP) followed by either recombination of the cells with PRP or platelet poor plasma (PPP), and incubation of recombined mixtures with endotoxin, a significantly higher thromboplastin induced synthesis was found in the presence of platelets (23.6 $\pm$ 6.3 x $10^{-3}/10^{6}$ cells in the presence of platelets as compared to 9.0 $\mp$ 3.8 x $10^{-3}/10^{6}$ cells in the absence, $p < 0.01$).

In this way, we also showed that by recombining blood cells of a low responder with PRP of a high responder instead of its autologous PRP, the endotoxin response increased tremendously. Vice versa, when blood cells of a high responder was recombined with PRP of a low responder, a drastic reduction (up to 70%) in endotoxin response was observed as compared to the response obtained through the recombination with the autologous PRP. Intake of acetylsalcylic acid (ASA) caused a 50% enhancement of endotoxin stimulation of monocytes by endotoxin. In a high responder, intake of ASA resulted in a 250% enhancement (Osterud, to be published elsewhere).

Role of Fatty Acids in Endotoxin Induced Thromboplastin Synthesis of Blood Monocytes

In recent experiments we showed that liposomes prepared from soya lecithin and containing 60% of the fatty acid 18:2, amplified the thromboplastin synthesis in monocytes when blood was exposed to endotoxin. The liposomes had no stimulatory effect by themselves, but enhanced the thromboplastin synthesis in endotoxin stimulated monocytes 3-5 fold. The effect was maximal at 15 ug phospholipids per ml blood (Osterud et al., to be published elsewhere).

An important role of polyunsaturated fatty acids was also found in a study where we allowed 20 men and 20 women to drink 25 ml cod liver oil per day for 8 weeks. After 8 weeks the endotoxin stimulation of monocytes was reduced with 35% as expressed by induced thromboplastin synthesis (Hansen and Osterud, manuscript in preparation).

Table 5. The Effect of A Lipoxygenase Inhibitor (NDGA) on the Endotoxin Induced Synthesis of Thromboplastin in Monocytes of 6 Individuals

Conc. of inhib. (μM)	Thromboplastin Act. x $10^{-3}/10^6$ cells					
	Case 1	Case 2	Case 3	Case 4	Case 5	Case 6
0	51.5	29.7	18.9	18.0	8.2	7.5
10	46.2	13.6	15.2	15.0	8.6	8.0
50	8.7	9.8	12.0	8.5	8.5	7.5
100	18.2	15.0	12.5	10.4	7.8	8.7

The Enhancement of Endotoxin Induced Thromboplastin Synthesis in Monocytes by Granulocytes

The role of granulocytes on the stimulation of monocytes is scarce. In these experiments blood cells from a high responder was compared with blood cells of a low responder on 4 different occasions. The platelets appeared to only enhance the endotoxin stimulation of monocytes in high responders, whereas no significant effect of platelets was found on monocyte stimulation of the low responders as shown in Table 6.

Granulocytes isolated by the method where dextran is used to sediment the red cells, generated only minor amounts of thromboplastin when incubated with endotoxin as expected. The small amounts generated are probably due to some contamination of the PRP with a few monocytes. In contrast, when the granulocytes were added together with the monocytes a striking rise in endotoxin induced thromboplastin synthesis of the monocytes was observed (Table 6). This enhancement could not be a soluble product secreted from the dextran treatment of the blood, but might still reflect an intracellular product generated in the granulocytes as a result of the incubation with the dextran.

Table 6. The Effect of Granulocytes on Endotoxin Stimulation of Monocytes in "High Responder" and "Low Responder"

Endotoxin incubated with	Thromboplastin Act. x $10^{-3}/10^6$ Cells $\pm$ S.D.	
	High responder	Low responder
Monocytes + PRP	30.1 $\pm$ 14.2	7.8 $\pm$ 2.5
Granulocytes + PRP	3.2 $\pm$ 1.1	1.5 $\pm$ 0.8
Monocytes + granulocytes + PRP	61.7 $\pm$ 9.6	43.9 $\pm$ 13.9

DISCUSSION

Monocytes in cell cultures may be stimulated by endotoxin to produce thromboplastin activity also in the absence of complement factors (3). The failure of endotoxin to induce thromboplastin synthesis when freshly isolated monocytes are incubated with endotoxin in complement depleted plasma (Tables 2 and 3) suggest that the complement system at least is mandatory for endotoxin induced thromboplastin synthesis in monocytes of whole blood. This discrepancy may be accounted for by the ability of monocytes/macrophages in cell culture to produce the complement factors (8). Another discrepancy between experiments carried out in cell cultures as compared to an intact whole blood system or plasma system is the enormous difference in the concentration of the stimulating agent, endotoxin, required to induce the thromboplastin synthesis. Whereas, we in our whole blood systems are using 2-5 ng endotoxin/ml blood, up to 25-50 µg endotoxin/ml is used in cell cultures to obtain similar or even less thromboplastin activity of the monocytes (20).

Our observation that endotoxin added to whole blood only is bound or taken up by the monocytes in the presence of an intact complement system (Table 1), is further supporting the important role of complement system in the endotoxin stimulation of monocytes in blood. It has also been suggested by others that complement components may play a role in the specific binding of endotoxins to the monocyte/macrophage membrane (7). In our studies, both the classical and the alternative pathway seemed to be involved, as both C1q and D added back to plasma depleted of C1q and D, partially restored the ability of endotoxin to induce thromboplastin in the monocytes (Table 3). This confirms the earlier observation by Morrison and Cline (11), who showed that bacterial lipopolysaccharides activate both the classical and the alternative pathways of the complement system.

Recently there have been several reports on the intracellular signals involved in the activation of white cells. In this context, two pathways have emerged as central mechanisms for cell activation. One of the systems is the activation of phospholipase C system which utilizes phosphatidylinositol as substrate, whereupon IP3 is generated with resultant mobilization of Ca++. In addition diacylglycerol is formed, and this compound is known to activate protein kinase C which should result in protein phosphorylation. Both calcium mobilization and protein phosphorylation have been implicated in cellular activation in a variety of cells (2). The other phospholipase system involved is the activation of the phospholipase A2 enzyme followed by the release and further metabolization of arachidonic acid (20:4). This activation pathway has been suggested to also be important in several cell systems.

Our data imply an essential role of the arachidonic acid release in the endotoxin induced synthesis of thromboplastin in blood monocytes (Table 4). Interestingly is the observation that the lipoxygenase inhibitor, nordihydroguaiaretic acid, had no effect on the endotoxin stimulation of the monocytes in those with very nonsensitive monocytes, whereas an 80% inhibition was found in an individual with very active monocytes (high responder) (Table 5). This phenomenon is probably best explained by the tremendous enhancing effect of platelets on the endotoxin stimulation of monocytes. Apparently, a major reason for the very high sensitivity to stimuli of monocytes in some individuals is probably that these individuals also possess very active platelets.

Recently it has become evident that monocytes play a central role in the development of atherosclerosis, since the so called foam cells have been shown to be macrophages (6). Very active platelets have been associated with high risk of cardiovascular disease. Our results may therefore give another explanation to this phenomenon, since the atherogenic effect of the platelets may partially be exerted through their interaction with the monocytes in the circulating blood.

Although endotoxin has been used as the stimulating agent in our study, this may prove to be of great advantage, since it recently was suggested that endotoxin as a naturally occurring toxin bound to lipoproteins may be transported into the artery wall and initiate the atherosclerotic reaction (23). In that study it was also demonstrated that all lipoprotein classes bind endotoxin in direct proportion to their plasma cholesterol concentrations. We feel that the highly endotoxin sensitive monocytes are more susceptible to penetration of vessel walls, and therefore also more likely to induce an atherosclerotic reaction.

The effect of granulocytes on the endotoxin stimulation of monocytes might be due to the dextran incubation required for the red cell sedimentation. If so, at least no excretion product could account for the effect since the cells were separated and washed afterwards. Whatever the mechanism for the granulocyte enhancement of the endotoxin induced thromboplastin synthesis in monocytes is, it shows that granulocytes may generate products that have a significant effect on the stimulation of monocytes, specially in low responders. Further studies to explore the role of granulocytes in the monocyte activation are now being performed.

ACKNOWLEDGEMENT

This study was supported by grants from the Norwegian Cancer Society and the Norwegian Research Council for Science and the Humanities.

REFERENCES

1. Broze, Jr., G. J., 1982, Binding of human factor VII and VIIa to monocytes. J. Clin. Invest. 70: 526.

2. Dennis, E. A., 1987, Regulation of eicosanoid production: Role of phospholipases and inhibitors. Bio/Technology 5: 362.

3. Edwards, R. L., and Perla, D., 1984, The effect of serum on monocyte tissue factor generation. Blood 64: 707.

4. Friberger, P., Knos, M., and Mellstrom, L., 1982, in: "Endotoxins and their detection with the limulus amebocyte lysate test". S. W. Watson, J. Lewin and T. J. Novitsky, eds. Alan R. Liss Publishing, New York.

5. Garner, R., Chater, B. V., and Brown, D. L., 1974, The role of complement in endotoxin shock and dissemianted intravascular coagulation: experimental observations in the dog. Brit. J. Haematol. 28: 393.

6. Gerrity, R. G., 1981, The role of the monocyte in atherogenesis. I. Transition of blood borne monocytes into foam cells in fatty lesions. Am. J. Pathol. 103: 181.

7. Haeffner-Cavaillon, N., Cavaillon, J.-M., Etievant, M., Lebbar, S., and Szabo, L., 1985, Specific binding of endotoxin to human monocytes and mouse macrophages: serum requirement. Cellular Immunol. 91: 119.

8. Hetland, G., Johnson, E., and Aasebo, U., 1986, Human alveolar macrophages synthesize the functional alternative pathway of complement and active C5 and C9 in vitro. Scand. J. Immunol. 24: 603.

9. Lorenzet, R., Niemetz, J., Marcus, A. J., and Brockman, M. J., 1986, Enhancement of mononuclear procoagulant activity by platelet 12-hydroxyeicosatetraenoic acid. J. Clin. Invest. 78: 418.

10. McCartney, A. C., Banks, J. G., Clements, G. B., Sleigh, J. D., Tehrani, M., and Ledeingham, I. McA., 1j983, Endotoxinemia in septic shock: Clinical and post mortem correlations. Intensive Care Med. 9: 117.

11. Morrison, D. C., and Cline, L., 1977, Activation of the classical and properidin pathways of complement by bacterial lipopolysaccharides (LPS). J. Immunol. 48: 362.

12. Niemetz, J., and Marcus, A. J., 1974, The stimulatory effect of platelets and platelet membranes on the procoagulant effect of leukocytes. J. Clin. Invest. 54: 1437.

13. Osterud, B., Bogwald, J., LIndahl, U., and Seljelid, R., 1981, Production of blood coagulation factor V and tissue thromboplastin by macrophages in vitro. FEBS Letters 127: 154.

14. Osterud, B., and Bjorklid, E., 1982. Factor VII associated with monocytes in endotoxin stimulated blood. Biochem. Biophys. Res. Commun. 108: 620.

15. Osterud, B., and Eskeland, T., 1982, The mandatory role of complement in the endotoxin-induced synthesis of tissue thromboplastin in blood monocytes. FEBS Letters 149: 75.

16. Osterud, B., and Bjorklid, E., 1982, The production and availability of tissue thromboplastin in cellular populations of whole blood exposed to various concentrations of endotoxin. Scand. J. Haematol. 29: 175.

17. Osterud, B., and Flaegstad, T., 1983, Increased tissue thromboplastin activity in monocytes of patients with meningococcal infection related to an unfavourable prognosis. Thromb. Haemostas. 49: 5.

18. Osterud, B., 1984, Activation pathway of the coagulation system in normal haemostasis (Review). Scand. J. Haematol. 32: 337.

19. Pick, E., and Bromberg, Y., 1982, Quo Vadis macrophage activation. Role of phospholipids in the elicitation of the oxidative burst in macrophages. Transpl. Procd. 14: 570.

20. Prydz, H., and Lyberg, T., 1980, Effect of some drugs on thromboplastin (Factor III) activity of human monocytes in vitro. Biochem. Pharmacol. 29: 9.

21. Rivers, R. P. A., Hathaway, W. E., and Weston, W. L., 1975, The endotoxin-induced coagulant activity of human monocytes. Brit. J. Haematol. 30: 311.

22. Tenner, A. J., Leshavre, P. H., and Cooper, N. R., 1981, Purification and radiolabeling of human Clq. J. Immunol. 127: 648.

23. van Lenten, B. J., Fogelman, A. M., Haberland, M. E., and Edwards, P. E., 1986, The role of lipoproteins and rececptor-mediated endocytosis in the transport of bacterial lipopolysaccharide. Proc. Nat'l. Acad. Sci. 83: 2704.

COMPARATIVE STUDY OF LIPOPOLYSACCHARIDE-, LIPID IVa-, AND LIPID X-INDUCED TUMOR NECROSIS FACTOR PRODUCTION IN MURINE MACROPHAGE-LIKE CELL LINES

T. P. Birkland, R. D. Cornwell, D. T. Golenbock, and R. A. Proctor

Department of Medical Microbiology, University of Wisconsin Medical School, Madison, Wisconsin, U.S.A.

Tumor necrosis factor (TNF) was initially described in the sera of **Mycobacterium bovis** strain BCG infected mice treated with endotoxin (2) and defined by its ability to cause necrosis of tumors in mice. In addition to this potentially beneficial effect, TNF has been shown to be intimately involved in the pathophysiology of bacterial lipopolysaccharide (LPS)-induced shock and lethality in mice (1). In both instances, the primary sources of TNF are macrophages (5).

Macrophage-like cell lines are useful in the study of cytokine production, but few comparative studies exist that compare and contrast sensitivity to LPS-induced TNF production and the relative amount produced. This study assessed TNF production in the murine macrophage-like cell lines RAW 264.7, J774A.1, PU5-1.8 and P388D1.

All cells were obtained from the American Type Culture Collection and were grown as loosely adherent cells in petri dishes with low endotoxin RPMI 1640 medium (M.A. Bioproducts, Inc., Walkersville, MD) plus 10% heat-inactivated low endotoxin fetal bovine serum (Hyclone Laboratories, Logan, UT). Cells were plated either into 96 well tissue culture plates (7.5 x 10^4 cells/well) or 24 well plates (2 -3 x 10^5 cells/well). LPS (**Escherichia coli** 0111:B4, Difco Laboratories, Detroit, MI), the disaccharide tetraacyl lipid A precursor compound IVa (6) (a gift from Dr. C. R. H. Raetz), or the synthetically prepared monosaccharide precursor of lipid A, lipid X (6) (Sandoz Pharmaceutical Co., Basel, Switzerland), were added for various lengths of time. After incubation, supernatants were collected and frozen at -70°C until assayed for TNF content using a modification of the actinomycin-D sensitized L929 cell cytotoxicity assay of Flick (3). Briefly, 2 x 10^4 L929 cells in 100 µl were plated per well into 96 well plates, and incubated overnight before 100 µl of macrophage supernatant was added. Serial two-fold dilutions were performed on the plate, and actinomycin-D (1 µg/ml final concentration) added to achieve a final assay volume of 200 µl well. After 16 hr, cytotoxicity was quantified by MTT dye reduction of viable cells. In this study, one TNF unit is reported as the reciprocal of the dilution required to achieve a 50% reduction in MTT dye content/well compared to untreated control wells.

The minimal LPS concentration needed to obtain measurable levels of TNF production after 24 hr incubation is shown in Fig 1. RAW 264.7 cells were the most sensitive to LPS, with 0.1 ng LPS/ml eliciting 10 units of TNF

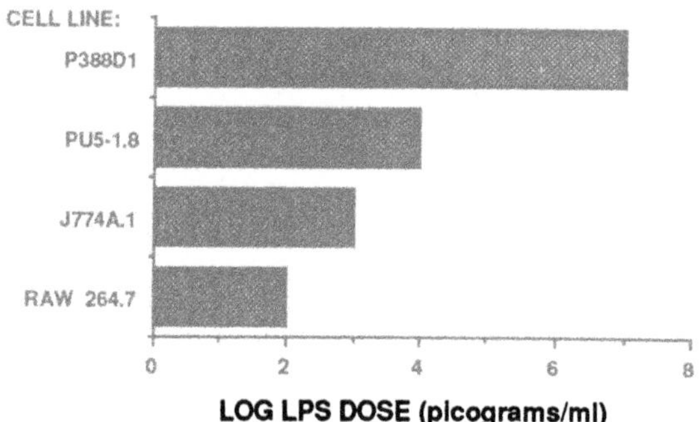

Fig 1. The minimal dose of LPS required to induce measurable TNF production. Cells were incubated 24 hr with varying concentrations of LPS in RPMI 1640 with 10% FBS, and TNF activity of the supernatant was determined. TNF-induced cytotoxicity was measured in actinomycin-D sensitized L929 cells as assessed by the ability of viable cells to reduce MTT dye. One unit of TNF causes a 50% decrease in reduced MTT measured. The minimum concentration of LPS required for TNF production is given in log10 picograms LPS per ml.

activity. The J774A.1 cell line produced measurable TNF at 1 ng LPS/ml; PU5-1. at 10 ng/ml; and P388D1 at 10,000 ng LPS/ml.

Maximal LPS-induced TNF production in RAW 264.7 cells is shown in Fig 2. Measurable TNF production is observed with 0.1 ng LPS/ml; increasing amounts of TNF are found with increasing concentrations of LPS, up to the highest LPS concentration tested, 10,000 ng LPS/ml.

The relative activity of LPS, lipid IVa, and lipid X to induce TNF production in RAW 264.7 and J774A.1 cells was studied (Fig 3). Lipid X induced TNF production only at the highest dose tested, 10,000 ng/ml, and only in RAW 264.7 cells. Compound IVa induced measurable TNF at 10 ng/ml in RAW 264.7 cells, and 1000 ng/ml in J774A.1 cells. Both cell lines produced large amounts of TNF in response to LPS. These results show that LPS is the best inducer of TNF, followed by compound IVa, and then lipid X.

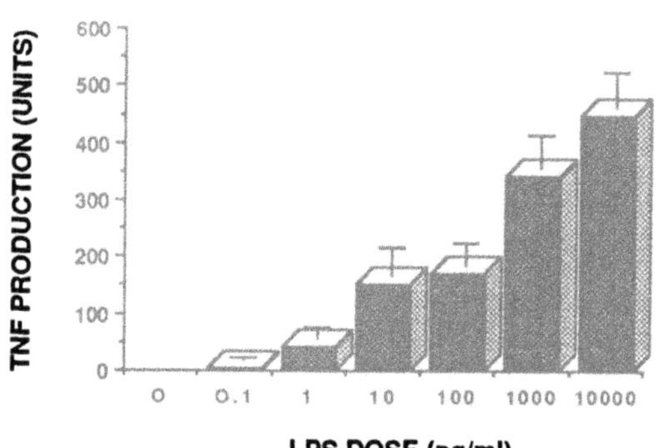

Fig 2. Dose-response curve of LPS-induced TNF production in RAW 264.7 cells. Cells were incubated 24 hr with varying concentrations of LPS in medium, and TNF activity of the supernatant was determined using L929 cell cytotoxicity. Error bars denote the standard error of the mean (SEM).

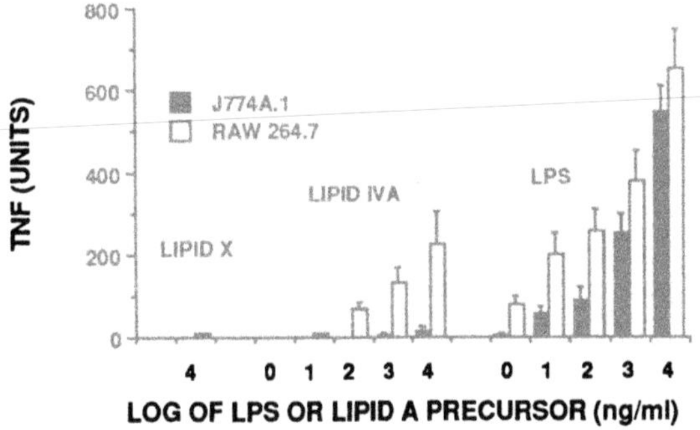

Fig 3. Induction of TNF production in J774A.1 and RAW 264.7 cells by lipid X, lipid IVA, or LPS. Cells were incubated with sonicated log10 dilutions, from 1 ng/ml to 10,000 ng/ml, of the different lipids and incubated 24 hr. Cell supernatants were assayed for TNF activity using the L929 cell cytotoxicity assay. Error bars denote the standard error of the mean (SEM).

TNF production in RAW 264.7 cells is relatively rapid, with detectable amounts observed after 2 hr incubation when treated with 1000 ng LPS/ml (Fig 4), and increasing amounts of TNF in the supernatants are observed with time. Maximal amounts are found at 24 hr, the last time point tested. A similar rapid production and increase with time was observed with J774A.1 cells, with maximal amounts at 18-24 hr (data not shown).

The cellular mechanisms for the differential susceptibilty of the macrophage cell lines for LPS-induced TNF production are not known. In vivo production of TNF can occur when LPS alone is injected into mice, but lower levels of LPS can induce TNF production in mice primed by BCG or **Corynebacterium parvum** (5). With respect to TNF production, the RAW 264.7 cell may possibly represent a cell in the "primed" state and produce TNF at low LPS concentrations of LPS and may represent cells arrested in a non-optimally primed stage. Continued study of these cell lines may provide insight into the control of LPS-induced TNF production and strategies to combat LPS-induced, TNF-mediated pathophysiology.

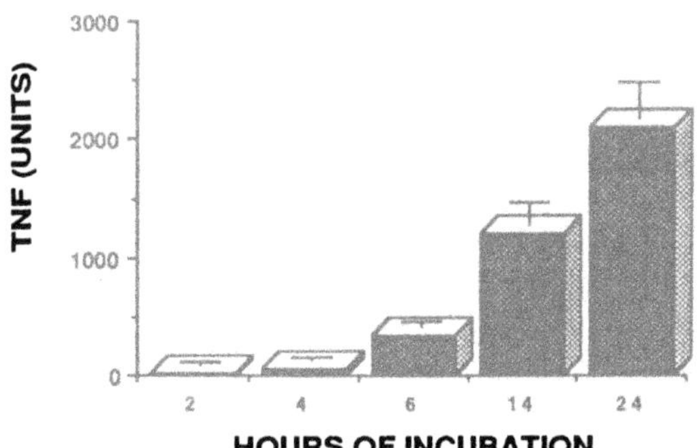

Fig 4. Time course of TNF production in RAW 264.7 cells. Cells were incubated with 1000 ng/ml LPS for varying lengths of time, and TNF activity quantified using the L929 cell cytotoxicity. Error bars denote the standard error of the mean (SEM).

REFERENCES

1. Beutler, B., Milsark, I. W., Cerami, A., 1985, Passive immunization against cachectin/tumor necrosis factor (TNF) protects mice from the lethal effect of endotoxin. Science 229: 869.

2. Carswell, E. A., Old, L. J., Kassel, R. L., Green, S., Fiore, N., Williamson, B., 1975, An endotoxin-induced serum factor that causes necrosis of tumors. Proc. Natl. Acad. Sci. 72: 3666.

3. Flick, D. A., Gifford, G. E., 1984, Comparison of in vitro cell cytotoxicity assays for tumor necrosis factor. J. Immunol. Methods 68: 167.

4. Gifford, G. E., Flick, D. A., 1987, Natural production and release of tumor necrosis factor, in: "Tumour necrosis factor and related cytokines", G. Bock and J. Marsh, eds., Wiley Publishing, New York, NY, Ciba Foundation Symposium 131.

5. Mannel, D. N., Falk, W., Meltzer, M. S., 1981, Inhibition of nonspecific tumoricidal activity by activated macrophages with antiserum against a soluble cytotoxic factor. Infect. Immun. 33: 156.

6. Strain, S. M., Armitage, I. M., Anderson, L., Takayama, K., Quereshi, N., and Raetz, C. R. H., 1985, Location of polar substituents and fatty acyl chains on Lipid A precursors from a 3-deoxy-D-manno-octulosonic acid-deficient mutant of **Salmonella typhimurium**. J. Biol. Chem. 260: 16089-16098.

LIPOPOLYSACCHARIDE-INDUCED PRIMING OF THE MURINE MACROPHAGE-LIKE CELL LINE J774A.1 FOR ENHANCED PRODUCTION OF REACTIVE OXYGEN INTERMEDIATES IS BLOCKED BY ANTISERUM TO MURINE INTERFERON β

T. P. Birkland and R. A. Proctor

Department of Medical Microbiology, University of Wisconsin
Medical School, Madison, Wisconsin, USA

Previously, we have shown that lipopolysaccharide (LPS) can prime murine macrophage-like J774A.1 cells for an enhanced production of reactive oxygen intermediates (ROI) in a dose- and time-dependent manner. The goal of this study was to determine if cytokines produced and secreted by LPS-treated J774A.1 cells were involved in priming for enhanced production of ROI. This was accomplished by neutralizing cytokine activity using specific anti-cytokine antiserum added to the LPS-treated J774A.1 cells.

J774A.1 cells were obtained from the American Type Culture Collection and grown as loosely adherent cells in plastic petri dishes using RPMI 1640 with 10% fetal bovine serum as medium. Purified murine interferon (IFN) β, rabbit anti-MuIFN β antiserum, and rat anti-MuIFN γ monoclonal antibody were obtained from Lee Biomolecular Inc., San Diego, CA. Recombinant MuIFN was a gift from Dr. Ernest Borden. Recombinant Human Tumor Necrosis Factor α (TNF) and rMuIFN γ were gifts of Dr. Douglas Golenbock and were obtained from Dr. Michael Shepard of Genentech Inc., San Francisco, CA. Rabbit anti-recombinant-Mu-TNF α antiserum was obtained from Genzyme Co., Boston, MA. Matched pre-immune sera were obtained from the same sources. All glassware was baked overnight at 180°C and endotoxin content of solutions was monitored using a chromogenic **Limulus** amoebocyte lysate assay.

Adherent J774A.1 in 96 well plates were treated with sonicated dilutions of LPS (**Escherichia coli**) 0111:B4, phenol-water extracted, Difco Labs, Detroit, MI) and allowed to incubate for at least 24 hr. LPS and various antisera were added concurrently unless otherwise noted. Monolayers were then washed and ROI production initiated using 500 ng/ml phorbol myristate acetate and quantified by nitroblue tetrazolium dye (NBT) reduction using a modification of the method of Pick (2).

Ten nanograms LPS/ml resulted in maximal priming of J774A.1 cells. Priming by 24 hour LPS incubation can be markedly inhibited in a dose-dependent manner by anti-IFN β added concurrently with LPS (Fig 1). Maximal inhibition occurred with 50 neutralizing units anti-IFN β/ml(1:200 dilution). Pre-immune serum had no effect on priming. In Fig 2, cells were incubated a total of 39 hours; inhibition of priming by anti-IFN β is dependent on the time of addition of the antisera. Maximal inhibition occurred when anti-IFN β was added concurrently with 10ng/ml LPS, and lessened with increasing time

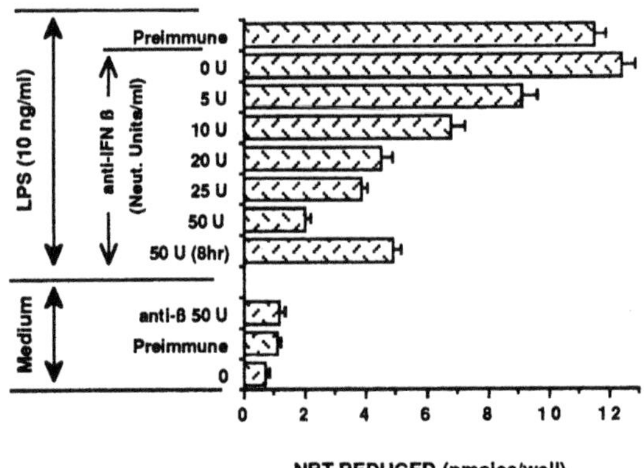

Fig 1. Dose-dependent of inhibition of LPS priming by antiserum to anti-IFN β. Various doses of anti-IFN β antiserum were added concurrently with 10 ng/ml LPS, except for 50 U (8 hr), which indicates antiserum added 8 hr after LPS was added, and NBT reduction determined 24 hr after LPS was added. Protein content per well for all treatment groups was not significantly different from untreated controls.

after LPS addition. No significant inhibition was observed when anti-IFN β was added 36 hr after LPS treatment.

Antiserum to murine TNF α partially inhibited LPS priming of J774A.1 cells in a dose-dependent manner (Fig 3). Maximal inhibition occurred with 4000 neutralizing units anti-TNF α/ml. Pre-immune serum had no effect on priming (data not shown).

The ability of cytokines to prime J774A.1 cells was tested. Recombinant IFN γ, natural purified IFN β and recombinant IFN β all can prime J774A.1 cells after a 24 hr incubation (data not shown). Recombinant human TNF α can also prime J774A.1 cells (Fig 3); in this experiment, antiserum to murine TNF, which does not cross react with human TNF, does not inhibit priming,

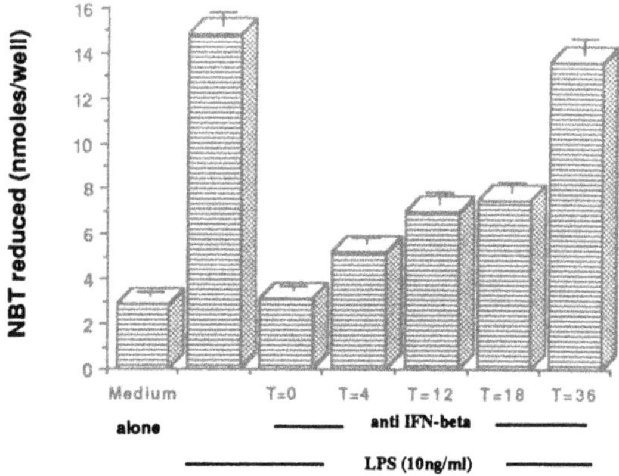

Fig 2. Time dependence of inhibition of LPS priming by anti-IFN β. 50 IFN neutralizing Units/mL was added at various hours (T=0,4,12,18, or 36 hr) after LPS treatment of J774A.1 cells. T=0, antiserum was added concurrently with LPS. Total incubation time was 39 hr. No significant difference in protein content per well was detected for any treatment group.

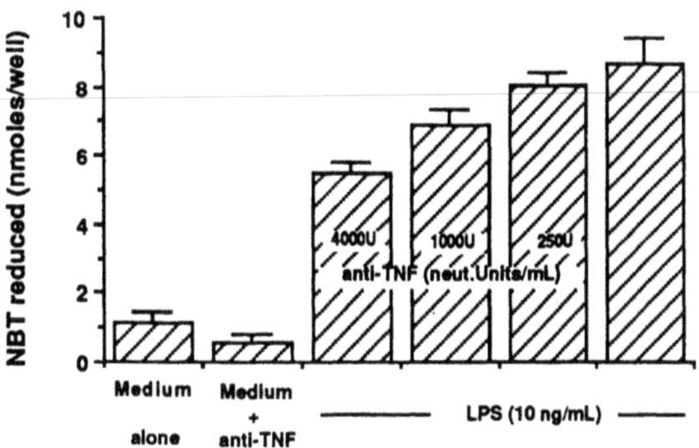

Fig. 3 Dose-dependent decrease of LPS induced priming by anti-TNF α. Antiserum was added concurrently with LPS (10 ng/ml), and NBT reduction determined 24 hr later. Protein content of treatment groups and untreated controls did not differ.

indicating that rHuTNF priming is not due to TNF-induced endogenous TNF production. Anti-IFN β blocked rHuTNF priming (Fig 4), indicating that at least part of the priming observed may be due to rHuTNF-induced IFN β acting in an autocrine fashion.

The activity of anti-IFN β on priming by IFN γ was tested. Anti-IFN β does not inhibit IFN γ priming of J774A.1 cells, while anti-IFN γ antibody does, indicating the effect of anti-IFN β is not a toxic effect on J774A.1 cells themselves (data not shown).

Finally, the ability of J774A.1 cells to produce anti-IFN β and TNF α was determined. IFN β was quantified by using inhibition of vesicular stomatitis virus-induced cytopathic effect on L929 cells and TNF α was quantified by L929 cell cytotoxicity assay; specificity of the assays was determined using anti-IFN β and anti-TNF α respectively. Both IFN β and TNF α are rapidly secreted into the culture supernatants of LPS-treated J774A.1 cells, with significant amounts present 3 hr after LPS treatment.

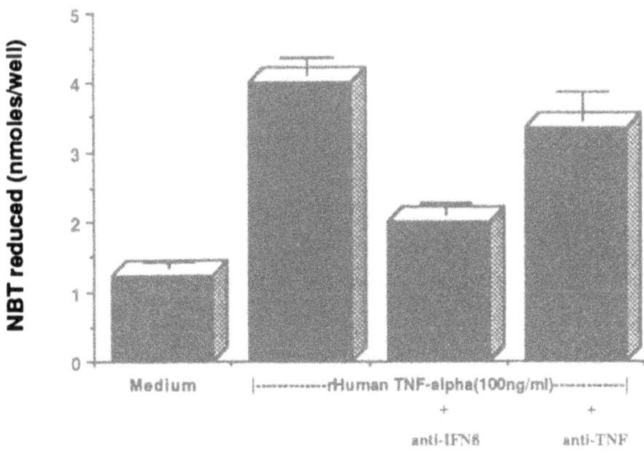

Fig. 4 Priming of J774A.1 cells by 24 hr incubation with recombinant human TNF α. Priming by 100 ng rHuTNF α/ml is inhibited by anti-IFN β antiserum at 50 IFN β neutralizing Units/ml when added concurrently with TNF, but not by rabbit anti-murine recombinant TNF α (4000 neutralizing units/ml).

Although autocrine effects of cytokines has been hypothesized previously, these results are the first direct evidence that LPS-induced priming of J774A.1 cells for enhanced production of ROI is due to the action of endogenously produced cytokines and not due to a direct effect of LPS on the cell itself. For J774A.1 cells, IFN β is of primary importance, as indicated by the marked inhibition of priming by antibody to IFN β. TNF α can induce priming, and at least part of the priming is due to TNF-induced IFN β production. IFN β has resulted in priming in human cells (3) and a decrease in ROI production in mouse macrophages (1). The effects of IFN β on macrophages may be a function of the particular macrophage population being studied.

At low doses, LPS-induced release of endogenous mediators results in augmentation of macrophage function, as observed here. At higher doses, the deleterious consequences of LPS-induced shock in vivo are also due to endogenous mediators. Further study of the positive-feedback system described here may provide insight into control of macrophage endogenous mediators involved in LPS-induced pathophysiology.

REFERENCES

1. Borashi, D., Ghezzi, P., Salmona, M., and Tagliabue, A., 1982, IFN-β-induced reduction of superoxide anion generation by macrophages. Immunol. 45: 621.

2. Pick, E., Mizel, D., 1981, Rapid microassays for the measurement of superoxide and hydrogen peroxide production by macrophages in culture using an automatic enzyme immunoassay reader. J. Immunol. Methods 46: 211.

3. Yoshida, R., Murray, H. W., and Nathan, C. F., 1988, Agonist and antagonist effects of interferon α and β on activation of human macrophages. J. Exp. Med. 167: 1171.

LIPOPOLYSACCHARIDE-CONTAINING CYTOPLASMIC MEMBRANES AS IMMUNOSTIMULATORS OF THE PERITONEAL MACROPHAGES

E. Ivanova[1], J. Gumpert[2], and A. Popov[3]

[1]Institute of Microbiology, Bulgarian Academy of Sciences Sofia 1113, [2]Central Institute of Microbiology and Experimental Therapy, 6900 Jena, DDR, [3]Scientific Medico-Biological Institute, Medical Academy, Sofia 1431, Bulgaria

During the last years we established that the stable L-forms of S. aureus, L. monocytogenes and E. coli were able to survive and multiply inside peritoneal macrophages of experimental animals (11). Our recent studies showed that the cytoplasmic membranes of L-form cells of E. coli WF+ contained lipopolysaccharide (LPS) (8) and induce more pronounced immunostimulating effect on antigen-binding spleen T-lymphocytes compared to cells of the parent bacterium (6) and also compared to an equivalent amount of E. coli lipopolysaccharide (7).

Having in mind the immunoadjuvant and immunostimulant activities of intracellular bacteria and LPS (12), our aim in the present study was to examine the influence of cytoplasmic membranes of E. coli WF+ L-forms on the number and on bactericidal activity of mouse peritoneal macrophages. Another task was to study by electron microscopy the process of phagocytosis of membranes by rat peritoneal macrophages.

The stable protoplast type L-form of E. coli WF+ was induced by subinhibitory concentrations of penicillin G (4) and cultivated in Tryptic soy broth "Difco" supplemented with 1% Yeast extract "Difco", 10% inactivated horse serum, 3% sodium chloride and 1000 E/ml penicillin G. The cytoplasmic membranes were isolated from L-form cells according to our method described earlier (5).

The immunological experiments were performed with 412 male mice weighing 18-20 g. Wistar male rats weighing 80-100 g were used as sources of peritoneal macrophages for electron microscopic investigations.

The number of the peritoneal exudate cells 7, 14, 21 and 30 days after i.p. inoculation of 0.5 mg L-form cytoplasmic membranes was estimated. The number of the same cells 1 or 24 hr after i.p. infection with cells of the parent strain, as well as one or six days after infection with L-form cells was determined up to 30 days after membrane treatment.

Bactericidal activity of peritoneal macrophages on cells of E. coli WF+ was estimated also once in a week 30 days after membrane injection. Bactericidal activity is expressed as a percentage of the number of colony-forming units (CFU) isolated from macrophages of experimental animals related to the number of CFU isolated from macrophages of control animals. RPMI 1640

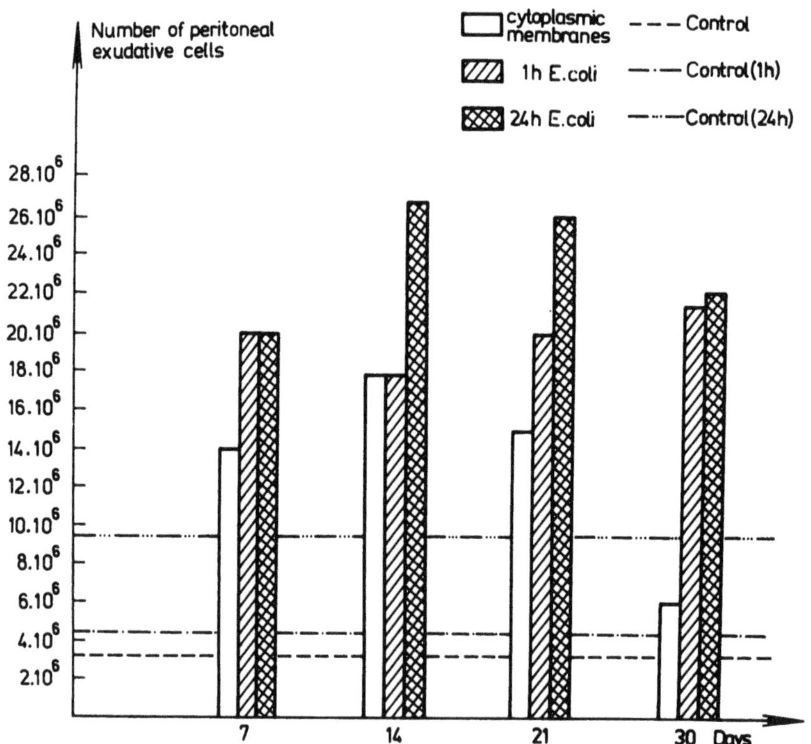

Fig 1. Number of the peritoneal exudate cells: a) in mice, inoculated i.p. with L-form cytoplasmic membranes; b) in membrane treated mice 1 hr and 24 hr after i.p. infection with E. coli WF+ cells; c) in mice 1 hr and 24 hr after i.p. infection with E. coli WF+ cells.

(Difco) medium supplemented with 10% fetal calf serum (Difco) was used for macrophage cultivation.

Electron microscopic investigations of rat peritoneal macrophages after 24 hr in vitro interaction with L-form cytoplasmic membranes were performed. The prefixation procedure was in 2.5% glutaraldehyde dissolved in 0.2M Na-cacodylate buffer. After incorporation of cells in 2% agar fixation of agar pieces by 1% OsO_4 for 18 hr at 4°C was done. The embedding in Vestopal was performed. The ultra thin sections were prepared by ultra cut "Reichert". Hitachi S500 instrument was used for electron microscopic observations.

It was established that the i.p. inoculation with cytoplasmic membranes induced a 4-5 fold increase of the number of peritoneal exudative cells compared to the control mice lasting for 30 days (Fig 1). The animals pre-treated with cytoplasmic membranes were able to react by 4-5 fold larger number of their peritoneal exudative cells after i.p. infection with E. coli WF+ cells, compared to the infected nontreated mice. Maximal increase was found by the 14th day of investigation (Fig 1).

The animals pretreated by L-form cytoplasmic membranes react by 2.5-3.5 fold larger increase of the number of peritoneal exudate cells after i.p. infection with L-form cells of E. coli WF+ compared to the infected non-treated mice (Fig 2).

It was observed that the macrophages of membrane-treated mice had 6-10

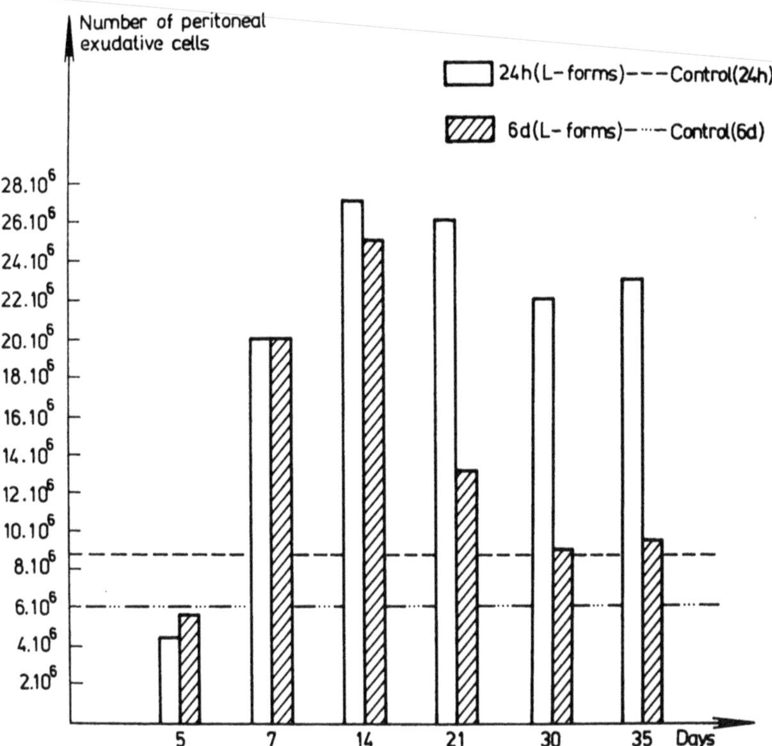

Fig 2. Number of the peritoneal exudate cells: a) in membrane treated mice 24 hr and 6 days after i.p. infection with L-form cells of E. coli WF+; b) in mice one and six days after i.p. infection with L-form cells of E. coli WF+.

fold increased bactericidal activity compared to the controls. The bactericidal activity in mice, primarily injected with cells of E. coli WF+ was less increased and lasted for a shorter period compared to the macrophages of membrane treated mice (Fig 3).

Our electron microscopic observations of rat peritoneal macrophages which reacted in vitro for 24 hr with cytoplasmic membranes showed that the adhesion processes were still going on (Fig 4a) and macrophage surfaces were activated (Fig 4a-d). Aggregates of membranes and their remnants were ingested and phagosomes formed could be seen in the peripheral part of cytoplasm (Fig 4b,c) or near the nucleus (Fig 4d) without the presence of lysosomes. Phagolysosome fusion was observed occasionally.

The established immunostimulating activity of L-form cytoplasmic membranes could be explained by the presence of LPS in them (8) as well as by their increased phospholipid contents (2). The unusual location of LPS in the cells of bacterial L-forms could be due to the location of the enzymes responsible for synthesis of LPS in the membrane (10). Because of the absence of cell wall in the stable L-form cells (4) this antigen remain bound to the cytoplasmic membrane (8).

Two of the features of LPS seem to be responsible for the immunostimulating activity of L-form cytoplasmic membranes. One of them is the ability of LPS to increase the secretion of a colony-stimulating factor from macrophages. On the other hand this antigen is able to induce formation of secondary lysosomes in macrophages, which interact with its own nucleus, leading to mitogenic response. Thus an enhanced synthesis of lysosomal enzymes is achieved (1). The increased bactericidal activity of membrane-stimulated macrophages could be due to such a mitogenic activity exhibited by the LPS.

The electron microscopic observations have shown a delayed digestion of membranes. We have established inhibition of phagolysosome fusion during phagocytosis of whole L-form cells too (11). It is known that the classical immunoadjuvant Mycobacterium cells survive within cytoplasm of macrophages

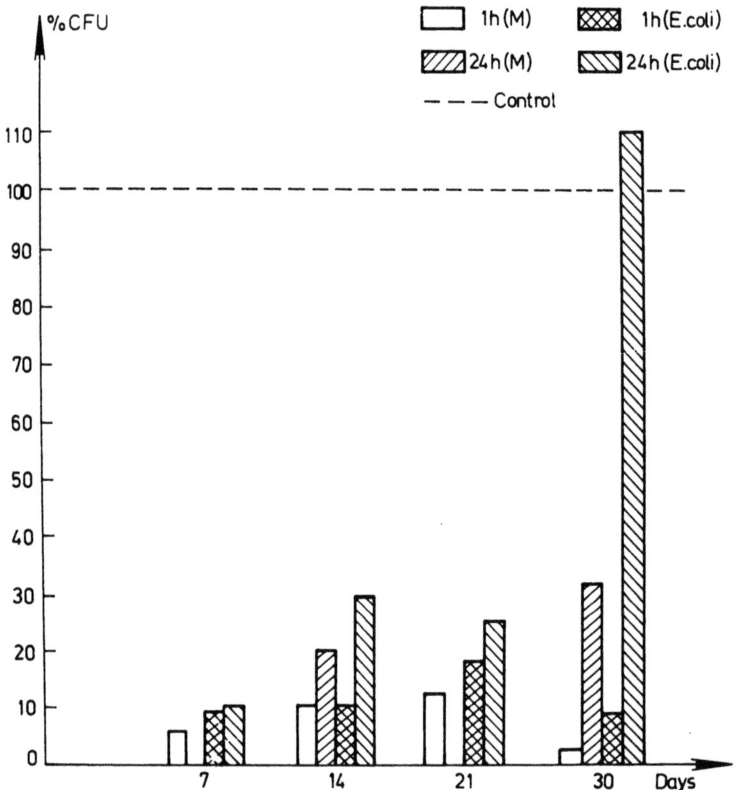

Fig 3. Bactericidal activity of peritoneal macrophages: a) in membrane treated mice estimated after 1 hr and 24 hr interaction with cells of E. coli WF+ (1hM, 24hM); b) in mice preliminary inoculated with 10^9 suspensions of cells of E. coli WF+ (1hr E. coli, 24h E. coli).

(3). According to the present knowledge the delay of metabolic processes of some bacterial antigens represents a mechanism of their immunostimulating activity (12).

Bearing in mind the large spectrum of action of macrophages on regulation of immune response (9), as well as the decreased toxicity of LPS after its incorporation as a component of L-form cytoplasmic membranes (7) we can make an optimistic prognosis for their use as stimulators of cellular immune response.

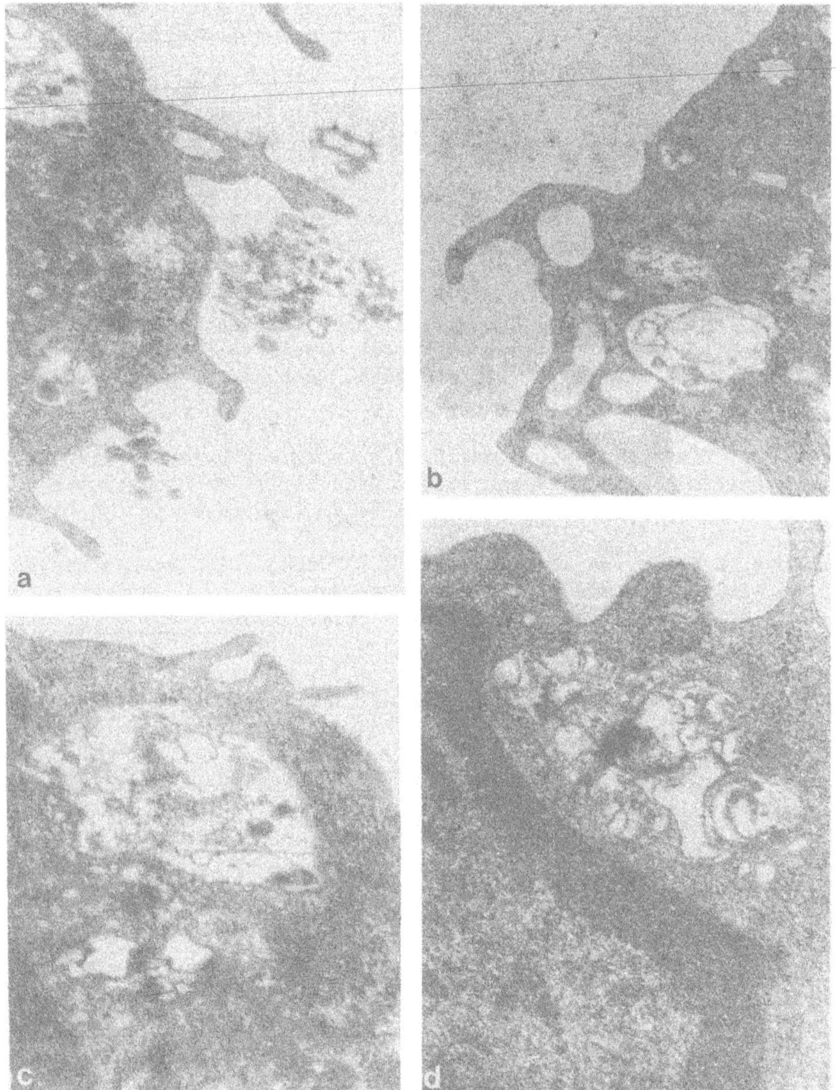

Fig 4. Ultrathin sections of rat peritoneal macrophages after 24 hr in vitro interaction with L-form cytoplasmic membranes: a) adhesion of a membrane and L-form cell ghost, phagolysosome fusion; b,c) phagosome, containing membranes and its remnants in the peripheral part of cytoplasm; d) phagosome, containing membranes and its remnants near the nucleus. Magnification: a,b-34000x, c-51000x, d-45000x.

REFERENCES

1. Bradley, S. G., 1979, Cellular and molecular mechanisms of action of bacterial endotoxins. Ann. Rev. Microbiol. 33: 67-94.

2. Baykousheva, S., Ivanova, E., Gumpert, J. and Toshkov, As., 1980, On the lipid composition of a stable L-form of Escherichia coli W 1655 F+. Acta Microbiol. Bulg. 6: 11-16.

3. Frehell, C., de Chastellier, C., Lang, T. and Rastogi, N., 1986,

Evidence for inhibition of fusion of lysosomal and prelysosomal compartments in macrophages infected with pathogenic Mycobacterium avium. Infect. Immun., No. 1, 52: 252-262.

4. Gumpert, J. Schuhmann, E. and Taubeneck, U., 1971, Ultrastruktur der stabilen L-Formen von Escherichia coli B and W 1655 F+. Z. Allg. Mikrobiologie 11: 19-33.

5. Ivanova, E. and Gumpert, J., 1986, Use of cytoplasmic membranes of bacterial L-forms as immunostimulators. Invention Reg. No. 75653, 8. 07.

6. Ivanova, E., Slavcheva, E., Gumpert, J. and Georgiev, D., 1988, Cytoplasmic membranes as activators of T-cell population, VIth Congress of Immunol., Toronto, Canada, 6-11 July 1986. Abstracts, p. 332; Epidemio, Microbiol. and Inf. Dis. (in press).

7. Ivanova, E., Slavcheva, E., Gumpert, J., Georgiev, D. and Stojanova, P., 1988, Cytoplasmic membranes and lipopolysaccharide of Escherichia coli as immunostimulators. Acta Microbiol. Bulg. (in press).

8. Michailova, L., Ivanova, E., Gumpert, J., Toshkov, As. and Jordanova, M., 1984, Immunoelectron microscopic determination of O-antigen localization in stable L-forms of Escherichia coli. C. R. Acad. Bulg. Sci. No. 1, 37: 77-80.

9. Nathan, C. F., Murray, H. W. and Cohn, Z. A., 1980, The macrophage as an effector cell. N. Engl. J. Med. 303: 622.

10. Osborn, M. J., Gander, J. E., Parisie, E. and Carson, J., 1972, Mechanism of assembly of the outer membrane. II. Site of synthesis of lipopolysaccharide. J. Biol. Chem. 247: 3973-3986.

11. Schmitt-Slomska, J., Michailova, L., Ivanova, E. and Toshkov, As., 1986, Adhesion and phagocytosis of Staphylococcus aureus L-forms. J. Basic Microbiol. No. 7, 26: 429-440.

12. Toshkov, As. and Dimov, V., Immunostimulation and immunostimulators, actual problems in science. Bulg. Acad. Sci., XII, No. 8.

EFFECTS OF LIPOPOLYSACCHARIDE OR RECOMBINANT HUMAN-INTERLEUKIN-1β ON CHEMILUMINESCENCE BY PERITONEAL MACROPHAGES FROM NORMAL AND MRL-**lpr/lpr** MICE

C. Damais[#], L. Friteau, D. Lando and B. Dugas[#]

[#]U313 INSERM, Hôpital Pitié-Salpêtrière, Paris, France
Laboratoire d'Immunologie, Roussel-Uclaf, Romainville, France

INTRODUCTION

Mononuclear phagocytes, under physiological conditions in a resting state, can be functionally activated by a number of stimuli (singly or in combination) both **in vitro** and **in vivo**. Amongst stimuli, some are known to prime macrophages for enhancing their level of oxidative metabolism revealed by luminol-dependent chemiluminescence (LDCL). Macrophage activation is a multi-step phenomenon which culminates to tumoricidal activity (5). This activation process is accompanied by synthesis of a variety of biologically active molecules such as Interleukin-1 (IL-1). Interleukin-1 released by macrophages can be induced **in vitro** by natural and synthetic bacterial immunoadjuvants such as lipopolysaccharide (LPS) (7) and Muramyl dipeptide (1). IL-1 is a polypeptide displaying a broad spectrum of biological activities (3). In this work, we compared the ability of LPS and recombinant human Interleukin-1β (rHu-IL-1β) (Roussel-Uclaf) to prime **in vivo** murine peritoneal macrophage-LDCL of both normal (Balb/c and MRL-+/+) and MRL-**lpr/lpr** mice. MRL-**lpr/lpr** mice develop a systemic lupus erythematosus-like syndrome characterized by numbers of cellular and humoral abnormalities (6), such as an increase in absolute number of lymphocytes and macrophages as function of age (2, 4, 6). Peritoneal macrophages from this strain of mice spontaneously showed an increased expression of class II antigen, expression of Interleukin-2 receptor and exhibited an enhanced oxidative metabolism triggered by phorbol-ester (PMA) (2, 4).

Characterization of Peritoneal Cells from LPS- or rHu-IL-1β-treated normal and MRL-**lpr/lpr** Mice

Injection by the i.p. route of an optimal dose of rHu-IL-1β (1 ng) to Balb/c and MRL-+/+ mice induced 24 hr later, in the peritoneal cavity, an increase in cellular number (Table 1), which was mostly related to an increase in absolute number of polymorphonuclear cells (both neutrophil and eosinophil), macrophages and lymphocytes. This enhancement was not due to a local cell division but resulted from a positive indirect chemotaxis. The cellular increase was not observed with 20 week-old MRL-**lpr/lpr** mice. Likewise, treatment with an optimal dose of LPS (10 μg/mouse) did not induce an increase in peritoneal cell number 24 hr later, administration neither in MRL-**lpr/lpr** nor, in that case, in normal mice (Table 1).

Table 1. Peritoneal cell count (x10^6) 24 hr after rHu-IL-1β or LPS injection to normal (4 and 20 week-old) and 20 week-old MRL-**lpr/lpr** mice[a].

Strains of mice	In vivo treatment with		
	vehicle	rHu-IL-1β	LPS
Balb/c	2.0 ± 0.5	7.0 ± 1	2.4 ± 5
MRL-+/+	2.2 ± 0.2	8.0 ± 1	2.0 ± 0.4
MRL-**lpr/lpr**	4.0 ± 1.0	4.0 ± 1	4.5 ± 0.5

[a]Values represent mean ± SEM from 8 experiments.

Effect of i.p. Injection of rHu-IL-1β and of LPS on LDCL by Peritoneal Macrophages from Normal and MRL-**lpr/lpr** Mice

When injected **in vivo**, rHu-IL-1 and LPS primed, in a dose dependent manner, peritoneal macrophages from normal Balb/c and MRL-+/+ mice to undergo LDCL-responses induced by PMA (Table 2). The priming effect of rHu-IL-1 or LPS reached maximum after 24 hr and then declined until 72 hr (data not shown). Although, LPS and rHu-IL-1β seemed to be uneffective to stimulate MRL-**lpr/lpr** mice (see Table 1), LPS injection to young adult stimulate peritoneal macrophages but PMA-triggered responses lowered as a function of age (Table 3) showing that status of activation of peritoneal macrophages changed according to appearance of the disease. By contrast, rHu-IL-1β was able to prime peritoneal macrophages to undergo LDCL responses upon PMA-triggering (Table 3) suggesting that activated macrophages from MRL-**lpr/lpr** mice were still able to respond to appropriate signal.

Table 2. LDCL response by peritoneal macrophages from normal and MRL-**lpr/lpr** mice 24 hr after i.p. injection of various doses of rHu-IL-1β or of LPS[a].

Dose injected[b]	LDCL (mV ± SEM) after injection of	
	rHu-IL-1β	LPS
0.01	16 ± 2	10 ± 2
0.1	19 ± 3	22 ± 1
0.3	32 ± 5	31 ± 3
1.0	40 ± 7	34 ± 6
3.0	45 ± 2	47 ± 8
10.0	44 ± 9	50 ± 3

[a]Peritoneal macrophages were stimulated **in vitro** with 200nM PMA. Similar results were obtained with Balb/c and MRL-+/+ mice and vehicle-treated mice did not exhibit an increase in PMA-triggered LDCL (10 ± 1 mV).
[b]μg/mouse for LPS and ng/mouse for rHu-IL-1β.

Table 3. LDCL response by peritoneal macrophages from LPS- (10 μg) or rHu-IL-1β (1ng) injected MRL-**lpr/lpr** mice as a function of age[a].

Age (weeks)	LDCL (mV ± SEM) after injection of		
	vehicle	rHu-IL-1β	LPS
4	8 ± 1	39 ± 7	44 ± 2
12	11 ± 3	42 ± 3	25 ± 6
20	18 ± 2	44 ± 5	20 ± 1

[a]Peritoneal macrophages were stimulated **in vitro** with 200nM PMA.

DISCUSSION

Data presented herein provide further evidence for abnormalities of peritoneal macrophage function in MRL-**lpr/lpr** mice. The decreasing ability of macrophages to be primed **in vivo** by LPS underlined the progressive emergence of hyperactivated cells in these mice.

LPS is an efficient first and/or second signal (i.e., synergistically with Interferon-g) in normal macrophage stimulation. LPS was uneffective to stimulate activated macrophages from 20 week-old MRL-**lpr/lpr**. By contrast, rHu-IL-1β could stimulate normal and/or activated macrophages showing that this monokine could act as a paracrine molecule capable to modulate cell metabolism at different stages of differentiation.

REFERENCES

1. Damais, C., Riveau, G., Parant, M., Gerota, J. and Chedid, L., 1982, Production of lymphocyte activating factor in the absence of endogenous pyrogen by rabbit or human leukocytes stimulated with muramyl dipeptide derivatives. Int. J. Immunopharmac. 4: 451.

2. Dang-Vu, A. P., Pisetsky, D. S. and Weinberg, J. B., 1987, Functional alterations of macrophages in autoimmune MRL-**lpr/lpr** mice. J. Immunol. 138: 1757.

3. Dinarello, C. A., 1984, Interleukin-1. Rev. Infect. Dis. 6: 51.

4. Dugas, B., Lecaque, D., Lando, D., Secchi, J and Damais, C., 1988, Effect of **in vivo** injection of recombinant human Interleukin-2 on peritoneal macrophages from MRL-**lpr/lpr** mice. J. Autoimmunity in press.

5. Nathan, C. F., Murray, H. W. and Cohn, Z. A., 1980, The macrophage as an effector cell. N. Engl. J. Med. 303: 622.

6. Theofilopoulos, A. N. and Dixon, F. J., 1981, Etiopathogenesis of murine SLE. Immunol. Rev. 55: 179.

7. Weinberg, J. B., Chapman, H. A. and Hibbs, J. B., 1978, Characterization of the effects of endotoxin on macrophage tumor cell killing. J. Immunol. 121: 72.

LPS-MEDIATED TRIGGERING OF T LYMPHOCYTES IN IMMUNE RESPONSE AGAINST GRAM-NEGATIVE BACTERIA

E. Jirillo, C. De Simone*, V. Covelli**, H. Kiyono°, J. R. McGhee°° and S. Antonaci***

Immunologia, **Neuroanatomia Clinica and ***Fisiopatologia Medica, University of Bari Medical School, Bari and *Malattie Infettive, University of dell'Aquila degli Abruzzi Medical School, L'Aquila, Italy and Departments of °Oral Biology and Preventive Dentistry and °°Microbiology, University of Alabama at Birmingham, Birmingham, AL, USA

INTRODUCTION

Penetration of pathogens into a susceptible host triggers an array of immune responses which involve all the immunocompetent cells (T and B lymphocytes, phagocytes and Natural Killer (NK) cells). However, in the case of bacteria, phagocytosis seems to be the most effective function in order to neutralize invading organisms. At the same time, until recently the role of lymphocytes in "processing" entire bacteria has been poorly investigated, even if bacterial components are able to activate lymphocytes (21).

An important step in the knowledge of the relationship between bacteria and lymphocytes has been represented by the discovery of Teodorescu and his associates (30) that bacteria can spontaneously bind to lymphocytes. Therefore, these investigators used the property of several species of gram-negative and gram-positive bacteria to bind to lymphocytes as a tool for defining human T and B lymphocyte populations with different functional capacities (30).

In the light of the above cited studies, our group has reexamined the adherence of bacteria to lymphocytes with the aim to better understand the characteristics and biological significance of the binding phenomenon.

For all the series of experiments which will be described below, we have employed a rough (R) mutant of Salmonella minnesota, the R345 (Rb) strain, because of its capacity to bind human and murine lymphocytes in a higher percentage than that observed with other R or smooth (S) Salmonella organisms (12, 14).

In this framework, we will report experiments on the role of lipopolysaccharide (LPS) in the binding to lymphocytes. Moreover, the characteristics of receptor site(s) for Salmonella on lymphoid cells will be illustrated.

Over the past few years, Tagliabue and colleagues (29) have described an antibacterial activity against S. typhi Ty 21a exerted by human peripheral blood lymphocytes (PBL). This activity has been ascribed to $CD4^+$ lymphocytes which are armed by IgA.

Here, we will provide evidence that in endemic areas for Salmonellosis (Bari, Italy) the above activity is higher than that detected in non-endemic areas (9). Furthermore, antibacterial activity is sustained by either T helper (TH) cells armed with IgA or T suppressor (TS) lymphocytes armed with IgG. Finally, some evidence on the role of LPS in the antibacterial activity will be discussed.

MATERIALS AND METHODS

Bacterial Strains

Salmonella minnesota Rb, Salmonella minnesota R595 (Re) and Salmonella typhimurium LT-2 from our collection were used in these studies.

PBL Isolation

PBL were isolated by Ficoll-Hysopaque density gradient centrifugation (8). Monocyte concentration in purified PBL was less than 3%, as assessed by nonspecific esterase criteria (31). In the murine system, lymphocytes were also isolated from other anatomical sites, as previously described (16).

$CD4^+$ and $CD8^+$ Cell Purification

Enriched $CD4^+$ and/or $CD8^+$ cell suspensions were obtained from purified PBL by complement-mediated lysis (25).

Bacterial Binding

Heat-killed Salmonella strains were used at different ratios to evaluate their cytoadherence to lymphocytes, as elsewhere described (12).

Antibacterial Activity

The test was performed by mixing Salmonella typhi with untreated or antibody-treated lymphoid cells. For details, see Tagliabue et al. (29).

RESULTS

Bacterial Structures Involved in the Binding

Enterobacteriaceae possess on the outer membrane of their cell wall a large molecule, the so-called LPS. LPS consists of three main regions, the O-polysaccharide chain, the core and the lipid A exhibiting many immunobiological activities (10). In particular, endotoxin acts as potent stimulator of B lymphocytes and macrophages (21).

Reasoning on the possible structures of Salmonella responsible for spontaneous adherence to human PBL or murine lymphoid cells, LPS has been taken into consideration for its large molecular weight and location on the outermost part of the cell wall.

In order to verify whether LPS plays a role in the binding to lymphocytes, the following experiments were performed. Either human PBL (12) or splenic lymphocytes from the C3H/HeJ murine strains (14) have been pretreated with Rb-LPS. Such a procedure leads to an inhibition of Salmonella Rb binding, even if one hundred per cent of adherence inhibition has never been obtained. In addition, isolated core from Rb-LPS leads to a similar degree of inhibition, this indicating that lymphocytes possess receptor binding site(s) for this structure, as also supported by Lehman and coworkers in their experiments (17). Moreover, studies have been undertaken to investigate whether the O-polysaccharide chain and the lipid A participate to the binding. In fact, pretreating human PBL with either Salmonella typhimurium-LPS (S strain) or with S. minnesota Re-LPS, we found that inhibition of binding is specific for the homologous Salmonella (12).

Altogether, these results point out that lymphocytes bear on their membrane binding site(s) for the three major components of LPS, even though receptors for core structures seem to be more expressed on lymphocyte surface.

The presence of protein components in the constitution of the cell wall such as porins of lipoproteins (10) led to further studies to ascertain the possible participation of these substances in the cytoadherence. Thus, Salmonella Rb organisms have been pretreated with thiol compounds such as Mersalyl or N-Ethyl-Malemeide which compete with the SH groups of proteins (23). This treatment gives rise to an inhibition of Rb cytoadherence to human PBL suggesting the involvement of bacterial proteins in the attachment to lymphocytes (23).

Receptors for Salmonella Rb on Lymphoid Cells

Quantitative analysis of Rb binding has been allowed by the use of new parameters such as the Binding Lymphocytes (BL) and the Bound Bacteria (BB) (22). BL expresses the percentage of lymphocytes which are coated by bacteria, while BB is the number of bound bacteria per lymphocyte. By varying the Salmonella/lymphocyte ratio in a range between 2 and 30, we have obtained saturation kinetics of BL and BB which are suggestive for the presence of receptors for bacteria on human PBL (22).

Concerning the nature of the receptors, experiments conducted by trypsin treatment of human PBL and murine splenic lymphocytes have demonstrated that the receptor is a protein (12, 14). In fact, trypsin cleavage of receptorial site(s) causes a dramatic reduction of Rb binding. However, overnight incubation of these lymphocyte suspensions at 37°C in 5% CO_2 allows the expression of receptors as supported by Rb binding recovery (12, 14).

The protein nature of the receptor is also confirmed by using the above thiol reagents which can compete with SH groups of cysteine on lymphocytes (23). Results show that thiol pretreatment of lymphoid cells inhibits cytoadherence, this supporting the proteinaceous nature of the receptor (23).

Role of Environmental LPS in the Expression of Rb Salmonella Receptors

Studies of Rb binding to murine lymphocytes brought very interesting results. In fact, in preliminary experiments it was striking to observe that splenic lymphocytes from the LPS-hyporesponsive murine strain, the C3H/HeJ mouse, underwent Rb binding in a higher percentage than that noted in the LPS-responsive counterpart, the C3H/HeN mouse strain (14). However, when adherence experiments were performed with lymphoid cells isolated from Peyer's Patches (PP), mesenteric lymph nodes (MLN) and peripheral blood, Rb binding was more elevated than that detected in their spleen (14). Since PP, MLN and PBL are under continuous exposure of LPS from gut flora (19), we reasoned that endotoxin may contribute to the expression of receptors for Salmonella on lymphocytes. This assumption is supported by other experimental evidences. For instance, in germ-free mice splenic lymphocytes seem to be completely devoid of receptors for Salmonella, this supporting the role of gut flora bacterial antigens in the development of the above receptors (15). Additionally, in vitro pretreatment of splenic C3H/HeN lymphoid cells with lipid A led to a significant enhancement of adherence (15). Due to the short period of time (1 hr) required for the expression of the receptor, we thought that lipid A can act causing earlier membrane modifications. In this respect, in parallel studies neuraminidase treatment of C3H/HeN splenic lymphocytes was able to enhance the Rb binding to a similar extent observed in the case of lipid A induction (14). Neuraminidase, as also demonstrated by Lehman, et al. (17) can act digesting the sialomucines of the membrane, thus unmasking possible receptor site(s) for Salmonella. Finally, in vivo administration of S-LPS in C3H/HeN mice significantly augments the in vitro binding of S. typhimurium LT-2 organisms to splenic lymphoid cells (ASM Meeting, 1985 - abstract).

Taken together, these results support the contention that LPS may regulate the expression of its own receptor.

Biological Significance of Bacterial Binding

Some hints on the in vivo function of bacterial adherence are provided by the observation that in patients with typhoid fever cytoadherence spontaneously occurs. In fact, in blood smears of these patients it is possible to enumerate a certain number of lymphocytes (from 5 to 10%) which are coated by bacteria. This occasional finding is also confirmed by more precise experiments in which cultures of bacteria-lymphocyte complexes led to the isolation of S. typhi, which was the same agent responsible for typhoid (13). Quite interestingly, the in vivo binding decreased with the time paralleling the end of the clinical course of the disease.

In this regard, antibiotic treatment is likely involved, since in vitro experiments point out that these agents compete with LPS for bacterial receptor structures on PBL surface (5).

These experiments suggest that during the course of infectious diseases the bacteria/lymphocyte complexes can be transported to the spleen where their engulfment by macrophages can occur.

The presence of receptors for Salmonella has been investigated in cancer patients undergoing chemo- and/or radiotherapy. At the end of the therapeutic regimen, the BB number on PBL was significantly reduced in comparison with values obtained at the beginning of the treatment (unpublished results). This fact may explain the increased frequency of bacterial infections (mostly gram-negative organisms) in cancer, which represents one of the major complications of the disease. In a group of cancer patients matched for age, sex and stage of neoplasia, we have administered a thymic hormone (timostimolina, Serono, Rome, Italy) in order to evaluate its effects on the binding. Results show that in these individuals the number of BB on PBL was not decreased at the end of the therapeutic treatment but rather significantly increased. Since bacterial binding is an energy-dependent phenomenon it is possible that timostimolina acts supplying energy to cells. In fact, previous experiments of our group have shown that addition of external ATP to PBL increases the BL and BB, while inhibitors of the electron transfer chain cause a decrease of BL and BB (23).

Bacterial binding has been also studied in old rats since aging is a condition associated with a deterioration of immune function. Actually, our results provide evidence that in aged rats splenic lymphocytes display a reduced capacity to undergo binding (11). However, in old human beings the bacterial binding is not dissimilar from that observed in the younger counterpart (6).

Recently, great emphasis has been given to the bidirectional communication between the neuroendocrine system and the immune system (24). In this regard, a role has been attributed to neuropeptides released from the central nervous system (CNS) and the vegetative nervous system (VNS) in the modulation of immunity (24). Among various neuropeptides, we have considered Met-Enkephalins (a CNS product) and substance P (a VNS product) for their putative capacity to influence bacterial adherence. While Met-Enkephalins do not display any effect on BL and BB in human PBL, substance P dramatically decreases binding (mostly acting on CD8 lymphocytes) (unpublished results). Since it is known that LPS can act on the neuroendocrine immune axis (18), substance P release in the course of infectious processes may modulate the bacterial adherence in terms of a possible noxious effect for the host.

Antibacterial Activity Exerted by Human PBL

Salmonella Rb adherence is restricted to 50% of human PBL and this evidence led us to carry out investigations on the phenotypic and functional characteristics of the remainder lymphocyte populations. Actually, the Rb-unbound fraction is enriched for NK and K cells and TH and TS lymphocytes bearing Fc receptors for IgA, IgG and IgM (1, 4, 26). In the light of these data, it became evident that Salmonella Rb binding does not occur casually, and at the same time certain categories of lymphocytes or other cell types such as NK and K cells do not actively participate to the binding.

What is the role of the Rb-unbound fraction in the bacterial adherence? A possible answer to this question is provided by a series of experiments conducted on human PBL from volunteers belonging to an endemic area for salmonellosis. Using enriched popoulations of $CD4^+$ and $CD8^+$ cells respectively, we have found that anti-Salmonella typhi or anti-Salmonella minnesota Rb activity is maintained by both lymphocyte subsets (9). In addition, competition experiments with anti-IgA and anti-IgG antibodies have led to the conclusion that TH cells are armed by IgA and TS cells are armed by IgG. This finding provides further support to the observation made by Tagliabue, et al. (29) according to which in non-endemic areas antibacterial activity is mediated by only IgA-armed $CD4^+$ cells.

In view of these data, we run experiments on the antibacterial capacity of the Rb-unbound cell fraction. Therefore, human PBL from an endemic area for salmonellosis were divided into Rb-bound and -unbound fractions by using a monolayer of adherent to plastic S. minnesota Rb organisms. Now, antibacterial activity was almost completely confined to the Rb-unbound fraction, while little activity was contained in the Rb-bound population. Thus, these experiments provide evidence that human PBL can be divided into two populations in terms of anti-Salmonella activity: one fraction undergoes binding, while another fraction enriched in $CD4^+$ and $CD8^+$ cells perform the actual antibacterial activity (9).

In this framework, we have also analyzed the role of LPS (lipid A) in the antibacterial activity. Then, pretreatment of human PBL with lipid A leads to a dramatic inhibition of antibacterial activity (unpublished observations). This may suggest that blocking of receptor site(s) for lipid A on lymphocytes functionally impairs the capacity of effector cells to perform their antibacterial activity.

Further experiments are required to elucidate the mechanism of the antibacterial activity (or killing?) and the exact role of LPS in the antibacterial function.

DISCUSSION

Our data emphasize a novel function of lymphoid cells, namely their ability to interact with entire bacteria. Up until now, a large body of evidence has been provided on the lymphocyte activation by bacterial antigens (e.g., LPS, lipoproteins or gram-positive components such as peptidoglycan, lipothecoid acid, etc.) (7, 10, 21). However, the relationship between immunocompetent cells and bacteria has been considered for a long time as a prerequisite of professional phagocytes. The findings reported here are focused on gram-negative organisms and, in particular, on Salmonella. Nevertheless, it is worth mentioning that in terms of bacterial binding other Enterobacteriaceae adhere to lymphocytes, such as E. coli, Yersinia enterocolitis, Campylobacter jejuni, etc. (unpublished results). Due to its higher capacity of binding, we have extensively employed for these experiments an R strain of Salmonella, the Rb, but we have evidence that in the course of infectious diseases other Salmonella strains acquire a more elevated binding capacity (unpublished results).

The role of LPS in the binding phenomenon is remarkable. In fact, LPS itself mediates the adherence to lymphocyte membrane, even if, to a less extent, proteins participate to the binding. On the other hand, environmental LPS from the gut flora may play an important function in the expression of receptor site(s) for Enterobacteriaceae on lymphoid cells. In this respect, activation of T lymphocytes from PP by endotoxin could lead to a migratory pathway of these cells from GALT to blood via lymphatic vessels. The fact that germ-free mice do not possess receptors on their splenic lymphocytes for bacteria may support our working hypothesis. In addition, in these mice induction of receptors mediated by lipid A fails to occur as it happens in conventional mice. In fact, only under prolonged incubation period of time (over 24 hr) Rb binding becomes evident in germ-free mice (unpublished results).

The biological significance of bacterial binding is provided by the observation of in vivo occurrence of binding in typhoid fever patients (13) and in septicaemic patients (unpublished results). In the absence of other experimental evidences, we have postulated that bacterial adherence to lymphocytes can represent a way of transporting bacteria from the bloodstream to distant organs such as spleen. However, it is likely that lymphoid cells from other anatomical sites such as Mucosal-Associated Lymphoreticular Tissues (MALT) can be more effective in the in situ adherence of bacteria. This has been found in bursa of Fabricius in chickens where it is possible to detect lymphocytes surrounded by bacteria (20). This may represent a protective function of bursa in birds.

As far as the role of mucosal lymphocytes is concerned, recent studies on the regulatory mechanisms of the mucosal immune system have led to the finding that contrasuppression plays a very important role in IgA secretion. In fact, PP contain effector T contrasuppressor cells (TCS) which favor the IgA response (27). These results stem from the evidence that C3H/HeJ mice contain PP TCS which transferred to orally tolerized syngeneic C3H/HeN mice reversed tolerance and supported secondary-type antibody responses (28). Now, the phenotype of these TCS cells has been defined and is the following: Lyt-1^+, 2^-, L3T4^- (16). Furthermore, this T cell subset contains a T3-T cell receptor complex. In prospective studies it would be very interesting to analyze the capacity of binding of Salmonella organisms to this cell subset and evaluate whether specific activation of the above TCS leads to a systemic immunoresponsiveness to these bacteria.

The protective role of bacterial adherence is also supported by the fact that S and R Salmonella share the ability to stimulate lymphokine (LK) release from human PBL. In fact, in vitro experiments have clearly shown that S and R Salmonella induce production of the LK Lymphocyte-Derived Chemotactic Factor (3) and Leukocyte-Inhibiting Factor (2). In the course of inflammatory processes, these LK may promote phagocytosis of bacteria contributing to their clearance from the host.

Antibacterial activity exerted by PBL seems also to be correlated to the bacterial adherence if one looks at the two events in a logical sequence. In fact, our data clearly evidence that lymphocytes which do not undergo binding instead are able to perform the antibacterial activity. Therefore, bacteria which have been trapped by one category of lymphocytes can be killed by effector cells such as IgA-armed TH and IgG-armed TS cells. The analogies between these two functions also support a sort of cooperative performance between them. In fact, antibacterial activity is inhibited by pretreatment of lymphocytes with LPS and, in particular, lipid A. In addition, the more elevated antibacterial activity in endemic areas for salmonellosis may indicate that the antigenic pressure present in the environment (especially gram-negative bacteria) activate lymphocytes in the expression of a more potent antibacterial function sustained also by $CD8^+$ cells armed by IgG.

In conclusion, the experiments reported here provide an update report on the relationship between LPS and immunocompetent cells.

ACKNOWLEDGMENTS

This work was supported by grants from Consiglio Nazionale delle Ricerche, Rome and Regione Puglia, Bari, Italy and by United States Public Health Service grants AI 19674, AI 21032, AI 18958, DE 04217, P60 AM 20614, DE 02670, a grant from the Procter and Gamble, Co. and a grant from the Alberta Heritage Foundation, USA.

REFERENCES

1. Antonaci, S., Jirillo, E., Ventura, M. T., Michalek, S. M., Bonomo, L. and McGhee, J. R., 1984, Relationship between immune system and gram-negative bacteria. II. Natural Killer cytotoxicity of Salmonella minnesota Rb 345-unbound human peripheral blood lymphocytes. J. Immunol. 133: 729.

2. Antonaci, S., Brandonisio, O., Ventura, M. T., Serlenga, E., Sansone, L. and Bonomo, L., 1985, Leukocyte Inhibitory Factor production by human peripheral blood lymphomonocytes stimulated with lipopolysaccharides from smooth and rough Salmonella strains. IRCS Med. Sci. 13: 261.

3. Antonaci, S. and Jirillo, E., 1985, Relationship between immune system and gram-negative bacteria: monocyte chemotaxis induced by supernatants from human peripheral blood $OKT8^+$ lymphocytes stimulated with smooth and rough Salmonella strains. Cell Immunol. 95: 258.

4. Antonaci, S., Jirillo, E., Kiyono, H., Williamson, S. I., Michalek, S. M. and McGhee, J. R., 1985, Relationship between immune system and gram-negative bacteria. III. Functional analysis of human peripheral blood lymphocyte subpopulations separated by cytoadherence with Salmonella minnesota Rb. Clin. Exp. Immunol. 62: 248.

5. Antonaci, S., Stasi, D., Gallitelli, M. and Jirillo, E., 1986, Inhibition by antibiotics of Rb Salmonella binding to human peripheral blood lymphocytes. Immunopharmacology 12: 23.

6. Antonaci, S., Gallitelli, M., Garofalo, A. R. and Jirillo, E., 1987, Functional properties of Salmonella minnesota Rb-bound and Rb-unbound cell fractions in elderly donors. Diagn. Clin. Immunol. 5: 1.

7. Beackey, E., Dale, J., Grebe, S., Ahmed, A., Simpson, W. and Ofek, I., 1979, Lymphocyte binding and T cell mitogenic properties of group A streptococcal lipoteichoic acid. J. Immunol. 122: 189.

8. Boyum, A., 1968, Isolation of mononuclear cells and granulocytes from human blood. Scand. J. Clin. Lab. Invest. 21: 77.

9. Cedola, M. C., Caretto, G., Nencioni, L., Tagliabue, A. and Jirillo, E., 1986, Natural antibacterial activity in individuals from an endemic area for Salmonellosis. EOS Riv. Immunol. Immunofarmacol. 6: 248.

10. Galanos, C., Luderitz, O., Rietschel, E. T. and Westphal, O., 1977, Newer aspects of the chemistry and biology of bacterial lipopolysaccharides with special reference to their lipid A components, in: "International Review of Biochemistry. Biochemistry of lipids II, vol. 14," T. W. Goodwin, ed., University Park Press, Baltimore.

11. Guanti, G., Porsia, R. and Jirillo, E., 1986, Salmonella adherence to rat lymphocytes and aging effect on the binding. EOS Riv. Immunol. Immunofarmacol. 6: 244.

12. Jirillo, E., Antonaci, S., Michalek, S. M., Colwell, D. E., McGhee, J. R. and Bonomo, L., 1984, Relationship between immune system and gram-negative bacteria. I. Spontaneous binding of smooth and rough Salmonella to human peripheral blood lymphocytes. Clin. Exp. Immunol. 58: 167.

13. Jirillo, E. and Antonaci, S., 1985, Spontaneous adherence of Salmonella typhosa to human peripheral blood lymphocytes in typhoid fever. Infection 13: 157.

14. Jirillo, E., Antonaci, S., Kiyono, H., Michalek, S. M. and McGhee, J. R., 1985, Relationship between immune system and gram-negative bacteria IV. T lymphocytes from Lps^d mice possess binding site(s) for Rb S lmonella. J. Immunol. 135: 3473.

15. Jirillo, E. and Antonaci, S., 1986, Relationship between immune system and gram-negative bacteria. Lipid A enhances Salmonella Rb cytoadherence to C3H/HeN splenic T lymphocytes, in: "Bacteria and the Host," M. Ryc and J. Franek, eds., Avicenum, Prague.

16. Kitamura, K., Kiyono, H., Fujihashi, K., Eldridge, J. H., Green, D. R. and McGhee, J. R., 1987, Contrasuppressor cells that break oral tolerance are antigen-specific T cells distinct from T helper ($L3T4^+$), T suppressor ($Lyt\text{-}2^+$) and B cells. J. Immunol. 139: 3251.

17. Lehmann, V., Streck, H., Minner, I., Krammer, P. H. and Ruschmann, E., 1980, Selection of bacterial mutants from Salmonella specifically recognizing determinants on the cell surface of activated T lymphocytes. A novel system to define cell surface structures. Eur. J. Immunol. 10: 685.

18. McCann, S. M., Ono, N., Khorram, O., Kentrati, S. and Aguila, C., 1987, The role of brain peptides in neuroimmunomodulation, in: "Neuroimmune Interaction," B. D. Jankovic, B. M. Marcovic, and N. I. Spector, eds., Annals of the New York Academy of Sciences.

19. McGhee, J. R. and Mestecky, J., 1983, The Secretory Immune System. Ann. NY Acad. Sci. 409: 1.

20. Monno, R. A., Manodoro, V., Di Carlantonio, M. E., Ianieri, A., Di Modugno, G. and Jirillo, E., 1986, Relationship between immune system and gram-negative bacteria. Binding of Salmonella pullorum-gallinarum to chicken lymphocytes. Eur. J. Epidemiol. 2: 294.

21. Morrison, D. C. and Ryan, J. L., 1979, Bacterial endotoxins and host immune responses. Advanc. Immunol. 28: 293.

22. Passarella, S., Casamassima, E., Quagliarello, E., Caretto, G. and Jirillo, E., 1985, Quantitative analysis of lymphocyte-salmonella interaction and effect of lymphocyte irradiation by helium neon laser. Biochem. Biophys. Res. Commun. 130: 546.

23. Passarella, S., Barile, M., Quagliarello, E., Caretto, G., Cedola, M. C. and Jirillo, E., 1986, Lymphocyte-salmonella interaction: energy dependence and thiol group involvement. Biochem. Biophys. Res. Commun. 137: 222.

24. Payan, D. G., McGillis, J. P. and Goetzl, E. J., 1986, Neuroimmunology. Advanc. Immunol. 39: 299.

25. Perlmann, P. and Wahlin, B., 1983, Characterization of human K cells by surface antigens and morphology at the single cell level. J. Immunol. 131: 2340.

26. Serlenga, E., Antonaci, S., Gallitelli, M., Garofalo, A. R., Jirillo, E. and Bonomo, L., 1985, Salmonella minnesota R345 (Rb) binding to human peripheral blood lymphocytes as a useful tool for the enrichment of cells mediating antibody-dependent cellular cytotoxicity in the Rb-unbound fraction. Ital. J. Med. 1: 17.

27. Suzuki, I., Kitamura, K., Kiyono, H., Kurita, T., Green, D. R. and McGhee, J. R., 1986, Isotype-specific immunoregulation: evidence for a distinct subset of T contrasuppressor cells for IgA responses in murine Peyer's patches. J. Exp. Med. 164: 501.

28. Suzuki, I., Kiyono, H., Kitamura, K., Green, D. R. and McGhee, J. R., 1986, Abrogation of oral tolerance by contrasuppressor T cells suggests the presence of regulatory T cell networks in the mucosal immune system. Nature 320: 451.

29. Tagliabue, A., Villa, L., Boraschi, D., Peri, G., De Gori, V. and Nencioni, L., 1985, Natural antibacterial activity against Salmonella Typhi by human $T4^+$ lymphocytes armed with IgA antibodies. J. Immunol. 135: 4178.

30. Teodorescu, M. and Mayer, E. P., 1982, Binding of bacteria to lymphocyte subpopulations. Advanc. Immunol. 33: 307.

31. Yam, L. T., Li, C. Y. and Crosby, M. H., 1971, Cytochemical identification of monocytes and granulocytes. Am. J. Clin. Pathol. 55: 283.

INVOLVEMENT OF I-A-RESTRICTED B-B CELL INTERACTION IN THE POLYCLONAL B CELL DIFFERENTIATION INDUCED BY LIPOPOLYSACCHARIDE*

Y. Takahama+, S. Ono#, K. Ishihara, M. Muramatsu and T. Hamaoka

Division of Oncogenesis, Biomedical Research Center, Osaka University Medical School, Fukushimaku, Osaka 553, Japan

SUMMARY

The present study has examined a functional role of Ia molecules expressed on murine B cells in polyclonal B cell differentiation induced by lipopolysaccharide (LPS). Reverse IgM PFC responses of unprimed B cells induced by LPS in the apparent absence of T cells and adherent accessory cells were markedly inhibited in a haplotype-specific manner by Fab monomer fragment of anti-class II (Ia) but not anti-class I MHC monoclonal antibody (mAb). However, the degree of inhibition of LPS responses of H-2-heterozygous F1 B cells expressing both parental I-A products by either one of anti-I-A mAb was at best half that of the parental B cells. Interestingly, when (B10 x B10.-BR)F1 ($H-2^{b/k}$) B cells were fractionated into adherent and nonadherent populations by their ability to bind to parental B10 B cell monolayers, LPS responses of F1 B cells adherent to and nonadherent to the B10 B cell monolayers were selectively inhibited by anti-I-A^b and anti-I-A^k mAb, respectively.. These results suggest that LPS-responsive F1 B cells comprise at least two separate populations with restriction specificity for only one of the parental I-A products expressed on B cells. In addition, it was demonstrated that the I-A-restriction specificity of LPS-responsive B cells is "plastic" and determined by H-2-genotype of bone marrow cells present during B cell ontogeny but not by that of radiation-resistant host elements. Namely, the LPS responses of B10-derived B cells from (B10 + B10.BR) ($H-2^b$ x $H-2^k$)F1 radiation bone marrow chimeras but not from B10 ($H-2^b$ x $H-2^k$)F1 chimeras became sensitive to the inhibition of anti-I-A^k mAb in the presence of mitomycin C-treated I-A^k-positive B cells, supporting a notion of receptor-Ia molecules interactions rather than like-like interactions. Thus, the present results provide evidence indicating that B-B cell interaction via recognition of self-I-A products is a crucial event in the polyclonal B cell differentiation induced by LPS.

+Fellowship of the Japan Society for the Promotion of Science for Japanese Junior Scientists.

*This work was supported by Grant-in-Aids from the Ministry of Education, Science and Culture, and the Osaka Foundation for Promotion of Clinical Immunology.

#Correspondence address - Dr. Shiro Ono

INTRODUCTION

The role of class II major histocompatibility complex (MHC)-encoded molecules (Ia molecules) in lymphocyte activation has been the subject of a great deal of investigation. Their function as restriction elements for T cells in the cellular interaction with B cells and the accessory cells such as macrophage/dendritic cells and their importance in the control of the immune response (Ir) gene have been well established (9, 10, 12, 19, 20, 27). In addition, many investigators have suggested that the Ia molecules are also involved in the T cell-independent B cell activation processes (2, 3, 7, 8, 14, 17, 18, 21, 22, 24, 26). For example, Forsgren et al., (7) reported that monoclonal antibodies (mAb) against class II MHC molecules are capable of inhibiting B cell activation induced by bacterial lipopolysaccharide (LPS). However, mechanism underlying such inhibition of the B cell activation by anti-class II MHC mAb is not obvious.

Our recent studies (6, 8, 11, 16-18, 24) have been focused on the mechanism of polyclonal B cell differentiation induced by a murine T cell hybridoma-derived lymphokine B151-TRF2. In previous work, we demonstrated that the B151-TRF2 acts on murine resting B cells to induce IgM-producing cells without any additional stimuli in the apparent absence of T cells and accessory cells (16, 17). In addition, this B cell activation process was markedly inhibited by mAb specific for class II MHC but not for class I MHC molecules (17). Interestingly, when MHC-heterozygous (P1 x P2)F1 ($H\text{-}2^{P1/P2}$) B cells were fractionated by their ability to bind to P1 B cell monolayers, the B151-TRF2 responses of the F1 B cells adherent to the P1 monolayer were inhibited by anti-I-A^{P1} but not by anti-I-A^{P2} mAb, whereas those of the nonadherent F1 B cells were inhibited only by anti-I-A^{P2} mAb (17, 24). Moreover, the B151-TRF2 responses of P1-derived B cells from lethally irradiated (P1 x P2)F1 or P1 mice reconstituted with P1 and P2 bone marrow cells (designated (P1 + P2) → (P1 x P2)F1 and (P1 + P2) → P1 chimeras, respectively) but not from P1 → P2 and P1 → (P1 x P2)F1 chimeras became sensitive to the inhibition of not only anti-I-A^{P1} but also anti-I-A^{P2} mAb only when the culture was conducted in the presence of mitomycin C-treated P2 B cells as auxiliary cells, demonstrating that they adaptively differentiate to recognize as self-structure allogeneic as well as syngeneic Ia molecules expressed on B cells (18). Taken together, these results strongly support the notion that the B-B cell interaction process via recognition of self-Ia molecules is involved in the B151-TRF2-induced B-cell activation and that their self-recognition specificity is dictated by the MHC haplotype of bone marrow cells present during the B cell ontogeny but not by the MHC haplotype of a radiation-resistant host environment.

Therefore, it is of interest to examine whether this novel type of cellular interaction, Ia-restricted B-B cell interaction, is a general process involved in polyclonal B cell differentiation. LPS is known to be most potent B cell mitogen and activate 10 to 50% of total B cell population in different mouse strains (1, 7, 13). In this study, we have analyzed the mechanism by which the anti-class II MHC mAb inhibits LPS- induced polyclonal B cell differentiation, by utilizing the strategies of our previous study on B151-TRF2-induced B cell activation. Our results indicate that class II MHC molecules function as restriction elements for B-B cell interaction in the early step of the LPS-induced polyclonal B cell activation.

MATERIALS AND METHODS

Animals

C57BL/10 (B10), B10.BR, (B10 x B10.BR)F1 and (C57BL/6 x C3H/He)F1 (B6C3-F1) mice were obtained from the Shizuoka Agricultural Cooperative Association for Laboratory Animals, Hamamatsu, Japan. Male mice were used at age 5 to 8 wk.

Radiation Bone Marrow Chimeras

Radiation bone marrow chimeras are denoted as bone marrow donor → irradiated recipient. Recipient (B10 x B10.BR)F1 or B6C3F1 mice were lethally x-irradiated with 925 rad and reconstituted 8-12 hr later with T cell-depleted B10 bone marrow cells (1 x 10^7) and/or T cell-depleted B10.BR bone marrow cells (1 x 10^7). The overall long-term survival of the used chimeras was 75%. Chimeras were rested at least 3 mo before use. These chimeric spleen cells were virtually all of donor origin. In the case of (B10 + B10.BR) → (B10 x B10.BR)F1 double bone marrow chimeras, their spleen cells were found to be roughly equal ratio of each donor-type. The chimeric spleen cells were unresponsive to host- and donor-type stimulating cells but responsive to third party allogeneic stimulating cells in mixed leukocytes reaction, as described previously (18).

mAbs

Anti-H-2 reagents used in this study are Protein A-purified mouse IgG mAbs as described previously (17, 18, 24).

LPS

Trichloroacetic acid (TCA)- and phenol-extracted Escherichia coli 0111: B4 LPS and TCA-extracted E. coli 0127:B8 LPS were purchased from Difco Laboratories, Detroit, MI. Phenol-chloroform-petroleum ether (P-C-PE)-extracted E. coli EH100 (Ra mutant) LPS, P-C-PE-extracted E. coli J5 (Rc mutant) LPS, phenol-extracted Serratia marcescens LPS, phenol-extracted and gel filtration-purified E. coli p26:B6 LPS were obtained from Sigma Chemical Co., St. Louis, MO. Phenol-extracted Salmonella minnesota LPS and P-C-PE-extracted S. minnesota R595 (Re mutant) LPS were obtained from Calbiochem, Behling Diagnosis, La Jolla, CA, and List Biological Lab. Inc., Campbell, CA, respectively. Butanol (BuOH)- and phenol-extracted E. coli K235 LPS, which were prepared by Dr. David C. Morrison, Emory University, Atlanta, GA (13, 15) were kindly provided by Drs. John L. Ryan and Alfred Singer, National Institutes of Health, Bethesda, MD. In most experiments, TCA-extracted E. coli 0111:B4 LPS were used unless otherwise indicated.

Other B Cell Activators

Lipid A prepared from S. minnesota R595 and the lipoprotein from the outer cell wall of S. typhimurium Re mutant were purchased from List Biological Lab. and Ribi Immunochem. Res., Inc., Hamilton, MT, respectively. 8-bromoguanosine (8BrGuo) and 8-mercaptoguanosine (8MGuo) were obtained from Sigma Chemical Co. Purified protein derivatives from Mycobacterium tuberculosis Aoyama B (PPD) was kindly provided by Dr. Kiyoshi Takatsu, Kumamoto University, Kumamoto, Japan. B151-TRF2 is a T cell hybridoma B151K12-derived B cell differentiation factor and was prepared as described (11, 16).

Preparation of $F(ab')_2$ and Fab Fragment of Anti-I-A mAb

Protein A-purified anti-I-A^k mAb 10-3.6 (IgG2ak; 8 mg) was digested with beads-immobilized pepsin (0.5 mg enzyme) or papain (0.1 mg enzyme), which were obtained from Pierce Chemical Co., Rockford, IL, for 2 and 5 hr at 37°C in 1 ml of 20 mM sodium acetate buffer, pH 4.5 and 20 mM sodium dihydrogenphosphate/20 mM cystein hydrocholoride/10 mM tetrasodium EDTA, pH 6.2, respectively. $F(ab')_2$ and Fab fragments were purified over a Protein A-Sepharose (Pharmacia Fine Chemicals, Uppsala, Sweden). The purity of these materials was ascertained by SDS-PAGE under the nonreducing condition.

Cell Preparation

T cell-depleted spleen cells were prepared from unprimed mice spleen cells by treatment of anti-Thy1.2 mAb + rabbit complement, and used routinely as B cells unless otherwise indicated. Purified B cells were prepared from unprimed mice spleen cells by Sephadex G10-passage and then treatment of anti-Thy1.2 + rabbit complement (17, 18, 24). Fractionation of F1 B cells on cell monolayers, treatment of anti-H-2^k mAb + complement and mitomycin C-treatment were previously described in detail (17, 18, 24).

Other Materials and Methods

Cell culture, reverse plaque-forming cell (PFC) assay for the detection of IgM-producing cells and other materials and methods used in this paper have all been described in our previous publications (6, 8, 11, 16-18, 24).

RESULTS

Ia-Dependent Activation Process Are Involved in the Early Step of LPS-induced Polyclonal B Cell Differentiation

To investigate the effect of anti-MHC mAbs on LPS-induced B cell differentiation, T cell-depleted B10 (H-2^b) or B10.BR (H-2^k) spleen cells were cultured with TCA-extracted LPS from E. coli 0111:B4 (herein after referred to as LPS) in the presence or absence of anti-class I or class II MHC mAb for 5 days. As can be seen in Fig 1A, polyclonal IgM PFC responses of B10.BR B cells induced by LPS were markedly inhibited by anti-I-A^k (10-3.6 or 10-2.16) and anti-I-E^k (14-4-4S) mAbs but not by anti-H-$2K^k$ (11-4.1) mAb. In addition, anti-I-A^b (34-5-3S) and anti-I-A^k mAb inhibited the LPS-induced responses of B10 and B10.BR B cells in a haplotype-specific manner, whereas anti-K^bD^b (28-8-6S) and anti-K^k mAb did not exhibit any inhibitory effect on the responses of both B cells (Fig 3). Because these anti-K^bD^b and anti-K^k mAbs were shown to bind to more than 97% of B10 and B10.BR B cells, respectively (18), it seems unlikely that the lack of inhibitory effects of anti-class I MHC mAbs is due to no binding of these mAbs to the corresponding B cells.

The anti-class I MHC mAbs used (11-4.1 and 28-8-6S, IgG2ak) are the same Ig subclass as most anti-class II MHC mAbs (34-5-3S, 10-3.6, and 14-4-4S) except 10-2.16 (IgG2bk). Therefore, it seemed unlikely that the inhibition by anti-Ia mAbs is mediated by secondary interaction of the mAbs with Fc-receptors after specific binding to the Ia molecules on B cells. To further exclude this possibility, we prepared $F(ab')_2$ and Fab fragments of anti-I-A^k mAb, which are known to lack the ability to interact with Fc-receptors. As shown in Fig 1B, both $F(ab')_2$ and Fab fragments of anti-I-A^k mAb inhibited the LPS-induced response of B10.BRB cells in the same degree as the intact anti-I-A^k mAb, demonstrating that anti-I-A-mediated inhibition of LPS-induced B cell responses is not resulted from Fc-receptor-mediated transduction of negative signals. It should be emphasized that Fab monomer fragment of the anti-I-A^k mAb has the ability to inhibit the B cell differentiation induced by LPS (Fig 1B), indicating that crosslinking of I-A molecules is not essential for the inhibition of the response. Because purified B cells depleted of T cells and adherent macrophage/dendritic cells were used as the responding B cells in this experiment (Fig 1B), these results indicate that Ia molecules expressed on B cells play a crucial role in the LPS-induced B cell differentiation.

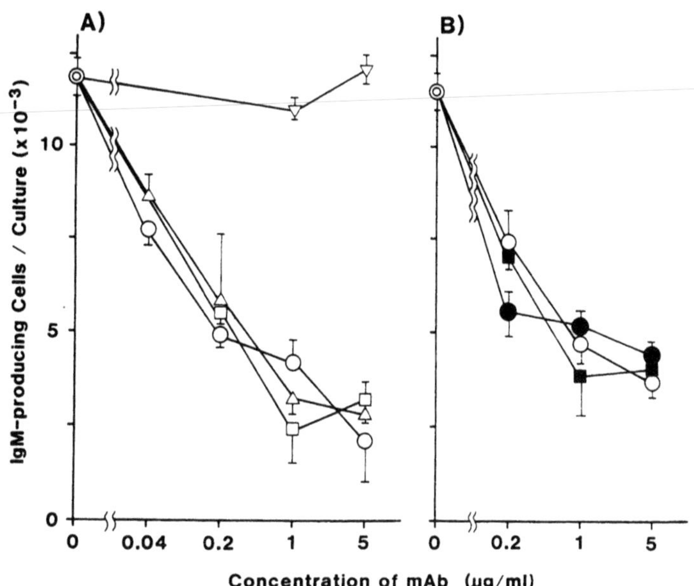

Fig 1. A) Inhibition of LPS-induced polyclonal B cell differentiation by anti-class II but not anti-class I MHC mAbs. T cell-depleted (anti-Thy1.2 mAb + complement-treated) B10.BR spleen cells (1×10^5) were cultured with 5 ug/ml LPS in the absence (◎) or presence of graded concentrations of anti-H-2 mAb. Protein A-purified 10-3.6 (anti-I-A β^k, O), 10-2.16 (anti-I-A β^k, □), 14-4-4S (anti-I-E α^k, △), or 11-4.1 (anti-K^k, ▽) were used. IgM-producing cells were enumerated on day 5 by the reverse IgM PFC assay. B) Inhibition of the LPS-induced B cell responses by $F(ab')_2$ and Fab fragments of anti-I-A mAb. Purified B10.BR B cells (G10-passed and anti-Thy1.2 mAb + complement-treated spleen cells) were cultured with 5 ug/ml LPS in the absence (◎) or presence of graded concentrations of intact IgG (O), $F(ab')_2$ fragment (●), or Fab fragment (■) of anti-I-A^k mAb (10-3.6).

To explore the time sequence with which the Ia-dependent activation process proceeds, anti-I-A^k mAb was added to the culture of T cell-depleted B10.BR spleen cells at different times over a 5-day culture period, in which LPS was present from the initiation of culture. As shown in Fig 2A, when anti-I-A mAb was added on day 2, LPS-induced B cell responses were not apparently inhibited, although the responses were indeed inhibited by the anti-I-A mAb if added on day 0. These results led us to the possibility that Ia-dependent activation process might be involved in the early step of LPS-induced B cell response. To further examine this possibility, an experiment of two-step culture was set up. T cell-depleted B10.BR spleen cells which had been cultured without LPS in the absence or presence of anti-MHC mAb for 2 days were washed extensively and cultured with LPS in the absence or presence of anti-MHC mAbs for an additional 3 days (Fig 2B). The polyclonal differentiation of B10.BR B cells was markedly inhibited when anti-I-A^k mAb was exposed to the responding B cells during the first 2 days of the 5-day culture, whereas the presence of the anti-I-A^k mAb during day 2 to 5 in the second culture did not affect the responses. Anti-H-2K^k mAb was unable to inhibit the responses, even when added to either culture step. Thus, it can be interpreted that polyclonal B cell differentiation induced by LPS involves an early activation process which is inhibitable by anti-Ia mAb.

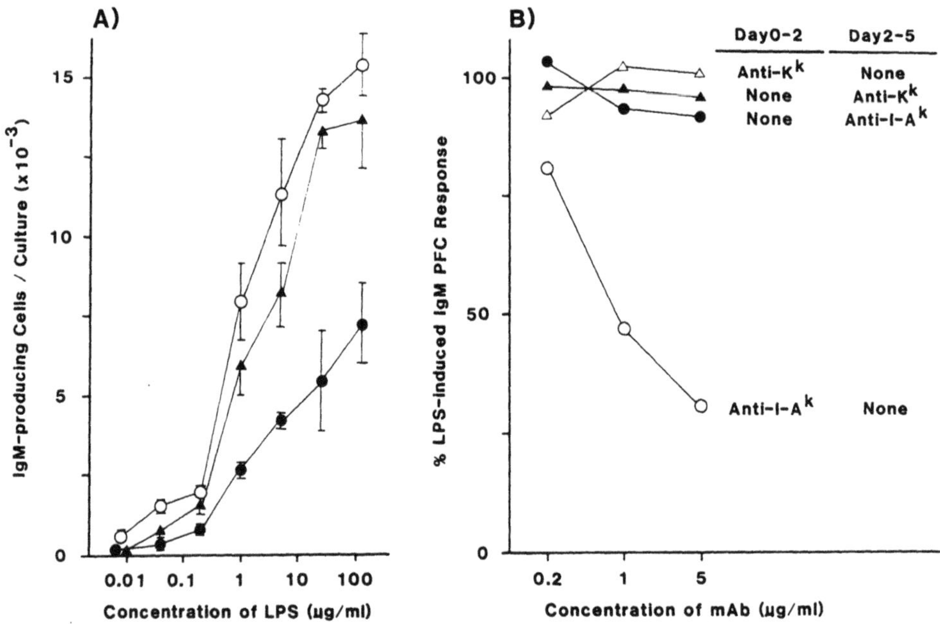

Fig 2. Anti-I-A mAb inhibits early events of the LPS-induced polyclonal B cell differentiation. A) The B cell responses are not inhibited by delayed addition of anti-I-A mAb. T cell-depleted B10.BR spleen cells (1×10^5) were cultured with the graded concentrations of LPS for 5 days. The B cell-culture was conducted in the absence (O) or presence of anti-I-A^k mAb (10-3.6; 5 μg/ml) which was added on day 0 (●) or day 2 (▲). B) Anti-I-A mAb inhibits the early but not the late phase of the LPS-induced B cell differentiation. T cell-depleted B10.BR spleen cells (1×10^6/2 ml) were cultured without LPS in the absence (● , ▲) or presence of graded concentrations of anti-I-A^k mAb (10-3.6; O) or anti-K^k mAb (11-4.1; Δ). Two days later, recovered cells (1×10^5) were cultured with 5 ug/ml LPS for an additional 3 days in the absence (O , Δ) or presence of graded concentrations of the anti-I-A^k (●) or anti-K^k (▲) mAb. Percent control PFC responses are calculated by the following formula: % response = 100 x (LPS-induced PFC in the presence of mAb/LPS-induced PFC in the absence of mAb).

The Ia-Dependent Activation Process Involved in LPS-Induced Polyclonal B Cell Differentiation is Mediated by the Recognition by B Cells of Self-Ia Molecules on B Cells

To gain insight into the mechanism of the Ia-dependent activation process in the early step of LPS-induced B cell differentiation, the inhibitory effect of anti-Ia mAbs on the LPS-induced responses of H-2-heterozygous F1 B cells, which codominantly express both parental Ia molecules on their surface, was examined. As shown in Fig 3, the responses of the parental B10 and B10.BR B cells were specifically inhibited by anti-I-A^b and anti-I-A^k mAbs, respectively. Interestingly, the degree of inhibition of the LPS-induced responses of (B10 x B10.BR)F1 B cells was at best half that of the parental B cells, indicating that anti-Ia mAb-mediated inhibition of LPS responses is not due to the transmission of negative signal to the responding B cells by virtue of its binding to the Ia molecules. These results raised a possibility that B-B cell interaction process via recognition of self-Ia molecules is involved in LPS-induced response and that the LPS-responsive F1 B cells

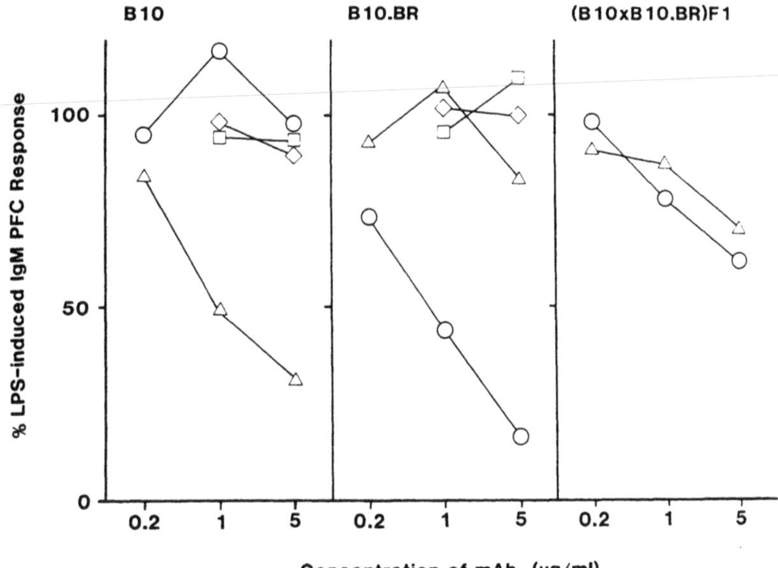

Fig 3. H-2-heterozygous F1 B cells are less susceptible to the inhibitory effects of anti-parental I-A mAbs on LPS-induced polyclonal B cell differentiation. T cell-depleted B10, B10.BR or (B10 x B10.BR)F1 spleen cells (1 x 10^5) were cultured with 5 ug/ml LPS in the absence or presence of graded concentrations of anti-I-A^b (34-5-3S; Δ), anti-I-A^k (10-3.6; O), anti-K^bD^b (28-8-6S; ◇) or anti-K^k (11-4.1; □) mAb for 5 days.

consist of two separate populations capable of recognizing only one of the parental I-A molecules expressed on B cells.

To examine this possibility, F1 B cells were fractionated into adherent and nonadherent cell populations by panning onto either one of parental B cell monolayers, and haplotype specificity of the inhibition of their LPS-induced responses by the respective anti-parental Ia mAbs was examined. As shown in Table 1, the responses of unfractionated F1 B cells were marginally inhibited by either anti-I-A^b or anti-I-A^k mAb, which was demonstrated in the same experiment to inhibit strikingly the responses of corresponding parental B10 or B10.BR B cells in a haplotype-specific manner. To be noted, the responses of F1 B cells adherent to the B10 B cell monolayer now became inhibitable by anti-I-A^b but not by anti-I-A^k mAb, whereas those of F1 B cells nonadherent to the B10 B cell monolayer were inhibited only by anti-I-A^k but not by anti-I-A^b mAb. Reciprocally, the responses of F1 B cells adherent and nonadherent to the B10.BR B cell monolayer were selectively inhibited by anti-I-A^k and anti-I-A^b mAbs, respectively. These results demonstrate that the LPS-responsive F1 B cells consist of at least two distinct subpopulations, of which the responses are selectively inhibited by either one of the anti-parental Ia mAbs, when fractionated by their ability to bind to the respective parental B cell monolayers. It should be noted that the responses of (B10 x B10.BR)F1 B cells nonadherent to the B10 and B10.BR B cell monolayers were selectively inhibited by another parent-specific anti-I-A^k and anti-I-A^b mAbs, respectively. This excludes a possibility that the Ia-restricted B cell activation observed here attributes to the irradiated parental cell contamination released from the monolayers. Rather, these results imply that F1 B cells already contain two independent populations with restriction specificity for only one of the parental Ia molecules before monolayer fractionation. In addition, as reported previously (24), the flow cytofluorometric analysis revealed that F1 B cells adherent and nonadherent to only one of the parental B cell monolayers expressed both parental Ia molecules almost equally. This result also excludes the possibility that the restriction specificity of F1 B cells might reflect quantitative variation in the expression of either parental Ia molecules.

Thus, these results strongly support the notion that the Ia-dependent activation process in the early step of LPS-induced polyclonal B cell differentiation is mediated by the B-B cell interaction via recognition of self-Ia molecules.

The Ia-Restriction Specificity of LPS-Responsive B cells is Dictated by the H-2 Haplotype of Bone Marrow Cells Present During the B Cell Ontogeny but not by the H-2 Haplotype of a Radiation-Resistant Host Environment

Because the LPS-responsive B cells were shown to recognize self-Ia molecules, it was of interest to investigate how their Ia-restriction specificity was determined. To examine this question, B10 → B6C3F1 ($H\text{-}2^{b/k}$) and (B10 + B10.BR) → (B10 x B10.BR)F1 ($H\text{-}2^b + H\text{-}2^k \rightarrow H\text{-}2^{b/k}$) radiation bone marrow chimeras were constructed. Table 2. shows that the LPS-induced responses of B10-derived B cells from B10 → B6C3F1 chimeras were inhibited by anti-I-A^b but not by anti-I-A^k mAb even when MMC-treated B10.BR B cells expressing I-A^k molecules were present in the culture as auxiliary cells. On the other hand, when B10-derived B cells were isolated from (B10 + B10.BR) → (B10 x B10.BR)F1 chimeras by treating the T cell-depleted spleen cells with anti-$H\text{-}2^k$ mAbs + complement, the LPS-induced responses of these B10-derived B cells were inhibited not only by anti-I-A^b mAb but also by anti-I-A^k mAb in the presence of allogeneic B10.BR auxiliary B cells. However, these anti-I-A^k-mediated inhibition of the responses of the chimeric B10-derived B cells was not observed when the cell cultures were conducted in the absence or presence of B10 auxiliary B cells. Although data are not shown, IgM PFC generated from the culture of anti-$H\text{-}2^k$ + complement-treated (B10 + B10.BR) → (B10 x B10.BR)F1 chimeric B cells in the presence of B10.BR auxiliary B cells were almost completely eliminated by the treatment with anti-$H\text{-}2^b$ mAb + complement but not with anti-$H\text{-}2^k$ mAb + complement, excluding the possibility that the newly acquired self-Ia-recognition specificity of one parental B cells from double bone marrow chimeras is due to the activity of contaminating another parental B cells. These results demonstrate that B10-derived B cells from (B10 + B10.BR) → ($H\text{-}2^b$ x $H\text{-}2^k$)F1 but not from B10 → ($H\text{-}2^b$ x $H\text{-}2^k$)F1 bone marrow chimeras can differentiate to recognize allogeneic Ia^k molecules as self-structures. Moreover, B10-derived B cells isolated from (B10 + B10.BR) → B10 chimeras were also able to acquire the self-recognition specificity for allogeneic Ia^k molecules, in which the B10-derived B cells had been confronted with $H\text{-}2^k$ alloantigens exclusively expressed by bone marrow-derived cells but not by host environment (data not shown). Thus these results provide evidence indicating that Ia-recognition specificity of LPS-responsive B cells is not influenced by the radiation-resistant host environment but determined by the H-2 haplotype of the radiation-sensitive bone marrow-derived cells present during B cell ontogeny.

The Ia-Dependent Activation Process Is Involved In the Induction of IgM-Producing Cells by Various Polyclonal B Cell Activators

Results described above provided evidence for the involvement of Ia-restricted B-B cell interaction in the polyclonal B cell differentiation induced by a TCA-extracted LPS from E. coli 0111:B4. It is known that there exist various LPS prepared from different bacterial strains and the immunologic properties of LPS are depending upon the method of extraction (13, 15). Therefore, attempt was made to examine the involvement of Ia-dependent activation process in the polyclonal B cell differentiation by various LPS pre-

Table I

Fractionation of LPS-responsive F1 B cells into two subpopulations by their ability to bind to parental monolayers.

Responding B Cells*			Reverse IgM PFC Induced by LPS §			% Response ‡	
Strain	Fractionation by Monolayer: Strain of Monolayer	Fractionation by Monolayer: Fraction	No mAb	Anti-I-A^b #	Anti-I-A^k ¶	Anti-I-A^b	Anti-I-A^k
B10	-	-	9,748 ± 487	3,170 ± 634 ‖	10,151 ± 1,523	33	104
B10.BR	-	-	11,670 ± 467	10,048 ± 804	4,134 ± 496	86	35
(B10x B10.BR)F1	-	-	10,619 ± 743	8,400 ± 504	8,812 ± 529	79	83
	B10	Adherent	1,820 ± 18	852 ± 77	1,779 ± 53	47	98
		Nonadherent	12,560 ± 628	12,220 ± 733	4,472 ± 581	97	36
	B10.BR	Adherent	2,261 ± 113	2,966 ± 148	567 ± 96	102	25
		Nonadherent	13,670 ± 1,094	4,477 ± 179	12,182 ± 731	33	89

* T cell-depleted (B10xB10.BR)F1 spleen cells were fractionated on parental T cell-depleted spleen cell monolayers as described previously (17,24), and these fractionated F1 B cells ($1x10^5$) were cultured with 5μg/ml LPS for 5 days in the absence or presence of anti-I-A mAbs.

§ Numbers of PFC responses listed are the values subtracted from the respective background responses in the absence of LPS. The background PFC responses were less than 50. The values shown are the arithmetic means ± standard errors of triplicate determinations.

‡ Percent responses are calculated as in Figure 2B.

\# 34-5-3S 5μg/ml.

¶ 10-3.6 5μg/ml.

‖ Underlines indicate significant inhibition ($P<0.01$ by student's *t*-test) of the PFC responses.

Table II

LPS-responsive B cells from double bone marrow chimera but not from semiallogeneic bone marrow chimera acquire the self-recognition specificity for the other parental I-A molecules.

Responding B Cells*		Auxiliary B Cells	Reverse IgM PFC Induced by LPS §			% Response ‡	
Mice	Treatment	Added †	No mAb	Anti-I-A^b #	Anti-I-A^k ¶	Anti-I-A^b	Anti-I-A^k
B10	-	-	10,412± 625	4,631± 602 ‖	11,191± 336	44	107
B10.BR	-	-	13,752± 1,788	11,329± 1,586	4,121± 701	82	30
B10→B6C3F1	-	-	7,719± 463	3,030± 758	7,224± 1,950	39	94
		B10	8,208± 657	2,994± 329	6,888± 2,204	36	84
		B10.BR	8,192± 10	3,036± 152	8,492± 127	37	104
(B10+B10.BR) → (B10x B10.BR)F1	Anti-H-2^k+C	-	7,198± 144	2,662± 80	7,593± 304	37	105
		B10	7,252± 653	3,126± 515	7,499± 600	43	103
		B10.BR	6,880± 69	3,003± 150	2,549± 255	44	37

* T cell-depleted spleen cells from (B10+B10.BR)→(B10xB10.BR)F1 chimeras were further treated with mixture of anti-H-2^k mAbs (11-4.1, anti-K^k; 12-2-2S, anti-K^{k}D^k; 10-2.16, anti-I-A^k; 14-4-4S, anti-I-E^k) and rabbit complement as described previously (18), and these B cells (1×10^5) were cultured with 5μg/ml LPS for 5 days in the absence or presence of anti-I-A mAbs.

† Mitomycin C-treated spleen cells which had been depleted of T cells were used as the auxiliary B cells. The auxiliary cells alone did not give rise to PFC upon stimulation with LPS.

§ See Table I. Background PFC responses were less than 30.

‡ See Table I.

See Table I.

¶ See Table I.

‖ See Table I. $P<0.01$.

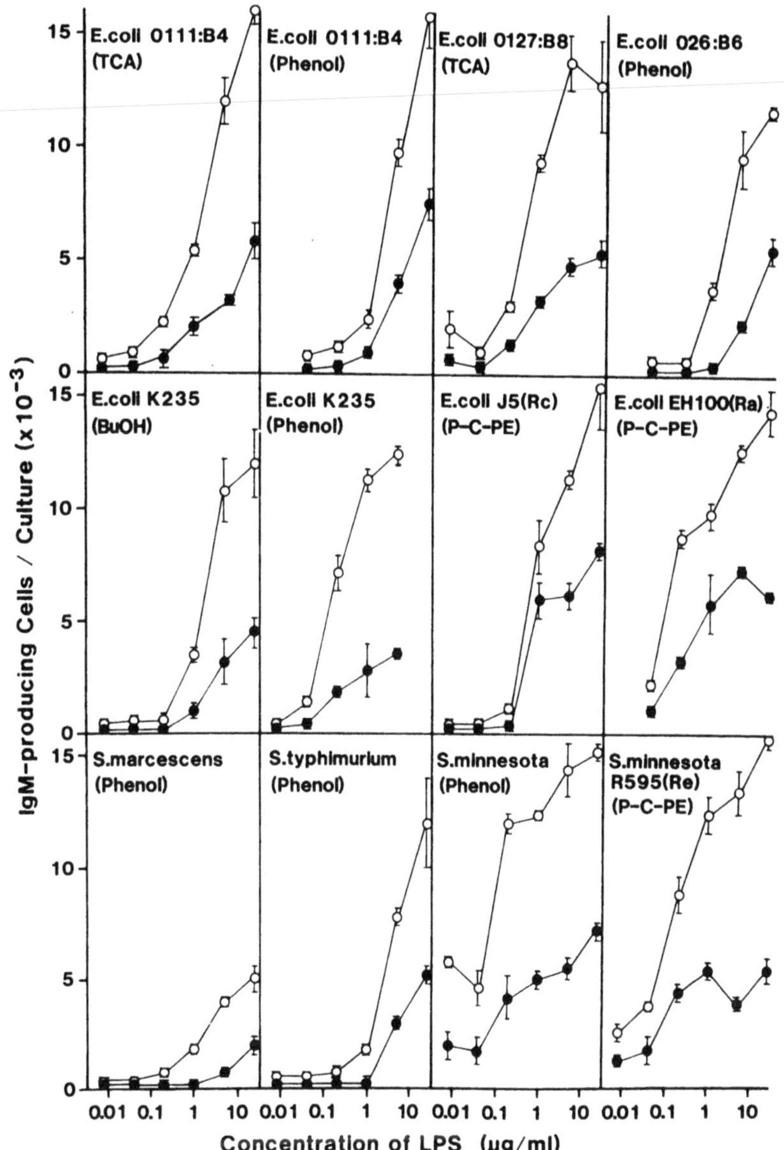

Fig 4. Anti-I-A mAb inhibits polyclonal B cell differentiation induced by various LPS preparations. LPS used are described in Materials and Methods. T cell-depleted B10.BR spleen cells (1×10^5) were cultured with graded concentrations of the indicated LPS in the absence (O) or presence (●) of anti-I-A^k mAb (5 μg/ml 10-3.6) for 5 days.

parations. As shown in Fig 4, anti-I-A^k mAb consistently inhibited the polyclonal B cell responses of T cell-depleted B10.BR spleen cells induced by LPS extracted with different methods from different bacterial strains. In addition, such an anti-I-A mAb-mediated inhibition was also observed in the polyclonal B cell differentiation induced by lipid A, lipoprotein (LPS-associated proteins), PPD, and C_8-substituted guanosines as well as a T cell-derived B cell differentiation factor B151-TRF2 (Fig 5).

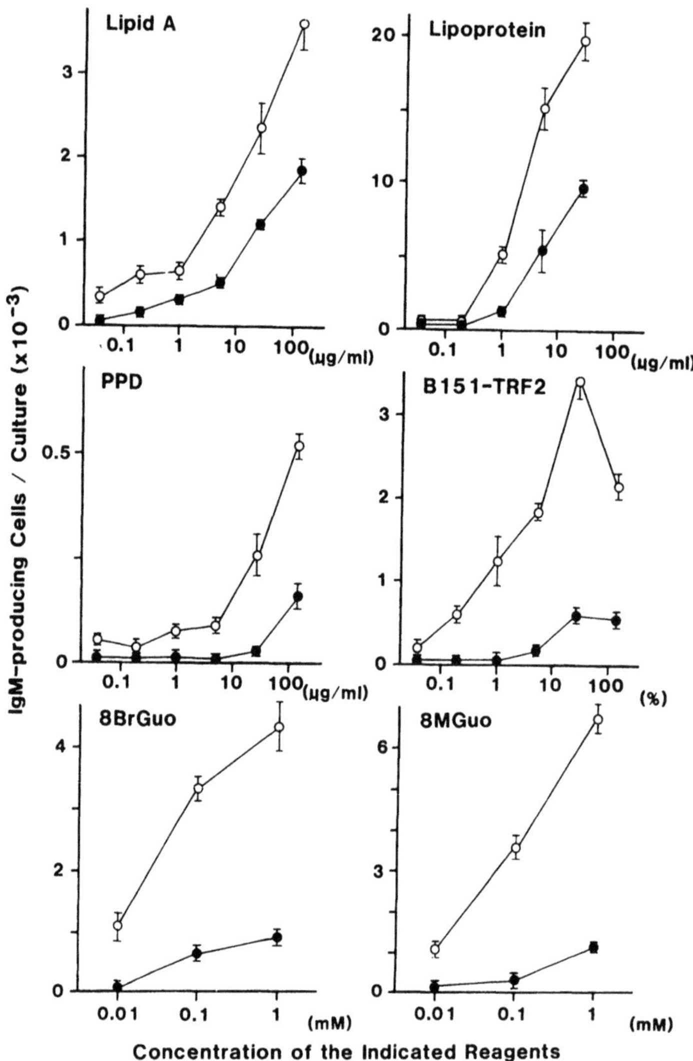

Fig 5. Anti-I-A mAb inhibits polyclonal B cell differentiation induced by various B cell stimulating reagents. Polyclonal B cell activators used are described in Materials and Methods. 1×10^5 T cell depleted B10.BR spleen cells (1×10^6 in the case of B cell stimulation by C8-substituted guanosines) were cultured with graded concentrations of the indicated polyclonal B cell activator in the absence (O) or presence (●) of anti-I-A^k mAb (5 μg/ml 10-3.6) for 5 days.

Thus, collectively, the present experiments provide evidence indicating that a novel type of cellular interaction, Ia-restricted B-B cell interaction, exists in the polyclonal B cell differentiation pathways in general.

DISCUSSION

Results described in this study can be interpreted as indicating that Ia-restricted B-B cell interaction is involved in the differentiation of resting B cells into IgM-producing cells by LPS capable of activating a large fraction of B cells. In addition, it is suggested that the specificity of the putative self-Ia-recognizing receptors on B cells is "plastic" and determined by the H-2 haplotype of bone marrow cells present during B cell ontogeny but not by that of radiation-resistant host elements.

The notion that the self-Ia-recognition is mediated by B cells is supported by the following lines of evidence. 1) LPS inducing the polyclonal B cell differentiation is known to have no ability to activate T cells directly (1, 13). 2) LPS-responsive F1 B cells prepared from athymic nude mice could be fractionated into two subpopulations with the restriction specificity for either one of parental Ia molecules (data not shown). 3) The MHC haplotype of host environment including thymus, which predominantly dictates the self-recognition specificity of T cells, was not responsible for the determination of self-recognition specificity expressed by the LPS-responsive B cells (Table 2). 4) The LPS-induced polyclonal B cell differentiation was not inhibited by anti-L3T4 (GK1.5) and anti-LFA-1 (M17/5.2) mAbs (our unpublished observations), both of which could almost completely inhibit the Ia-restricted T cell responses (4, 5, 18, 24). Thus, it is unlikely that the self-Ia recognition is due to the activity of small numbers of Ia-restricted T cells contaminating in the responding B cell populations.

Indeed, our recent experiments have provided further convincing evidence for the involvement of Ia-restricted B-B cell interaction. Namely, a number of clusters were formed when purified small B cells from athymic nude mice were cultured without any stimulation for 2 or 3 days. The clustered and nonclustered cells were purified by a recently devised cell sorter ACAS470 which can sort out desired cells in a tissue cultured plate in situ. Only B cells from the clusters but not from nonclusters gave rise to IgM-producing cells when stimulated with LPS or B151-TRF2 for an additional 2 days. Moreover, the ability of clustered B cells to respond to the stimuli was inhibited by anti-I-A but not anti-H-2K mAb (25). These results also visualized the Ia-restricted B-B cell interaction in the early process of polyclonal B cell differentiation.

It remains to be determined, however, whether the recognition by LPS-responsive B cells of self-Ia molecules expressed on B cells is mediated by their surface immunoglobulin (sIg) or, alternatively, occurs via yet unidentified cell interaction molecules distinct from sIg. Recently, we have found that removal of sIg from the responding F1 B cells by capping using rabbit anti-mouse Ig antibody does not affect the subsequent fractionation by their ability to bind to the parental B cell monolayer into two separate populations with restriction specificity for only one of the parental Ia molecules (Ono, Takahama, and Hamaoka, manuscript in preparation). Thus, the Ia-restricted recognition by LPS-responsive B cells does not appear to be mediated by sIg.

The present study does not address the question of whether the I-E molecules are also involved in the Ia-restricted B-B cell interaction. We have recently shown, however, that F1 B cells are fractionated with the restriction specificity for the parental I-A but not I-E molecules, and the acquisition of self-recognition specificity for I-E molecules are not observed in double bone marrow chimeras. In addition, the polyclonal B cell responses were inhibited by Fab fragment of anti-I-A but not by anti-I-E mAb (Takahama, Ono, Ishihara, Muramatsu, and Hamaoka, submitted for publication). These results are compatible with the idea that only I-A molecules are involved in the B-B cell interaction, whereas I-E molecules function as a receptor transducing regulatory signals.

We have previously shown that Ia-restricted B-B cell interaction is involved in polyclonal B cell differentiation induced by a T cell-derived lymphokine B151-TRF2 (17, 18, 24). The results described in this study provide further evidence indicating that the Ia-restricted B-B cell interaction also exists in polyclonal B cell differentiation induced by various stimuli including LPS from various bacterial strains, lipid A, lipoproteins (LPS-associated proteins), PPD, and C8-substituted guanosines (Fig 5). Because LPS is known to activate 10-50% of total B cell population in the mouse spleens (1, 7), it is likely that the Ia-restricted B-B cell interaction is a general process involved in the polyclonal B cell differentiation.

The present study do not necessarily rule out the existence of Ia-independent B cell activation processes. Indeed, polyclonal B cell differentiation induced by LPS could not be perfectly inhibited by the addition of high concentration of anti-I-A mAb (Figs 1, 2, 3 and 4). This incompleteness of anti-I-A mAb-mediated inhibition was more obvious in the B cell differentiation induced by LPS or lipid A as compared to the B cell differentiation induced by B151-TRF2 or C8-substituted guanosines (Figs 4 and 5). Analyses to discriminate whether these Ia-dependent and independent B cell activation processes reflect different activation stages or different subsets of responding B cells are currently in progress.

Concerning the biological significance of the I-A-restricted B-B cell interaction, we have recently found that LPS- or B151-TRF2-induced IgM PFC responses against bromelain-treated mouse erythrocytes (BrMRBC) was controlled by I-region-linked genes, purely operating at the B cell level. Namely, B cells from mice bearing I^s haplotype exhibited low anti-BrMRBC PFC response, whereas they gave rise to reverse IgM PFC, anti-TNP PFC and other autoantibodies reactive with ssDNA and collagen type II comparable in magnitude to those of the other high responder strains. This selective low response was shown to be resulted from low frequency of BrMRBC-specific precursor B cells by limiting dilution analysis. The B cells of (high responder B10 x low responder SJL)F1 ($H-2^{b/s}$) exhibited intermediate anti-BrMRBC PFC responses, and their responses were preferentially inhibited by anti-$I-A^b$ mAb. Moreover, when (B10 x SJL)F1 B cells were fractionated by their ability to bind to parental B cell monolayers, the F1 B cells adherent to SJL ($H-2^s$) monolayers exhibited selective low anti-BrMRBC responses (8). Thus, these results provide evidence indicating that self-Ia recognition specificity expressed by B cells importantly influences the generation of anti-BrMRBC precursor B cells.

Collectively, the present study shows a novel type of MHC-restricted cellular interaction, Ia-restricted B-B cell interaction, exists in the polyclonal B cell differentiation in general and provide a new insight into the mechanism underlying the MHC-linked Ir-gene control of B cell repertoire selection including autoantibody generation.

ACKNOWLEDGEMENT

We thank Mr. Ryoichi Ikegami for his expert technical assistance in PFC assay.

REFERENCES

1. Andersson, J., Coutinho, A., and Melchers, F., 1977, Frequencies of mitogen-reactive B cells in the mouse. Frequencies of B cells producing antibodies which lyse sheep or horse erythrocytes, and trinitrophenylated sheep erythrocytes. _J. Exp. Med._ 145: 1520.

2. Bonagura, V. R., Agostino, N., Crow, M. K., and Pernis, B, 1985, Anti-immunoglobulin stimulation of human B lymphocytes is inhibited by anti-class II major histocompatibility complex antibodies. Cell. Immunol. 96: 442.

3. Clement, L. T., Tedder, T. F., and Gartland, G. L., 1986, Antibodies reactive with class II antigens encoded for by the major histocompatibility complex inhibit human B cell activation. J. Immunol. 136: 2375.

4. Davignon, D., Martz, E., Reynolds, T., Kurzinger, K., and Springer, T. A., 1981, Monoclonal antibody to a novel lymphocyte function-associated antigen (LFA-1): mechanism of blockade of T lymphocyte-mediated killing and effects on other T and B lymphocyte functions. J. Immunol. 127: 590.

5. Dialynas, D. P., Wilde, D. B., Marrack, P., Pierres, A., Wall, K. A., Havran, W., Otten, G., Loken, M. R., Pierres, M., Kappler, J., and Fitch, F. W., 1983, Characterization of the murine antigenic determinant, designated L3T4a, recognized by monoclonal antibody GK1.5: expression of L3T4a by functional T cell clones appears to correlate primarily with class II MHC antigen-reactivity. Immunol. Rev. 74: 29.

6. Dobashi, K., Ono, S., Murakami, S., Takahama, Y., Katoh, Y., and Hamaoka, T., 1987, Polyclonal B cell activation by a B cell differentiation factor, B151-TRF2. III. B151-TRF2 as a B cell differentiation factor closely associated with autoimmune disease. J. Immunol. 138: 780.

7. Forsgren, S., Pobor, G., Coutinho, A., and Pierres, M., 1984, The role of I-A/E molecules in B lymphocyte activation. I. Inhibition of lipopolysaccharide-induced responses by monoclonal antibodies. J. Immunol. 133: 2104.

8. Hamaoka, T., Murakami, S., Dobashi, K., Takahama, Y., Hirayama, F., Ishihara, K., and Ono, S., 1988, I-A-restricted B-B cell interaction and its relation to autoimmunity, in: "B cell development". O. Witte, M. Howard, and N. Klinman, eds. Alan R. Liss Publishing, New York p. 215.

9. Hodes, R. J., Ahmann, G. B., Hathkock, K. S., Dickler, H. B., and Singer, A., 1978, Cellular and genetic control of antibody responses in vitro. IV. Expression of Ia antigens on accessory cells required for responses to soluble antigens including a response under Ir gene control. J. Immunol. 121: 1501.

10. Kappler, J. W., and Marrack, P., 1978, The role of H-2 linked genes in helper T cell function. IV. Importance of T-cell genotype and host environment in I-region and Ir gene expression. J. Exp. Med. 148: 1510.

11. Katoh, Y., Ono, S., Takahama, Y., Miyake, K., and T. Hamaoka, 1986, Polyclonal B cell activation by a B cell differentiation factor, B151-TRF2. II. Evidence for interaction of B151-TRF2 with glycoprotein on B cell membrane via recognition of terminal N-acetyl-D-glucosamine residue(s). J. Immunol. 137: 2871.

12. Katz, D. H., Hamaoka, T., and Benaceraff, B., 1973, Cell interaction between histoincompatible T and B lymphocytes. II. Failure of physiologic cooperative interactions between T and B lymphocytes from allogeneic donor strains in humoral response to hapten-protein conjugates. J. Exp. Med. 137: 1405.

13. Morrison, D. C., and Ryan, J. L., 1979, Bacterial endotoxins in host immune responses. Adv. Immunol. 28: 293.

14. Niederhuber, J. E., Frelinger, J. A., Dugan, E., Coutinho, A., and Shreffler, D. C., 1975, Effects of anti-Ia serum on mitogenic responses. I. Inhibition of the proliferative response to B cell mitogen, LPS, by specific anti-Ia sera. J. Immunol. 115: 1672.

15. Ono, S., Yaffe, L. J., Ryan, J. L., and Singer, A., 1983, Functional heterogeneity of the Lyb-5 B cell subpopulation: mutant xid B cells and normal Lyb-5$^-$ cells differ in their responsiveness to phenol-extracted lipopolysaccharide. J. Immunol. 130: 2014.

16. Ono, S., Hayashi, S. I., Takahama, Y., Dobashi, K., Katoh, Y., Nakanishi, K., Paul, W. E., and Hamaoka, T., 1986, Identification of two distinct factors, B151-TRF1 and B151-TRF2, inducing differentiation of activated B cells and small resting B cells into antibody-producing cells. J. Immunol. 137: 187.

17. Ono, S., Takahama, Y., and Hamaoka, T., 1986, Polyclonal B cell activation by B cell differentiation factor B151-TRF2. I. Involvement of self-Ia recognition process mediated by B cells. J. Immunol. 137: 1149.

18. Ono, S., Takahama, Y., and Hamaoka, T., 1987, Ia-restricted B-B cell interaction. I. The MHC haplotype of bone marrow cells present during B cell ontogeny dictates the self-recognition specificity of B cells in the polyclonal B cell activation by a B cell differentiation factor, B151-TRF2. J. Immunol. 139: 3213.

19. Rosenthal, A. S., and Shevach, E. M., 1973, Function of macrophages in antigen recognition by guinea pig T lymphocytes. I. Requirement for histocompatible macrophages and lymphocytes. J. Exp. Med. 138: 1174.

20. Schwarts, R. H., and Paul, W. E., 1976, T-lymphocyte-enriched murine peritoneal exudate cells. II. Genetic control of antigen-induced T-lymphocyte proliferation. J. Exp. Med. 143: 529.

21. Sherr, D. H., and Dorf, M. E., 1985, H-2 restricted helper activity mediated by immunoglobulin-bearing lymphocytes. J. Immunol. 134: 2084.

22. Singer, A., and Hodes, R. J., 1983, Major histocompatibility complex-restricted self-recognition in responses to trinitrophenyl-Ficoll. Adaptive differentiation and self-recognition by B cells. J. Exp. Med. 156: 1415.

23. Spieker-Polet, H., Hagen, K., and Teodorescu, M., 1985, The role of intercellular contacts in the activation of B lymphocytes by anti-immunoglobulin antibodies. J. Immunol. 134:2827.

24. Takahama, Y., Ono, S., Glimcher, L. H., and Hamaoka, T., 1987, Polyclonal B cell activation by a B-cell differentiation factor B151-TRF2. IV. B151-TRF2-responsive F1 B cells consist of two separate populations capable of recognizing only one of the parental I-A products expressed on B cells. J. Mol. Cell Immunol. 3: 177.

25. Takahama, Y., Ono, S., Ishihara, K., and Hamaoka, 1989, Cluster formation among small resting B lymphocytes leading to B cell activation. Int. Immunol. 1: 36.

26. Yamamoto, H., Bitoh, S., and Fujimoto, S., 1984, Regulation of immune responses via genetically restricted cellular interactions. I. Augmentation of antibody responses by idiotype-specific enhancing B lymphocytes. J. Immunol. 133: 2882.

27. Zinkernagel, R. M., and Doherty, P. C., 1974, Immunological surveillance against altered self components by sensitized T lymphocytes in lymphocytic choriomeningitis. Nature 251: 547.

IDENTIFICATION AND CHARACTERIZATION OF LIPOPOLYSACCHARIDE RECEPTOR MOLECULES ON MAMMALIAN LYMPHOID CELLS

M.-G. Lei, L. Flebbe, D. Roeder and D. C. Morrison

Department of Microbiology
University of Kansas Medical Center
Kansas City, KS 66103

INTRODUCTION

Since the discovery by Neter in the late 1950's that bacterial endotoxic lipopolysaccharides (LPS) will bind readily to cells of mammalian origin (reviewed in 15), the concept of specific receptors for LPS has intrigued endotoxin researchers. A variety of immunologic, biochemical and morphologic approaches have been adopted in order to demonstrate experimentally the existence of such LPS receptors; in general however, such efforts have been confounded by relatively high levels of nonspecific binding to mammmalian cell membrane components (reviewed in 16). A specific membrane localized high affinity LPS binding lipoglycoprotein present on human erythrocytes was identified by Springer and his colleagues in 1970 (24, 25), although efforts to extend these observations to human platelets and leukocytes or murine lymphocytes were less successful (26, 27). More recent efforts by several investigators have provided strong evidence for receptors on distinct cell subpopulations for carbohydrate components of specific preparations of LPS, (reviewed in 7), but the specific receptor for the structurally conserved, biologically active lipid A component of LPS has, to date, not been defined.

The seminal paper of Sultzer, in 1968, reporting the existence of an endotoxin unresponsive C3H/HeJ inbred mouse strain (28), allowed the development of powerful new experimental approaches to the question of the mechanism of action of bacterial endotoxins, and more specifically, the possible existence of defined LPS/lipid A receptors. Since virtually all cells of lymhoid (and nonlymphoid) origin from this endotoxin-unresponsive mouse were reported to be refractory to the stimulatory effects of lipid A, (reviewed in 17) the postulate that this C3H/HeJ mouse strain failed to express functional LPS receptors appeared to be a rational and testable hypothesis. Early reports by Coutinho and his colleagues (2, 4, 5) provided strong immunological evidence that the lymphoid cells from these endotoxin unresponsive mice could be characterized by their lack of reactivity with a xenogeneic antiserum which bound to B-cells of all normal mice and displayed all of the predicted characteristics of an antibody to a receptor molecule. On the basis of these results, it was concluded that LPS responsive cells from the C3H/HeJ mouse lacked a specific surface antigen defined by Coutinho and his colleagues as an LPS receptor. Studies by other investigators, unfortunately did not confirm these exciting results (30). In our own laboratory, experiments have suggested that, if an antigenic difference does exist between endotoxin unresponsive C3H/HeJ mice and histocompatible C3H normal mouse strains, that antigenic difference is less immunogenic than a minor histocompatibility antigen (6).

In the past several years, our laboratory has developed an alternative approach for the potential identification and characterization of specific LPS receptors. Based upon the success in other experimental systems of the use of photoaffinity probes to identify receptor molecules, we first developed specific, radiolabeled, photoactive LPS derivatives for these studies. The availability of disulfide linked photoaffinity probes was instrumental in circumventing the potential problem of LPS heterogeneity in subsequent interpretation of binding data. The results of our initial studies demonstrated that LPS, derivatized with the photoaffinity probe sulfosuccinimidyl-2-(p-azidosalicyl-amino)-1,3',-dithiopropionate (SASD), quantitatively substituted phosphorylethanolamine groups on LPS, and that the resulting ASD-LPS could be radioiodinated to high specific activity with ^{125}I (31). Of importance in those studies, specific binding of LPS to monoclonal antibody (both heavy and light chain) could be readily demonstrated by SDS-PAGE and autoradiography. Finally, as assessed by a variety of **in vitro** assays, the derivatized ASD-LPS was shown to be indistinguishable from control LPS preparations in a variety of **in vitro** biological assays. These combined studies suggested that the ASD-LPS derivative would be a suitable probe by which to explore the concept of LPS receptors.

We have recently begun a series of experiments, using this photoaffinity LPS probe, to define specific LPS binding proteins on preparations of mammalian lymphoid cells. The results of our published and unpublished results to date are summarized here, and suggest that a specific membrane localized protein of approximate molecular mass of 80 kDa and pI of 6.5 may serve as a receptor for LPS/lipid A on murine lymphoid cells. This 80 kDa protein is the dominant LPS binding protein present on murine B-cells, T-cells and splenic macrophages, and is also readily detected on the murine pre B-cell line 70Z/3 and T-cell line YAC-1 (12). Binding is saturable and appears to be specific for lipid A (13). We have not detected either qualitative or quantitative differences in this LPS binding protein when splenocytes form C3H/HeJ and C3HeB/FeJ mice have been compared. Of interest, an LPS binding protein with equivalent electrophoretic mobility properties is also readily detected on peripheral blood mononuclear cells of a variety of species, including man and rabbits, but is not detectable on peripheral blood mononuclear cells of the chicken (21). Preliminary results have suggested that chicken antiserum raised against two-dimensional-gel purified homogenates of the 80 kDa LPS binding protein will modulate the immunostimulatory activity of LPS in an **in vitro** mitogenic assay. These combined results would support the concept of specific LPS/lipid A receptors on mammalian cells of lymphoid origin, and suggest that such receptors may be conserved surface antigens of a variety of mammalian lymphoid cells.

MATERIALS AND METHODS

Lipopolysaccharides and Derivatives

The LPS from **E. coli** 0111:B4 was extracted and purified exactly as described earlier (19) and was used for all photocrosslinking derivatizations. The preparation of the radioiodinated ^{125}I-ASD-LPS derivative was exactly as described by Wollenweber and Morrison (30), and had a specific activity of approximately 1-5uCi/μg of LPS. All ASD-LPS preparations were stored at -70° until used for experiments.

Animals

Mice of the C3Heb/FeJ and C3H/HeJ strains were purchased from Jackson Laboratories (Bar Harbor, ME) and were of both sexes. Mice of the athymic

Balb/c (Nu/nu) strain were the gift of Dr. David Morris (Dept. Pathology, KU Medical Center). All mice used in these experiments were between 3-8 months of age. New Zealand white rabbits were purchased from White Hare Rabbitry (Stark City, MO) and were 2-3 kg in weight. White leghorn chickens were purchased from Colonial Poultry Farm (Pleasant Hill, MO) and were approximately six months of age. All animals were maintained in the animal facility at the University of Kansas Medical Center and were provided food and water ad libitum.

Cells and Cell Lines

Single cell suspensions of murine splenocytes were isolated from spleen cells of several inbred mouse strains and partially purified subpopulations of B-cells (Nu/nu), T-cells and adherent macrophages prepared as previously described (6, 10). Peripheral blood mononuclear cells were isolated from the blood obtained from normal healthy human volunteers using standard Ficol-Hypaque purification procedures. Rabbits were bled from the central ear artery into acid citrate dextrose anti-coagulant and chickens from the central wing vein. Peripheral blood mononuclear cell preparations from these latter species were also prepared by Ficol-Hypaque gradient purification with minor modification. The murine pre B-cell line 70Z/3 was obtained from the American Type Culture Collection. The T-cell line, YAC-1, was the generous gift of Dr. Linda L. Perry (Rocky Mountain Labs, Hamilton, MT). The undifferentiated murine Sp2/0 myeloma cell line was kindly provided by Dr. Balachandran Narayanaswamy, (Univ. of Kansas Med. Ctr). The cell lines were maintained in RPM1-1640 culture medium supplemented with 2-mercaptoethanol, 10% fetal bovine serum, glutamine, penicillin and streptomycin (2 mM, 100 U/ml and 100 μg/ml respectively).

Photoaffinity Crosslinking

For all of the described experiments, cell preparations were crosslinked with ^{125}I-ASD-LPS using LPS from **E. coli** 0111:B4. Following crosslinking, all preparations were reduced with 2-mercaptoethanol. Since the iodinatable group and the photoactive azido group are distal to the disulfide linkage of the ASD-LPS, reduction after crosslinking effectively transfers radiolabel from the derivatized ASD-LPS to the LPS binding sites on the cells with coincident elimination of LPS from subsequent two-dimensional gel analyses. In most experiments, 100 μl of 10^8 cells/ml in RPMI-1640 were incubated with 5 μg of ^{125}I-ASD-LPS for 30 min at 37°C, irradiated with short wavelength UV light (4 watts maximum emission at 254 nm), washed three times by centrifugation and analyzed by two-dimensional isoelectric focusing/SDS-PAGE.

Two Dimensional (2-D) Electrophoresis

2-D gel electrophoresis was carried out as described by O'Farrell (20). A pH range of 3-10 ampholytes was used in the first (isoelectric focusing) dimension and the equilibrium pH values of individual gel segments determined as described (13). The second dimension (SDS-PAGE) employed 11% polyacrylamide gels and was calibrated using Biorad (Richmond CA) molecular weight standards for electrophoresis. Gels were stained with 0.2% Coomassie blue R250/50% methanol/12% acetic acid and destained with 20% ethanol/10% acetic acid. Autoradiography was carried out as described (31) using Kodak X-Omat XK-1 film and Dupont cassettes with two Dupont Cronex lighting plus intensifying screens for 1-3 days at -70°C.

Preparation of Antiserum

For the preparation of antiserum against the murine 80 kDa LPS binding protein, the protein was partially purified by 2-D electrophoresis on SDS-PAGE. A region of about 10 mm^2 corresponding to the 80 kDa LPS binding protein, identified by autoradiography, was excised from gels, homogenized with complete Freund's adjuvant and used to immunize white leghorn chickens intramuscularly (approximately ten gels per chicken). After two weeks, animals were boosted with antigen in incomplete Freund's adjuvant. Chickens were bled by the central wing vein five days following secondary immunization and the antiserum obtained heated at 56°C for 30 min prior to use. Sera from unimmunized chickens served as controls for these studies.

Lymphocyte Proliferation Assays

Stimulation of B-lymphocyte mitogenesis was carried out exactly as described previously (6). Briefly 5 x 10^5 murine splenocytes, prepared as described above were cultured in 200 µl of media in flat bottom microtiter plates with LPS and/or other additives. ^{3}H-thymidine was added at 24 hr and the cells harvested on a multiple automated sample harvester 18 hr later. Counts are the average of triplicate determinations and individual determinations are routinely within 10% of the mean.

RESULTS

Determination of LPS Binding to Murine Splenocytes

For our initial experiments, C3Heb/FeJ spleen cells were incubated with ^{125}I-ASD-LPS for 30 min at 37°, photocrosslinked by ultraviolet irradiation, washed by centrifugation, reduced by 2-mercaptoethanol, solubilized by detergent and urea and the solubilized lysates subjected to 2-D electrophoresis. The gels were then autoradiographed to detect LPS binding proteins. A repre-

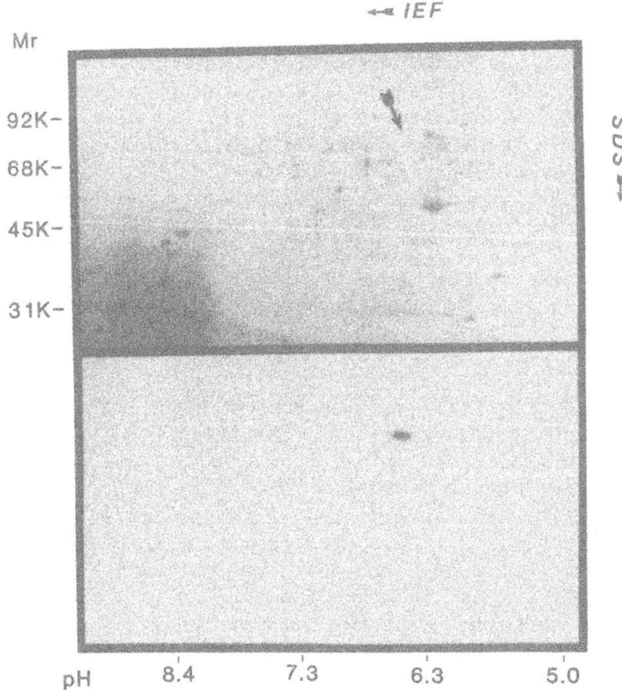

Fig 1. 2-D gel electrophoresis of photocrosslinked, iodinated and reduced C3HeB/FeJ mouse splenocytes. Top panel: Coomassie blue R-250 stain of the 2-D gels. The arrow indicates the position of the LPS specific binding protein. Bottom panel: autoradiograph of the 2-D gel.

sentative profile of the Coomassie blue stained protein distribution of the splenocyte lysate and resulting autoradiograph is shown in Fig 1. A dominant LPS binding protein with molecular mass of approximately 80 kDa and pI of about 6.5 is readily detected in the latter. Analysis of the protein distribution staining pattern in the region of the autoradiograph hot-spot suggests that this 80 kDa LPS binding protein is not a major protein species in the soluble extract.

We have carried out control experiments in which electrophoresis in the first dimension was performed for periods of time less than that required for equilibrium, in order to assess potential binding of LPS to cationic proteins which might migrate off the gel. We have not detected any such LPS binding proteins. Further, we have not detected LPS binding to proteins of less than 30 kDa in any experiments. (In our hands, the ampholytes in the low molecular weight (<20 kDa) cationic region of the 2-D gels do not readily elute from the polyacrylamide and stain relatively intensely with Coomasie blue. Since this staining detracts from the presentation of these data we have excluded this region of the gel in the Figures shown in this manuscript.

Expression of the 80 kDa LPS Binding Protein on Lymphoid Cell Subpopulations

It is well recognized that a variety of lymphoid cell subpopulations in splenocytes have the capacity to be functionally responsive to LPS (reviewed in 18). Experiments were therefore carried out to assess the expression of the 80 kDa LPS binding protein on B and T lymphocytes, and macrophages. Splenocytes enriched for B cells were prepared as the nonadherent subpopulation of cells from athymic (Nu/nu) splenocytes. Splenocytes enriched for T-cells were from non-adherent normal splenocytes in which B cells were selectively depleted by adsorption to goat antimouse Ig-coated petri dishes. Splenic macrophages were obtained as the two hr plastic adherent splenocyte subpopulation, and were greater than 97% esterase positive.

Experiments identical to those described above for the unfractionated splenocytes were carried out on these partially purified cell populations and the results are shown in Fig 2A-C for B-cells, T-cells and macrophages respectively. The major salient feature of these autoradiographs is the presence, in each, of the dominant 80 kDa LPS binding protein. Of interest, two additional LPS binding proteins of approximately 30 kDa are detected in the T-cell enriched splenocytes (denoted by "b" in Fig 2B). These latter LPS binding proteins appear to have similar molecular weights but differ significantly in pI. Additionally, two secondary LPS binding proteins are detected in the macrophage enriched splenocyte populations, both of which have higher molecular weight than the major 80 kDa LPS binding protein (denoted by "b" in Fig 2C). These data would suggest that this protein may be conserved on many lymphoid cell subpopulations.

Since the enriched splenocyte subpopulations are, however, not homogeneous, the possibility that binding to a minor cell contaminant present in each preparation cannot be totally excluded. To address this concern, equivalent experiments were carried out on the murine 70Z/3 pre B-cell line, and the murine YAC-1 T-cell line. We have also examined specific LPS binding to the Sp2/0 undifferentiated murine myeloma cell line. The results of these studies are shown in Fig 3A-C respectively. In confirmation of the results shown in Fig 2A and 2B, both the murine B-cell and T-cell lines demonstrate the presence of a dominant 80 kDa LPS binding protein, in spite of the fact that the overall protein distribution patterns, as assessed by Coomassie blue staining, are clearly distinct. It is noteworthy that the two 30 kDa LPS binding proteins detected in the splenocyte T-cells (Fig 2B) are not readily detectable in the YAC-1 cell line. As shown in Fig 3C, the undifferentiated myeloma cell line fails to express the 80 kDa LPS binding protein. Exposure of the 2-D gels to the X-ray film for periods of time up to four fold greater

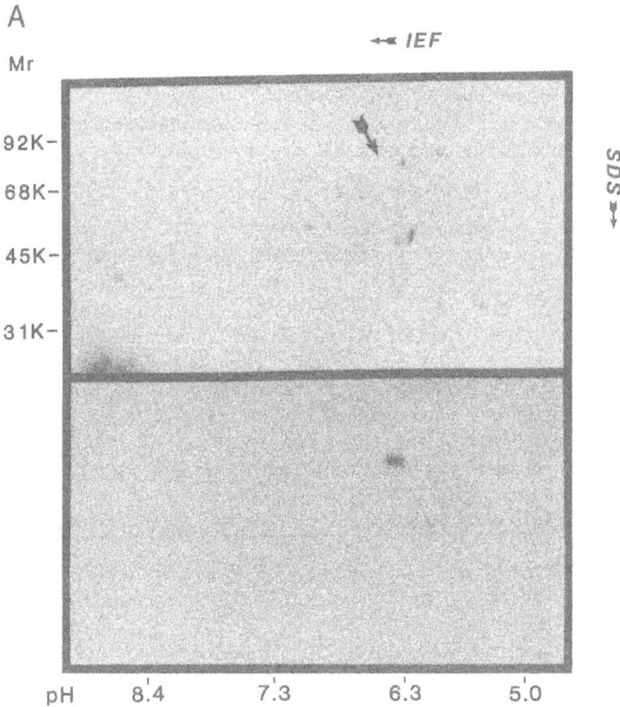

Fig 2A. 2-D gel electrophoresis of photocrosslinked, iodinated and reduced splenocyte subpopulations. (A) Nonadherent splenocytes from athymic (Nu/nu) mice (B cell enriched splenocytes). Top Panel: Coomassie blue R-250 stain pattern. Bottom Panel: Autoradiograph of the 2-D gel.

than that required to give high intensity hotspots on the B-and T-cell lines, failed to reveal any specific LPS binding proteins.

In addition to the intrinsic value of this observation, this latter result with Sp2/0 myeloma cells would suggest that the observed 80 kDa LPS binding protein is not the result of some technical artifact generated during the experimental protocol. It might be noted, in this respect, that we have also failed to detect the 80 kDa LPS binding protein on erythrocytes or several additional cell lines. Finally we have carried out rigorous control experiments to exclude potential contributions of culture media components, such as fetal calf serum, to the observed specific LPS binding profiles. Pertinent to this latter statement, results identical to those presented here are obtained when splenocytes are prepared and crosslinked in the absence of fetal calf serum.

Conservation of the 80 kDa LPS Binding Protein

Since many species manifest deleterious pathophysiological responses to LPS, it was of interest to query the expression of the 80 kDa LPS binding protein on peripheral blood mononuclear cells of species other than the mouse. To this end, peripheral blood mononuclear cells were obtained from rabbits and from normal human volunteers. Experiments identical to those described above were carried out to assess LPS binding and the results are

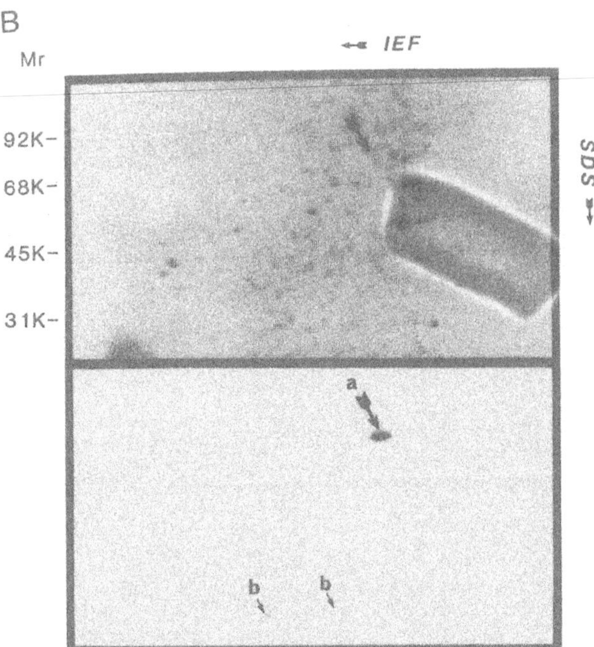

Fig 2B. Mouse T-lymphocytes. Top panel: Coomassie blue stain pattern. Bottom panel: autoradiograph of the 2-D gel. "a" indicates the major LPS specific binding protein.

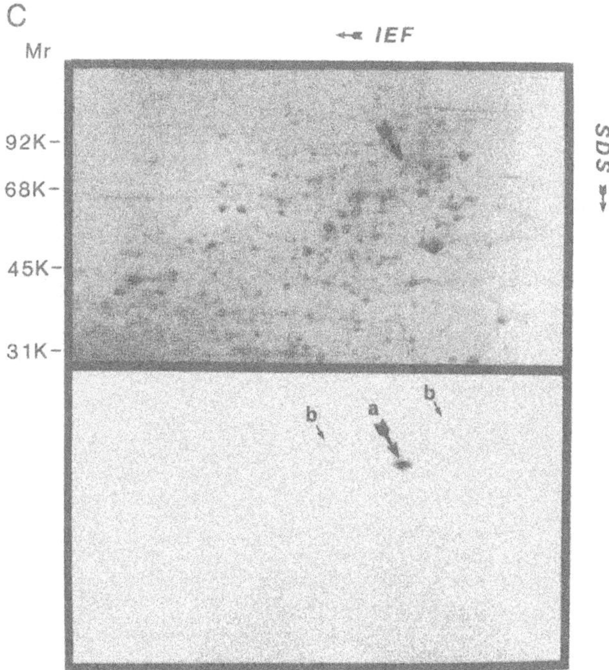

Fig 2C. Mouse macrophages. Top panel: Coomassie blue stain pattern. Bottom panel: autoradiograph of the 2-D gel. "a" indicates the major LPS specific binding protein. "b" indicates the minor LPS specific binding proteins.

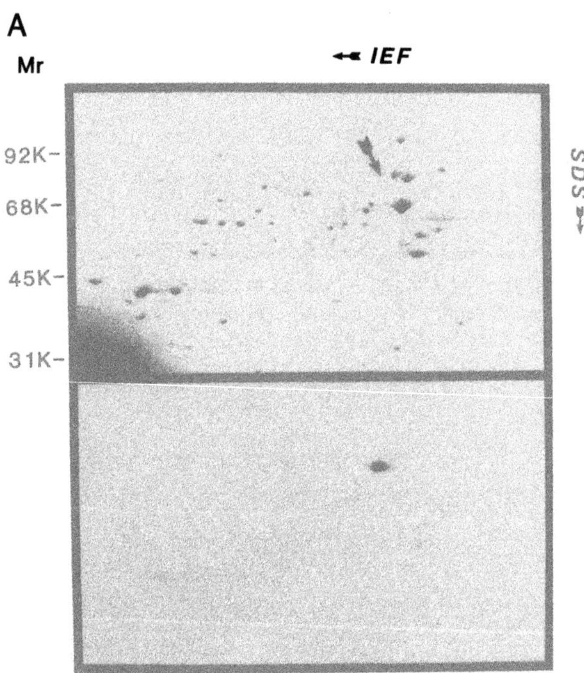

Fig 3A. 2-D gel electrophoresis of photocrosslinked, iodinated and reduced mouse cell lines. Pre-B-lymphocyte 70Z/3 line. Top panel: Coomassie blue stain. Bottom panel: autoradiograph of the 2-D gel. Arrow on the top panel indicates the position of the LPS specific binding protein.

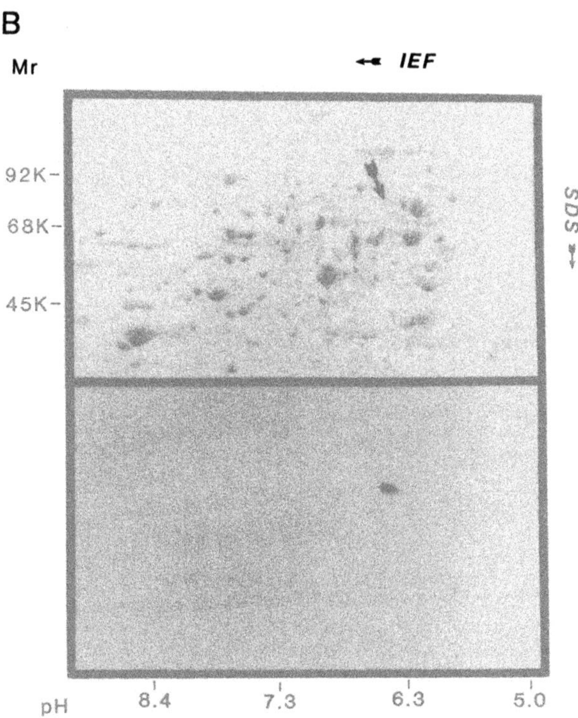

Fig 3B. YAC-1 murine T-cell line. Top panel: Coomassie blue stain pattern. Bottom panel: autoradiograph of the 2-D gel.

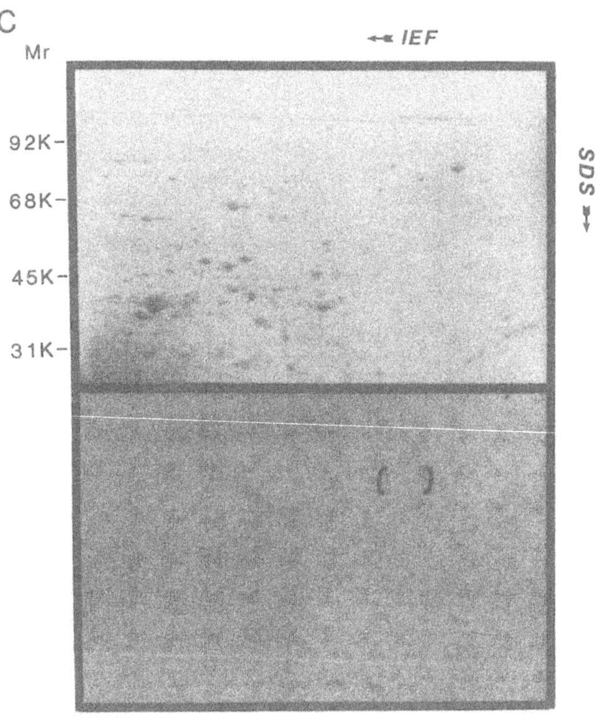

Fig 3C. Mouse myeloma Sp2/O cell line. Top panel: Coomassie blue stain pattern. Bottom panel: autoradiograph of the 2-D gel. Bracket indicates the region missing the major 80 kDa LPS specific binding protein.

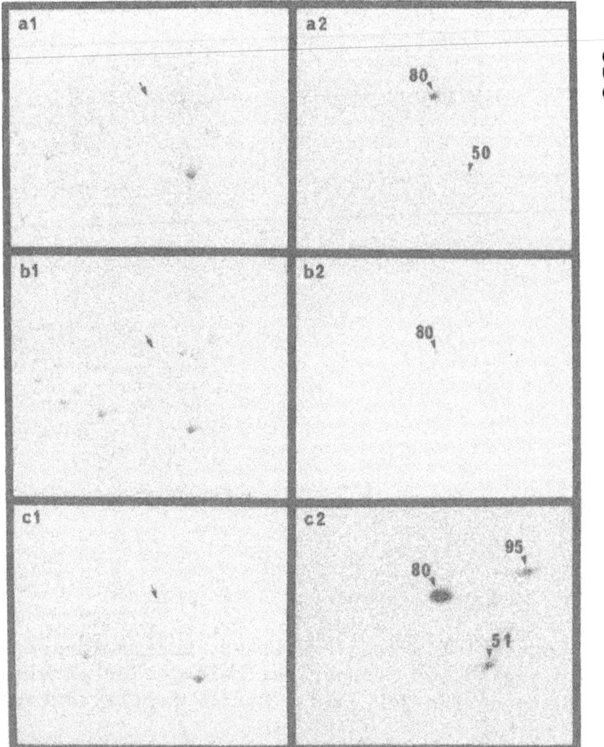

Fig 4. 2-D gel electrophoresis of photocrosslinked iodinated and reduced (a) human peripheral blood mononuclear cells, (b) mouse splenocytes (c) rabbit peripheral blood mononuclear cells. a1, b1, and c1 show the Coomassie blue R-250 stain patterns of the 2-D gels; a2, b2, and c2 show the autoradiographs of the 2-D gels of a1, b1, and c1, respectively.

shown in Fig 4a-c. In each of these cell preparations, the 80 kDa LPS binding protein is readily detected with essentially the same pI as that found for the murine splenocytes. In the human peripheral blood mononuclear cells, a second LPS binding protein with approximate molecular mass of 50 kDa is also detected. In rabbit peripheral blood mononuclear cells, two additional LPS binding proteins with molecular mass of 95 kDa and 51 kDa are also readily detected. In studies not reported here, we have also demonstrated the presence of the 80 kDa protein on peripheral blood mononuclear cells of the cow, goat, pig, sheep and horse (21). We would thus suggest that this protein may be highly conserved among mammalian species.

The chicken has been reported to be refractory to many of the immunostimulatory and pathophysiological effects of endotoxic LPS (23). It was therefore of some interest to assess the expression of LPS binding proteins on peripheral blood mononuclear cells of this species. The results of one such experiment are shown in Fig 5, and suggest that the presence of the 80 kDa LPS binding protein is not readily detectable on chicken mononuclear cells even when autoradiographs are exposed for periods of time up to one week. The significance of this observation within the framework of sensitivity/resistance to endotoxin remains to be elucidated.

Fig 5. 2-D electrophoresis of photocrosslinked, iodinated and reduced chicken peripheral blood mononuclear cells. Top panel: Coomassie blue R-250 stain of the 2-D gels. Bottom panel: autoradiograph of the 2-D gel.

Characteristics of LPS Binding to the 80 kDa Protein

For the majority of the experiments described above, a period of incubation of 30 min at 37°C has been employed to detect binding. Experiments carried out at 4°C, in the presence of sodium azide, also allow detection of binding to the 80 kDa protein; however, as assessed by relative intensity of the autoradiograph, binding is reduced in comparison to the 37°C control.

Experiments to determine the kinetics of LPS binding to the 80 kDa protein at 37°C were also performed. For these studies, duplicate samples of murine splenocytes were incubated with ^{125}I-ASD-LPS at 37°C for various lengths of time, UV irradiated and then analyzed by 2-D electrophoresis. The region of the polyacrylamide gel corresponding to the 80 kDa protein identified by autoradiography was then excised from the gel and counted by scintillation spectroscopy. The results of this study are summarized in Fig 6 and indicate that binding increases rapidly over the first 5-10 min and is essentially complete by 20-30 min. We have not observed any qualitative differences (i.e., appearance of dominant LPS binding species other than the 80 kDa protein) at earlier time periods.

Experiments have also been carried out to determine the relationship between concentration of LPS and binding to the 80 kDa protein. The experimental protocol was essentially that as described above and the results are shown in Fig 7. At low concentrations of LPS (Fig 7a), the binding to the 80 kDa protein is directly proportional to the amount of LPS added to the splenocytes; at high concentrations, binding appears to be saturable (Fig 7b). Based upon the approximate specific activity of the LPS, the saturation level of binding observed in Fig 7b, the number of cells employed, and assuming a

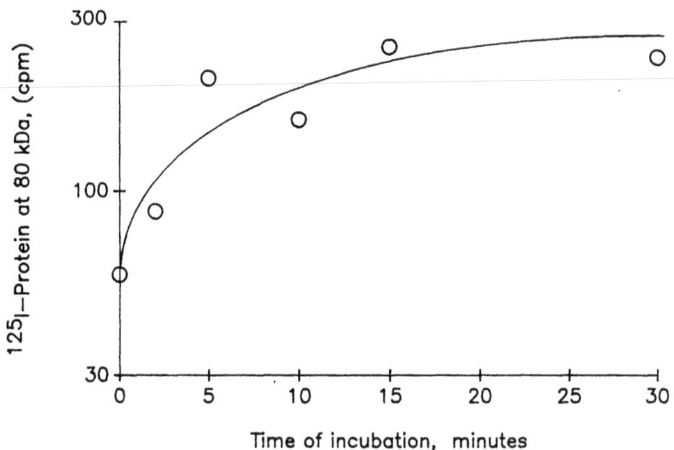

Fig 6. Time course of the binding of ^{125}I-ASD-LPS to the 80 kDa protein. Mouse splenocytes and ^{125}I-ASD-LPS were incubated at 37°C for various times. After photocrosslinking, reduction and 2-D gel electrophoresis, the LPS binding sites (the 80 kDa protein) were excised from the gels and their radioactivity were determined in a gamma spectrometer.

monomer LPS molecular weight of 10,000, it is possible to calculate approximately 5,000-10,000 80 kDa LPS binding sites per cell.

Subcellular Localization of the 80 kDa LPS Binding Protein

The data present above showing binding of ASD-LPS to the 80 kDa protein at 4°C in the presence of sodium azide suggest that this protein may be expressed on the cell membrane of murine splenocytes. To provide additional support for this hypothesis, splenocytes were crosslinked with ^{125}I-ASD-LPS and washed three times to remove unbound LPS. Cells were then lysed and a purified membrane fraction prepared by isopycnic sucrose density gradient ultracentrifugation as described by Jett et al. (9). Membrane markers for the purification included cell surface prelabeled with peroxidase conjugated goat antimouse Ig at 4°C and assessed by standard peroxidase reactions. The 2-D electrophoresis pattern and autoradiography of the purified, solubilized splenocyte membranes are shown in Fig 8 and clearly indicate the presence of the 80 kDa LPS binding protein.

Inhibition of Binding by Heterologous LPS and Lipid A

The data presented above suggest that LPS binding is saturable with respect to the 80 kDa protein. Experiments were, therefore, carried out to assess the capacity of homologous and heterologous underivatized LPS (i.e., LPS which does not have the ASD crosslinking group) to inhibit binding of ASD-LPS to the 80 kDa protein. A fifty fold excess of underivatized LPS from **E. coli** 0111:B4, 055:B5 or **S. minnesota** wild type, reduced binding of ASD-LPS to the 80 kDa protein by 65%, 55% and 32% respectively. In contrast the ASD-crosslinker coupled to an irrelevant protein carrier, human gamma globulin, inhibited binding of ASD-LPS to the 80 kDa protein by less than 5%, suggesting that the ASD crosslinking group does not contribute significantly to the binding interaction. Finally the addition of one hundred fold excess of either purified Ra-LPS or purified lipid A reduced binding ASD-LPS to less than detectable levels (13). These combined data indicate that binding specificity of the 80 kDa protein is most probably for the conserved lipid A region of the LPS macromolecule.

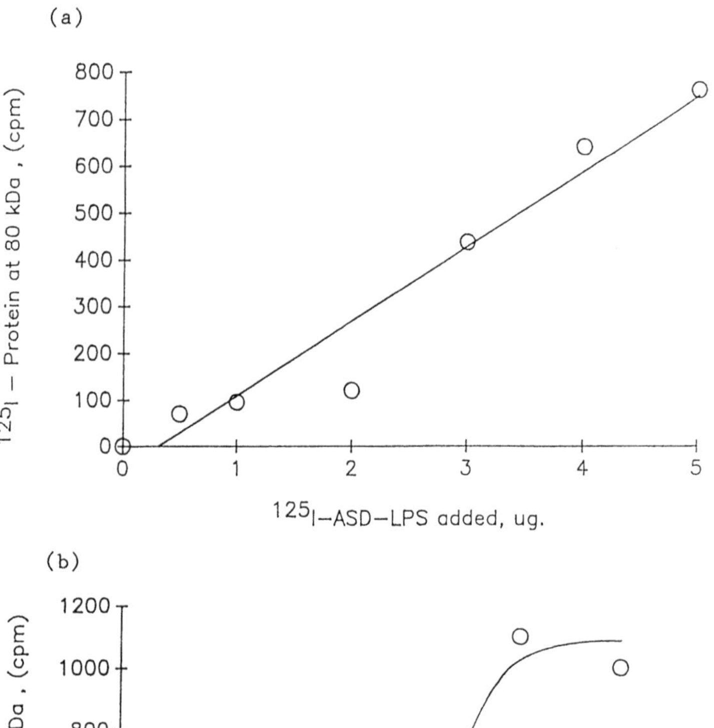

Fig 7. Dose response of the binding of the LPS specific 80 kDa LPS binding protein. **E. coli** 0111:B4 ^{125}I-ASD-LPS 0.5 to 5 μg (Fig 1a) or 1 to 50 μg (Fig 1b) were added to 1 x 10^7 mouse splenocytes in a final volume of 200 μl (Fig 1a) or 1.1 ml (Fig 1b) in the photoaffinity labeling study. After photocrosslinking and 2-D gel electrophoresis, the LPS binding sites (the 80 kDa protein) were excised from the 2-D gels and their radioactivity determined in a gamma spectrometer (Packard Multiprias 1, Packard Instrument Company, Downers Grove, IL).

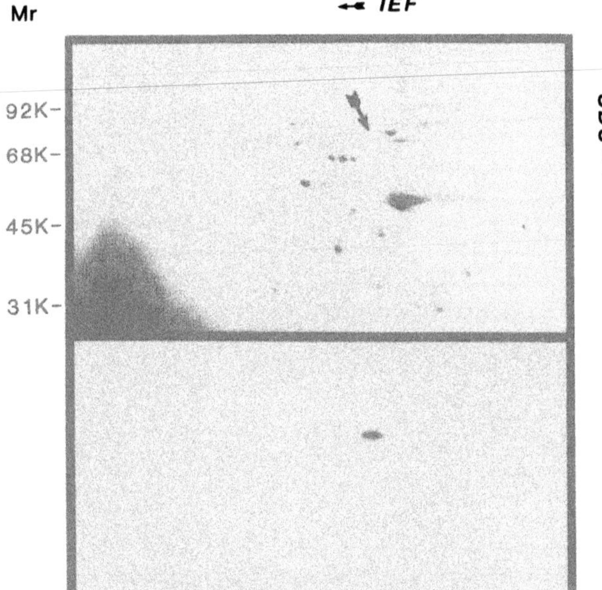

Fig 8. 2-D gel electrophoresis of isolated mouse splenocyte membranes. Splenocytes were first photoaffinity labeled with ^{125}I-ASD-LPS, then isolated using gradient ultracentrifugation. Top panel: Coomassie blue stain pattern. Bottom panel: autoradiograph of the 2-D gel.

Expression of the 80 kDa Protein on Splenocytes of C3H Responder and Non-responder Mice

The C3H/HeJ mouse has been well characterized for its genetically defined refractory state to the immunostimulatory and pathophysiologic effects of endotoxic LPS (reviewed in 17). Since it is possible that the 80 kDa LPS protein serves as a specific receptor for LPS, and since the C3H/HeJ mouse has been reported to lack specific LPS receptors (2, 4, 5), it was of relevance to query the level of 80 kDa LPS binding protein on splenocytes of C3H responder and non-responder mice. A summary of the results of these experiments are shown in Fig 9, which depict an enlargement of the region of the autoradiograph containing the 80 kDa hotspot. Several closely migrating species can be resolved, each of molecular mass of 80 kDa but slightly differing pI values. Of importance, no significant qualitative or quantitative differences have been detected in the binding of the ASD-LPS to the 80 kDa protein of either splenocyte population.

Effect of Antiserum Raised Against the 80 kDa LPS Binding Protein

While the collective data presented above are clearly consistent with the hypothesis that the 80 kDa LPS binding protein may serve as a receptor for LPS on cells of immunologic interest, they present no definitive evidence for a functional role for this protein. In an effort to address this issue we have recently undertaken studies to generate immunologic reagents with specificity for this protein. In view of the fact that chickens appear not to express the 80 kDa LPS binding protein, adult white leghorn chickens were immunized with polyacrylamide gel homogenates prepared from 2-D gels and the

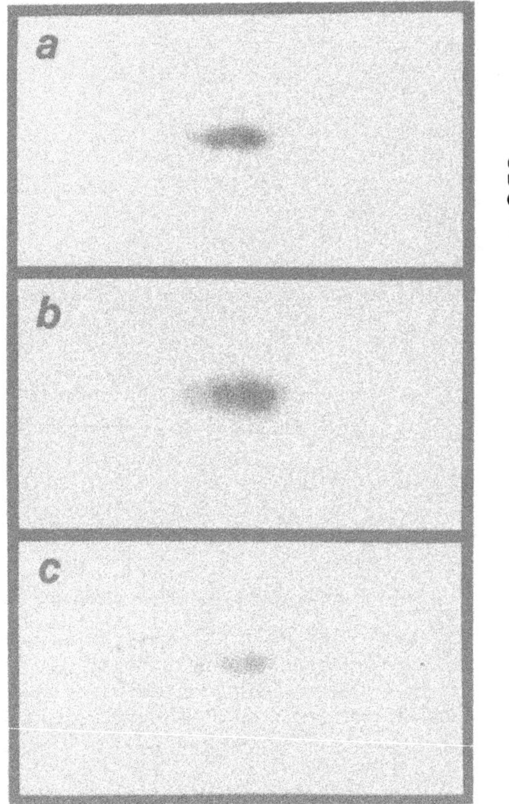

Fig 9. 2-D gel electrophoretic analysis of the 80 kDa LPS binding protein from C3H/HeJ and C3HeB/FeJ mouse splenocytes. The figure shows the enlarged profile of the 80 kDa, pI 6.5 region of the autoradiographs of the 2-D gels. (a) C3H/HeJ mouse splenocytes. (b) C3HeB/FeJ mouse splenocytes. (c) C3H/HeJ and C3HeB/FeJ spleen cells mixtures (1:1 ratio).

80 kDa, pI 6.5 hotspot identified by autoradiography. Chickens were bled five days following a second injection of antigen and serum (termed anti-80 kDa CS) prepared.

Our preliminary efforts to characterize this antiserum have involved an assessment of its effects on LPS induced B-cell proliferation in **in vitro** cultures of murine splenocytes. Sera from unimmunized chickens (NCS) have served as a control for these experiments. The results of several such experiments are shown in Fig 10a and 10b, in which various concentrations of either anti-80 kDa CS or NCS have been added to LPS stimulated C3Heb/FeJ splenocytes. While, at the concentrations examined, NCS had little detectable effect on LPS induced proliferation, the anti 80 kDa serum had a highly significant biphasic effect on LPS induced mitogenesis. This biphasic enhancement was observed at cell concentrations of LPS examined, with optimal enhancement observed at about 1:160 antiserum dilution. When the collective data are examined at dilutions of antisera where the net effect is an enhancement of mitogenesis (1:160 to 1:640) and the effects determined as a function of LPS concentration, the results shown in Fig 11a are obtained. These results indicate an anti 80 kDa CS dose-dependent shift in the response to LPS mitogenic stimulation. In contrast, no such shift in the dose

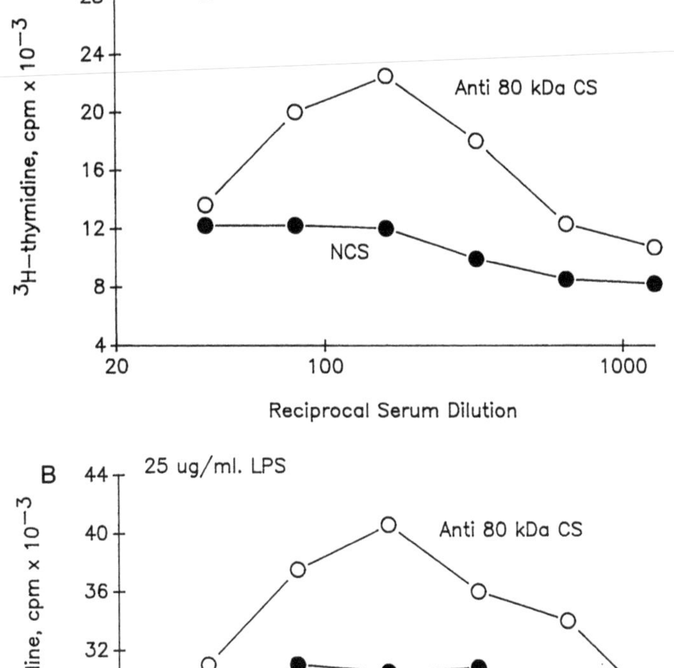

Fig 10. Effect of anti 80 kDa CS and NCS on LPS mitogenic activity. Various dilutions of chicken sera were prepared in complete culture media (RPMI 1640 with supplements) and added to individual wells of microtiter plates along with various concentrations of LPS. Then C3Heb/FeJ splenocytes were added and ^{3}H-Thymidine incorporation determined as described in Materials and Methods. a) 0.8 µg/ml LPS b) 25 µg/ml LPS

response curve with NCS is observed (Fig 11b) except for a very modest increase in the background level of ^{3}H-thimidine incorporation. It is noteworthy that, in the absence of LPS, the antiserum itself does not manifest the capacity to induce B-cell mitogenesis.

DISCUSSION

The results described in this manuscript provide evidence for the existence of an endotoxic lipopolysaccharide binding protein which is expressed on the cytoplasmic membrane of mammalian lymphoid cells. This protein has a molecular mass of 80 kDa and an approximate pI of 6.5. Binding of LPS to this protein is both time and temperature dependent, is linear with respect to LPS at low LPS concentrations and is saturable at high LPS concentrations. Binding of LPS is specific for the lipid A component of LPS and is inhibited by both heterologous LPS and by purified lipid A. The 80 kDa LPS binding protein is expressed on both T-cell enriched and B-cell enriched

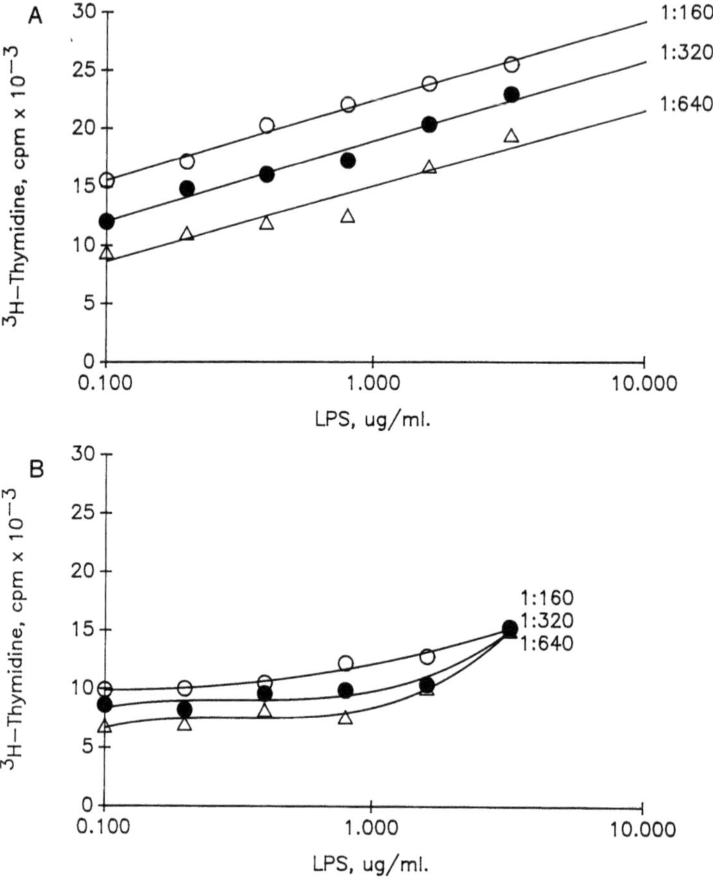

Fig 11. The effect of anti 80 kDa CS (11a) or NCS (11b) on the proliferation response of spleen cells to LPS. The experimental protocol is as described in the legend to Fig 10.

murine splenocytes as well as murine splenic macrophages. It is also expressed on murine B and T cell lines but is absent from an undifferentiated murine myeloma cell line. There appears to be no major qualitative or quantitative differences in the expression of the 80 kDa LPS binding protein on splenocytes of the C3H/HeJ and C3Heb/FeJ mouse strains. A dominant 80 kDa LPS binding protein with electrophoretic properties remarkably similar to that observed on murine cells is readily detectable on peripheral blood mononuclear cells of a variety of mammalian species. This protein is, however, absent from adult chicken peripheral blood mononuclear cells. Antiserum to the murine 80 kDa protein raised in chickens appears to modulate the **in vitro** mitogenic activity of LPS on murine splenocytes. These collective data are consistent with the 80 kDa LPS binding protein functioning as a specific receptor for LPS initiated cellular responses.

The observed pattern of expression of the 80 kDa LPS binding protein on murine splenocytes subpopulations is of interest and merits further comment. We find this protein expressed on B cells, T cells and macrophages, and these results are confirmed by the appropriate experiments carried out in homogeneous murine B- and T-cell lines. While the presence of LPS binding proteins on B cells and macrophages is certainly not surprising, and are to be anticipated, the presence of this protein on T cells might, at first, seem inconsistent with the inability of LPS to induce mitogenic responses in these cells (1). The fact that LPS does, in fact, induce proliferation in a subpopulation of murine T cells notwithstanding (29), there is considerable experimental evidence in the literature for direct LPS mediated effects on T cell function. Perhaps the best evidence, in this respect, is the now well documented requirement for LPS responsive T-cells in the manifestation of the adjuvant activity of LPS. As elegantly shown by Michalek, McGhee and their colleagues using C3H LPS-responder and nonresponder cell popoulations (14), the **in vitro** enhancement of immune responses to antigen by LPS requires that both T-cells and macrophages be of the LPS responder phenotype--thus dictating that T-cells manifest an appropriate cellular recognition system for LPS. Given that LPS also promotes changes in surface antigen expression in murine thymocytes (22) the existence of LPS binding proteins on T-cells would, therefore, appear as a reasonable hypothesis. Support for this hypothesis is provided by the data presented here.

A second result which merits additional comment is the observation that the 80 kDa LPS binding protein appears to be equivalently expressed on splenocytes of both normal and LPS-nonresponder inbred mouse strains. Earlier results from a number of laboratories (reviewed in 17) have provided considerable experimental data which would either support or refute the concept that the genetic difference between the endotoxin unresponsive C3H/HeJ and histocompatible C3H strains is the absence of a structural gene which encodes a specific LPS receptor. The best evidence in support of this concept is the immunologic data of Coutinho et al., (2, 4, 5) discussed earlier in this manuscript. Consistent with this hypothesis is the observation of Jakobivitz et al., (8) that responsiveness or unresponsiveness to LPS appears to be embodied in a membrane fraction of LPS responder B-cells; however the issue of whether the responsible element in such membrane preparations is a specific membrane receptor, or some critical component of the transmembrane signaling apparatus distinct from an LPS receptor and defective in C3H/HeJ lymphocytes was not addressed. On the other hand, there is growing experimental evidence that C3H/HeJ cells are not refractory to immunostimulation with all protein-free LPS preparations (3). In addition, as shown by Ulevitch et al., (11), reconstitution of mitogenic activity in C3H/HeJ B cells can be accomplished by addition of trypsin to LPS stimulated cultures. Since it is unlikely that trypsin serves to create an LPS-receptor on cells for which the normal structural gene is purportedly somehow altered, it is most reasonable, as postulated by Ulevitch, that the trypsin is providing some essential secondary triggering signal subsequent to occupancy of the receptor by the LPS ligand. Our results reported here would be in accord with the concept that the genetic defect in the C3H/HeJ mouse which renders lymphoid cells from this mouse refractory to LPS stimulation is not the alteration of a structural gene encoding for an LPS receptor.

The evidence in support of the 80 kDa LPS binding protein as a specific receptor for LPS in the initiation of LPS induced cellular responses is compelling; this protein is membrane localized, specific for all LPS and lipid A, and binding is saturable with about 10,000 binding sites per cell. Unequivocal evidence that the 80 kDa LPS binding protein is, in fact, a true functional receptor has been more difficult to obtain. Our experimental approach to this question has been to generate antisera to the 80 kDa protein in order to demonstrate modulation of expression of LPS mediated cellular responses. Early efforts to generate antiserum to the protein by immunization of rabbits and rats were disappointing, in large part we believe, because of the existence of electrophoretically similar LPS binding proteins expressed on mononuclear cells of these species (see below). Our more recent and still preliminary efforts have involved hyperimmunization of chickens, which appear not to express the 80 kDa LPS binding protein. Chicken antisera raised to 2-D gel purified 80 kDa protein significantly alter LPS mediated **in vitro** mitogenic activity although the antisera, by itself, is without immunomodulatory activity except by suppressing background thymidine incorporation at the highest concentrations tested. We have, to date, not been successful in demonstrating by Western blot analysis, specific binding to the LPS photocrosslinked 80 kDa binding protein; however, the relative amount of protein detected by Coomassie blue staining in the region of the autoradiograph hotspot appears to be extremely low and its efficiency of transfer to nitrocellulose is not known. As a consequence, formal proof that the anti 80 kDa serum is directed against the LPS binding protein remains as a primary objective of our current research efforts.

We believe it to be of considerable potential significance that an 80 kDa protein can be defined on the surface of peripheral blood mononuclear cells of a wide variety of mammalian species which has the property of specific binding to LPS and/or lipid A. Whether lipid A binding is the primary function of this membrane protein, or whether it participates in some cellular activity critical to maintenance of the cell's integrity and only fortuitously binds LPS/lipid A is, at present, unclear. The extent of immunologic cross reactivity of this antigen between species will also be of interest.

In summary, our results presented here provide some of the first biochemical evidence for the existence of specific LPS binding sites on the cell membranes of mammalian lymphoid cells. The elucidation of the biochemical structure of these LPS binding proteins and how they function within the framework of LPS mediated immunostimulation and release of biologically active monokines and other cytokines will provide important new information on mechanisms of LPS host responses. This understanding, in turn may well contribute to unique new therapeutic approaches to immunomodulation and/or intervention in endotoxin mediated shock and multiorgan failure.

ACKNOWLEDGEMENTS

The authors acknowledge the collective contributions of our laboratory and others in many useful and informative discussions during the course of this work, particularly Drs. Stanley Vukajlovich, James Killion, John Ryan and Richard Silverstein, also Mr. Stuart Bright, Vernon Tesh and David Travis. We acknowledge the outstanding secretarial assistance of Ms. Janet Hollands. This research was supported by research grant AI-23447 from the NIH.

REFERENCES

1. Chiller, J. M., Skidmore, B. M., Morrison, D. C. and Weigle, W. O., 1973, Relationship of lipopolysaccharide structure to its function in mitogenesis and adjuvanticity. Proc. Nat. Acad. Sci. 70: 212.

2. Coutinho, A., Forni, L. and Watanabe, T., 1978, Genetic and functional characterization of an antiserum to the lipid A specific triggering receptor of murine B lymphocytes. Eur. J. Immunol. 8: 63.

3. Flebbe, L., Morrison, D. C. and Vukajlovich, S. W., 1989, Immunostimulation of C3H/HeJ Lymphoid Cells by R-Chemotype Lipopolysaccharide Preparations. J. Immunol. 142: 642.

4. Forni, L. and Coutinho, A., 1978, An antiserum which recognizes lipopolysaccharide-reactive B cells in the mouse. Eur. J. Immunol. 8: 56.

5. Forni, L. and Coutinho, A., 1978, Receptor interactions on the membrane of resting and activated B cells. Nature (London) 273: 304.

6. Goodman, S. A. and Morrison, D. C., 1985, Lipopolysaccharides receptors on lymphocytes. I. Lack of immunologic recognition of a putative LPS

receptor on LPS responder lymphocytes by LPS non-responder mice. J. Immunology 135: 1906.

7. Haeffner-Cavaillon, N., Cavaillon, J. M. and Szabo, L., 1985, Cellular receptors for endotoxin, in: "The Cellular Biology of Endotoxin," Handbook of Endotoxon, Vol. 3, L. J. Berry, ed., Elsevier Publ. Comp., Amsterdam, p.1.

8. Jakobovits, A., Sharon, N. and Zan-Bar, I., 1982, Acquisition of mitogenic responsiveness by non-responding lymphocytes upon insertion of appropriate membrane components. J. Exp. Med. 156: 1274.

9. Jett, M., Seed, T. M. and Jamieson, G. A., 1977, Isolation and characterization of plasma membranes and intact nuclei from lymphoid cells. J. Biol. Chem. 252: 2134.

10. Killion, J. W. and Morrison, D. C., 1988, Mechanisms of murine Salmonellosis immunity induced by immunization with lipopolysaccharide-lipid A-associated protein complexes in C3H/HeJ mice. FEMS Microbiology Immunology 47: 41.

11. Kuus, K., Johnston, A. R. and Ulevitch, R. J., 1985, Enhancement of C3H/HeJ B-cell responsiveness to lipopolysaccharide (LPS) with Trypsin. Fed. Proc. (Abst.) 44: 974.

12. Lei, M-G and Morrison, D. C., 1988, Specific endotoxic lipopolysaccharide-binding proteins on murine splenocytes. I. Detection of lipopolysaccharide-binding sites on splenocytes and splenocyte subpopulations. J. Immunology 141: 996.

13. Lei, M-G and Morrison, D. C., 1988, Specific endotoxic lipopolysaccharide-binding proteins on murine splenocytes. II. Membrane localization and binding characteristics. J. Immunology 141: 1006.

14. McGhee, J. R., Farrarr, J. J., Michalek, S. M., Mergenhagen, S. E. and Rosenstreich, D. L., 1979, Cellular requirements for lipopolysaccharide adjuvanticity: a role for both T lymphocytes and macrophages **in vitro** responses to particular antigens. J. Exp. Med. 149: 793.

15. Morrison, D. C., 1985, Nonspecific interactions of bacterial lipopolysaccharides with membranes and membrane components, in: "Cellular Biology of Endotoxins," L. J. Berry, ed., Elsevier North Holland, Amsterdam, p. 25.

16. Morrison, D. C. and Raziuddin, S., 1981, Endotoxin-cell membrane interactions leading to transmembrane signals, in: "Contemporary Topics in Molecular Immunology," Vol. 8, W. J. Mandy and F. P. Inman, eds., Plenum Pub. Co., New York, p. 187.

17. Morrison, D. C., 1986, The C3H/HeJ mouse strain: Its role in the elucidation of host response to bacterial endotoxin, in: "Microbiology, 1985," P. Bonventre, ed., ASM Publications, Washington, D. C., p. 23.

18. Morrison, D. C. and Ryan, L. J., 1979, A Review - Bacterial endotoxins and host immune function, in: "Advances in Immunology," Vol. 28, F. J. Dixon and H. G. Kunkel, eds., Academic Press, New York, p. 293.

19. Morrison, D. C. and Leive, L., 1975, Isolation and characterization of two fractions of lipopolysaccharides from **E. coli** 0111:B4. J. Biol. Chem. 250: 2911.

20. O'Farrell, P. H., 1975, High resolution two-dimensional electrophoresis of proteins. J. Biol. Chem. 250: 4007.

21. Roeder, D. J., Lei, M.-G. and Morrison, D. C., 1989, Endotoxic-lipopolysaccharide-specific binding proteins on lymphoid cells of various animal species: association with endotoxic susceptibility. Infec. and Immun. 57: 1054.

22. Scheid, M. P., Goldstein, G., Hammerling, U. and Boyse, E. A., 1975, Induction of T and B lymphocyte differentiation **in vitro**, in: "Membrane Receptors of Lymphocytes," M. Seligman, J. L. Prud'homme, and F. M. Kourilsky, eds., North-Holland Publ., Amsterdam, p. 353.

23. Skjorten, F. and Evensen, S. A., 1973, Induction of disseminated intravascular coagulation in the factor XII-deficient fowl. Thromb. Diath Haemorrh. 30: 25.

24. Springer, G. F., Adye, J. C., Bezkorovainy, A. and Jirgensons, B., 1974, Properties and activity of the lipopolysaccharide-receptor from human erythrocytes. Biochemistry 13: 1379.

25. Springer, G. F., Adye, J. C., Bezkorovainy, A. and Murthy, J. R., 1973, Functional aspects and nature of lipopolysaccharide-receptor of human erythrocytes. J. Infect. Dis. 128: S202.

26. Springer, G. F. and Adye, J. C., 1975, Endotoxin-binding substances from human leukocytes and platelets. Infect. Immun. 12: 978.

27. Springer, G. F., Adye, J. C., Mergenhagen, S. E. and Rosenstreich, D. L., 1977, Endotoxin interaction with phosphatides from human leukocytes and platelets, and with lymphoid cells of susceptible and resistant mice, in: "Microbiology, 1977," D. Schlessinger, ed., ASM Publications, Washington, D. C., p. 326.

28. Sultzer, B. M., 1968, Genetic control of leukocyte responses to endotoxin. Nature (London) 219: 1252.

29. Vogel, S. N., Hilfiker, M. L. and Caulfield, M. J., 1983, Endotoxin-induced T-lymphocyte proliferation. J. Immunol. 130: 1744.

30. Watson, J., Kelly, K. and Whitlock, C., 1980, Genetic control of endotoxin sensitivity, in: "Microbiology, 1980," D. Schlessinger, ed., Amer. Soc. Microbio. for Washington, D. C., p. 4.

31. Wollenweber, H. W. and Morrison, D. C., 1985, Synthesis and biochemical characterization of a photoactivatable, iodinatable, cleavable bacterial lipopolysaccharide derivative. J. Biol. Chem. 260: 15068.

REGULATORY MECHANISM OF EXPRESSION OF LPS BINDING SITE(S) AND SIGNALING EVENTS BY LPS IN MACROPHAGES

K. S. Akagawa, K. Kamoshita, T. Tomita*, T. Yasuda*, and T. Tokunaga

Department of Cellular Immunology, National Institute of Health, 2-10-35, Kamiosaki, Shinagawa-ku, Tokyo 141, and The Medical Institute, University of Tokyo*, 4-6-1 Shiroganedai, Minato-ku, Tokyo 108, Japan

INTRODUCTION

Lipopolysaccharide (LPS) from gram-negative microorganisms is a potent activator of macrophages. LPS induces macrophages to secrete immunoregulatory substances including interleukin 1 (IL 1), tumor necrosis factor (TNF), interferon, colony stimulating factors (CSFs) and, prostaglandins. Furthermore LPS activates tumor cytotoxicity of macrophages by itself or in combination with interferon.

We showed that murine alveolar macrophages (AM) were unresponsive to activation for tumor cytotoxicity by LPS, while peritoneal macrophages (PM) were responsive, because of the lack of binding with LPS on the cell surface of AM (4). These results suggest that there is a binding site(s) for LPS on the cell surface of macrophages and the binding of LPS to them is necessary for the induction of tumor cytotoxicity of macrophages. However, the molecular basis of this reactivity or the signaling events initiated by LPS in macrophage activation are not yet resolved.

In the present paper, we show our recent results concerning the LPS binding site(s) on the cell surface of macorophages and the signaling events deduced by LPS.

MATERIALS AND METHODS

Animals

Specific pathogen-free female C3H/HeSlc (6 to 8 wk) and C3H/HeJ (4 to 6 wk) mice were obtained from the Shizuoka Experimental Animal Cooperative (Hamamatsu, Japan).

Reagents

Proteose peptone and Brewer's thioglycollate medium were obtained from Difco Laboratories. (Detroit, MI). LPS (**Escherichia coli** 055:B5) conjugated with fluorescein isothiocyanate (FITC-LPS, molar ratio 24:1) was obtained from List Biological Laboratories, Inc. (Campbell, CA). LPS (**E.**

coli 0111:B4), Dibutyryl cAMP, indomethacin, pertussis toxin (PT) and actinomycin D were obtained from Sigma Chemical Co. (St. Louis, MO).

Culture Medium

RPMI 1640 medium was prepared from powdered stock (Nissui Seiyaku Co., Ltd., Tokyo, Japan) and supplemented with 100 U of penicillin G potassium (Banyu Seiyaku Kabushiki Kaisha, Tokyo) per ml and 100 μg of streptomycin sulfate (Meiji Seika Kaisha, Yokohama, Japan) per ml. Fetal bovine serum (FBS) (Z. L. Bockneck Laboratories Inc., Ontario, Canada) was inactivated by heating at 56°C for 30 min before use. The FBS contained 0.003 ng of LPS per ml, according to the Limulus amebocyte lysate test. RPMI 1640 medium was further supplemented with 10% FBS and used as culture medium unless otherwise stated.

Preparation of Macrophages

AM were prepared as described previously (3). Peritoneal resident cells (PC) and peritoneal exudate cells (PEC) were obtained from normal mice and mice that had received an intraperitoneal injection of 2 ml of 10% proteose-peptone or Brewer's thioglycollate medium 3 days before. AC, PC and PEC were washed three times by centrifugation and resuspended in ice-cold RPMI 1640 medium. Total cell counts were made with a hemocytometer and cells were differentiated on cytocentrifuge preparations (Cytospin centrifuge, Shandon Southern Instruments, Inc., Sewickley, PA) stained with diff-Quick (Kokusai Siyak Kabushiki Kaisha, Koube, Japan). These cells were pipetted into wells of 96-well flat-bottom tissue culture plates (Falcon No 3072; Becton Dickinson & Co., Oxnard, CA), or spotted onto coverslips (13-mm diameter) and were incubated at 37° C for 2 hr, and nonadherent cells were removed by repeated washing with physiological saline solution. At least 96% of the adherent cells were macrophages as judged by morphologic and phagocytic criteria, and they were used as AM, resident peritoneal macrophages (PRM), peptone induced peritoneal exudate macrophages (P-PEM) or thioglycollate induced peritoneal exudate macrophages (T-PEM).

Recombinant CSFs

Recombinant murine granulocyte-macrophage colony stimulating factor (rmGM-CSF)(10) was kindly provided by Dr. N. Minato (Jichi Medical School, Toochigi-ken, Japan) and Dr. T. Sudo (Toray Basic Research Institute, Kanagawa-ken, Japan). Recombinant human (rh)CSF-1 was kindly donated by Dr. M. Takahashi (Otsuka Pharmaceutical Co., Ltd., Tokushima, Japan). These recombinant CSFs were obtained as culture supernatants of Cos-1 cells transfected with the expression vector containing the cDNA clone of each of the genes. Stock solutions of 5×10^4 U of rmGM-CSF per ml and of 6000U of rhCSF-1 per ml, respectively, contained < 0.5 ng of LPS per ml according to the Limulus amebocyte lysate test, respectively. Medium conditioned by Cos-1 cells transfected with the same vector but not containing any CSF gene was used as a control (mock-CSF).

Interferon-γ (IFN-γ)

Recombinant murine (rm)IFN-γ, obtained from gene expression in **E. coli** (12) was a gift from Toray Industries, Inc. (Tokyo). Specific activity of the IFN-γ was 8.3×10^6 U/mg, and a stock solution of 1×10^5 U/ml contained < 0.05 ng of LPS per ml as determined by the Limulus amebocyte lysate test.

Antibody

$F(ab')_2$ fragment of rabbit anti-asialo GM antibody (IgG) was prepared as described previously (4). Monoclonal antibody F4/80 was kindly provided by Dr. S. Gordon (Sir William Dunn School of Pathology, Oxford University, England). Monoclonal antibody M1/70HL against Mac-1 antigen was obtained from Hybritech Inc. (San Diego, CA). FITC-labeled $F(ab')_2$ fragments of goat anti-rabbit IgG and goat anti-rat IgG were obtained from Cooper Biomedical Inc. (Malverm, PA). These antibodies were diluted appropriately with PBS containing 0.1% NaN_3.

Assay for Tumor Cytotoxicity

The assay method was described previously (4). Two hundreds μl of ^{51}Cr labeled EL4 cell suspension containing 1×10^4 cells were added to the macrophage monolayers, and incubated for 20 hr. The plates were then centrifuged and 100 μl of the supernatant was removed from each well for counting radioactivity on an automatic gamma spectrometer. Cytotoxicity was expressed as percent specific ^{51}Cr release calculated from the average of triplicate samples as follows: percent specific release= (experimental release - spontaneous release) / (maximum release - spontaneous release).

TNF Assay

The activity of TNF was assayed as follows. L929 cells (30,000/0.1 ml) were cultured with serially diluted test samples in 96-well flat-bottomed microtiter plates at 37° C for 18 hr in the presence of actinomycin D (5 μg/ml). After incubation, the plates were washed and cell lysis was determined by staining the plates with crystal violet for about 15 min, rinsed with running tap water, and allowed to dry in air. Absorbance of the cells in each well was read with a Sjeia Auto Reader (LModel ER-8000, Sanko Junyaku Co., Ltd., Tokyo) using the 570 nm filter. The machine was blanked (zero absorbance) with wells showing maximal killing. Absorbance of the cells incubated with medium alone was considered as 100% survival. Absorbance readings were converted to percentage survival and dose-response curves generated. One unit of TNF is defined as the reciprocal of the dilution of a preparation which resulted in 50% survival of cells.

Preparation of ^3H-labeled LPS

LPS from **E. coli** F515 (Re-LPS) was treated first with $NaIO_4$ and then treated with $NaB3H_4$. The specific activity of the ^3H-Re-LPS was 10,400 cpm/μg.

LPS Binding Assay

The assay was a modification of the method described previously (12). Macrophages were plated at a final density of 5×10^5 cells per well (24-well culture plate), and were incubated with ^3H-Re-LPS (200 μl/well) in the presence of 0.1% NaN_3 at 4° C for various periods of time. After the incubation, the radioactive supernatant was discarded and the unbound material was rapidly removed by washing the plates with PBS. The cells were then solubilised by 0.1% triton x 100 and radioactivity was measured with a liquid scintillation counter. For the binding-inhibition studies increasing amounts of unlabeled ligand were added to the radio labeled Re-LPS, keeping the total volume at 200 μl.

Measurements of Cellular cAMP

Macrophages (2×10^6) were seeded into each well of 6-well plates and the cells were incubated with LPS (10 μg/ml) for various periods of time at 37° C. The cells were washed and cyclic AMP was extracted with 0.2M HCl. Concentrations of cAMP were determined by using the cAMP ^{125}I-RIA Kit (Yamasa Shoyu Kaboshiki Kaisha, Chiba, Japan).

RESULTS

Lack of LPS Binding Site(s) on the Surface of Murine AM

Previously we found that AM obtained from various mouse strains were refractory to activation by LPS (5), while PM from the same strains of mice were responsive to LPS. Treatment of AM with lymphokines or rmIFN-γ rendered AM responsive to LPS. AM treated with rmIFN-γ showed tumor cytotoxicity by LPS stimulation and became sensitive to direct toxicity of LPS(5). We also found that rmIFN-γ rendered C3H/HeJ macrophages responsive to LPS (5). In these points, AM are phenotypically similar to PM of C3H/HeJ mice which defect of LPS responsiveness is controlled by a single, co-dominantly inherited, autosomal gene located in chromosome 4. Since LPS or lipid A can bind to B cells and macrophages from C3H/HeJ mice, it was suggested that the unresponsiveness of C3H/HeJ mice to LPS is due to a factor(s) other than a defect in binding (8).

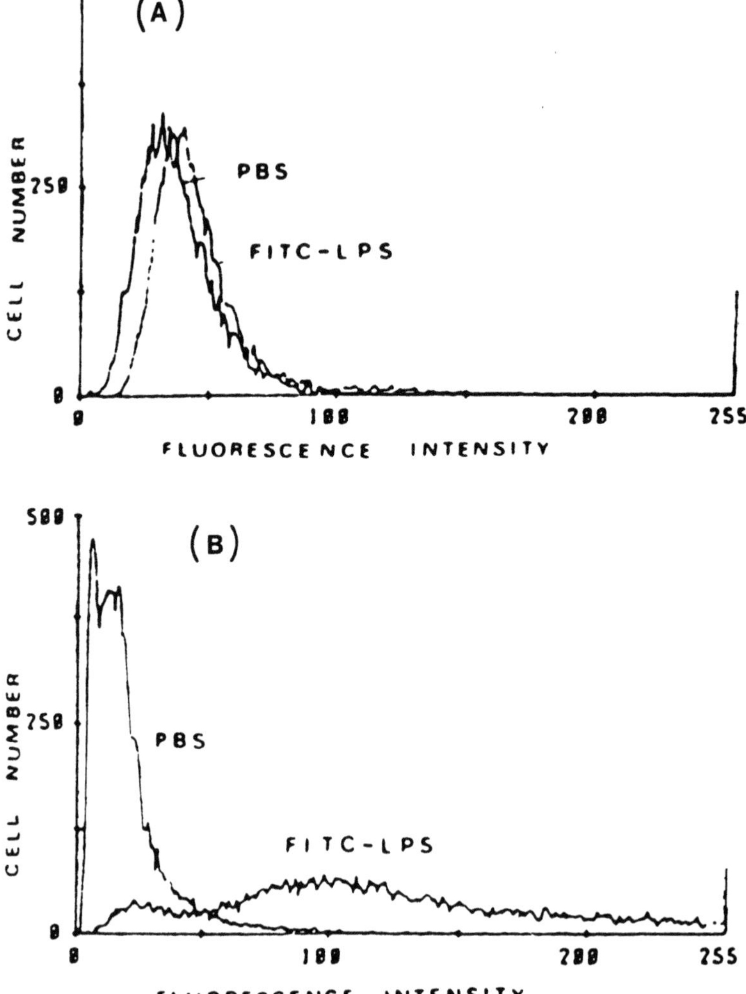

Fig 1. Fluorescence histogram from FACS analysis of AM and PRM labeled with FITC-LPS. AM (A) and PRM (B) were incubated with FITC-LPS (100 μg/ml) or with PBS at 0° C for 60 min and washed.

To test the possibility that the unresponsiveness of AM to LPS was due to the lack of LPS binding site, we examined the binding of LPS to AM by using FITC-labeled LPS. The binding of FITC-LPS to AM was analyzed by flow cytometry. Almost all PM were stained with FITC-LPS, while < 5% of the AM were stained (Fig 1). Furthermore about 60% of AM treated with lymphokines or rmIFN-γ were stained with FITC-LPS (5). These results suggest that the defective responsiveness of AM to LPS is due to the lack or very low expression of LPS binding sites on the surface and that in vitro treatment with lymphokines or rmIFN-γ brings about the expression of them and renders AM responsive to LPS.

As shown in Table 1, binding of FITC-LPS to PM and rmIFN-γ treated AM was inhibited in the presence of unlabeled LPS or polymixin B which is known to form a stable molecular complex with the lipid A region of LPS and block the effect of LPS. These results suggest that the binding of LPS to these macrophages is not due to nonspecific attachment but rather a specific binding to LPS or lipid A receptor.

Effects of CSFs on the Expression of LPS Binding Site(s) of Macrophages

Previously we reported that in mice, AM and PM differ markedly not only in the expression of LPS binding site(s), but also in the expression of cell surface glycosphingolipid, asialo GM1 (3, 4). Almost all AM express asialo GM1, while most of PM do not express asialo GM1, though there are exceptions: expression of high asialo GM1 in Brewer's thioglycollate medium induced PM (10) and in PM activated with lymphokines or LPS in vitro or with BCG or Heat-killed Corynebacterium parvum in vivo (4). However the origin of such heterogeneity of AM and PM is not yet known.

Table 1. Binding of FITC-LPS in the Presence or Absence of Unlabeled LPS or Polymixin B on the Surface of Macrophages

Cells	Presence of unlabeled LPS or polymixin B		Cells stained with FITC-LPS (%)
AM	-		3.9
	LPS	10 μg/ml	2.8
	Polymixin B	100 μg/ml	3.1
		200 μg/ml	1.2
AM treated	-		60.8
with IFN-γ	LPS	10 μg/ml	3.0
	Polymixin B	100 μg/ml	2.2
		200 μg/ml	1.5
PM	-		98.0
	LPS	10 μg/ml	22.0
	Polymixin B	100 μg/ml	39.2
		200 μg/ml	4.7

Macrophages on the coverslips were stained with FITC-LPS (100 μg/ml for 60 min at 0° C in the presence or absence of unlabeled LPS or polymixin B.

Recently, we found that not only can murine AM proliferate and generate colonies in vitro after exposure to either CSF-1 or GM-CSF, but also they are bipotential cells whose choice of differentiation is determined by the level of the distinct CSF (2). The phenotype of the cells in the colonies formed by AM incubated with rmGM-CSF was AM-like as shown in Table 2; more than 90% of the cells were stained by anti-asialo GM1 but not by FITC-LPS, and had AM-like morphology. Moreover expression of Mac-1 antigen in these cells as well as original AM was very low. However, the phenotype of the cells in the colonies formed by AM incubated with rhCSF-1 was PM-like; more than 90% of the cells were stained by FITC-LPS and M1/70HL, but not by anti-asialo GM1, and showed PM-like morphology. The cells in all colonies formed by AM were macrophages, because they were F4/80 positive. The cells in the colonies formed by AM incubated with rmGM-CSF changed their phenotype after treatment with rhCSF-1; the percentage of cells stained by anti-asialo GM1 decreased, and that of cells stained by FITC-LPS increased. The cells in the colonies formed by AM incubated with rhCSF-1 never changed their phenotype after incubation with rmGM-CSF.

More than 90% of P-PEM expressed LPS binding site(s) and less than 20% of them expressed asialo GM1. On the other hand, more than 90% of T-PEM expressed LPS binding site(s) and about 80% of the cells also expressed asialo GM1. However, both P-PEM and T-PEM became asialo GM1 negative after incubation with rmGM-CSF, rhCSF-1. P-PEM and T-PEM as well as AM proliferated and formed colonies in the presence of rmGM-CSF or rhCSF-1. In contrast to AM, more than 90% of the cells in all colonies formed by P-PEM or T-PEM incubated with either rmGM-CSF or rhCSF-1 were stained by FITC-LPS but not by anti-asialo GM1 (2).

Characterization of LPS Binding Site(s) of Macrophages by Using ^{3}H-Re-LPS

Above results suggest strongly the existence of LPS binding site on the surface of macrophages. Therefore we tried to analyze further the nature of the LPS binding site(s) of macrophages by using isotope labeled Re-LPS from *E. coli* F515 strain. PRM were incubated with various concentrations of ^{3}H-Re-LPS in the presence or absence of excess amount of unlabeled Re-LPS at 4° C for 5 hr. As shown in Fig 2, ^{3}H-Re-LPS binding to PRM was depended on the concentrations of ^{3}H-Re-LPS and was inhibited by the presence of excess amount of unlabeled LPS. The amount of ^{3}H-Re-LPS bound to PRM depended on

Table 2. Surface Markers of Cells in the Colonies Formed by AM

Incubated with	No. of colonies[a] / $2x10^{4}$ cells	% Cells stained with [b]			
		Anti-asialoGM1	FITC-LPS	M1/70HD	F4/80
rmGM-CSF	86+8.3	92.6+3.7	3.1+1.5	25.4+3.0	95.9+0.2
rhCSF-1	82+14.9	5.7+3.5	88.6+0.8	98.6+0.6	97.9+1.1

AM (2 x 10^{4}/coverslip) were incubated with rmGM-CSF (20 U/ml) or rhCSF-1 (1000 U/ml) for 14 days and the cells were stained by the indicated antibodies or by FITC-LPS. The medium was changed every 4 days.

[a]Data are expressed as the mean + SD of triplicate cultures.

[b]Data are expressed as the mean + SD of 100-300 cells counted in at least 10 colonies.

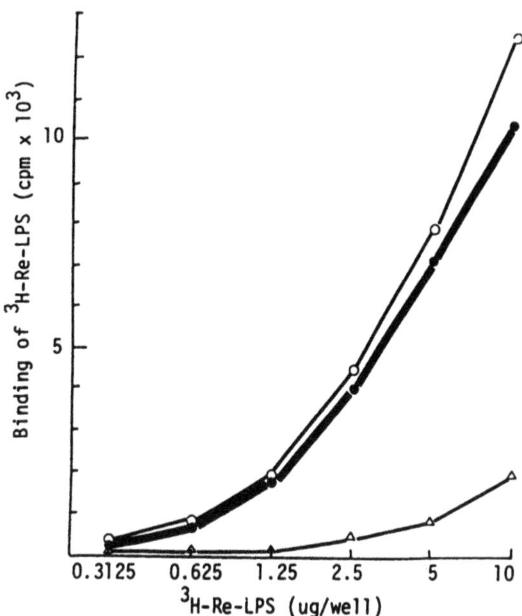

Fig 2. Binding of ^{3}H-Re-LPS to macrophages as a function of ^{3}H-Re-LPS concentration. PRM (5 x 10^{5} cells/well) were incubated at 4° C for 5 hr with increasing amounts of labeled Re-LPS in the absence (O) or presence (Δ) of unlabeled Re-LPS (500 μg/well). (●) represent the specific binding of ^{3}H-Re-LPS to PRM.

cell number. Kinetic study showed that specific binding reached a plateau after 5 hr at 4° C.

To investigate the specificity of ^{3}H-Re-LPS binding to macrophages, we examined the ability of various agents to compete in this binding assay. Unlabeled LPS competed for binding in a dose response manner. The same level of inhibition was obtained with synthetic lipid A as shown in Fig 3. However LPS from **E. coli** 0111:B4 appeared to be a far less efficient competitor than Re-LPS or lipid A: it takes about 20-fold higher concentrations to reach the same level of inhibition shown by Re-LPS or lipid A. These results suggest that the lipid A moiety is important for the binding of LPS to macrophages.

Macrophages pretreated with pronase not only lost their ability to bind ^{3}H-Re-LPS but also failed to produce TNF by LPS stimulation (Table 3). When pronase-treated macrophages were incubated with medium at 37° C for 16 hr, the cells restored the ability to bind ^{3}H-Re-LPS and produced TNF by LPS stimulation as shown in Table 3.

Effects of Dibutyryl cAMP or Indomethacin on the Activation of Macrophages by LPS

P-PEM were incubated with various concentrations of LPS and dibutyryl cAMP for 18 hr and then tested for cytotoxic activity. As shown in Fig 4, P-PEM incubated with LPS developed cytotoxicity for EL4 cells, depending upon the concentration of LPS. P-PEM incubated with dibutyryl cAMP alone did not evoke cytotoxicity. However P-PEM incubated with LPS plus dibutyryl cAMP induced enhanced cytotoxicity. By contrast, if indomethacin at a concentration of 5 x 10^{-5} M was added to the activation phase, cytotoxic activity was nearly completely abolished as shown in Fig 4. We tested the dibutyryl cAMP

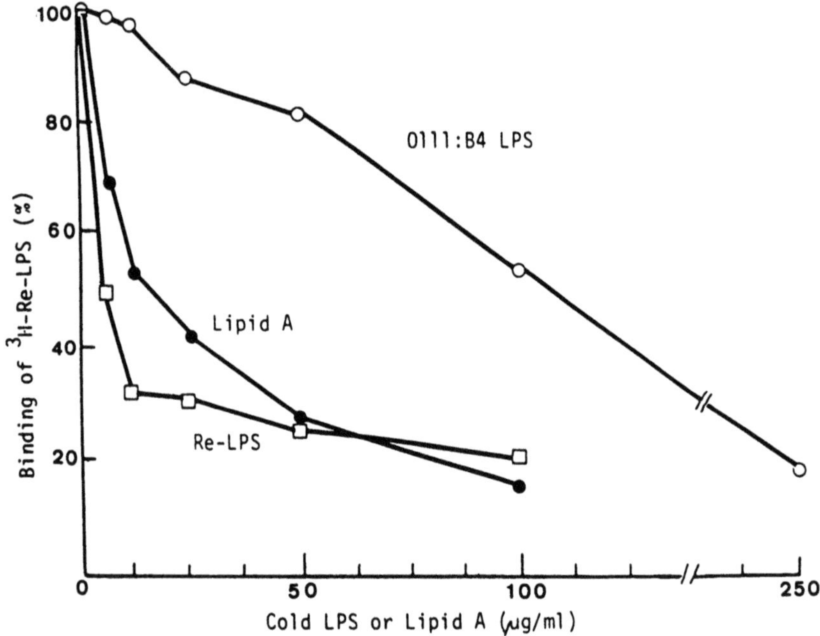

Fig 3. Inhibition of binding of ^{3}H-Re-LPS to macrophages by unlabeled Re-LPS, synthetic lipid A and LPS from E. coli 0111:B4. PRM (5 x 10^5 cells/well) were incubated with ^{3}H-Re-LPS (2.5 µg/well) plus various concentrations of unlabeled Re-LPS (□), synthetic lipid A (●) or LPS from E. coli 0111:B4 (O) at 4° C for 5 hr. Data was expressed as a percentage of the binding measured in the absence of added unlabeled LPS.

Table 3. Effects of Pronase Treatment on the LPS Binding and TNF Production of Macrophages

Macrophages[1]	TNF production[2] LPS (ng/ml)				Binding of[3] ^{3}H-Re-LPS (cpm)
	0	1	10	100	
Untreated	< 10	< 10	37	198	3804 (100%)
Pronase treated	< 10	< 10	< 10	< 10	810 (21.3%)
Pronase treated (16 hr before)	< 10	< 10	1	73	3035 (79.8)

[1]Brewer's thioglycollate medium induced PEM (5 x 10^5/well) were treated with pronase (2 mg/ml) for 60 min just before or 16 hr before the addition of LPS.

[2]The cells were washed, incubated with LPS for 5 hr, and the culture supernatants were harvested for the assay of TNF production.

[3]Macrophages were incubated with 200 µl of ^{3}H-Re-LPS (12.5 µg/ml) for 5 hr at 4° C. The data have been corrected for nonspecific binding (total counts minus number of counts bound to PEM in the presence of a large excess [200 µg/well] of unlabeled LPS).

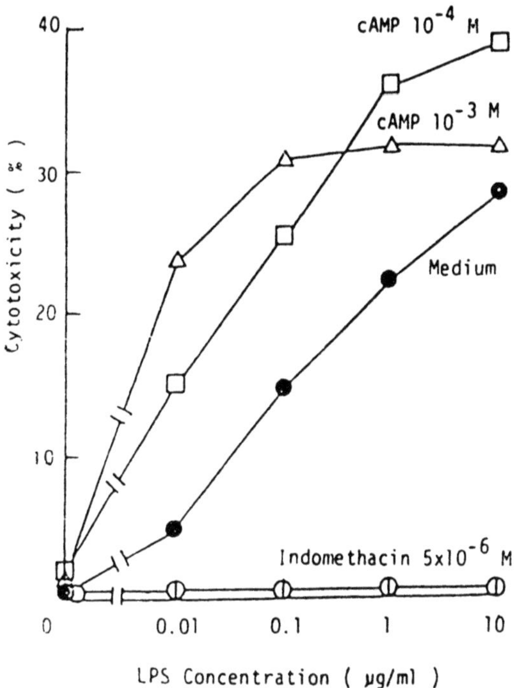

Fig 4. Effects of indomethacin and dibutyryl cAMP on the activation of tumor cytotoxicity by macrophages. Peptone induced PEM were incubated with various concentrations of LPS in the presence (△□) or absence (●) of dibutyryl cAMP or indomethacin (O) for 18 hr. The cells were washed and then assayed for their cytotoxicity against ^{51}Cr labeled EL4 cells.

for the ability to reverse the inhibition by indomethacin. As shown in Fig 5, addition of dibutyryl cAMP resulted in significant restoration of cytotoxic activity.

We examined the intracellular levels of cAMP in macrophages stimulated with LPS. Intracellular level of cAMP of P-PEM incubated with LPS (10 μg/ml) increased 2 to 3 times within 30 min, while that of P-PEM incubated with medium alone did not change significantly (data not shown). These results suggest that increase of intracellular level of cAMP which is caused by PGE_2 produced by LPS is important for the activation for cytotoxicity of macrophages.

Effects of Pertussis Toxin on the Activation of Macrophages by LPS

As described above, increase of intracellular level of cAMP augment the induction of cytotoxicity of macrophages stimulated with LPS, we examined the effects of PT which is known to inactivate Gi of adenylate cyclase and increase the intracellular level of cAMP on the activation of macrophages by LPS. P-PEM were incubated with various concentrations of PT for 4 hr and then stimulated with LPS for an additional 18 hr. Pretreatment of macrophages with PT significantly augmented the cytotoxicity as shown in Fig 6. PT pretreated P-PEM produced increased amount of TNF by stimulation with LPS as shown in Fig 7. However addition of dibutyryl cAMP inhibited the production of TNF by P-PEM stimulated with LPS (Table 4). These results suggest that PT, apart from its actions on Gi, also modifies other G proteins involved in the activation cascade of macrophages stimulated by LPS.

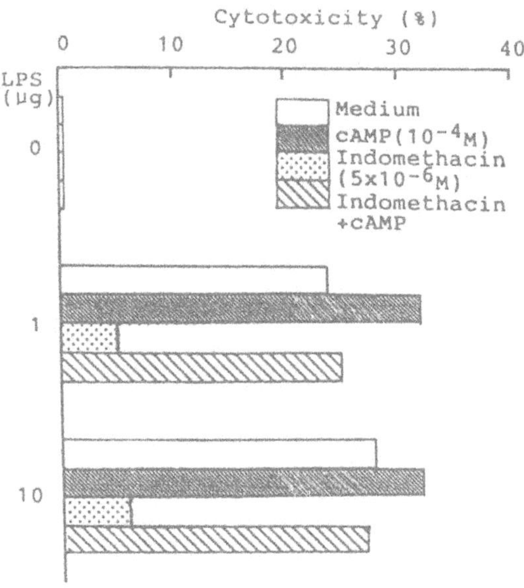

Fig 5. Effect of dibutyryl cAMP on the inhibition of LPS mediated tumor cytotoxicity of macrophages by indomethacin. P-PEM were incubated with LPS in the presence of indomethacin (5×10^{-5} M) and dibutyryl cAMP (10^{-4} M) for 18 hr. The cells were washed and then assayed for cytotoxicity against ^{51}Cr labeled EL4 cells.

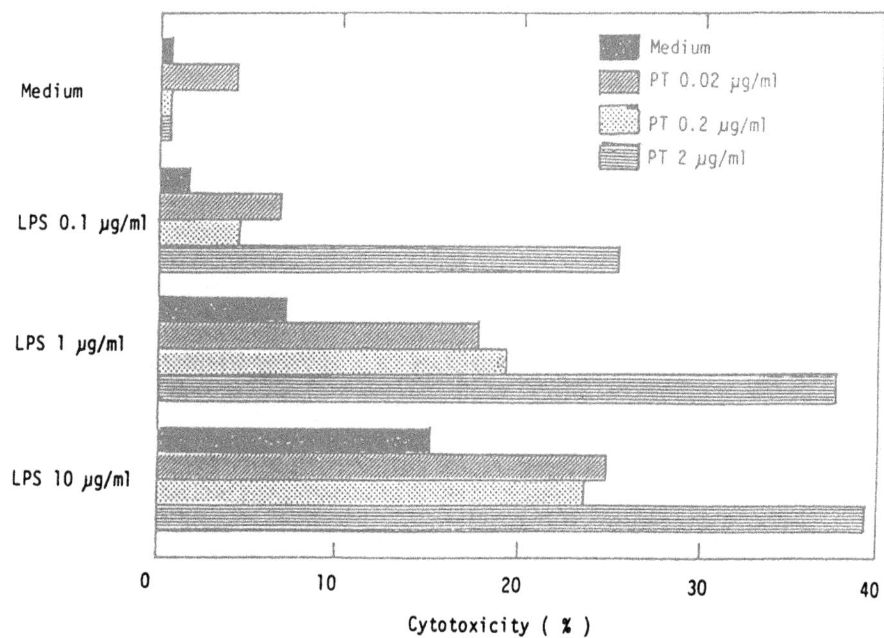

Fig 6. Effect of pertussis toxin on the activation for tumor cytotoxicity of macrophages by LPS. P-PEM induced PEM were incubated with various concentrations of PT for 4 hr. The cells were washed and then incubated with various concentrations of LPS for 18 hr. The cells were washed again and assayed for their cytotoxicity against ^{51}Cr labeled EL4 cells.

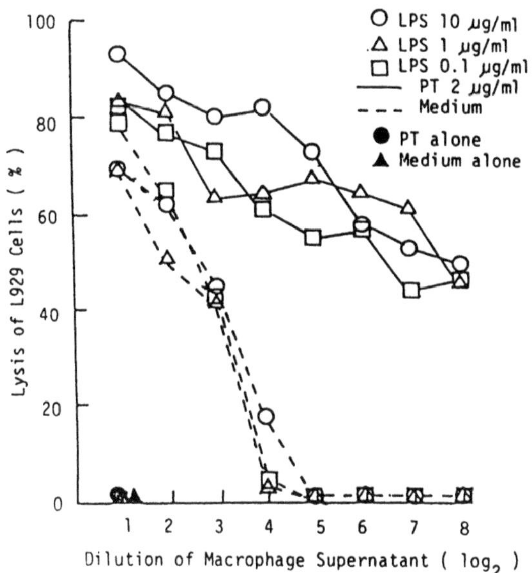

Fig 7. Effect of PT on TNF production by macrophages stimulated with LPS. P-PEM were incubated with PT for 4 hr. The cells were washed and then incubated with LPS for 16 hr. The supernatants were obtained for the assay of TNF.

DISCUSSION

Our data presented here suggest the existence of LPS binding site(s) on the surface of macrophages. The binding site(s) may be protein or glycoprotein. Because macrophages treated with pronase lost the ability to bind LPS. Unlabeled synthetic lipid A and Re-LPS showed the same level of inhibition in the binding assay using ^{3}H-Re-LPS, while LPS from **E. coli** 0111:B4 showed a far less efficient inhibition. Therefore the binding site(s) may recognize lipid A portion of LPS.

AM did not bind LPS and did not respond to LPS. However after treatment of AM with IFN-γ, the cells expressed the binding site(s) and became responsive to LPS. Moreover, pronase-treated PM not only lost their LPS binding site(s), but also failed to respond to LPS. However pronase-treated PM expressed LPS binding site(s) again after the incubation with medium for 16 hr and the cells became sensitive to LPS. Thus the expression of the binding site(s) on the surface of macrophages correlates with the responsibility of the cells to LPS.

Our observations suggest that CSF also affect the expression of LPS binding site(s) of macrophages (5). We have shown that AM and PM proliferate and generate colonies after exposure to CSF-1 or GM-CSF. More than 90% of the cells in the colonies formed by AM incubated with GM-CSF expressed asialo GM1 but not LPS binding site(s). However more than 90% of the cells formed by AM incubated with CSF-1 expressed LPS binding site(s) but not asialo GM1. On the other hand, more than 90% of the cells in the colonies formed by PM incubated with GM-CSF or CSF-1 expressed LPS binding site(s) but not asialo GM1. These results suggest that expression of LPS binding site(s) on the surface of macrophages is regulated by the state of differentiation of the cells.

The mechanism of activation of macrophages by LPS is not yet clear. In the present study, we have shown that LPS induces the elevation of intra-

Table 4. Inhibition of TNF Production by Dibutyryl cAMP in Macrophages Stimulated with LPS

Macrophages	TNF Production (U/5 x 10^5 cells)			
	LPS (μg/ml)			
treated with	0	0.1	1	10
Medium	<10	46	65	85
Dibutyryl cAMP				
10^{-3} M	<10	<10	<10	<10
10^{-4} M	<10	<10	<10	<10
10^{-5} M	<10	30	30	37

Peptone induced PEM were incubated with various concentrations of LPS or medium alone in the presence or absence of dibutyryl cAMP for 16 hr. TNF activity of the supernatants was measured as described in Materials and Methods.

cellular level of cAMP through the production of PGE_2, and this pathway is required for the activation for cytotoxicity of macrophages by LPS. This conclusion is based on the following findings. Addition of dibutyryl cAMP during the activation phase of macrophages by LPS augmented the cytotoxicity. Indomethacin inhibited the cytotoxicity and dibutyryl cAMP restored the cytotoxicity of the indomethacin-inhibited macrophages. LPS induced the elevation of cAMP level of macrophages within 30 min. Our results are consistent with those of earlier study (7). In that study, indomethacin inhibited the activation for cytotoxicity of starch induced PEM by LPS and PGE_2 restored the inhibition. Our findings are different from those of another earlier study (15). In that study indomethacin augmented and PGE_2 inhibited the cytotoxicity of PRM by LPS. The reason for the discrepancies among these studies can be attributed to differences in the assay system used; the source of the macrophages, the target cell type, and the time course of the assay, particularly with respect to the addition of LPS and drugs. In this point, we found that dibutyryl cAMP and indomethacin had a negative and positive effects, respectively, on the cytotoxicity, if these drugs were added during the effector phase of cytotoxicity of LPS-activated macrophages.

As the dibutyryl cAMP alone was not sufficient to activate cytotoxicity of macrophages, LPS may induce other signaling pathway which is also necessary for the activation for cytotoxicity. Several studies indicate some of the effects of LPS on macrophages and B cells may be mediated by hydrolysis of PIP2 (13, 14), translocation of protein kinase C (6) and activation of protein kinase C (16). Studies to clarify the relationship between those observations and ours are underway.

We have shown that PT, which affect several members of the G protein family of signaling components, augmented the activation for cytotoxicity and TNF production of macrophages stimulated with LPS. As stated above, increase of intracellular level of cAMP augmented the activation for cytotoxicity. Therefore the effects of PT on cytotoxicity may depend on the inhibition of Gi protein coupled to adenylate cyclase. However it is unlikely that the effects of PT on the response of macrophages to LPS are simply due to the inhibition of Gi protein. That is, addition of dibutyryl cAMP inhibited the production of TNF by LPS stimulation. Taken together, these observations suggest that PT, apart from its action on Gi, also modifies other G proteins involved in the activation cascade stimulated by LPS. Our data are different from those of earlier study (9). In that study, PT inhibited the biological responses induced by LPS. The reason for the discrepancies may depend on the differences in the assay system and the cell type used.

ACKNOWLEDGMENTS

This work was supported in part by a grant for cancer research from the Ministry of Education, Science and Culture of Japan and a grant from Japan Health Sciences Foundation.

REFERENCES

1. Akagawa, K. S., Kamoshita, K., Onodera, S., and Tokunaga, T., 1987, Restoration of lipopolysaccharide-mediated cytotoxic macrophage induction in C3H/HeJ mice by interferon- γ or a calcium ionophore. Jpn. J. Cancer Res. (Gann) 78: 279.

2. Akagawa, K.S., Kamoshita, K., and Tokunaga, T., 1988, Effects of granulocyte-macrophage colony-stimulating factor and colony-stimulating factor-1 on the proliferation and differentiation of murine alveolar macrophages. J. Immunol. 141: 3383.

3. Akagawa, K. S., Maruyama, Y., Takano, M., Kasai, M., and Tokunaga, T., 1981, A cell surface antigen expressed on mouse lung macrophages. Microbiol. Immunol. 25: 1215.

4. Akagawa, K. S., and Tokunaga, T., 1982, Appearance of a cell surface antigen associated with the activation of peritoneal macrophages in mice. Microbiol. Immunol. 26: 831.

5. Akagawa, K. S., and Tokunaga, T., 1985, Lack of binding of bacterial lipopolysaccharide to mouse lung macrophages and restoration of binding by interferon. J. Exp. Med. 162: 1444.

6. Chen, Z. Z., Coggeshall, K. M., and Cambier, J. C., 1986, Translocation of protein kinase C during membrane immunoglobulin-mediated transmembrane signaling in B lymphocytes. J. Immunol. 136: 2300.

7. Drysdale, B. E. and Shin, H. S., 1981, Activation of macrophages for tumor cytotoxicity: identification of indomethacin sensitive and insensitive pathways. J. Immunol. 127: 760.

8. Gregory, S., Zimmerman, D. H., and Kern, M., 1980, The lipid A moiety of lipopolysaccharide is specifically bound to B cell subpopulations of responder and nonresponder animals. J. Immunol. 125: 102.

9. Jakway, J. P, and DeFranco, A. L., 1986, Pertussis toxin inhibition of B cell and macrophage responses to bacterial lipopolysaccharide. Science 234: 743.

10. Kajigaya, S., Suda, T., Suda, J., Saito, M., Miura, Y., Iizuka, M., Kobayashi, S., Minato, N., and Sudo, T., 1986, A recombinant murine granulocyte/macrophage (GM) colony-stimulating factor derived from an inducer T cell line (IH5.5). J. Exp. Med. 164: 1102.

11. Mercurio, A. A., Schwarting, G. A., and Robbins, P. W., 1984, Glyco-

lipids of the mouse peritoneal macrophages. Alterations in amount and surface exposure of specific glycolipid species occur in response to inflammation and tumoricidal activation. J. Exp. Med. 160: 1114.

12. Nicole, H. C., Chaby, R., Cavaillon, J. M., and Szabo, L., 1982, Lipopolysaccharide receptor on rabbit peritoneal macrophages. 1. Binding characteristics. J. Immunol. 128: 1950.

13. Prpic, V., Weiel, J. E., Somers, S. D., Diguiseppi, J., Gonias, S. L., Pizzo, S. V., Hamilton, T. A., Herman, B., and Adams, D. O., 1987, Effects of bacterial lipopolysaccharide on the hydrolysis of phosphatidylinositol-4,5-bis-phosphate in murine peritoneal macrophages. J. Immunol. 139: 526.

14. Rosoff, P. M., and Cantley, L. C., 1985, Lipopolysaccharide and phorbol esters induce differentiation but have opposite effects on phosphatidylinositol turnover and Ca^{2+} mobilization in 70Z/3 pre-B lymphocytes. J. Biol. Chem. 260: 9209.

15. Taffet, S. M., and Russell, S. W., 1981, Macrophage-mediated tumor cell killing: Regulation of expression of cytolytic activity by prostaglandin E. J. Immunol. 126: 424.

16. Wightman, P. D., and Raetz, C. R. H., 1984, The activation of protein kinase C by biologically active lipid moieties of lipopolysaccharide. J. Biol. Chem. 259: 10048.

ENDOTOXIN AND KUPFFER CELLS IN LIVER DISEASE

K. Tanikawa and M. Sata

The 2nd Department of Medicine, Kurume University, School of Medicine, 830 Kurume, Japan

INTRODUCTION

Endotoxin, originating from the intestinal tract is mainly taken up by the Kupffer cell in the liver. Thus, endotoxemia is not seen in normal individuals. However, if the Kupffer cell is depressed in its function in various hepatic diseases, endotoxin appears in the general circulation causing various symptoms, signs and other clinical states seen in liver diseases. Clinical management for endotoxemia has become extremely important because endotoxin has various biological activities, some of which cause fatal outcome. In addition, almost all kinds of experimental liver injuries are more or less associated with endotoxemia (3). Therefore, endotoxin has been an important subject to study, especially by hepatologists. In this presentation, endotoxemia often seen in acute hepatitis type A, alcoholic hepatitis and cholestasis was studied in association with Kupffer cell function in regard to elucidation of the causes of various clinical manifestations occurring in hepatic diseases.

MATERIALS AND METHODS

Acute Hepatitis Type A

Biopsy specimens, taken from patients with acute hepatitis type A in the acute phase, were examined by electron microscope with special attention to the changes in Kupffer cells. Detection of HAV particles was carried out by immunoperoxidase technique using anti-HAV antibody.

The incidence of endotoxemia was examined by the Limulus lysate test in acute viral hepatitis including type A. Circulating immune complexes of IgM, IgA and IgG classes in the serum were measured by the Raji cell assay in acute viral hepatitis including type A. IgM-anti Lipid A antibody and IgM-anti HAV antibody levels in the serum were assayed by ELISA tests in acute hepatitis type A. Total counts of fecal microflora were studied in the stool taken from patients with acute viral hepatitis including type A.

Alcoholic Hepatitis

The incidence of endotoxemia was examined by the Limulus lysate test in alcoholic hepatitis. Hepatic uptake of ^{99m}Tc colloids was studied by liver scanning in alcoholic hepatitis. Clearance of CSFe particles in the general circulation was determined in controls and alcoholic individuals. Cultured Kupffer cells taken from rats and fed Lieber's liquid diet (36% of total calorie as alcohol for 6 wk) were used for endocytosis studies in which particles of various sizes were tested. In addition, Fc receptors on the cell surface of the cultured Kupffer cells were examined by using peroxidase-anti peroxidase Ig. Furthermore, uptake of endotoxin into the cultured Kupffer cell was also studied. Dimeric and monomeric IgA were measured by HPLC and IgA class anti-lipid A antibody levels were assayed by ELISA in alcoholics and patients with alcoholic liver injuries, and IgA containing cells in the colonic mucosa demonstrated by immunohistochemistry were counted.

Cholestasis

Biopsy specimens taken from cholestatic patients were examined by electron microscope with special attention to changes in Kupffer cells. Clearance studies of CSFe particles in the general circulation were performed in patients with obstructive jaundice. Cultured Kupffer cells taken from rats a week after ligation of the common bile duct were studied for endocytosis activities. In addition, effects of various bile acids on the endocytosis of these cells were also examined.

RESULTS AND DISCUSSION

Acute Hepatitis Type A

Acute hepatitis type A is clinically characterized by high fever (over 38°C) at onset, occasional occurrence of extrahepatic manifestations such as renal failure, and a high level of IgM in comparison with other types of acute viral hepatitis. However, it has not been clear why type A has such characteristic clinical features. Biopsy specimens taken from patients with type A in the acute phase show a remarkable mononuclear cell infiltration in the portal tract and prominent changes of hepatocytes and Kupffer cells in the periportal area of the lobule (1). Immunoperoxidase study revealed HAV to be preferentially found in hepatocytes and Kupffer cells in the periportal area. Under the electron microscope the Kupffer cell appeared to be remarkably enlarged with distorted organelles, flattened cell membrane without pseudopodia and full of electron dense lipofuscin-like lysosomes containing numerous HAV particles (Fig 1). These fine structural features suggest dysfunction of Kupffer cells in the acute phase of hepatitis type A (4).

Endotoxin was positive by Limulus lysate test in 71% of hepatitis type A, 18% of type NANB and no endotoxemia was found in type B in the acute phase (Table 1). Endotoxin has been known as a pyrogenic factor and thus endotoxin seen in the serum at the acute phase seems to be spilled over into the general circulation due to dysfunction of Kupffer cells. The pyrogenic factor release from Kupffer cells stimulated by HAV before dysfunction of these cells may be another explanation for high fever at onset.

Circulating immune complexes are more frequently detected and higher in titer in the acute phase of hepatitis type A in comparison with other types of acute viral hepatitis (Fig 2). Since immune complexes are also mainly taken up by the Kupffer cell, such high incidence of immune complexes in the circulation correlates with dysfunction of the Kupffer cell in type A and occasionally extrahepatic manifestations such as renal failure. This is partly explained by the high incidence of immune complexes in the general circulation. High titers of serum IgM are one of the characteristic laboratory findings in hepatitis type A as well as primary biliary cirrhosis. Miller et al., (2) reported an increase in IgM class antibody against gut bacteria. We have studied the changes of total serum IgM, IgM class anti-LPS antibody and IgM class anti HAV-antibody levels. Total IgM levels correlated

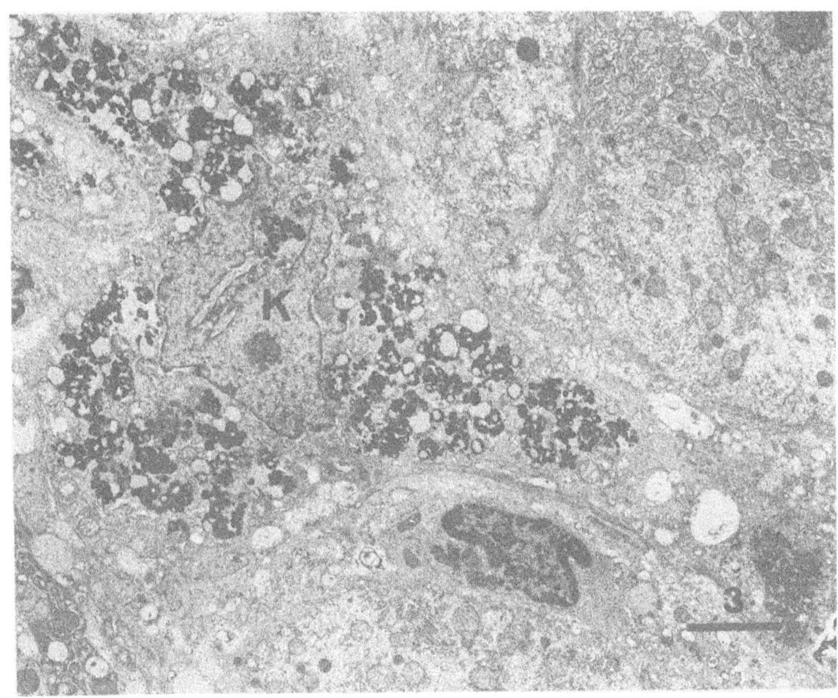

Fig 1. Electron micrograph of a Kupffer cell in acute hepatitis type A. The Kupffer cell appears to be markedly enlarged with numerous electron dense materials and distorted organelles.

Table 1. Incidence of endotoxemia in acute viral hepatitis. Endotoxemia is seen highly in hepatitis Type A.

Type	No.of Pt.	Clinical day after onset < 14 days	> 14 days
A	7	5 (71.4%)	0
B	8	0	0
NANB	11	2 (18.0%)	0

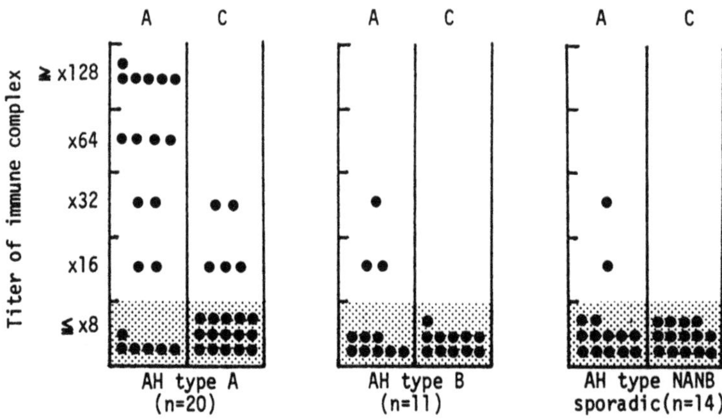

Fig 2. IgM-immune complex in three types of acute viral hepatitis by Raji cell assay. A = acute phase; C = convalescent phase

well with those of IgM class anti-LPS in the clinical course, but not with IgM class anti-HAV antibody levels (Fig 3). IgM class anti-LPS antibody levels were also significantly higher in hepatitis type A, compared to type B. In addition, studies on fecal microflora showed no increase in any type of acute viral hepatitis. These results indicate that intestinal factors such as endotoxin spill over to the general circulation are important in the production of IgM.

Summarizing these data, characteristic clinical features seen in acute hepatitis type A are related to transient dysfunction of Kupffer cells, resulting in endotoxemia. In addition, it can be speculated that endotoxemia in the acute phase is associated with pathogenesis of hepatocyte damage by hepatitis type A virus.

Alcoholic Hepatitis

Alcoholic hepatitis, especially its severe form, is clinically characterized by fever, granulocytosis and multiple organ failure such as renal failure, and concomitant infection. The clinical features suggest a defect in defense mechanisms, such as dysfunction of Kupffer cells. In fact, our studies showed that endotoxin is detected in serum by the Limulus lysate test in 21% of alcoholic hepatitis cases and endotoxemia was seen in all 7 severe cases examined (Table 2).

Clearance study of CSFe particles in the general circulation showed a remarkable delay in alcoholics in comparison with controls (Fig 4), indicating depressed endocytosis by Kupffer cells. Indeed, ^{99m}Tc-liver scanning showed a marked decrease in uptake into Kupffer cells in alcoholic hepatitis. An experimental study was made using cultured Kupffer cells to clarify the effect of alcohol on endocytosis of Kupffer cells. Cultured Kupffer cells isolated from rats fed a liquid diet for 6 weeks were found to have flattened cell membranes without pseudopodia, swollen mitochondria and decreased amounts of microtubules in the cytoplasm (Fig 5). In addition, Fc receptors were found to be remarkably decreased in number (Fig 6).

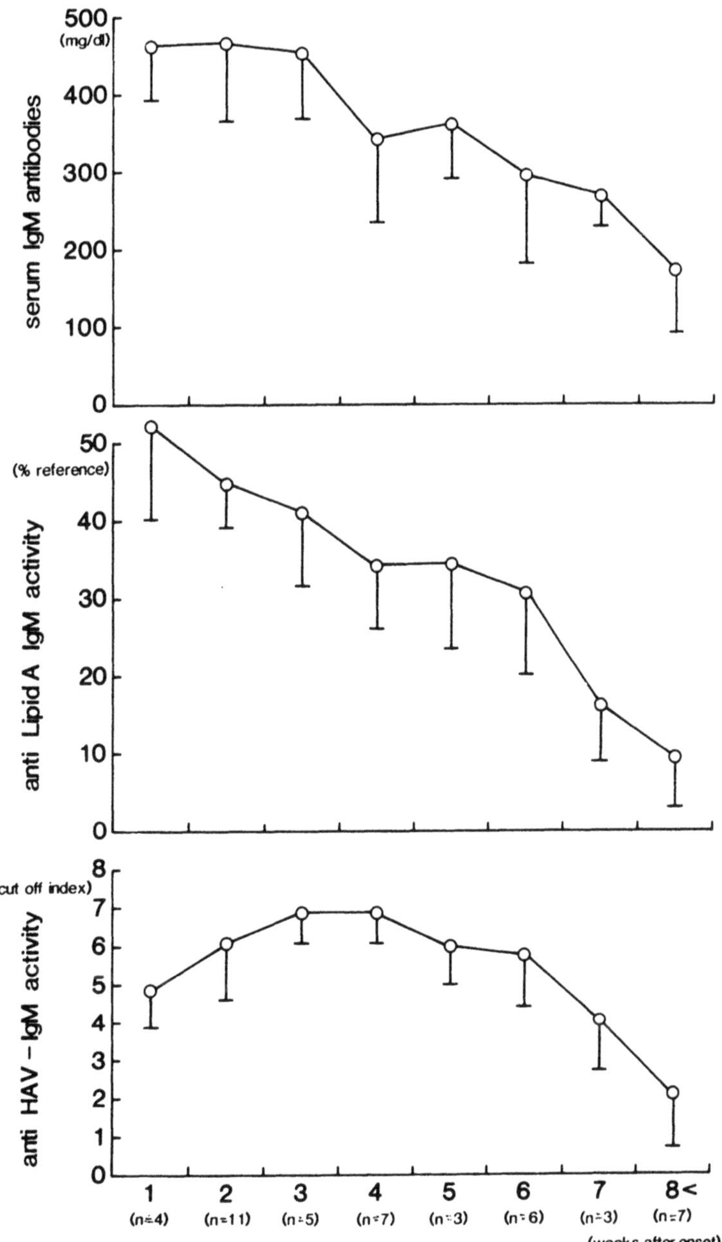

Fig 3. Time course of serum IgM antibodies, anti-Lipid A - IgM activity and anti-HAV - IgM activity in patients with acute hepatitis A. Serum IgM, anti-Lipid-IgM and anti-HAV-IgM in the clinical course of acute hepatitis type A. Titers of serum IgM are shown to be well correlated with those of anti Lipid A-IgM.

Table 2. Endotoxemia is often observed in alcoholic hepatitis, especially its severe cases.

Incidence of endotoxemia in SAH and AH

Et	++	+	±	-	rate of endotoxemia
SAH	2	5	0	0	7/7 (100%)
AH	0	1	3	15	4/19 (21.0%)

SAH = severe alcoholic hepatitis
AH = alcoholic hepatitis

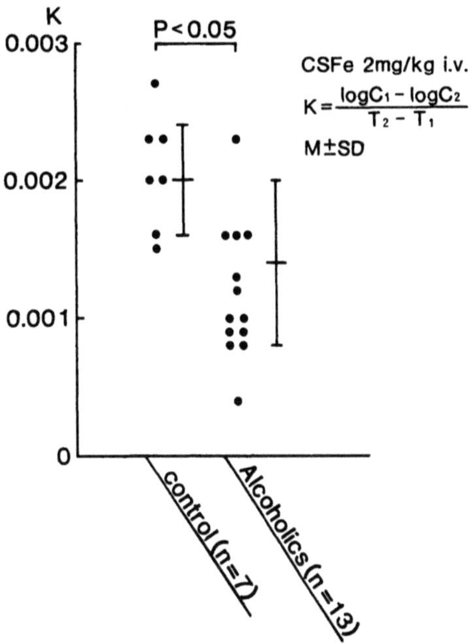

Fig 4. CSFe clearance in the general circulation shows to be markedly delayed in alcoholics.

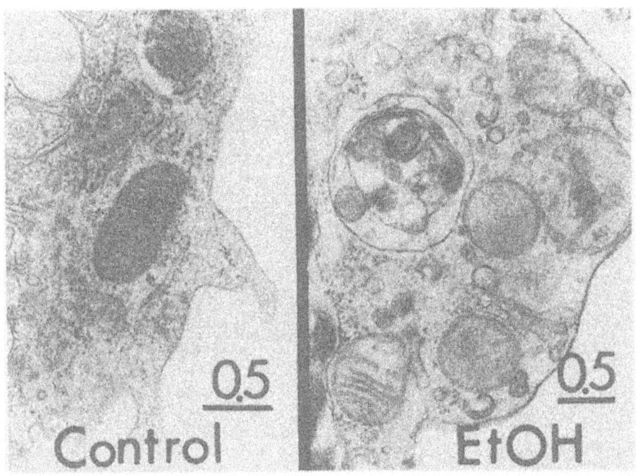

Fig 5. Electron micrograph of a cultured Kupffer cell (right), taken from the rat, fed Lieber's liquid diet for 6 wk, shows to have distorted organelles.

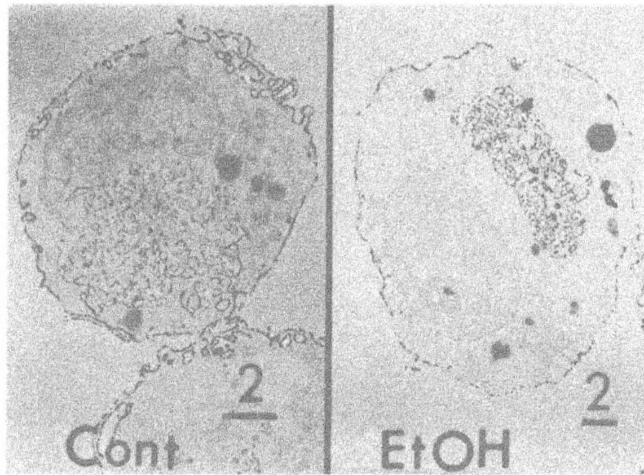

Fig 6. Electron micrograph of a cultured Kupffer cell (right), taken from the rat, fed Lieber's liquid diet for 6 wk, shows a decreased number of Fc receptors on the cell membrane.

Marked depression in endocytosis was also noted in cultured Kupffer cells taken from chronic alcohol fed rats (Figs 7, 8). In addition, uptake of endotoxin in the medium into the cultured Kupffer cell was also found reduced (Fig 9). The clinical and experimental studies indicate that depressive effects of alcohol on Kupffer cell are evident and such depressed functions are characteristic in alcoholics and alcoholic liver injuries. Thus a high incidence of endotoxemia in alcoholic liver injuries could be explained by alcohol induced Kupffer cell dysfunction.

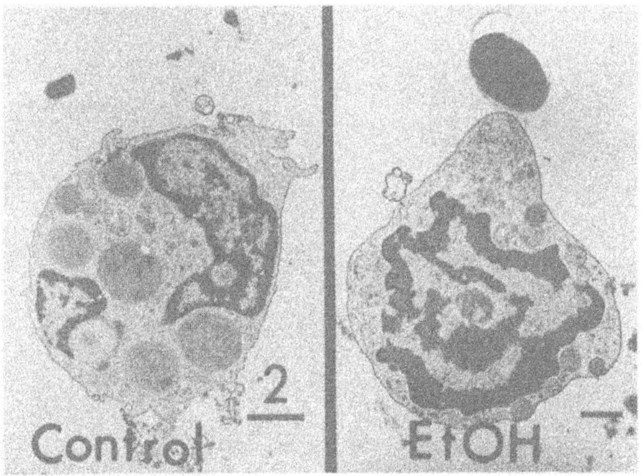

Fig 7. Electron micrograph of a cultured Kupffer cell (right), taken from the rat, fed Lieber's liquid diet for 6 wks. No latex particles in the medium are taken up into the cell comparing with the control (left).

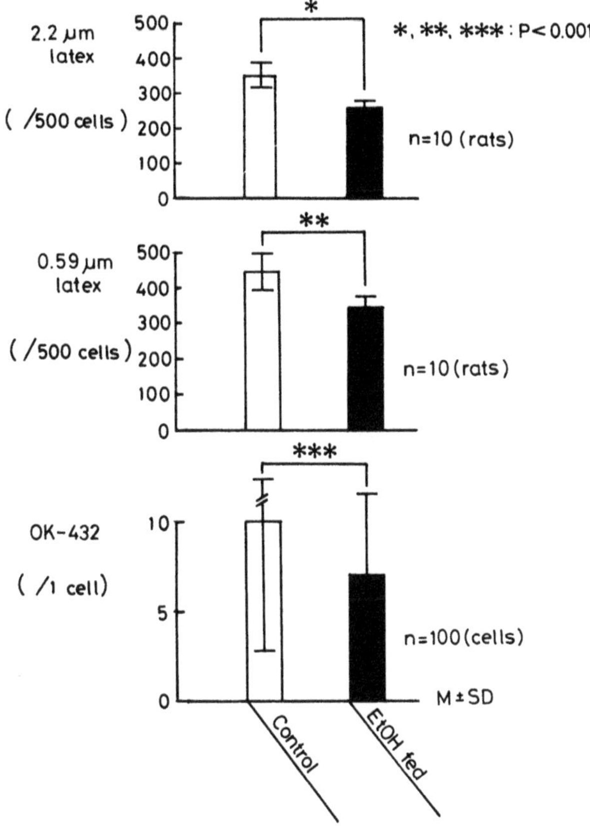

Fig 8. Effect of chronic ethanol feeding on endocytosis of particles of various sizes into the cultured Kupffer cells, taken from rats, fed Lieber's liquid diet for 6 wk. The endocytosis shows to be significantly depressed.

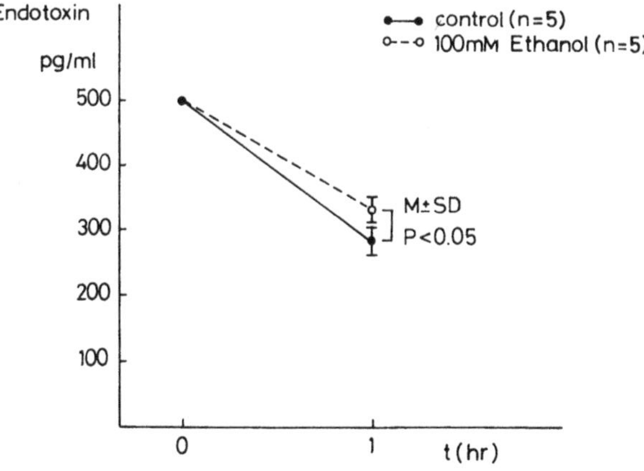

Fig 9. The effect of ethanol on the clearance of endotoxin by cultured Kupffer cells (n = 5)
Uptake of endotoxin into the cultured Kupffer cells in the medium containing 100 mM ethanol reveals to be significantly depressed.

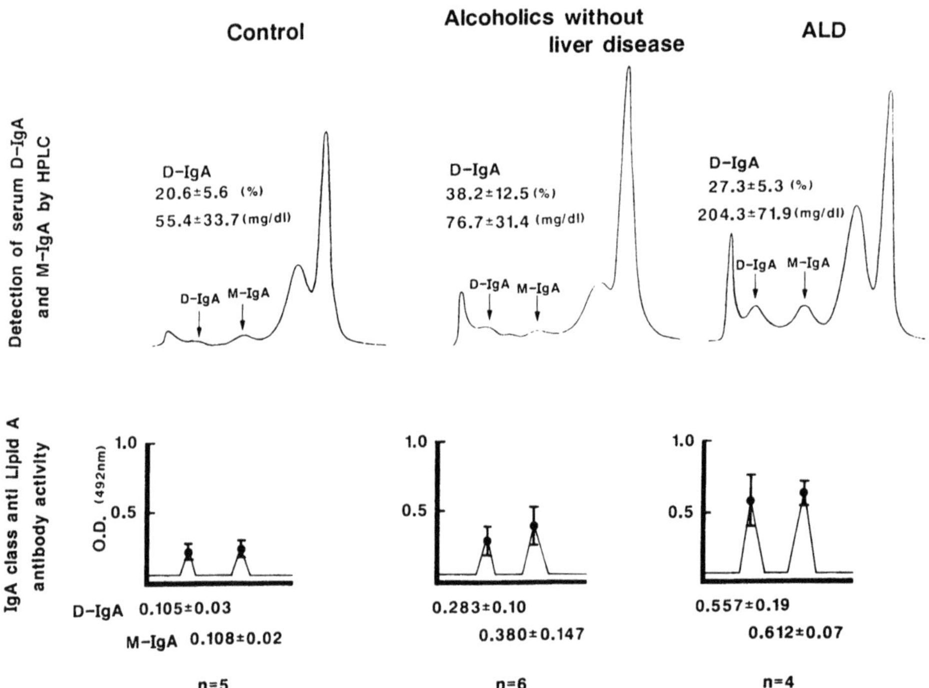

Fig 10. Correlation of the Dimeric IgA, Monomeric IgA and IgA class anti Lipid A antibody activity of the alcoholics and alcoholic liver disease.
Dimeric IgA and IgA class anti Lipid A antibody in the serum showed to be increased in alcoholics and patients with alcoholic liver injuries.

It has been reported that daily ethanol ingestion increases intestinal permeability to macromolecules in experimental animals (5). Thus, in alcoholics or alcoholic liver injuries, absorption of endotoxin into the intestinal mucosa and finally into the portal vein seems to be increased. This could promote higher incidence of endotoxemia in alcoholic liver injuries with depressed function of Kupffer cells.

Dimeric IgA level in the serum was shown to be increased in both alcoholics and patients with alcoholic liver injuries by HPLC and a marked increase in IgA class anti-Lipid A antibody levels was also noted (Fig 10). Immunohistological examination revealed a remarkable increase in number of the IgA containing cell in the colonic mucosa of alcoholic liver injuries (Fig 11).

Titers of total IgA, dimeric IgA and IgA class anti-LPS antibody in the serum were decreased gradually after abstinence (Fig 12). Since dimeric IgA is produced mainly in the plasma cell located in the intestinal mucosa, an increase in serum dimeric IgA and IgA containing cells in the colonic mucosa indicates an increased production of dimeric IgA in the intestinal mucosa in alcoholic liver injuries. The increase in IgA class anti-LPS antibody in the serum suggests that endotoxin taken up into the intestinal mucosa is one of the factors in stimulating production of dimeric IgA. Both depressed Kupffer cell function and an increased uptake of endotoxin into the intestinal mucosa

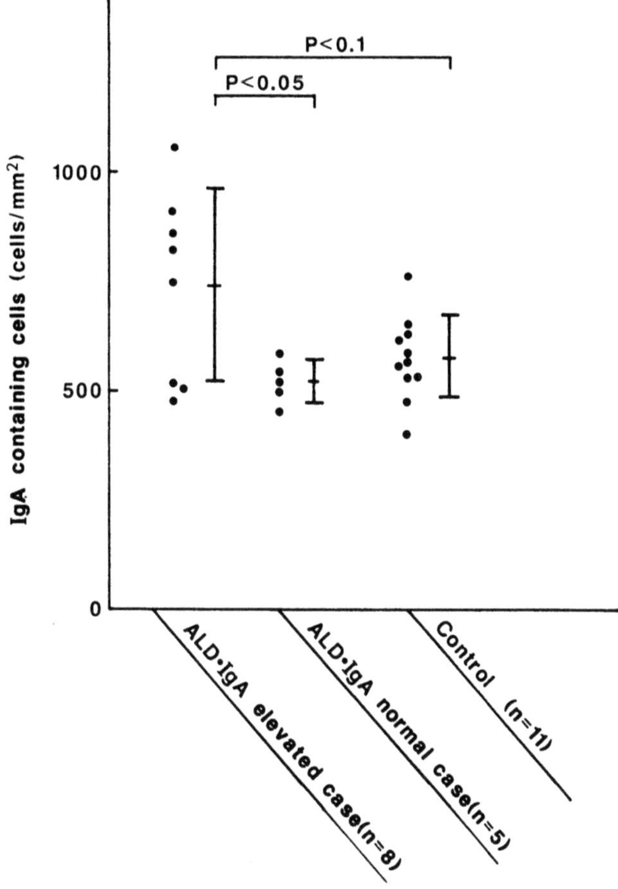

ALD : Alcoholic liver disease

Fig 11. IgA containing plasma cells in the colonic mucosa are significantly increased in number in patients with alcoholic liver disease.

would be the main explanation for the high incidence of endotoxemia in alcoholic liver injuries.

Cholestasis

In cholestasis of long duration, sepsis, shock or renal failure, all of which are frequently fatal, are occasionally seen and are accompanied by endotoxemia. The prevention of such complications is important clinically. The causes of such complications in cholestasis have partly been explained, but mostly remain unknown.

By electron microscopy, Kupffer cells were found to be markedly enlarged with flattened cell membrane without pseudopodia and contained numerous electron dense materials and distorted mitochondria in the cytoplasm (Fig 13). Those fine structural features suggest dysfunctions of the cell.

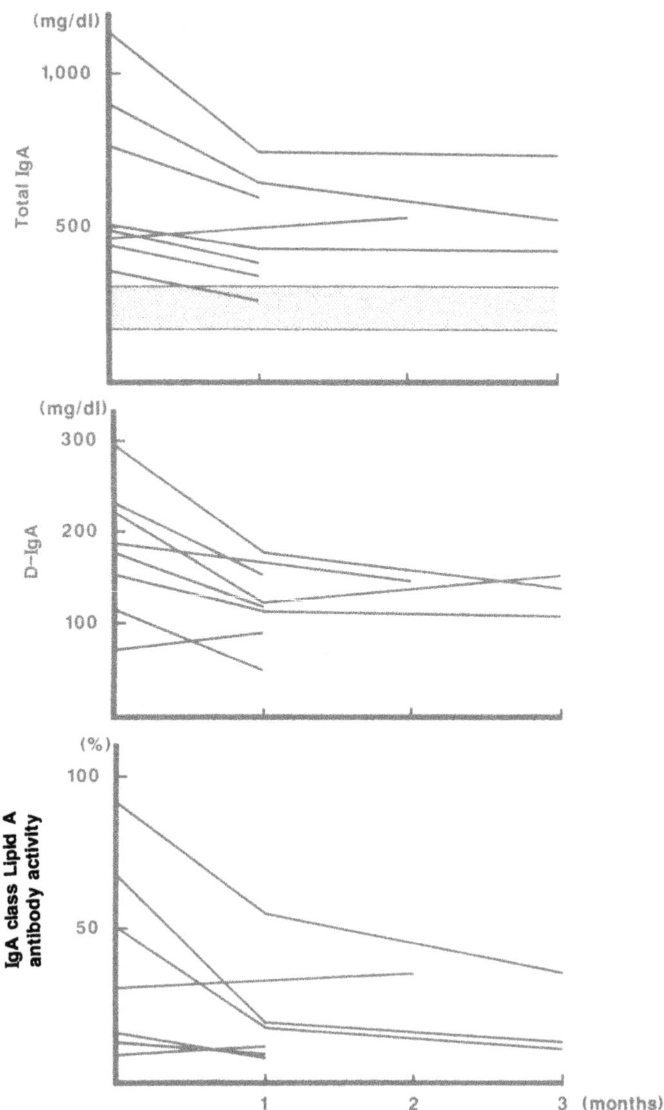

Fig 12. Changes of the total IgA, dimeric IgA and IgA class Lipid A antibody in the serum showed to be gradually decreased in patients with alcoholic liver disease after abstinence

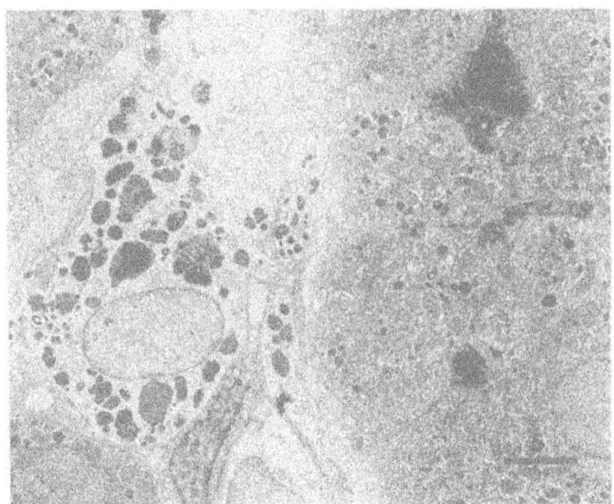

Fig 13. Electron micrograph of the Kupffer cell in obstructive jaundice.

Clearance studies of CSFe in the circulation showed a marked delay in cholestasis (Fig 14). Most colloidal particles infused intravenously are taken up into Kupffer cells. Thus, depressed endocytosis of this cell is evident. Cultured Kupffer cells taken from rats with common bile duct ligation for a week revealed marked fine structural changes (Fig 15) and also depression of endocytosis.

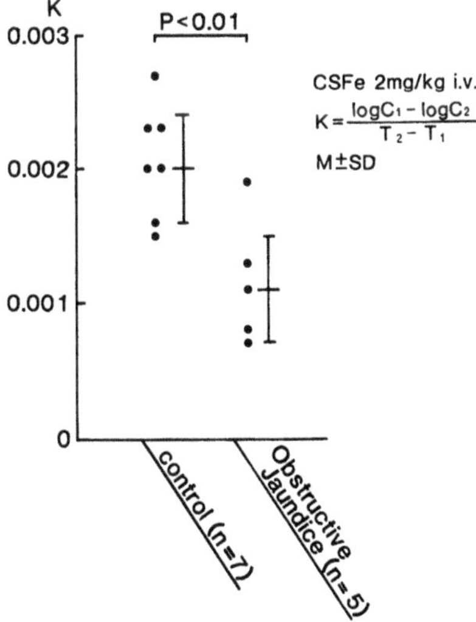

Fig 14. CSFe clearance in the general circulation showed to be significantly delayed in obstructive jaundice.

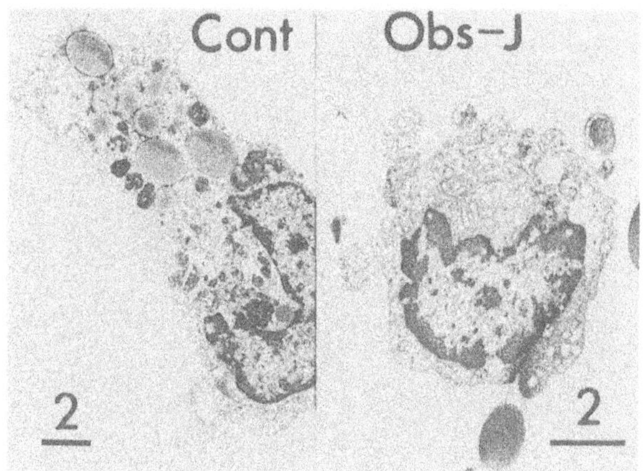

Fig 15. Electron micrograph of a cultured Kupffer cell (right), isolated from the rat with obstructive jaundice for a week. Remarkable changes are observed in the Kupffer cell which also shows no endocytotic activities comparing with the control Kupffer cell (left).

Bile acids would be the main causative factors to damage Kupffer cell function in regard to many agents stagnating in the blood in cholestasis. CDCA was found to have the most depressive effect on endocytosis of cultured Kupffer cells among various bile acids (Fig 16). Those findings suggest that Kupffer cell dysfunction is one of the most important factors for appearance of endotoxemia and serious complications in cholestasis.

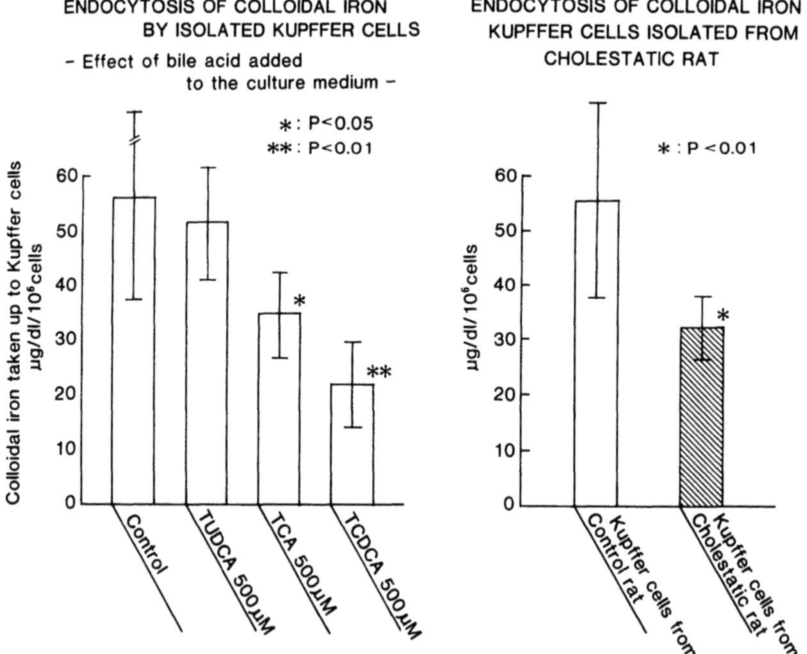

Fig 16. Endocytosis of cultured Kupffer cells taken from cholestatic rats and effects of various bile acids. CDCA showed to have the most depressive effects on the endocytosis of the Kupffer cell.

CONCLUSION

Symptoms, sign and other clinical and laboratory findings seen in acute hepatitis type A, alcoholic hepatitis and cholestasis are probably partly explained by endotoxemia due to Kupffer cell dysfunction occurring in these hepatic diseases. Because of such clinical and experimental evidences, management or prevention of depressed Kupffer cell function is important, especially in patients with these liver diseases.

REFERENCES

1. Abe, H., Beninger, P. R., Ikejiri, N., Setoyama, H., Sata, M., and Tanikawa, K., 1982, Light microscopic findings of liver biopsy specimens from patients with hepatitis A and comparison with type B. Gastroenterology 82: 938.

2. Miller, H. F. A., Legler, K., and Thomssen, R., 1983, Increase in immunoglobulin M antibodies against good bacteria during acute hepatitis A. Infect. Immun. 40: 542.

3. Nolan, J. P., and Camara, D. S., 1982, Endotoxin, sinusidal cells and liver injury, in: "Progress in liver disease Vol. VII", Popper, H. and Schaffner, F., eds., Grune & Stratton, New York.

4. Tanikawa, K., Sata, M., Setoyama H., and Abe, H., 1986, Changes of the Kupffer cell and clinical manifestations in acute hepatitis type A, in: "Cells of the hepatic sinusoid, Vol. I,", A. Kirn, D. L. Knook and E. Wisse, eds. Kupffer Cell Foundation, The Netherlands.

5. Worthington, B. S., Meserole, and Syrotuck, J. A., 1978, Effect of daily ethanol ingestion on intestinal permeability to macromolecules. Digestive Diseases 23: 23-32.

SECTION V.

HOST RESPONSES

METABOLIC FATE OF ENDOTOXIN IN RAT

M. Freudenberg and C. Galanos

Max-Planck-Institut für Immunobiologie
Freiburg, FRG

INTRODUCTION

Endotoxins (lipopolysaccharide, LPS) of gram-negative bacteria induce numerous biological activities which, depending on concentration of endotoxin and reactivity of the host may be either harmful or beneficial (for review see 12, 23). The pathophysiological effects of endotoxin drew much attention in the past and classical endotoxin activities like pyrogenicity, leucopenia or Shwartzman reaction were studied extensively. On the other hand, questions concerning the endotoxin itself, its pathway through the organism and its ultimate fate drew little attention and remained virtually unexplored. Thus for many years it was generally believed that the organism possesses mechanisms for detoxifying endotoxin (1, 3, 17-19, 22, 30-34, 36). Evidence for this, however, was never presented.

We became interested in the fate of endotoxin in the host because we believed that the knowledge of its distribution in blood and tissues, and the possible alteration in its chemical structure, as well as the route of its excretion from the body would disclose important information on its humoral and cellular targets, its possible detoxification, and the host-dependent mechanisms of its action.

The biological properties of LPS are embedded in the lipid part of the molecule, the lipid A. For this reason S- and R-form LPS and free lipid A are generally found to exhibit comparable toxic and other biological activities despite the large differences in the quality and quantity of sugars they contain (12). Lipopolysaccharides are heterogeneous mixtures of molecules, the heterogeneity being especially apparent in S-form LPS. SDS polyacrylamide gel electrophoreses revealed that S-form LPS exhibit numerous bands of different O-polysaccharide chain-length, and that they always contain variable amounts of R-form LPS (15, 28).

Consequently the biological activity of S-form preparations is the combined effect of both types of LPS. Despite the similarities in the biological behavior of S- and R-form LPS, differences do however exist. These concern, e.g., the rate at which they are cleared from the blood (2, 4, 16), their affinity for cell-membranes and their interaction with the complement system (24). For this reason the investigation on the fate of LPS **in vivo** described in this report was carried out in parallel on both types of LPS (S and R). The smooth form LPS of Salmonella abortus equi (S-LPS) and Re-form

LPS of S. minnesota R595 and of E. coli F515 (Re-LPS) were used throughout the study.

RESULTS AND DISCUSSION

Clearance

Clearance of LPS was measured using biosynthetically radiolabeled LPS preparations (4). It was found that the rate of clearance of LPS is independent of the amount injected. S- and Re-LPS in amounts of 0.05-10.0 mg in rats (5) and of 0.01-4.0 mg in mice were cleared at the same rate in both species.

The results obtained revealed that the rate of LPS clearance is dependent on its chemical and physicochemical properties. S-LPS injected intravenously into rats persisted in the circulation much longer (T1/2 = hr) than the Re-LPS (T1/2 = min) (4). For both types the rate of clearance was dependent on the state of molecular aggregation. Higher aggregation sodium salts of the S- and R-LPS were cleared faster than their respective less aggregated triethylamine salts (Fig 1) (6). In conventional LPS preparations phosphate and carboxylic groups of the LPS molecule are neutralized by a mixture of different metal cations and amines, the composition of the mixture varying from batch to batch. Therefore different batches of LPS may exhibit different clearance times. The use of uniform salt forms of LPS prepared by electrodialysis (13) in clearance studies has the advantage that more reproducible results are obtained. In the studies described here uniform salts of LPS were used.

Differences in the rate of clearance between smooth and rough LPS were also observed by others (2, 16). Therefore, in general, rough LPS, due to their chemical structure, are removed from the circulation of injected animals faster than smooth LPS. It should be noted, however, that smooth LPS preparations do not consist of chemically identical molecules. They are always mixtures of true smooth and of rough molecules, in ratios varying from preparation to preparation (15, 28). It is not known at present whether smooth and rough molecules present in the preparation are removed from the circulation at a different rate of clearance because these may be present as mixed miscelles. To study the clearance of smooth and rough molecules present in S-LPS we injected large amounts of ^{14}C-labeled S-LPS in C3H/HeJ mice (4 mg/mouse) intravenously and measured circulating LPS by radioactivity measurement and by estimation of abequose. Abequose is one of the sugars of the O-repeating unit of the S-LPS used (S. abortus equi, see Fig 1) (14) and is therefore present only in smooth-form molecules. The ^{14}C-isotope in LPS (32×10^4 cpm/mg) was incorporated into glucosamine and therefore present in smooth and rough molecules. In the original S-LPS preparation 4.05 ug abequose per 10^3 cpm was present. Two hr after injection the amount of abequose/10^3 cpm in circulating blood increased to 5.98 ug and then remained constant (followed up to 6 hr after injection) which indicated that at least in C3H/HeJ mice during first 2 hr after injection molecules lacking abequose (rough) were cleared at a higher rate than molecules containing abequose (smooth). This makes it evident that R-form LPS is cleared faster than S-form, even when the two types of LPS are present as a mixture.

Binding to HDL in Plasma

Analysis of the distribution of LPS among blood components after its i.v. injection revealed that, in rats, from the second minute onward LPS is present exclusively in plasma, with the cellular compartment of blood free of LPS. In plasma the LPS undergoes complex formation with high density lipoprotein (HDL) and circulates in this complex-form until it is cleared from the circulation (4). This was found when plasma samples of rats injected

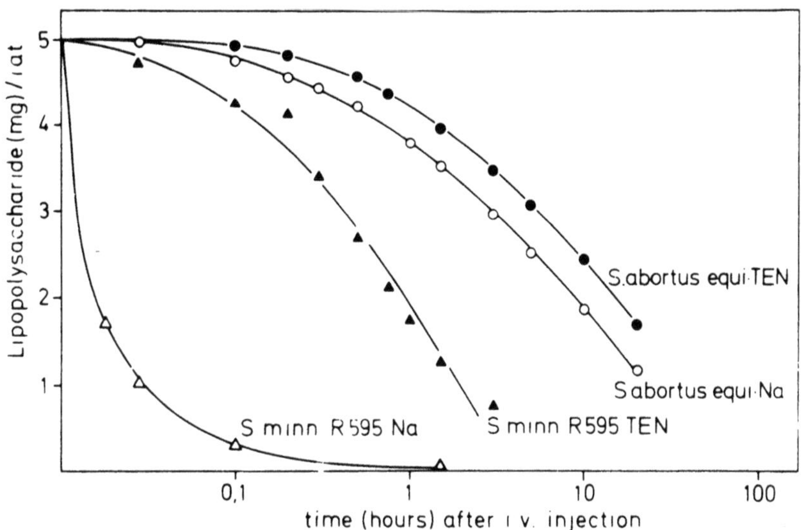

Fig 1. Blood clearance of LPS in low (triethylamine) and high (Na) molecular weight. ^{14}C uniformly labeled LPS preparations were injected in AS2 rats intravenously. At different times thereafter blood samples were collected and remaining radioactivity measured.

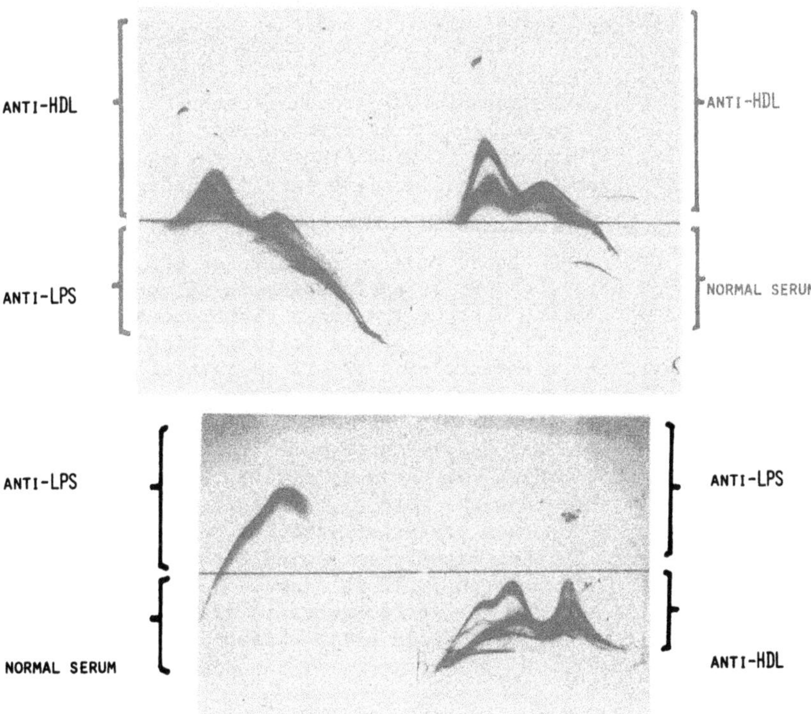

Fig 2. Cross-immunoelectrophoresis with intermediate gel of rat plasma 1 hr after intravenous injection of S-LPS (5 mg/rat) showing a co-precipitation of LPS with HDL.

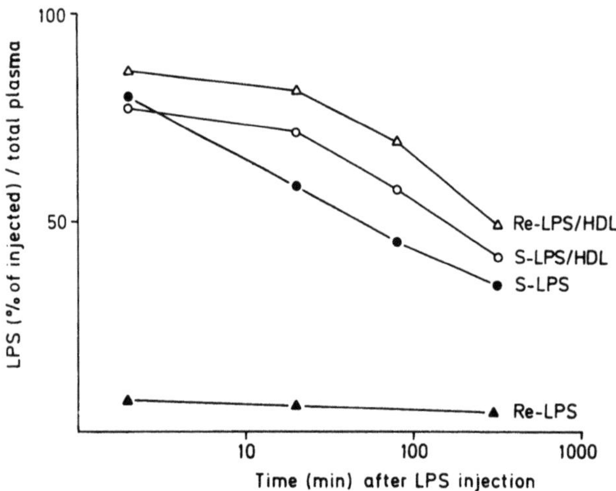

Fig 3. Blood clearance of free and HDL-pre-complexed S- and Re-^{14}C-LPS in Lewis rats. For precomplexation LPS was incubated with normal rat serum (400 μg/ml) at 37°C for 2 hr. Free LPS in 0.5 ml distilled water or HDL-bound LPS in 0.5 ml serum in a concentration of 200 μg LPS/rat were injected i.v.. At different times thereafter blood samples were collected and radioactivity measured.

with LPS were analyzed by cross immunoelectrophoresis with antisera to plasma proteins and to LPS which revealed that HDL and LPS co-precipitate (Fig 2). Using a different method Ulevitch and coworkers came to the same results (21, 35).

The binding of LPS to HDL has biological consequences. It inhibits the nonspecific binding of LPS to cells such as erythrocytes (7) and lymphocytes (own unpublished data). This makes it understandable why in the circulation blood-cells remain LPS-free, although **in vitro** in the absence of serum they readily bind LPS.

The binding of LPS to HDL leads to a retardation of LPS clearance (21) and to a lower rate of uptake of LPS by macrophages **in vitro** (6). We were therefore interested in knowing whether the large differences between the clear ance times of S- and R-form LPS may be related to their binding to HDL. For this reason we compared the clearance of free LPS to that of LPS bound to HDL by preincubation with rat serum for 2 hr/37°C **in vitro.** In rats free Re-LPS disappeared from the circulation with a half life (T1/2) of less than 2 min whereas HDL-bound Re-LPS was removed much more slowly (Fig 3). In contrast, pre-complexing of S-LPS to HDL had only a relatively weak effect on its rate of clearance. Therefore the rate of clearance of S- and R-LPS becomes very similar when they are present in complex form with HDL. The results indicate that the bulk of Re-LPS is removed from the circulation before the LPS binds to HDL, whereas S-LPS is removed mainly as a complex with HDL. They support the idea that differences in clearance times of smooth and rough LPS in general are based on the effectiveness of their binding to HDL **in vivo.**

Distribution

The content of LPS in rat organs was measured using radiolabeled LPS preparations (6, 8). The measurements showed differences in the distribution of S- and Re-LPS. Re-LPS was accumulated mainly in the liver, where the maximum LPS concentration (80% of injected radioactivity) was found 5 hr

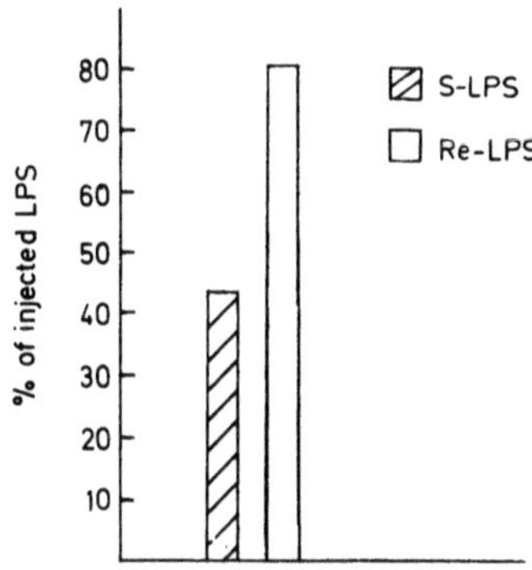

Fig 4. Amounts of LPS in the liver at the time of highest accumulation. The highest accumulation of Re-LPS in tissue was found at 5 hr, that of S-LPS on day 3 after i.v. injection and was independent of the dose of LPS.

after injection (Fig 4). The highest tissue concentration of LPS was measured in liver and spleen (Fig 5). In all other organs the LPS concentration was much lower or not detectable. The cells participating in LPS uptake were identified by immunohistochemistry (9). In the liver, the cells involved in the primary uptake of Re-LPS were sinusoidal macrophages, granulocytes and hepatocytes, in other organs macrophages and granulocytes. After injection of S-LPS, the amount of radioactivity in rat organs increased with time up to 72 hr. By this time most of the LPS (on average 43% of injected) was found in the liver (Fig 4) (8). Highest tissue concentration was measured in the spleen followed by the liver and adrenal gland (Fig 5). In other organs the S-LPS-concentration was at least 5 times lower, but in general not as low as Re-LPS. In the liver and in other organs the LPS was taken up by macrophages and granulocytes. Hepatocytes were not involved in the primary uptake of S-LPS. However, both LPS, S- and Re-, pass ultimately from sinusoidal cells

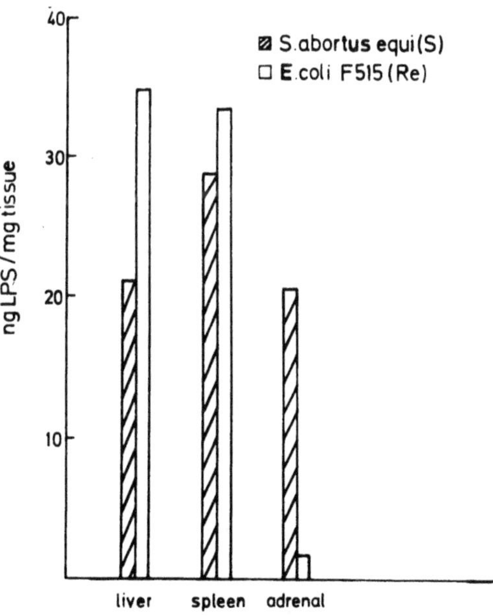

Fig 5. Concentration of tissue-bound LPS after i.v. injection (100 μg/rat) at the time of highest accumulation.

to hepatocytes (9). In experiments carried out in mice it was shown that also here only Re-LPS and not S-LPS has direct access to hepatocytes (29). In the initial period, after LPS injection autophagocytosis of LPS-positive granulocytes by liver sinusoidal cells was observed (10). It is assumed that the differences in the organ distribution between S- and Re-LPS are due at least partly to their differential binding to HDL **in vivo**. This would at least explain the difference in their uptake by the adrenal gland. It was shown earlier that HDL bound LPS in contrast to unbound LPS, is taken up by the adrenal gland via HDL receptors (21, 25). Therefore it is reasonable that S-LPS which easily binds to HDL concentrates in the adrenal gland, whereas Re-LPS, which in vivo mainly bypass this binding, do not.

Degradation

Degradation of bacterial endotoxins has often been assumed to proceed in the host organism and several mechanisms of detoxification alleged to begin in the blood stream were proposed (17-19, 22, 32, 33, 36). However, conclusive evidence for degradation and detoxification of LPS was never presented. In our experiments, no evidence for chemical detoxification or degradation of LPS in blood was found (5), not even with LPS preparations that persist in the blood for a long time. A first hint for **in vivo** alterations in the structure of LPS was obtained when the persistence of LPS in the liver and other organs was studied using two different methods of detection. These were radioactivity measurements after injection of ^{14}C uniformly radiolabeled LPS, and immunohistochemistry using antibodies directed against the radioactive LPS used (8, 9). By the former method LPS persisting in organs was detectable regardless of whether it was present in an intact or chemically altered form, whereas by the latter method the LPS was detectable only as long as its antigenic reactivity was intact. These studies showed that the detectability of S- and Re-LPS antigens in the liver was lost 5-9 days after injection, despite the fact that large amounts of radioactive LPS continued to be present beyond this time. The S-LPS persisted here for more than 5 wks, Re-LPS for more than 8 wks. The discrepancy in the data obtained by the two methods indicated that chemical changes responsible for loss of immunodetectability of LPS had occurred. Further evidence for chemical alteration of LPS was obtained when radioactive S-LPS, in which sugars and fatty acids were labeled with 2 distinct isotopes (^{3}H, ^{14}C) was injected in rats and its fate followed. The LPS present in liver and other organs three days after its injection exhibited a lower fatty acid to carbohydrate ratio than the original LPS (8). The same was true for Re-LPS. Direct evidence that degradation of LPS had occurred was obtained when the S-LPS was reisolated from the rat liver 3 days after its injection and chemically analyzed (8). The core and O-polysaccharide sugars (see Fig 6), dOclA, heptose, galactose, mannose and rhamnose were found in similar ratios as in the intact LPS. The lipid A was still present covalently bound to the polysaccharide, showing that the overall macromolecular structure of LPS had remained unaltered. However, the analysis revealed a significant decrease in the relative amounts of abequose and of fatty acids. Abequose represents the immunodominant sugar of the S-LPS (S. abortus equi) and understandably its loss was paralleled by a reduction in the antigenic activity of the reisolated material. The loss of abequose also explains the loss of immunodetectability of LPS present in the liver mentioned above. Further, abequose occupies a branched position along the O-specific chain which explains why the macromolecular structure of the reisolated LPS remained unaltered despite the loss of this sugar. The reduction in fatty acids involved 3-hydroxytetradecanoic-acid (by 40%), dodecanoic- (by 50%), hexadecanoic- (by 60%) and 2-hydroxytetradecanoic acid (almost absent).

The LPS-degradation product, reisolated from the liver was tested in several biological tests (pyrogenicity, lethal toxicity, local Shwartzman reaction and LAL gelation) and its activity compared to that of the intact

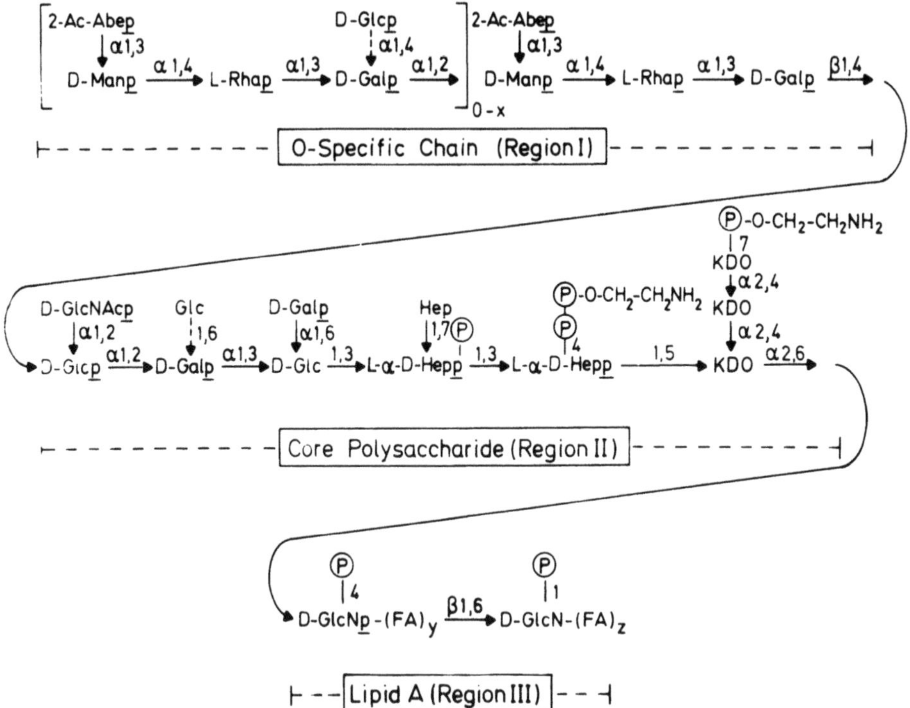

Fig 6. Structure of Salmonella abortus equi lipopolysaccharide.

LPS. Despite the significant reduction in fatty acids the endotoxic properties of the degraded LPS were fully preserved. This was not necessarily expected because changes in lipid A, especially cleavage of fatty acids by, e.g., alkali treatment are known to lead to detoxification of LPS (26, 27).

The original position of the missing fatty acids is not known. We assume however that unlike alkali treatment, which leads to a random cleavage of ester-bound fatty acids in the lipid A, the **in vivo** degradation involves sites of acylation that are not essential for expression of the biological activities investigated here. These findings are additional evidence that an underacylation of lipid A does not necessarily result in loss of biological activity provided the minimum requirements regarding number and position of acyl residues are fulfilled by the remaining fatty acids.

Excretion

The removal of LPS from the body takes place at a very slow rate, over many weeks. LPS that has undergone degradation in the liver and other organs is subsequently excreted mainly through the gut (6, 20). Fig 7 shows the pattern of excretion of radioactivity in feces of double-labeled S- and R-form LPS during the first 14 days after their intravenous administration in rats. The total amount of S- and R-form LPS excreted during this time amounted to 32% and 22% of the injected amount respectively. A shift in the ratio of ^{14}C (sugars) to ^{3}H (fatty acids) in the excreted material revealed that in both LPS partial deacylation had occurred. The degraded LPS excreted in the gut is very similar to that re-isolated from the liver 3 days following LPS injection, retaining the overall macromolecular structure of the original LPS and exhibiting a similar loss of fatty acids. Biliary excretion has been identified as one route by which degraded LPS reaches the gut.

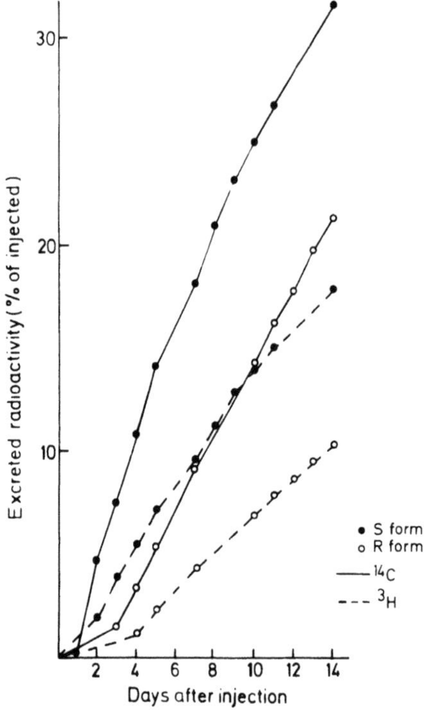

Fig 7. Excretion of ^{3}H (fatty acids) and ^{14}C (sugars) in feces of rats injected with ^{3}H, ^{14}C-LPS preparations.

During our studies another as yet unknown route of LPS excretion, its removal via the lungs, has been identified. In this route of excretion, the transportation of LPS into the alveolar and bronchiolar space is effected by macrophages. Using immunohistochemistry it could be shown that macrophages already carrying LPS migrate to the lung and ultimately leave this organ by passing through the alveolar and bronchial walls (9, 11). After LPS-injection the lung remains free of LPS for several hours. Migration of LPS positive macrophages then begins and their number in the lung increases with time. Between days 3 and 14 after LPS injection all macrophages obtained by bronchoalveolar lavage were LPS-positive. Many of the macrophages present in bronchoalveolar space between the second and eighth day were identified morphologically as activated macrophages. There was a striking correlation between the appearance of LPS-positive macrophages and lung tissue injury. The LPS present in alveolar macrophages was also identified as partially deacylated and we believe that in rats this LPS later reaches the gut and forms part of the LPS excreted in feces.

Small amounts of LPS are excreted in the urine (6, 20). This material, however, represents low molecular-weight metabolic products of LPS which are detectable on account of the radioactivity they contain. This route of excretion involves 4 to 7% of the injected radioactivity for the 14 day period after LPS injection.

ACKNOWLEDGEMENTS

The technical assistance of H. Stübig, C. Steidle, I. Minner, M. L. Gundelach and C. Strohmeier is gratefully acknowledged. This work was partly supported by the Deutsche Forschungsgemeinschaft through Sonderforschungsbereich 154 to C.G.

REFERENCES

1. Bertok, L., 1980, Role of bile in detoxification of lipopolysaccharide, in: "Microbiology," D. Schlesinger, ed., Am. Soc. Microbiol., Washington D.C.

2. Chedid, L., Parant, F., Parant, M. and Boyer, F., 1966, Localization and fate of ^{51}Cr-labeled somatic antigens of smooth and rough Salmonellae. Ann. N.Y. Acad. Sci. 133: 712.

3. Farrar, W. E., Jr. and Corwin, L. M., 1966, The essential role of the liver in detoxification of endotoxin. Ann. N. Y. Acad. Sci. 133: 668.

4. Freudenberg, M. A., Bøg-Hansen, T. C., Back, U. and Galanos, C., 1980, Interaction of lipopolysaccharides with plasma high-density lipoprotein in rats. Infect. Immun. 28: 373.

5. Freudenberg, M. A., Kleine, B. and Galanos, C., 1984, The fate of lipopolysaccharide in rats: evidence for chemical alteration in the molecule. Rev. Infect. Dis. 6: 483.

6. Freudenberg, M. A. and Galanos, C., The metabolic fate of endotoxins, in: "Bacterial Endotoxins: Pathophysiological effects, clinical significance and pharmacological control," A. R. Liss, Inc., New York, in press.

7. Freudenberg, M. A., Bøg-Hansen, T. C., Back, U., Jirillo, E. and Galanos, C., 1980, Interaction of lipopolysaccharides with plasma high density lipoprotein in rats, in: D. Eaker and T. Wadstrom, eds., Natural Toxins, Pergamon Press, New York.

8. Freudenberg, M. A. and Galanos, C., 1985, Alterations in rats in vivo of the chemical structure of lipopolysaccharide from Salmonella abortus equi. Eur. J. Biochem. 152: 353.

9. Freudenberg, M. A., Freudenberg, N. and Galanos, C., 1982, Time course of cellular distribution of endotoxin in liver, lungs and kidneys of rats. Br. J. Exp. Path. 63: 56.

10. Freudenberg, N., Freudenberg, M. A., Bandara, K. and Galanos, C., 1985, Distribution and localization of endotoxin in the reticuloendothelial system (RES) and in the main vessels of the rat during shock. Path. Res. Pract. 179: 517.

11. Freudenberg, N., Freudenberg, M. A., Guzman, J., Mittermayer, C., Bandara, K. and Galanos, C., 1984, Identification of endotoxin-positive cells in the rat lung during shock. Virchows Arch [Pathol. Anat.] 404: 197.

12. Galanos, C., Lüderitz, O., Rietschel, E. T. and Westphal, O., 1977, Newer aspects of the chemistry and biology of bacterial lipopolysaccharides, with special reference to their lipid A component. Intern. Rev. Biochem., Biochemistry of Lipids II 14: 239.

13. Galanos, C. and Lüderitz, O., 1975, Electrodialysis of lipopolysaccharides and their conversion to uniform salt forms. Eur. J. Biochem. 54: 603.

14. Galanos, C., Lüderitz, O. and Westphal, O., 1979, Preparation and properties of a standardized lipopolysaccharide from Salmonella abortus equi (Novo-Pyrexal). Zbl. Bakt. Hyg. 243: 226.

15. Goldman, R. C. and Leive, L., 1980, Heterogeneity of antigenic-side-chain length in lipopolysaccharide from Escherichia coli 0111 and Salmonella typhimurium LT2. Eur. J. Biochem. 107: 145.

16. Hofman, J. and Dlabac, V., 1974, The role of lipid A in phagocytosis of gram-negative bacteria and their lipopolysaccharides. J. Hyg. Epidemiol. Microbiol. Immunol. 18: 447.

17. Johnson, K. J. and Ward, P. A., 1972, The requirement for serum complement in the detoxification of bacterial endotoxin. J. Immunol. 108: 611.

18. Johnson, K. J., Ward, P. A., Goralnick, S. and Osborn, M. J., 1977, Isolation from human serum of an inactivator of bacterial lipopolysaccharides. Am. J. Pathol. 88: 559.

19. Keene, W. R., Landy, M. and Shear, M. J., 1961, Inactivation of endotoxin by a humoral component. VII. Enzymatic degradation of endotoxin by blood plasma. J. Clin. Invest. 40: 302.

20. Kleine, B., Freudenberg, M. A. and Galanos, C., 1985, Excretion of radioactivity in faeces and urine of rats injected with ^{3}H, ^{14}C-lipopolysaccharide. Br. J. Exp. Path. 66: 303.

21. Mathison, J. C. and Ulevitch, R. J., 1979, The clearance, tissue distribution, and cellular localization of intravenously injected lipopolysaccharide in rabbits. J. Immunol. 123: 2133.

22. May, J. E., Kane, M. A. and Frank, M. M., 1972, Host defense against bacterial endotoxemia - contribution of the early and late components of complement to detoxification of bacterial endotoxin. J. Immunol. 109: 893.

23. Morrison, D. C. and Ulevitch, R. J., 1978, The effects of bacterial endotoxins on host mediation systems. Am. J. Pathol. 93: 527.

24. Morrison, D. C. and Kline, L. F., 1977, Activation of the classical and properidin pathways of complement by bacterial lipopolysaccharides (LPS). J. Immunol. 118: 362.

25. Munford, R. S., Andersen, J. M. and Dietschy, J. M., 1981, Sites of tissue binding and uptake in vivo of bacterial lipopolysaccharide-high density lipoprotein complexes. Studies in the rat and squirrel monkey. J. Clin. Invest. 68: 1503.

26. Neter, E., Westphal, O., Lüderitz, O., Gorzynski, E. A. and Eichenberger, E., 1956, Studies of enterobacterial lipopolysaccharides. Effects of heat and chemicals on erythrocytes-modifying, antigenic, toxic, and pyrogenic properties. J. Immunol. 76: 377.

27. Niwa, M., Milner, K. C., Ribi, E. and Rudbach, J. A., 1969, Alteration of physical, chemical and biological properties of endotoxin by treatment with mild alkali. J. Bacteriol. 97: 1069.

28. Palva, T. and Mäkelä, H., 1980, Lipopolysaccharide heterogeneity in Salmonella typhimurium analyzed by sodium dodecyl sulfate/polyacrylamide gel electrophoresis. Eur. J. Biochem. 107: 137.

29. Ramadori, G., Hopf, U., Galanos, C., Freudenberg, M. A. and Meyer zum Büschenfelde, K. H., 1980, In vitro and in vivo reactivity of lipopolysaccharides and lipid A with parenchymal and non-parenchymal liver cells

in mice, in: "The reticuloendothelial system and the pathogenesis of liver disease," H. Liehr and M. Grün, eds., Elsevier, Amsterdam, North Holland.

30. Rudbach, J. A., Anacker, R. L., Haskins, W. T., Johnson, A. G., Milner, K. C. and Ribi, E., 1966, Physical aspects of reversible inactivation of endotoxin. Ann. N. Y. Acad. Sci. 133: 629.

31. Rutenburg, S. H., Smith, E. E., Rutenburg, A. M. and Fine, J., 1961, Degradation of endotoxin by splenic extracts. Antimicrob. Agents Chemother. 142.

32. Skarnes, R., Rutenburg, S. and Fine, J., 1968, Fractionation of an esterase from calf spleen implicated in the detoxification of bacterial endotoxin. Proc. Soc. Exp. Biol. Med. 128: 75.

33. Skarnes, R. C., 1970, Host defense against bacterial endotoxemia: mechanism in normal animals. J. Exp. Med. 132: 300.

34. Trapani, R. J., Waravdekar, V. S., Landy, M. and Shear, M. J., 1961, In vitro inactivation of endotoxin by an intracellular agent from rabbit liver. J. Infect. Dis. 110: 135.

35. Ulevitch, R. J., Johnston, A. R. and Weinstein, D. B., 1981, New function for high density lipoproteins. Isolation and characterization of a bacterial lipopolysaccharide-high density lipoprotein complex formed in rabbit plasma. J. Clin. Invest. 67: 827.

36. Yoshioka, M. and Konno, S., 1970, Characteristics of endotoxin-altering fractions derived from normal serum. III. Isolation and properties of horse serum α2-macroglobulin. Infect. Immunol. 1: 431.

BACTERIAL ENDOTOXIN AS A PROBE TO INVESTIGATE VIRAL INDUCED IMMUNE DEFICIENCIES

M. Bendinelli, D. Matteucci, P. G. Conaldi and E. Soldaini

Department of Biomedicine, Virology Section
University of Pisa, Pisa, Italy

INTRODUCTION

Viral Induced Immune Deficiencies

That viral induced immune deficiencies (VID) are a major medical problem is dramatically emphasized by the ongoing pandemic of acquired immune deficiency syndrome (AIDS). However, the ability to impair the immune system of the host is not limited to the human immune deficiency virus (HIV). The first report that viral infections may be the cause of clinically significant perturbations of immune reactivity was published long before AIDS was even dreamed of. Eighty years ago Clement von Pirquet reported that children with measles showed a transient anergy to tuberculin as evidenced by reduced skin tests. Since this pioneering work a vast array of human and animal viruses have been shown to suppress many parameters of immunological reactivity in infected hosts (for recent reviews, see 1, 27, 28, 32, 36).

It is now generally accepted that the clinical consequences of virus immune deficiencies (VID) may be many. First, VID may pave the way for other infecting agents which can cause susceptibility to these infections and represent a serious threat to life. Presently HIV is the prototype of viruses that predispose to opportunistic infections. However, much evidence has accumulated over the years that patients with or convalescent from measles, influenza, rubella, cytomegalovirus, and other viral infections can present an increased susceptibility to superinfection by a variety of exogenous or reactivated endogenous pathogens. Just to give a recent example, antecedent measles has been seen to substantially increase the mortality rate of otherwise generally benign adenoviral infections in infants (39).

Second, VID may decrease the resistance to tumors. Development of neoplasms that are much less frequent or progressive in the normal population is one of the hallmarks of AIDS. Although there is no unequivocal evidence that other VID of man are related to subsequent neoplasia, experimental infections with immunodepressive viruses in animals have been shown to facilitate the growth of grafted tumors (4).

Third, VID may influence the course of the inducing infection. Although this problem does not appear to have emerged in clinical settings, experimental infections have illustrated that viral perturbation of immune functions may reduce the host's ability to block the spread of infecting virus or facilitate the establishment of viral persistence (1, 27, 28, 32, 36). On the other hand, since immunopathologic processes play a key role in the genesis of many viral diseases, it can be convincingly argued that VID might also alleviate cell and tissue damage.

Last but not least, there is the related problem of the implications for the design of appropriate therapies. Antiviral drugs are presently so few that nonspecific immunostimulants have been considered as potentially useful, and have sometimes been used, for treating viral diseases. The attempt to alleviate the immunosuppressive effects of the infecting virus might represent a further incentive for this therapeutic strategy. However, as discussed more extensively elsewhere (1), until the mechanisms of disease production by viruses and the role played by VID are better understood, such an approach is grossly premature. Data obtained in well controlled models warn that, at least in certain infections, the use of nonspecific immunostimulants might be detrimental rather than beneficial to the patient (3).

Mechanisms of Immunosuppression by Viruses

Although the problems outlined above command for a detailed understanding of VID, investigations have so far been little rewarding. The great complexity of both the immune system and viral pathogenesis has prevented from scraping much beyond the mere surface. As a result, a great deal of information has accumulated but comprehension of the mechanisms involved is far from satisfactory.

It is now generally accepted that a major pathway to immune derangement is direct viral replication in the cells which compose the immune system. Indeed, many widely different viruses have been shown to replicate in one or more classes or subclasses of lymphocytes and/or macrophages, with effects that range from cytolysis to much more subtle changes, including the selective loss of specific differentiated functions. This is an important mechanism because 1) many viruses replicate preferentially in activated immunocytes such as those which proliferate and differentiate during specific and polyclonal responses to infection; 2) in spite of the fact that the proportion of cells supporting viral growth may be small, the effect can be destructive for immune functions owing to amplification phenomena which find an ideal substratum in the activation cascades peculiar to the functioning of immune networks; 3) viral variants with preferential tropism for lymphoid cells have been seen to emerge during certain infections (27).

It is, however, well recognized that direct invasion of immunocompetent cells is only one of several means whereby VID can be generated. Additional mechanisms may include the production of virus or host derived immunosuppressive factors by infected nonlymphoid tissues, antigenic competition, triggering of immunoregulatory events by antiviral immune responses, hormonal imbalances, etc. The problem is compounded because different pathophysiologic mechanisms may be intertwined, acting concomitantly or in sequence. Moreover, their relative contribution may vary not only with the inducing virus, but also with the route, multiplicity, duration and other variables that characterize each specific infectious event (1).

Bacterial endotoxin is a powerful inducer of adaptive biological responses and much is known about its mode of action (30, 37). It can therefore represent an ideal tool for analyzing specific aspects of the cellular and molecular basis of VID. In the following sections we review two different animal models of VID where the use of endotoxin has proved useful in dissecting the underlying mechanisms.

Immunosuppression by Murine Retroviruses

A number of oncogenic murine retroviruses induce generalized immunosuppressive effects which have interesting analogies to those seen in HIV infected patients. Such effects, first recognized in the early sixties, have been extensively investigated in an attempt to evaluate whether they influence tumor development and progression, as in most cases depressed immune responsiveness precedes tumorigenesis (4). Interest has, however, increased markedly after the discovery that highly immunosuppressive retroviruses also exist in humans.

Friend leukemia complex (FLC) is the best characterized among such models. It consists of two viruses, a replication competent chronic leukemia-inducing virus, named F-MuLV, and a defective virus, known as SFFV. The latter is responsible for the rapidly progressing erythroblastosis and erythroleukemia which develop in adult susceptible mice within a few days from injection with the entire viral complex. In contrast, F-MuLV, which can be easily propagated as an independent entity, when injected alone into mice, causes leukemias of varied histotype after a latency of several months.

Despite such differences in oncogenic potential, infecting adult mice with FLC or F-MuLV produces immunosuppressive effects that in the early stages are strikingly similar. F-MuLV represents 90 to 99% of the viral activity found in FLC preparations, and it is therefore likely that it plays a major role in the immunodepressive effects (4) as well as in other aspects of FLC pathogenicity (22).

Several lines of evidence argue against the interpretation that the general systemic immunosuppression caused by FLC is merely due to the massive splenomegaly which often occurs following infection (4, 29). However, in studying the mechanisms involved, we have constantly compared FLC with F-MuLV in order to distinguish better those directly associated with the viral infection from those which might be secondary to the ensuing proliferative disease.

Taken as a whole, our results and those of others indicate that FLC induced immunosuppression is a complex phenomenon involving many cell types of the immune system (4). Thus, understanding how much alterations are generated may be relevant to AIDS pathogenesis, which also appears to result from dysfunction of several immunocompetent cell types (19, 34). Existing evidence is indicative that bacterial endotoxin can substantially influence host response to FLC and vice versa (Table 1). Below we focus on the results obtained by using bacterial lipopolysaccharide (LPS; from E. coli 0127:B8, Westphal) to investigate FLC induced immunosuppression (Tables 2 and 3).

Table 1. Bacterial endotoxin can substantially influence host's response to viruses of the Friend leukemia complex and vice versa

LPS enhances spleen focus formation by FLC (35);
LPS enhances F-MuLV production by splenic B cells (10);
LPS is more toxic in FLC infected than normal mice (16);
LPS can prolong survival of FLC infected mice (16).

Table 2. Beneficial effects of bacterial endotoxin on immunosuppression by viruses of the Friend leukemia complex: synopsis

---

Proliferative response to LPS less reduced than response to other mitogens;

Antibody response to LPS less reduced than response to other antigens, including PS;

LPS restores the antibody responsiveness to other antigens in vivo and in vitro;

LPS restores the ability of macrophages to cooperate with lymphocytes.

LPS as a Mitogen

In these experiments we compared the lymphoproliferative response to various mitogens exhibited by normal and infected spleen cells of FLC susceptible BALB/c mice. As a rule the response to LPS was generally less affected than that to T cell mitogens. Resistance of LPS induced blastogenesis to suppression by FLC has been noted also by other workers (13, 17).

It is not known whether polyclonal B cell activation by retroviruses (4) contributes to such apparent resistance. In any case the phenomenon is of interest because B cells are considered much more susceptible than T cells to infection by viruses of the FLC (10). In addition, in vitro stimulation with LPS (but not with T cell mitogens) has been reported to specifically enhance F-MuLV replication in splenic lymphocytes, as detected by infectious center assay (10). Thus, it appears that B cells can support FLC replication and nevertheless respond normally or near normally to mitogens. Similar conclusions have been reached concerning antibody production (4).

LPS as an Immunogen

These studies were carried out in two inbred mouse strains which epitomize the extremes of susceptibility (BALB/c) and resistance (C57BL/6) to FLC. In both strains the antibody response to LPS proved considerably less affected affected than the response to several other immunogens tested, including

Table 3. Bacterial endotoxin and production of soluble mediators by spleen cells of mice infected with viruses of the Friend leukemia complex: synopsis

---

LPS pulsed macrophages release soluble factors which restore responsiveness;

LPS pulsed macrophages produce and release normal or enhanced levels of IL 1;

LPS pulsed macrophages express normal levels of membrane associated IL-1 activity;

LPS pulsed spleen cells release reduced amounts of IFN-gamma, but normal levels of IFN-alpha/beta .

---

thymus dependent antigens such as sheep red cells (SRC) and thymus independent antigens such as TNP-ficoll or pneumococcus polysaccharide. For example, in BALB/c mice FLC given 3, 6 or 10 days before the antigen depressed the anti-LPS PFC counts respectively by 68, 87, and 94% as compared to suppressions of over 90% at all three times in the anti-SRC response. In the same strain F-MuLV produced a transient impairment of the antibody response to LPS, whereas the response to SRC was permanently affected.

In C57BL/6 mice, no suppression of the antibody response to LPS was observed by either viral preparation regardless of the time interval between virus inoculation and immunization. In contrast, the response to alkaline treated LPS (alk-LPS) was markedly reduced also in C57BL/6 mice (5). This finding suggested that the relative resistance of LPS specific antibody responses to suppression by FLC is associated with the lipid moiety of this molecule.

LPS as an Immunostimulant

These studies evaluated the ability of LPS to restore the immune responsiveness of infected mice. The experiments were performed in vivo and in vitro.

Groups of mice infected with FLC or F-MuLV were immunized intravenously with SRC and simultaneously given LPS by the same route at doses from 10 to 100 μg/mouse. LPS enhanced the production of splenic SRC-specific antibody forming cells (PFC) to a much greater degree in infected than control animals. The difference was most evident in C57BL/6 mice, where the PFC response achieved by infected animals given LPS reached levels close to those observed in uninfected mice given the same dose of LPS. This trend was observed regardless of the SRC dose used to immunize the animals. In BALB/c mice the effect was less pronounced, but still significant (5).

Similar experiments were performed in vitro by adding graded doses of LPS to cultures of infected spleen cells immunized with optimal doses of SRC. Under these conditions the enhanced immunostimulation affected by LPS in infected mice was even more evident than in vivo and, most importantly, was quite impressive also with cells from BALB/c mice. For example, LPS added at doses of 10 μg/ml increased the numbers of anti-SRC PFC produced by infected BALB/c cells by a factor of 10 - 20, whereas the enhancements observed with normal cells rarely exceeded a two-fold factor. The effect was markedly reduced by the antibiotic polymyxin B, known to neutralize many activities of LPS. In keeping with evidence that most immunological effects of LPS are due to the lipid region, alk-LPS was inactive (5). It should be noted however that recent results have shown that detoxified LPS from S. marcescens is also capable of stimulating the antibody responsiveness of FLC infected mice (16).

Enhancement of humoral immune responses by LPS appears to result from direct interaction with various classes of immunocytes, such as polyclonal stimulation of B cells and macrophage activation, and from indirect mechanisms, including the production of soluble factors (30, 37). Dose-response experiments evidenced that in vitro doses of LPS too low to give a detectable mitogenic effect were still capable of reversing the immunodepressed state of infected spleen cells. This suggested that the reconstitutive activity of LPS for infected spleen cells was not necessarily related to its B cell mitogenicity (5).

LPS as a Macrophage Activator

The reduced antibody responsiveness of FLC and F-MuLV infected mice and spleen cells is partially or entirely cured by administering relatively small numbers of exogenous macrophages from normal syngeneic donors together with the immunizing antigen. This and other evidence discussed extensively elsewhere (4) has indicated that immunosuppression by these viruses is at least partly due to a defect(s) in accessory cells, most likely at the level of the functions needed for antigen presentation. Macrophages are among the earliest cells to be invaded by viruses of the FLC. Depression of bacterial killing and other important functions has also been described in retrovirus infected macrophages, although these results are sometimes controversial (2). Moreover, abnormalities of macrophages and other accessory cells are increasingly recognized as contributing factors to the immune disruption associated with HIV (19, 34).

We explored the possibility that the reconstitutive action of LPS is mediated by macrophages. The problem was approached in two ways. Macrophages vary in their ability to restore the antibody responsiveness of infected mice depending on the district of origin and pretreatment. As compared to proteose peptone elicited peritoneal macrophages, resident peritoneal and splenic macrophages have little, if any, activity (4). Thus we checked whether LPS could convert the latter cells to an active state. Indeed, a short preincubation with LPS, followed by extensive washings, rendered resident peritoneal and spleen macrophages very efficient in restoring the antibody response of infected spleen cells (5).

In a more direct approach we cross recombined adherent and nonadherent cells of infected and noninfected spleens and studied their ability to mount an antibody response to SRC. As expected, adherent splenoctes of infected mice were unable to serve as accessory cells, when cultured with control nonadherent cells, in the generation of a normal antibody response. In contrast, after a brief treatment with LPS and washings, such cells regained the ability to collaborate with nonadherent spleen cells as, or even more, efficiently than adherent spleen cells from normal mice. The activity was expressed also in the presence of polymyxin B in the medium at concentrations capable of blocking any residual LPS (5).

Factors released by macrophages have been repeatedly implicated in LPS adjuvanticity. Moreover, factors in the serum of LPS treated mice have been shown to enhance the antibody responsiveness of FLC infected animals (9). We, therefore, examined whether the restoration of antibody responsiveness brought about by LPS-pulsed macrophages of infected BALB/c mice was due to soluble factors. Supernatants conditioned by normal splenic and peritoneal macrophages pulsed with LPS (but not with alk-LPS) potentiated the antibody response much more effectively in infected than normal spleen cell cultures. Interestingly, the restoration affected by the supernatants was even higher than that achieved by direct addition of LPS (5).

LPS may be retained and processed by macrophages in such a way that its bioactivity is increased (15). However, restoration by supernatants of LPS pulsed macrophages was only marginally reduced by polymyxin B and was also observed in LPS-resistant C3H/HeJ mice (5). This seems to exclude that the effect is solely due to LPS or LPS fractions released by the macrophages.

Collectively, these results support the view that macrophages and factors produced by them play a crucial role in LPS induced reversal of the immunosuppressed state. At present it is, however, impossible to come to any firm conclusion on whether this beneficial effect is solely mediated by macrophages. LPS has an astonishing range of activities and might influence other immune cell types impaired by FLC viruses.

LPS as a Cytokine Inducer

Macrophages are versatile secretory cells. Following interaction with and/or endocytosis of LPS, they produce a variety of soluble factors suspected to play a central role in the pathophysiological changes induced by this substance (37). Several such factors provide important interactive signals to the cells involved in immune responses. Using LPS as a stimulant we compared the ability of macrophage cultures derived from normal and infected mice to accumulate selected factors.

In several experiments adherent splenocytes of FLC and F-MuLV infected BALB/c mice produced interleukin (IL) 1 levels much higher than normal cells. The effect peaked during the third week of infection with both viral preparations (26). Increased IL 1 production has been documented in other conditions associated with reduced immune responsiveness, including HIV infected patients (8), and might represent an attempt to compensate for reduced reactivity of other cell types.

The finding, however, was not consistent. In some experiments the difference between normal and infected cells was minimal or not significant. So far, the reasons for such variability have remained elusive. Inhibitors of IL 1 activity have been described in several situations including virus-infected hosts (31). A synthetic peptide homologous to retroviral envelope proteins has also been reported to inactivate IL 1 (24). Nevertheless, we found no indications that inhibitors might contribute to generate the observed inconsistency. In normal and infected spleen cell cultures extracellular IL 1 accumulation started within a few hours from LPS stimulation and followed similar kinetics. No significant release of IL 1 was found in cultures of spleen cells from infected mice or normal mice exposed in vitro to the viruses.

LPS pulsed macrophages express a surface membrane-associated IL 1 activity (mIL 1) which may be important in their accessory functions and is at least partly dissociated from secretion of soluble IL 1 (38). In the light of the reduced accessory cell function exhibited by macrophages of infected mice, we determined whether expression of mIL 1 activity is affected by infection. Adherent spleen cells obtained from normal and infected mice were stimulated with LPS, fixed with paraformaldehyde, and examined for ability to stimulate thymocyte proliferation. They released no IL 1 activity in the supernatant but expressed the expected mIL 1 activity, as shown by thymidine incorporation by thymocytes cultured in their presence. Adherent spleen cells of infected and control mice exerted comparable stimulatory activities indicating that mIL 1 expression is not grossly altered by infection (26).

We also examined the ability of LPS to elicit interferon (IFN) production by infected spleen cells. Murine splenocytes stimulated in vitro with LPS release both IFN-α/β, produced mainly by macrophages and B cells during the first hours of incubation, and IFN-γ produced by T lymphocytes at later times of culture (6). Results showed that IFN-α/β production is not significantly modified at least during the first two weeks of infection. In contrast, IFN-γ production was markedly reduced or entirely ablated early after infection. There was no detectable IFN in cultures of nonstimulated infected or normal cultures (unpublished results).

Collectively, these results confirmed that the ability of macrophages to produce the monokines studied remains essentially normal following FLC or F-MuLV infection, whereas lymphokine production by T cells is grossly impaired. Many aspects of IL 2 physiology, including IL 2 receptor expression, are drastically perturbed by FLC and F-MuLV infections (26). In turn, these changes might be related to the severe NK cell impairment observed in FLC-infected mice (33). Similar changes have been observed in AIDS patients (8, 19, 34).

IFN-γ production involved a number of discrete steps. Studies have shown that macrophages and IL 2 are important mediators and regulators of

IFN-γ induction by LPS and other stimuli (12). We presently do not know whether the deficit in LPS induced IFN-γ production observed in infected mice is secondary to other perturbations. Profound alterations of the dynamics and functions of T cells have been observed in susceptible mice infected with viruses of the FLC (4, 23). We have preliminary evidence that the mechanisms of transmembrane signal transduction are also altered by infection in these cells.

The addition at high doses of purified or recombinant IL 1 and/or IL 2 failed to restore the reduced antibody responsiveness of infected spleen cultures (26). We are presently investigating combined treatments with other cytokines. A recent report suggests that tumor necrosis factor, which mimics many effects of LPS, may have therapeutical value in FLC infected mice (21).

Immunosuppression and Lymphoid Involution Induced by Group B Coxsackieviruses

Group B coxsackieviruses (CVB) are widespread human enteroviruses. They cause a significant proportion of the acute meningeal and other neurological disorders that affect man. Other diseases associated with CVB range from acute gastrointestinal, respiratory and other mucocutaneous disorders to acute carditis and myositis. These forms often present a fulminant course in children under three months of age. CVB have also been implicated as candidate etiological agents of subacute or chronic diseases of obsecure etiology such dilated myocardiopathy, type 1 juvenile diabetes, and others.

The mechanisms whereby CVB produce such a vast array of diseases are poorly understood. The rapid cytolysis of infected cells caused by these viruses does not seem to explain their entire pathogenic potential. As a result of clinical investigations using newly developed diagnostic tools and of intensive studies in experimentally infected mice, it is becoming increasingly apparent that CVB share many pathogenetic complexities classically associated with enveloped viruses. For example, they can persist for a considerable time in infected patients, cause subtle changes of infected cells, and also trigger immunopathologic damage to infected and uninfected tissue. However, so far neither clinical studies nor murine models have clearly defined the role played by the host's immune system in CVB induced pathogenesis (3).

We have focused our attention on the interactions CVB establish with cells of the immune system. These studies have shown that CVB infect and actively replicate in lectin-stimulated human cordal blood mononuclear cells as well as in human immortalized lymphoid lines of B or T cell origin. In contrast, human adult peripheral blood mononuclear cells were only sporadically permissive even when preactivated with lectins and cultured in the presence of anti-IFN antibodies. Nevertheless, following CVB challenge adult blood mononuclear cells were functionally damaged, as shown by reduced ability to proliferate in response to mitogens (3, 11).

A somewhat similar situation is observed in experimentally infected adult mice. These animals show a reduced immune reactivity which can affect both humoral and cell mediated responses. In addition, infected mice may undergo a progressive, profound involution of central and peripheral lymphoid organs. Similar to the human situation, such detrimental effects on murine immune system occur in the absence of detectable viral replication in the affected tissues (3).

We have used LPS in a series of experiments aimed to understand the basis of the immunological disorders produced by type 3 CVB (CVB3) in adult BALB/c mice (Table 4).

Table 4. Bacterial endotoxin and immunosuppression by group B coxsackievirus type 3.

Lymphoproliferative response to LPS remains normal;
Antibody response to LPS remains normal;
LPS augments virus induced lethality;
LPS does not render lymphoid cells permissive to viral replication;
LPS treatment markedly exacerbates lymphoid involution;
LPS pulsed macrophages from atrophic spleens produce highly enhanced levels of selected monokines.

LPS as a Mitogen

The lymphoproliferative response to LPS of spleen cells of CVB3 immunosuppressed mice remained in the normal range. Since most viruses replicate preferentially in stimulated than in resting lymphoid cells, we have exploited the mitogenic action of LPS also to investigate whether the lymphoid cells of adult mice support CVB3 replication. All the attempts to propagate the virus on lymphoid cells derived from various organs, cultured alone or with mitogenic doses of LPS or other mitogens, failed. These studies excluded that even a tiny minority of short-lived permissive cells were present in the unstimulated or mitogen-stimulated lymphoid cell suspensions, thus disproving the assumption of previous authors that the high viral titers found in extracts of lymphoid organs obtained from CVB infected mice result from local viral replication. Such results helped establish that the deleterious effects of CVB3 on the immune system of mice do not stem from virus induced cytopathology.

LPS as an Immunogen

The antibody response to LPS and other thymus independent antigens was essentially spared by CVB3 as compared to the response to SRC and other thymus-dependent antigens. This confirmed that B lymphocytes are not a major target of immunosuppression by this virus, a conclusion born out by a number of additional data (3).

LPS as an Immunostimulant

We attempted to modify the progression of CVB3-induced lymphoid involution by administering LPS to mice at different times relative to infection. LPS was found to augment CVB3 induced lethality. LPS treated mice also showed a marked exacerbation of lymphoid involution (unpublished data), thus behaving as mice treated with other immunostimulants (3).

LPS as a Cytokine Inducer

Using protocols similar to those described for the FLC system, we have begun to investigate the ability of lymphoid cells from CVB3 infected mice to respond to LPS stimulation with the production of soluble mediators. Recent results have shown that the production of monokines is normal or near normal during the first weeek of infection but is substantially enhanced later on, concomitantly with the appearance of overt lymphoid involution (unpublished data). Such increase might be the expression of an attempt to counteract the infection triggered mechanisms which lead to lymphoid involution. However, we were unable to detect a spontaneous production of monokines by infected unstimulated cells. Thus, it is tempting to speculate that the increased production of monokines contributes to the genesis of lymphoid involution which is observed in CVB3 infected mice. We are presently investigating the role of tumor necrosis factor.

CONCLUSIONS

In spite of the considerable efforts of recent years, understanding of VID pathogenesis and of basic principles which regulate virus-lymphoreticular cell interactions in general is still in a rather primitive state. A better insight of such aspects may be relevant to the recognition of new mechanisms by which viruses escape immune defenses and produce disease, and is mandatory for the development of rational treatments aimed to circumvent the immunosuppressive consequences of viral infections. The two models discussed above illustrate how using LPS as an investigative tool can provide important leads to VID pathogenesis.

Discussed evidence also reemphasize that bacterial endotoxins can substantially modify host responses to viruses. In keeping with previous findings (7, 16, 18, 20), we have shown that LPS can both have a protective role against viral infections and exacerbate or be responsible for certain damages observed in virus infected hosts. The medical interest of these findings should not be underestimated. Viral infections can be accompanied by superinfections with endotoxin producing bacteria or might increase endotoxin absorption from the gut and there may be mutual consequences on the outcome of either infection, resulting in benefit or harm to the host (14).

The protective effects of LPS against viral infections has so far been attributed to the IFN inducing activity of this substance (20). The data discussed in section 3, suggest another possible mechanism, namely reversal of certain manifestations of VID. This may represent a further stimulus to the search for LPS derivatives and simpler related compounds with potential use in VID therapy. As we learn more on LPS biology and immunology, contribution of this area of research to ongoing work on VID will become more incisive and easier to interpret.

ACKNOWLEDGMENTS

The work discussed in this article was supported in part by the Special Projects "Oncology" and "Control of Infectious Diseases" and by a Bilateral Project of the Italian National Research Council and from the Ministry of Public Education. E. S. is the holder of a fellowship from the Italian Association for Cancer Research.

We are grateful to Lucia Barontini, Giulietta Cerretini and Annalisa Montagnani for skilled assistance.

REFERENCES

1. Bendinelli, M., 1984, Immunomodulation in viral infections: Virus or infection-induced? in: "Immunomodulation. New Frontiers and Advances," H. H. Fudenberg, H. D. Whitten and F. Ambrogi, eds., Plenum Press, New York.

2. Bendinelli, M., 1988, The reticuloendothelial system in infection with RNA tumor viruses, in: "The Reticuloendothelial System: A Comprehensive Treatise. Vol. 10. Infection," M. Escobar and J. P. Utz, eds., Plenum Press, New York.

3. Bendinelli, M. and Friedman, H., 1988, "Coxsackieviruses: A General Update," Plenum Press, New York.

4. Bendinelli, M., Matteucci, D. and Friedman, H., 1985, Retrovirus-induced acquired immunodeficiencies. Adv. Cancer Res. 45: 125.

5. Bendinelli, M., Matteucci, D., Giangregorio, A. M. and Conaldi, P. G., 1986, Restoration of antibody responsiveness by endotoxin in retrovirus-immunosuppressed mice: Role of macrophages, in: "Immunobiology and Immunopharmacology of Bacterial Endotoxins," A. Szentivanyi, H. Friedman and A. Nowotny, eds., Plenum Press, New York.

6. Blanchard, D. K., Djeu, J. Y., Klein, T. W., Friedman, H., and Stewart, W. E., 1986, Interferon-γ induction by lipopolysaccharide: Dependence on interleukin 2 and macrophages. J. Immunol. 136: 963.

7. Boggs, S. S. and Schwartz, G. N., 1978, Increased lethality after endotoxin in old or leukemic AKR mice. Proc. Soc. Exp. Biol. Med. 157: 424.

8. Bowen, D. L., Lane, H. C. and Fauci, A. S., 1986, Immunologic abnormalities in the acquired immunodeficiency syndrome. Prog Allergy 37: 207.

9. Butler, R. C., Frier, J. M., Chapekar, M. S., Graham, M. O. and Friedman, H., 1983, Role of antibody response helper factors in immunosuppressive effects of Friend leukemia virus. Infec. Immun. 39: 1260.

10. Cerny, J., Hensgen, P. A., Fistel, S. H. and Demler, L. M., 1976, Interactions of murine leukemia virus with isolated lymphocytes. II. Infection of B and T cells with Friend virus complex in diffusion chambers and in vitro: Effect of polyclonal mitogens. Int. J. Cancer 18: 189.

11. Conaldi, P. G., Matteucci, D., Soldaini, E. and Bendinelli, M., 1988, Interactions of group B coxsackieviruses with human lymphoid cells. Proc. 88th Annu. Meet. Amer. Soc. Microbiol. p. 132.

12. Croll, A. D. and Morris, A. G., 1986, The regulation of γ-interferon production by interleukins 1 and 2. Cell. Immunol. 102: 33.

13. Dracott, B. N., Wedderburn, N. and Doenhoff, M. J., 1978, The immunodepressive effect of Friend virus. IV. Effects on spleen B lymphocytes. Immunology 34: 679.

14. Dudding, L. R. and Garnett, H. M., 1987, Interactions of strain AD169 and a clinical isolate of cytomegalovirus with peripheral monocytes: The effect of lipopolysaccharide stimulation. J. Inf. Dis. 155: 891.

15. Duncan, R. L., Hoffman, J., Tesh, V. L. and Morrison, D. C., 1986, Immunologic activity of lipopolysaccharides released from macrophages after the uptake of intact E. coli in vitro. J. Immunol. 136: 2924.

16. Friedman, H. and Szentivanyi, A., 1986, Endotoxin and polysaccharide derivative induced enhanced antibody formation in leukemia virus infected mice, in: "Immunobiology and Immunopharmacology of Bacterial Endotoxins," A. Szentivanyi, H. Friedman and A. Nowotny, eds., Plenum Press, New York.

17. Genovesi, E. V., Livnat, D. and Collins, J. J., 1982, Immunotherapy of murine leukemia. VII. Prevention of Friend leukemia virus-induced immunosuppression by passive serum therapy. Int. J. Cancer 30: 609.

18. Gut, J. P., Schmitt, S., Bingen, A., Anton, M. and Kirn, A., 1984, Probable role of endogenous endotoxins in hepatocytolysis during murine hepatitis caused by frog virus 3. J. Inf. Dis. 149: 621.

19. Ho, D. D., Pomerantz, R. J. and Kaplan, J. C., 1987, Pathogenesis of infection with human immunodeficiency virus. N. Engl. J. Med. 317: 278.

20. Ho, M., 1983, Induction of interferon by endotoxin, in: "Beneficial Effects of Endotoxins," A. Nowotny, ed., Plenum Press, New York.

21. Johnson, C. S. and Furmanski, P., 1987, In vivo effects of tumor necrosis factor on normal and leukemic erythropoiesis. Proc. Annu. Meet. Am. Assoc. Cancer Res. 28: 399.

22. Jones, K. S., Ruscetti, S. and Lilly, F., 1988, Loss of pathogenicity of spleen focus-forming virus after pseudotyping with Akv. J. Virol. 62: 511.

23. Kitagawa, M., Matsubara, O. and Kasuga, T., 1986, Dynamics of lymphocytic subpopulations in Friend leukemia virus-induced leukemia. Cancer Res. 46: 3034.

24. Kleinerman, E. S., Lachman, L. B., Knowles, R. D., Snyderman, R. and Cianciolo, G. J., 1987, A synthetic peptide homologous to the envelope protein of retroviruses inhibits monocyte-mediated killing by inactivating interleukin 1. J. Immunol. 139: 2329.

25. Kurt-Jones, E. A., Beller, D. I., Mizel, S. B. and Unanue, E. R., 1985, Identification of a membrane-associated interleukin 1 in macrophages. Proc. Natl. Acad. Sci. USA 82: 1204.

26. Matteucci, D., Giangregorio, A. M., Lopez-Cepero, M., Specter, S., Bendinelli, M. and Friedman, H., 1989, Interleukins 1 and 2 production and responsiveness in the early stages of leukemogenic retrovirus infection of mice. Cell. Immunol. 119, in press.

27. McChesney, M. B. and Oldstone, M. B. A., 1987, Viruses perturb lymphocyte functions: Selected principles characterizing virus-induced immunosuppression. Ann. Rev. Immunol. 5: 279.

28. Mims, C. A., 1986, Interactions of viruses with the immune system. Clin. Exp. Immunol. 66: 1.

29. Morrison, R. P, Nishio, J. and Chesebro, B., 1986, Influence of the murine MHC (H-2) on Friend leukemia virus-induced immunosuppression. J. Exp. Med. 163: 301.

30. "Beneficial Effects of Endotoxins," 1983, Nowotny A., ed., Plenum Press, New York.

31. Roberts, N. J., Jr., Prill, A. H. and Mann, T. N., 1986, Interleukin-1 and interleukin-1 inhibitor production by macrophages exposed to influenza virus or respiratory syncytial virus. J. Exp. Med. 163: 511.

32. Rouse, B. T. and Horohov, D. W., 1986, Immunosuppression in viral infections. Rev. Inf. Dis. 8: 850.

33. Specter, S., Moody, D. J., Bendinelli, M. and Friedman, H., 1984, Suppression of natural killer cell activity by Friend murine leukemia virus. J. Nat. Cancer Res. 172: 1394.

34. Spickett, G. P. and Dalgleish, A. G., 1988, Cellular immunology of HIV infection. Clin. Exp. Immunol. 71: 1.

35. Steeves, R. A. and Grundke-Iqbal, I., 1976, Bacterial lipopolysaccharides as helper factors for Friend spleen focus-forming virus in mice. J. Natl. Cancer Inst. 56: 541.

36. Szentivanyi, A. and Friedman, H., 1986, "Viruses, Immunity and Immunodeficiency," Plenum Press, New York.

37. Szentivanyi, A., Friedman, H. and Nowotny, A., 1986, "Immunobiology and Immunopharmacology of Bacterial Endotoxins," Plenum Press, New York.

38. Unanue, E. R. and Allen, P. M., 1987, The basis for the immunoregulatory role of macrophages and other accessory cells. Science 236: 551.

39. Warner, J. O. and Marshall, W. C., 1979, Crippling lung disease after measles and adenovirus infection. Br. J. Dis. Chest 2: 89.

IMMUNOADJUVANTICITY OF ENDOTOXINS AND NONTOXIC DERIVATIVES FOR NORMAL AND LEUKEMIC IMMUNOCYTES

H. Friedman, T. Klein, S. Specter, C. Newton, and A. Nowotny

University of South Florida College of Medicine, Tampa, FL and University of Pennsylvania, Philadelphia, PA

Endotoxins from many Gram negative bacteria are known to be immunostimulators. For example, administration of crude or even purified lipopolysaccharide (LPS) endotoxin preparations into experimental animals challenged with various soluble and/or particulate antigens may result in altered immune responses, including enhanced responses, especially when the endotoxins are given shortly before or simultaneously with antigen (4, 10, 14, 15, 17, 19, 24, 25, 26). Studies in these laboratories have shown that a polysaccharide (PS)-rich derivative from endotoxins lacking the lipid A moiety and free of toxicity is a potent immunostimulant for normal mice (7, 8, 11). For example, the PS obtained from **Serratia marcescens** is equivalent to the intact endotoxin in enhancing the antibody response to a T cell dependent antigen such as sheep erythrocytes (SRBC) in vitro. In vivo the PS was less effective than LPS in enhancing the immune response to SRBC but still considerable adjuvant effect could be demonstrated (1, 2). Injection of SRBC into normal mice or addition of this antigen to cultures of splenocytes from non-immunized mice results in an antibody response readily detected by the hemolytic plaque assay in vitro. Furthermore, treatment of the animals or cell cultures with either LPS or its PS derivative results in enhanced antibody formation.

Previous studies in this laboratory have shown that mice infected with the retrovirus Friend leukemia virus (FLV) develop a marked immunodeficiency shortly after exposure to this RNA leukemia inducing virus (12, 13, 23, 25). Such immunodeficiency is similar to the acquired immunodeficiency seen in man infected with the human immunodeficiency retrovirus. Depression of antibody responsiveness, as well as cell mediated immunity, to a variety of test antigens accompanies such FLV infection. LPS-rich endotoxins, especially purified LPS from organisms such as Serratia or **E. coli**, are markedly adjuvantic in FLV infected animals, resulting in a marked restoration of antibody formation (6, 15, 23, 25). Addition of LPS to spleen cells from immunosuppressed FLV infected mice also restores immune responses, essentially to normal levels.

The present studies show that the PS-rich material from Serratia, when added to spleen cells from FLV immunosuppressed mice, also restores antibody plaque responses, similar to the intact LPS. Furthermore, administration of PS to mice infected with FLV markedly enhanced the antibody responsiveness of these animals, similar to the effects of LPS. However, the PS is essentially nontoxic for mice, both normal and FLV infected, as compared to LPS itself which is not only somewhat toxic for normal mice, especially at higher doses, but extremely toxic for the FLV immunosuppressed mice (13, 23). The relative absence of toxicity of the PS derivative for retrovirus infected mice offers a decided advantage because the animals do not become moribund when treated with this derivative. As shown in this report, both bacterial products, i.e., the intact LPS and the nontoxic PS, stimulated antibody response helper factor(s) in spleen cell cultures in a similar manner.

EXPERIMENTAL METHODS

Animals

Inbred male Balb/c mice, 6-8 wk of age, were used for these studies. They were obtained from Cumberland View Farms, Clinton, TN. The animals were infected by intraperitoneal injection of a 100 LD_{50} dose of FLV contained in 0.1 ml of a 1% clarified homogenate of infected mouse splenocytes. The virus was maintained by passage through adult normal Balb/c mice and contained both the spleen focus forming and lymphatic leukemia virus components of the Friend virus complex.

Lipopolysaccharides

Serratia LPS was prepared by the trichloroacetic acid extraction procedure of Boivin et al. (5, 21). The nontoxic PS derivative was obtained from the LPS by 0.2 N acetic acid hydrolysis. The chemical constituents and characteristics of both the LPS and PS have been described previously (1, 20).

Antigen

Sheep red blood cells and Elsevier's solution were obtained from Baltimore Biological Laboratories, Baltimore, MD. The RBCs were washed several times in medium and suspended to an 0.5% concentration.

Immunization

For in vivo immunization, mice were injected with 0.1 ml of the SRBC suspension. For in vitro immunization covered plastic Linbro plates were used as culture chambers (6, 13). Spleen cells from normal or FLV infected mice were washed in medium and the numbers of viable nucleated cells determined by the trypan blue dye exclusion technique with a hemocytometer. A suspension of 8 x 10^6 viable splenocytes in 2.0 ml complete tissue culture medium (RPMI 1640) enriched with a standard nutrient cocktail in 20% fetal calf serum was cultured in the Linbro plates as described previously. For immunization, 0.1 ml of the 0.1% suspension of SRBC was added to each culture (approximately 2 x 10^6 erythrocytes). All cultures were incubated for 5 days at 37° C in a humidified atmosphere containing 10% CO_2.

Assay for Antibody Forming Cells

The numbers of direct hemolytic antibody plaque forming cells (PFC) to the erythrocytes were determined by a standard micromethod (3, 6). The numbers of PFCs were enumerated for at least 8-24 cultures prepared from 2-4 spleen cell preparations and the average numbers of PFCs per million viable cells calculated. In all cases, only direct non-facilitated plaques were enumerated and these were considered due to IgM antibody producing cells.

In Vitro Production of the Antibody Response Helper Factor

Suspensions of 10^7 splenocytes per ml from normal mice were incubated in RPMI 1640 medium plus 10% fetal calf serum and antibiotics at 37° in CO_2.

Table 1. Effect of LPS on Antibody Response to SRBC by Spleen Cells from FLV Infected vs. Normal Mice

Dose LPS per mouse (μg)	PFC/10^6 Spleen Cells[b] FLV Infected	Normal Mice
None (control)	120 $\pm$ 18	836 $\pm$ 57
1.0	146 $\pm$ 26	892 $\pm$ 130
5.0	285 $\pm$ 18	1465 $\pm$ 210
10.0	973 $\pm$ 240	2261 $\pm$ 375
20.0	1860 $\pm$ 340	2640 $\pm$ 280
50.0	1810 $\pm$ 270	1976 $\pm$ 310
100.0	1265 $\pm$ 295	1895 $\pm$ 420

[a]Indicated dose of LPS injected i.p. into mice at time of challenge immunization with 4 x 10^6 SRBC.
[b]Average number of PFC/10^6 spleen cells for 3-4 mice 4-5 days after challenge immunization.
[c]Mice injected seven days earlier with 100 LD_{50} FLV.

Experimental cultures received 20 μg LPS or PS per ml at the time of culture initiation. Cell-free supernatants were collected after 5 days and either stored on ice or frozen until tested (6, 11).

Assay for Antibody Response Helper Factor

The presence of antibody response helper factor activity was determined by adding 0.1 ml of stimulated culture supernatants to in vitro antibody cultures at the time of sensitization with SRBC. The helper factor activity of each preparation was considered proportional to the degree of enhancement of the antibody response over that of untreated control cultures.

Interleukin 1 Assay

Interleukin 1 was assayed in culture supernatants by testing graded dilutions on cultures of C3He/HeJ mouse thymocytes which are unresponsive to LPS but respond in vitro to IL-1 (16). A standard murine peritoneal exudate culture supernatant was used as a control for IL-1 for comparative purposes. Purified antibody to IL-1 was used to neutralize IL-1 activity. In selected cases, gel filtration was used to size the material with IL-1 activity (16).

EXPERIMENTAL RESULTS

Previous studies in this and other laboratories had shown that susceptible strains of mice such as Balb/c infected with FLV show a marked and profound immunosuppression. Within a few days after infection with graded amounts of FLV the mice develop a marked immunodeficiency in terms of their ability to respond to sheep erythrocytes. As shown in Table 1, within a few days after infection with FLV there was a marked anergy in responsiveness of the mice to sheep RBCs. This is even more evident a wk after infection. When mice were injected with LPS one wk after infection with FLV, and tested 5 days later for responsiveness to sheep RBCs, a dose related enhancement of

Table 2. Effect of PS on Antibody Response to SRBC by Spleen Cells from FLV Infected vs. Normal Mice

Dose per mouse (μg)[a]	PFC/10^6 Spleen Cells[b]	
	FLV Infected[c]	Normal Mice
None (control)	138 ± 27	760 ± 49
1.0	159 ± 42	932 ± 72
5.0	297 ± 58	1260 ± 110
10.0	765 ± 180	1540 ± 132
20.0	1636 ± 285	1960 ± 275
50.0	1930 ± 310	2150 ± 310
100.0	1870 ± 290	2015 ± 295

[a]Indicated dose of PS injected i.p. into mice at time of challenge immunization with 4 x 10^8 SRBC.
[b]Average number of PFC/10^6 spleen cells for 3-4 mice 4-5 days after challenge immunization.
[c]Mice injected 7 days earlier with 100 LD_{50} FLV.

antibody formation of the spleen cells to SRBC was evident (Table 1). Although there was an even greater response by spleen cells from normal control mice, the ratio of increase as a percent increase of splenic PFCs in the LPS treated mice was much greater than that observed in the control animals, presumably because of the lower number of PFCs initially in the untreated FLV infected mice as compared to the controls.

Earlier studies had shown that this depression of antibody formation is not only due to a defect in immunocytes, i.e., B cells, producing antibody to sheep erythrocytes, but also a depression in the function or number of helper T cells as well as antigen processing macrophages. Regardless of the mechanism, it is clear that infection of mice with FLV results in a marked depression of antibody formation and this can be restored by injection of LPS at the time of infection. The enhancement is generally similar to that observed in untreated mice injected with the bacterial product. It is also quite apparent, as is evident in Table 2, that the nontoxic PS had similar effects. Injection of FLV infected animals with graded amounts of PS resulted in a marked increase in antibody forming cells in the spleen of these animals, essentially similar to that which occurred in normal mice treated with the LPS and immunized with sheep erythrocytes. Thus, both the LPS and PS were markedly stimulatory for in vitro antibody responsiveness of mouse spleen cells from either normal or FLV infected animals.

Immunocytes obtained one wk or longer after FLV infection of the donor mice were markedly deficient in their ability to respond to SRBC in vitro (Table 3). However, when these spleen cells from the FLV infected mice were treated with either LPS or PS in vitro they regained much of their ability to form PFCs to sheep erythrocytes. Thus, as indicated earlier, the LPS was a marked adjuvant for the anti-sheep RBC response by spleen cells from normal mouse spleens and the PS also had a similar effect.

In order to study the possible mechanisms involved LPS or PS induced splenocyte derived cell-free supernatants were examined for their ability to

Table 3. Effect of LPS or LPS on in Vitro Antibody Response of Mouse Spleen Cells to Sheep Erythrocytes

Dose per culture[a] (μg)	Antibody Response per 10^6 spleen cells[b]			
	PS Treatment		LPS Treatment	
	FLV Infected	Normal	FLV Infected	Normal
None (control)	97 ± 12	796 ± 48	82 ± 10	835 ± 65
5.0	386 ± 75	810 ± 60	360 ± 35	1170 ± 78
10.0	673 ± 195	1530 ± 184	862 ± 38	1730 ± 240
20.0	1310 ± 258	2650 ± 286	1470 ± 140	2970 ± 290
40.0	1830 ± 560	2970 ± 265	1630 ± 195	3100 ± 270

[a]Indicated dose of PS or LPS added to cultures of 5 x 10^6 spleen cells from normal or FLV-infected mice.
[b]PFC per 10^6 spleen cells from 3-4 cultures per group 4-5 days after in vitro immunization with 2 x 10^6 SRBC.
[c]Mice injected 10 days earlier with 100 LD_{50} FLV.

Table 4. Effect of LPS or PS Induced Cell Free Culture Supernatants on PFC Response of Spleen Cells from Normal or FLV Infected Mice

Culture Supernatant Added[a]		PFC/10^6 Spleen Cells[b]			
		FLV Infected[c]	Percent of Control	Normal mice	Percent of control
None		189 ± 15	--	912±38	--
LPS Induced	1:5	1630±48	862	1820±125	199
	1:10	1710±75	299	1938± 210	213
	1:20	730±36	386	1263±196	135
PS Induced	1:5	1430±40	757	1973±138	216
	1:10	1270±93	673	1494±173	164
	1:20	1020±65	540	1130±210	124

[a]Indicated dilution of 24 hr cell free culture supernatant from LPS or PS stimulated normal mouse spleen cell cultures added to cultures of 5 x 10^6 spleen cells from normal or FLV-infected mice.
[b]Average number of PFC 5 days after in vitro immunization of cultures with 2 x 10^6 SRBC.
[c]Mice injected 10 days earlier with 100 LD_{50} FLV.

Table 5. Induction of Antibody Helper Activity by LPS or PS in Cultures of Lymphoid Cells from Normal Mice

Cell Type Tested[a]	PFC/10^6 Spleen Cells[b]			
	LPS Treated		PS Treated	
	FLV Infected[c]	Normal mice	FLV Infected[c]	Normal mice
None	--	--	92 ± 18	930 ± 48
Spleen - intact	1260 ± 48	2630 ± 280	1430 ± 138	2760 ± 348
Adherent Spleen	1410 ± 156	2970 ± 270	1590 ± 230	3450 ± 460
Nonadherent Spleen	140 ± 29	1030 ± 76	136 ± 27	1140 ± 68
PE Cells	1370 ± 448	2435 ± 322	1510 ± 32	2560 ± 130

[a]Cultures of 5 x 10^6 spleen cells or separated adherent vs. nonadherent cells or peritoneal cells from normal mice treated in vitro with LPS or PS.
[b]Average PFC response, ± SE, for 3-4 cultures per group from normal or FLV infected mice 5 days after in vitro immunization with SRBC and treatment with 0.1 ml cell free supernatant from cells from normal mice incubated for 24 hr with 20.0 μg LPS or PS or, as a control, medium alone.
[c]Mice infected 10 days earlier with 100 LD_{50} FLV.

affect the antibody response of splenocytes from normal as well as FLV infected animals. As is apparent from Table 4, cell free culture supernatants from normal donor mouse spleen cells treated in vitro with LPS or PS for 24 hr had a varying ability to enhance the PFC response of spleen cell cultures derived either from normal control or FLV infected mice. The spleen cells from the FLV infected mice showed a marked immunosuppression in vitro when challenged with SRBC as compared to the responses of cells from normal mice. Supernatants from the LPS or PS treated normal spleen cells had a marked ability to enhance PFC responses by cells from the FLV infected as well as from normal mice. This occurred in a dose dependent manner in that higher dilutions of the culture supernatants were less effective. Nevertheless, it is evident that spleen cells from FLV infected mice showed enhanced PFC responses in vitro when treated with culture supernatants from either LPS or PS treated normal spleen cells. This response was generally similar to the enhanced responses of spleen cells from normal mice treated with the same supernatants (Table 4).

It was not clear from these experiments what was the cellular source of the immunoenhancing activity in the culture supernatants. In order to examine this question, immunoenhancing activity was assessed in culture supernatants of peritoneal exudate cells from normal mice treated with either LPS or PS, as well as in supernatants from nonadherent spleen cells consisting mainly of lymphocytes vs. adherent cells consisting mainly of macrophages (Table 5). The results obtained indicated that both LPS and PS induce an immunoenhancing factor mainly in macrophage rich cultures. LPS is known to induce various soluble mediators of immunity, especially interleukin 1. Thus it seemed likely that IL-1 was the active factor in these responses. Therefore, in additional experiments, it was found that specific anti-IL-1 antibody neutralized the immunoenhancing activity in culture supernatant (data not shown). Furthermore, gel filtration experiments indicated that the

Table 6. Effect of Bacterial Products on Spleen Weight and PFC Response of Normal or FLV-Infected Mice

Treatment[a]	Response of Mice[b]			
	FLV Infected Mice		Control Mice	
	Spleen Weight	PFC/10^6 Spleen cells	Spleen Weight	PFC/10^6 Spleen Cells
None (control)	878 ± 138	113 ± 32	119 ± 16	768 ± 45
LPS only	490 ± 156	960 ± 86	158 ± 32	1836 ± 120
PS only	526 ± 130	865 ± 72	130 ± 18	1640 ± 110
BCG only	310 ± 116	580 ± 40	199 ± 52	2140 ± 156
MDP only	638 ± 82	618 ± 83	138 ± 22	1809 ± 210
LPS + BCG	432 ± 72	1180 ± 130	289 ± 252	2965 ± 320
LPS + MDP	398 ± 63	1045 ± 72	171 ± 60	2760 ± 410
PS + BCG	420 ± 72	976 ± 68	286 ± 120	1132 ± 72
PS + MDP	486 ± 120	1132 ± 72	156 ± 40	2640 ± 210

[a]Groups of 5-6 mice injected i.p. with indicated stimulator on same day as injection i.p. with 100 LD_{50} FLV or, as control, with saline only; LPS, PS or MDP given at a dose of 10-20 μg/mouse or BCG given at a dose of 1.0 mg/mouse.
[b]Average response for 3-4 mice per group 10 days after injection.

active material in either the PS or LPS stimulated culture supernatants had the characteristics of IL-1 in terms of molecular size (data not shown).

The results of such experiments suggested that both the PS and LPS stimulated normal mouse spleen cells, presumably macrophages, to produce IL-1 which had immunorestorative activities for FLV immunosuppressed splenocytes. Thus it was possible that the nontoxic PS had properties quite similar to intact LPS not only for restoring antibody responsiveness of FLV infected spleen cells, but also affected the leukemic properties of the retrovirus as evident by altered splenomegaly. In this regard, both muramyl dipeptides (MDP) and bacillus Calmette Guerin (BCG) have been used as immunostimulants and adjuvants for antitumor activity in mice. Therefore, in the FLV infection system these substances were compared to LPS vs. PS as immunoadjuvants in FLV infected mice.

MDP, a small molecular weight adjuvant considered the smallest synthetic unit which has the immunostimulatory activity of intact BCG, had little effect in protecting mice from FLV induced immunodepression, but could serve synergistically in restoring antibody responsiveness of spleen cells from FLV infected mice when given together with either LPS or PS (Table 6). Only moderately enhanced PFC responses occurred with spleen cells from normal mice given MDP alone but much greater responses occurred when it was given together with LPS. A synergystic effect also occurred when PS was substituted for LPS in mice given either MDP or BCG (Table 6). Thus the smaller molecular weight PS had similar activities as the LPS in synergizing either with BCG or synthetic MDP in reducing both splenomegaly of FLV infected animals and increasing the PFC response to SRBC in these animals.

DISCUSSION AND CONCLUSIONS

Endotoxins have been studied for many decades as immunostimulants and as antitumor agents (4, 16, 19, 22, 26). Administration of endotoxin prior to an antigen usually results in an enhanced antibody response, especially when the antigen is given either in a suboptimal dose or when it is not a strong immunogen. Sheep erythrocytes are considered a very excellent immunogen but administraton of endotoxin in relatively small amounts simultaneously with the SRBCs shortly before immunization results in an enhanced immune response. Numerous studies the last few years, including those from this laboratory, have shown that LPS is a potent immunoenhancer, both in vitro and in vivo, to antigens such as sheep erythrocytes and the mechanism appears to be mediated, at least in part, by soluble mediators of immunity, especially IL-1 induced by LPS in macrophages activated with this stimulator (4, 11, 17, 24).

A nontoxic polysaccharide derivative from LPS has been found to have similar effects. Studies in this laboratory have shown that both LPS and PS are strongly immunomodulatory and induce not only IL-1 but also tumor necrotizing factor, tumor resistance enhancing factor, other immune factors and interferon.

Studies in which splenocytes were separated into adherent vs. nonadherent populations showed that the lymphocyte-rich nonadherent cell population did not have the capacity to produce antibody response enhancing activity when stimulated either with LPS or PS. In contrast, the macrophage-rich adherent cell population retained the antibody enhancing capacity of whole spleen cell suspensions when stimulated in vitro with either LPS or PS. This indicated that the macrophage is the cell type that responds directly to the bacterial products and these cells are stimulated to produce the immunoenhancing factor, presumably IL-1.

FLV is a retrovirus which induces an acquired immunodeficiency in mice evidenced by depressed antibody responses by their spleen cells. This is due to effects on lymphocytes but is also related to suppression of macrophage function as well as the function and number of helper T cells. Studies in this laboratory have shown that antibody response helper factor(s) has the ability to restore antibody formation by suppressed spleen cells from FLV infected mice. The antibody response helper activity is readily induced by PS as well as LPS. The effect of these bacterial products to enhance the antibody response of FLV suppressed mouse spleen cells is presumably due to production of IL-1 by those macrophages which had escaped impairment in the FLV infected mice.

The ability of macrophages to produce antibody helper activities, especially IL-1, was shown previously with spleen cells from normal mice and appears similar to that of spleen cells from FLV immunosuppressed mice (10, 11, 12). It is important to note, however, that PS, unlike LPS, has little if any toxicity and this is very important in the case of retrovirus infected mice which show increased susceptibility to toxicity by native LPS. Thus lack of toxicity by the PS in both normal and FLV-infected mice appears to have a major advantage in its potential use as an immunorestorative substance in retrovirus suppressed individuals. The ability to enhance antibody responsiveness in virus suppressed mice by the more toxic LPS is negated by its detrimental effects in retrovirus infection. Thus there appears to be an advantage in using a nontoxic substance with similar activity. Furthermore, the experiments on the possible mechanisms involved indicated that PS is potent in inducing spleen cells from FLV injected as well as from normal mice to produce the immunoenhancing factor IL-1. Supernatants from spleen cells from normal mice treated either with PS or LPS had the ability to restore antibody formation by spleen cells from either normal or FLV immunosuppressed mice. Further studies concerning the mechanism of action of the nontoxic PS derivative from endotoxin as a potential immunoenhancing adjuvant in retrovirus induced immunosuppression is certainly warranted.

SUMMARY

Studies with FLV infected mice, a model for retrovirus induced acquired immunodeficiency, showed that intact lipopolysaccharide rich extract from **Serratia marcescens** as well as the nontoxic polysaccharide derivative free of lipid A were equally adjuvantic in enhancing antibody formation to sheep erythrocytes, both in vivo and in vitro. The PS-rich endotoxin derivative had little or no toxic activity in leukemic animals as occurred with intact endotoxin. The adjuvanticity of both the nontoxic polysaccharide derivative as well as the intact endotoxin in enhancing antibody formation in FLV infected mice was evident also in vitro when spleen cells from infected animals were immunized with sheep erythrocytes simultaneously with the polysaccharide in comparison with the LPS. Supernatants from normal spleen cells treated in vitro either with the polysaccharide or the intact endotoxin showed immunoenhancing helper activity for both normal and FLV infected spleen cells and this enhancing activity was due to IL-1 induced by either bacterial product. Thus the immunoenhancing soluble mediator, i.e., IL-1, is induced equally by PS or LPS and has immunorestorative activity for FLV infected animals. The potential value of the nontoxic PS as an immunoadjuvant in retrovirus immunosuppressed lymphoid cells is evident. The results of these studies suggest that further investigations concerning the nature and mechanism involved in such adjuvancticity is warranted.

REFERENCES

1. Behling, U. H., and Nowotny, A., 1977, Immune adjuvancy of lipopolysaccharide and a nontoxic hydrolytic product demonstrating oscillating effect with time. J. Immunol. 118: 1905-1907.

2. Behling, U. H., Pham, P. H., Madani, F., and Nowotny, A., 1979, Components of lipopolysaccharide which induce colony stimulation, adjuvancy and radioprotection, in: "Microbiology," D. Schlessinger, ed., p. 103-107.

3. Bendinelli, M., Matteuci, P., and Friedman, H., 1986, Retrovirus-induced acquired immunodeficiencies. Ad. Canc. Res. 46: 78.

4. Berry, L. J., 1978, The mediation of endotoxemia effects, in: "Toxins," P. Rosenberg, ed., Pergamon Press, New York.

5. Boivin, A., Mesrobeanu, J., and Mesrobeanu, L., 1933, Extration d'un complexe toxique et antigenique a partier du bacille d'aertrycke. C.R. Soc. Biol. 114: 307.

6. Butler, R. C., Friedman, H., and Nowotny, A., 1980, Restoration of depressed antibody responses of leukemic splenocytes treated with LPS-induced factors. Adv. Exp. Med. Biol. 121: 315.

7. Butler, R. C., Friedman, H., Specter, S. and Eisenstein, T. K., 1981, Induction of immunoenhancing factors for murine splenocyte cultures by Salmonella typhosa ribosome and RNA extracts. Infect. Immun.

8. Frank, S. J., Specter, S., Nowotny, A., and Friedman, H., 1977, Immunocyte stimulation in vitro by nontoxic bacterial lipopolysaccharide derivatives. J. Immunol. 119: 855.

9. Friedman, H. and Specter, S., 1980, Virus induced immunomodulation, in: "Immunopharmacology," L. Chedid and J. Hadden, eds., Pergamon Press, New York.

10. Friedman, H., Klein, T. W., and Szentivanyi, A., eds., 1981, "Immunomodulation by Bacteria and their Products," Plenum Press, New York.

11. Friedman, H., Specter, S., and Butler, R. C., 1983, Stimulation of immunomodulatory factors by bacterial endotoxin and nontoxic polysaccharide, in: "Beneficial Effects of Endotoxins," A. Nowotny, ed., Plenum Press, New York.

12. Friedman, H., Specter, S., and Bendinelli, M., 1984, Viruses and the immune response, in: "Bacterial and Viral Inhibition and Modulation of Host Defenses," Academic Press, London.

13. Friedman, H., Szentivanyi, A., Specter, S. and Bendinelli, M., 1986, Virus interactions with the immune system, in: "Viruses, Immunity and Immunodeficiencies," Plenum Press, pp. 25.

14. Homma, J. Y., Kanegasaki, S., Luderitz, O., Shiba, T., and Westphal, O., eds., 1984, Bacterial Endotoxins, pp. 1-420, Verlag Chemie, Basel, Switzerland.

15. Klein, T. W., Specter, S., Friedman, H., and Szentivanyi, A., eds., 1983, "Biological Response Modifiers in Human Oncology and Immunology," Plenum Press, New York.

16. Lachman, L. L., 1983, Interleukin 1 release from LPS-stimulated mononuclear phagocytes, in: "Beneficial Effects of Endotoxins," A. Nowotny, ed., Plenum Press.

17. Nauts, H. C., 1946, The beneficial effects of bacterial injections on host resistance to cancer. N.Y. Cancer Res. Inst. Monograph 8.

18. Nowotny, A., 1963, Endotoxoid preparations. Nature 197: 721.

19. Nowotny, A., Golub, S., and Key, B., 1971, Fate and effect of endotoxin derivatives in tumor bearing mice. Proc. Soc. Exp. Biol. Med. 132: 26.

20. Nowotny, A., Behling, U. H., and Chang, H. L., 1975, Relation of structure to function in bacterial endotoxins. VIII. Biological activities in a polysaccharide-rich fraction. J. Immunol. 115: 199-203.

21. Nowotny, A., 1979, in: "Basic Exercises in Immunochemistry," 2nd edition, Springer Verlag Heidelberg, New York.

22. Prager, M. D., Ludden, C. M., Landy, W. J., Allison, J. P., and Kelto, G. B., 1975, Endotoxin stimulated immune response to modified lymphoma cells. J. Natl. Canc. Inst. 75: 773.

23. Specter, S. and Friedman, H., 1978, Viruses and immune responses. Pharm. Ther. A 2: 595.

24. Szentivanyi, A., Middleton, E., Williams, J. F., and Friedman, H., 1983, Effect of microbial agents on the immune network and associated pharmacologic reactivities, in: "Allergy: Principles and Practice," Second Edition, E. Middleton, C. E. Reed, and E. F. Ellis, eds., The C. V. Mosby Company, St. Louis, MO.

25. Szentivanyi, A. and Friedman, H., eds., 1986, "Viruses, Immunity and Immunodeficiency," Plenum Press, New York.

26. Yang, C. and Nowotny, A., 1974, Effect of endotoxin on tumor resistance in mice. Infect. Immun. 9: 95.

VARIOUS ASPECTS OF SYNERGISM BETWEEN ENDOTOXIN AND MDPs

M. Parant and L. Chedid*

Laboratory of Experimental Immunopharmacology, Institut Biomédical des Cordeliers, 75006 Paris, France and *University of South Florida, Tampa, FL, USA

INTRODUCTION

Muramyl dipeptide (MDP) is a synthetic glycopeptide analog of a part of bacterial peptidoglycan (13). It represents the minimal adjuvant-active structure and has also been shown to stimulate nonspecific resistance in animals subsequently infected (9). These effects have been demonstrated after injecting MDP in saline by different routes. The synthesis of MDP was followed by the preparation of a large number of derivatives with the hope of determining structure-activity relationships (12, 15), or at least of selecting immunostimulating compounds, which did not retain several side effects inherent to MDP administration (6, 24). Such an evaluation has allowed us to select an MDP derivative called Murabutide which is undergoing clinical trials with conventional vaccines after its safety has been established by animal toxicological studies, and in a phase I clinical trial.

The first observation concerned with a combined treatment with MDP and LPS has been reported in 1979 by Ribi et al. (28). They demonstrated an enhanced lethal effect of endotoxic preparations when MDP was administered simultaneously by the intravenous route into strain 2 guinea pigs. In this study they used MDP with Pseudogen vaccine (LPS from Pseudomonas aeruginosa) or with LPS from a rough strain, and found that very low doses of both MDP and an endotoxin preparation in combination led to a regression of a syngeneic hepatocellular carcinoma transplanted into guinea pigs (28). Since LPS is known to induce necrosis and regression of solid tumor transplants in syngeneic mice, this model was used by Bloskma et al. (3), to demonstrate a potentiating effect of MDP.

These data illustrate two aspects of the search for synergistic effects. The evaluation of adverse effects on the host that may occur during immunotherapeutic treatment, but also an increased efficiency resulting from a combined treatment. It is of interest to determine to which extent inflammatory reactions are part of local defense mechanisms of the host against bacterial agents.

MATERIALS AND METHODS

Animals

Swiss female mice (6 to 8 wk old) from Iffa Credo (Lyon, France) were used for toxicity experiments and infectious challenges. Balb/c female mice (12 wk old) were used for tumor necrosis, and nude and nu/+ Balb/c mice (8 wk old) were also obtained from Iffa Credo. Male Hartley guinea pigs weighing 300 to 400 g were obtained from Coblanbel (Roger Bellon, Paris, France).

Reagents

MDP (AcMur-L-Ala-D-iGln) and derivatives were kindly provided by Institut Choay, Paris, France. The following analogs were prepared by P. Lefrancier and M. Level who have reported their synthesis elsewhere: AcMur-L-Ala-D-Gln$^{\alpha}$-OnBu or murabutide, and MDP-1,2-dipalmitoyl-*sn*-glycerol or MDP-GDP (14, 17). *Salmonella enteritidis* LPS extracted by the phenol-water procedure was purchased from Difco Labs (Detroit, MI). Recombinant human THF (rHuTNF) was kindly provided by Biogen (Geneva, Switzerland) and Knoll AG (Ludwidshafen, FRA). Murine TNF (rMuTNF) and specific rabbit antiserum were generous gifts from Pr. W. Fiers (Ghent, Belgium).

Toxicity Assays

Toxicity of LPS or glycopeptides administered separately was evaluated in mice which had been adrenalectomized 48 hr before the intravenous challenge, or in mice given simultaneously by the intraperitoneal route 15 mg of D-galactosamine (hydrochloride, Sigma, Saint-Louis, MO, USA) and the solution to be tested. Toxic synergism was evaluated in guinea pigs or in mice by injecting LPS and MDP intravenously, either at the same time or at various time intervals.

Infectious Challenges

A *Klebsiella pneumoniae* strain of capsular type 2 (Institut Pasteur Collection n° 7832) was used in this study as in previous ones (8). LPS or muramyl peptides were administered in saline 24 hr before the bacterial challenge, and survivors were recorded for 15 days. The *p* values were obtained by the adjusted chi-square method.

In Vivo Tumor Assay

Methylcholantrene-induced fibrosarcoma (Meth A) was maintained in the ascite form by serial transplantations in Balb/c mice. For necrosis experiments, 10^6 tumor cells (in 0.1 ml) were injected intradermally into the depilated flank of female Balb/c mice. About 8 days later, tumor bearing mice (diameter of tumor mass around 8-10 mm) were treated intravenously and the necrosis was evaluated 48 hr later as described (5). Tumor regression was determined after 3 wk.

In Vivo TNF Production

For obtaining mouse serum containing a high level of TNF, BCG infection was used as priming agent (2×10^7 colony-forming units by the intravenous route) and mice were challenged 2 wk later with 25 μg LPS. In this case, and after priming with MDP, mice were exsanguinated 2 hr after LPS injection, and sera stored in liquid nitrogen until further use. The priming effect of MDP and derivatives was determined by injecting LPS at various time intervals after the glycopeptide.

The cytotoxic activity of the various sera was measured on mouse L929α cells in the presence of actinomycin D, essentially as described by Ruff and Gifford (31). The remaining adherent cells were stained for 15 min with a solution of 15% methanol with 0.5% crystal violet (Sigma). After washing, the dye was solubilized with SDS (1%) and absorbance read at 550 nm. The cytotoxicity in units per ml was defined as the reciprocal of the dilution resulting in 50% cytotoxicity which was determined by plotting the regression line of log dilution against absorbance. Under these conditions, the specific activity of rHuTNF was 1.6 x 10^7 U/mg protein.

RESULTS

Differences Between the Biological Effects of LPS and MDPs

LPS is a very strong immunostimulating agent either as an adjuvant of specific humoral responses to various antigens or as stimulant of nonspecific resistance to infectious challenges. Its efficiency makes often difficult to rule out an interference of LPS contamination when evaluating the capacity of any agent to enhance immunity. In contrast with LPS, MDP and analogs are characterized by the absence of immunogenicity except when they are linked to a carrier. As immunostimulating agent, synthetic MDPs are generally less potent than LPS, but marked differences have been underlined in several studies, namely immunostimulating properties of MDP were observed even after oral administration whereas LPS is ineffective by this route, and were established in animals unresponsive to LPS stimulation such as in very young mice (8, 26).

The side effects displayed by MDPs are extremely weak as compared with LPS, even when using animals made more susceptible to the lethal effect of gram negative bacteria preparations or to TNF. In BCG-treated mice known to be highly susceptible to the lethal effect of LPS (LD_{50} = 0.5 μg) and to produce large amounts of circulating TNF when challenged with LPS, MDP was very well tolerated at 1 mg per mouse. The LD_{50} of LPS (about 250 μg in normal mice) is increased 10,000 fold after adrenalectomy in mice, and at least 50,000 fold by treatment with galactosamine. These procedures have also been shown to sensitize animals to TNF toxicity. However, MDP and its analog murabutide did not provoke any mortality. On the same table, the minimal pyrogenic dose of MDP clearly indicate the difference with LPS which is 10,000 fold more pyrogenic, and also with murabutide devoid of any effect (Table 1). The effectiveness of the two glycopeptides as immunostimulating agents is quite comparable. However, the potentiation of their capacity by using conjugates containing MDP, or by using lipophilic derivatives may sometimes lead to the enhancement of pyrogenicity (10, 25). Various methods were used to eliminate or reduce toxicity of LPS and most of the detoxified preparations retained the ability to act as immunoadjuvants and to increase resistance to irradiation, but lost the protective effect against bacterial infections (7).

Sensitization to LPS Toxicity by some MDPs

Several examples of dissociation between the biological properties of MDP derivatives have been observed and it was therefore of interest to evaluate the effect of various MDP derivatives on LPS toxicity. Our results obtained in outbred guinea pigs have confirmed the data reported by Ribi et al. (28), showing an enhancement of LPS toxicity in animals given MDP at the same time. MDP and the nonpyrogenic murabutide were injected simultaneously to guinea pigs by the intravenous route with a nonlethal dose of LPS. As reported in Table 2, the mortality was increased in groups treated with MDP whereas murabutide did not enhance the host susceptibility to LPS. When the same experimental protocol was used in mice which are rather resistant to the lethal effect of LPS, a similar increase in sensitivity was found. The simultaneous administration of MDP elicited a high mortality rate in mice with a dose of LPS that did not kill any of the controls (8). In additional assays, MDP was unable to sensitize to LPS the low-responder C3H/HeJ mouse strain.

Table 1. Comparative toxic effects of LPS, MDPs and TNF

Compound	LD_{50} in Adx mice (μg)	LD_{50} in $GalNH_2$-treated mice (μg)	Minimal pyrogenic dose in rabbit (μg)
LPS	0.02	0.004	0.0016
MDP	>1,000	>1,000	23
Murabutide	>1,000	>1,000	>10,000
rHuTNF	4.7	0.47	1.1
rMuTNF	1.5	0.28	NT

Adx = adrenalectomized

The toxic synergism between LPS and MDP was established in both guinea pigs (28) and mice (8) with a single intravenous injection of the products. The route is important for LPS injection since the mortality is delayed by another route, but the small molecular weight MDP induced a similar effect on LPS toxicity when given by the subcutaneous or intraperitoneal route. By varying the time interval of administration, it was shown that the potentiation of LPS toxicity was lower a few hr after MDP injection and lost by 6 hr. However, the time schedule of a combined treatment was shown of importance in the potentiation of LPS-induced tumor necrosis by MDP (4), and in the priming effect of MDP on the production of circulating TNF in mice given an endotoxic preparation (see farther). In these studies an interval of some hours between injections of MDP and LPS was demonstrated to be more efficient, suggesting that the responses may be independent of an increased toxicity.

Table 2. Influence of MDP or Murabutide on LPS toxicity in guinea pig

Challenge by the intravenous route glycopeptide (μg)	LPS (150 μg)	No dead /total
MDP 500	-	0/10
Murabutide 500	-	0/10
-	+	0/10
MDP 50	+	2/10
MDP 150	+	7/10
MDP 500	+	10/10
Murabutide 150	+	1/10
Murabutide 500	+	0/10

Potentiation of LPS-Induced Tumor Necrosis by Pretreatment with MDP

Unlike LPS, MDP and the derivatives so far tested did not provoke any tumor necrosis in Balb/c mice having subcutaneous Meth A sarcoma implants. As already reported by Bloksma et al. (4), a previous injection of MDP injected a few hr before LPS potentiated the tumor damage. The MDP analogs that are inactive as immunoadjuvants did not enhance the LPS-induced response. Among hydrophilic adjuvant-active MDPs, differences in their potency have been observed and murabutide is slightly less effective than MDP. Lipophilic derivatives such as MDP-GDP appeared more efficient in potentiating the effect of a low dose of LPS (Table 3).

The results obtained with detoxified LPS such as SPLPS (7) are difficult to evaluate because a very low dose of residual toxic LPS may display a necrotic effect when given with MDP. However, bacterial vaccines which are relatively weak endotoxic products also represent potential agents to induce tumor necrosis in combination with MDPs. They were used successfully to produce high levels of circulating TNF in mice primed with MDP or derivatives.

The data obtained in the strain-2 syngeneic guinea pig line-10 tumor model showed that a small amount of endotoxic preparation when admixed with MDP sufficed to bring about optimal antitumor activity (29). It was concluded that a certain level of toxicity may be required to obtain the highest level of tumoricidal action although there is no direct correlation between endotoxic potency and tumor-regressive activity (29).

Effect of Combined Treatment with MDP and LPS on Nonspecific Resistance to Infections

Since 1956, the extraordinary potency of LPS as a stimulator of nonspecific resistance to numerous bacterial infections created excitement about this agent (reviewed in 22). The protective effect of nontoxic muramylpeptides against infectious challenges appeared weaker but was demonstrated under experimental conditions that make LPS ineffective, such as when admin-

Table 3. Influence of pretreatment with MDP or MDP-GDP on tumor necrosis induced by LPS in Balb/c mice bearing Meth A implants.

Pretreatment* i.v.	LPS i.v. (μg)	Sarcoma necrosis score +++	++	+	–	Regression*** No/Total
MDP	–	0	0	0	8	0/8
MDP-GDP	–	0	0	0	8	0/8
–	10	7	1	0	0	6/8
–	0.3	0	2	3	3	0/8
MDP	0.3	3	3	2	0	5/8
MDP-GDP	0.3	5	2	1	0	7/8

* 300 μg of MDP or of MDP-GDP 3 hr before LPS.

** Score was evaluated 48 hr after LPS injection.

*** Regression on day 30.

istered by the oral route or in young animals. In addition, MDPs are different from LPS because they do not produce a negative phase when given at the time of the bacterial challenge and do not elicit a refractory state (or "tolerance") after several injections.

The capacity of a small dose of LPS to enhance nonspecific immunity has often rendered difficult to measure the effectiveness of agents or of antibodies due to a possible contamination. To evaluate the role of a combined treatment with MDP and LPS against a bacterial infection, mice were treated intravenously 24 hr before a severe challenge with K. pneumoniae that killed all the controls within 1 day. Cumulative data from three identical experiments are reported in Table 4. They show that, in spite of the severity of this challenge, a dose of 10 ng LPS induced a significant protection whereas MDP had no effect with less than 100 μg per mouse. Nevertheless, ineffective doses of each agent were highly protective when administered together (Table 4).

In Vivo Priming Effect of MDPs on TNF Production Elicited by LPS

In BCG-infected mice, MDP alone did not induce the production of TNF activity in the serum, but slightly increased the response to a small dose of LPS. In untreated mice, MDPs did not cause the release of detectable levels of TNF in the blood although in vitro they were able to stimulate mouse macrophages to produce TNF. In our assays, the amount of TNF activity 2 hr after injection of 25 μg of LPS was about 400 U/ml of serum and a simultaneous injection of MDP induced a 10-fold increase in this level. As shown in Fig 1, the priming effect of MDP was more marked when it was injected a

Table 4. Anti-infectious effect of LPS and MDP in combined treatment against Klebsiella infection

Treatment (i.v.) MDP (μg)	LPS (μg)	Survivors/total
-	-	0/24
-	0.001	1/24
-	0.01	15/24**
-	0.1	24/24**
MDP 30	-	0/24
MDP 100	-	9/24**
MDP 30	0.001	14/24**
MDP-GDP 30	-	6/24
MDP-GDP 100	-	12/24**
MDP-GDP 30	0.001	17/24**

** = $p < 0.01$

Mice were infected with 6×10^4 K. pneumoniae organisms, corresponding to 5 LD_{100}.

few hr before LPS, reaching a TNF yield approximately 100-fold higher than in LPS-treated controls. In all groups, mice were bled two hr after LPS injection.

Another example shown in Fig 1 was obtained with mice given a lipophilic MDP derivative. The priming effect of MDP-GDP is comparable to that obtained with MDP but the level of TNF activity was still above that in control animals receiving LPS alone when they had received MDP-GDP 24 or 48 hr before LPS (Fig 1). Rabbit antibodies directed at rMuTNF and that do not cross react with lymphotoxin were used to confirm that the cytotoxicity found in the blood was indeed due to TNF.

Although the primary target cells for MDP are likely to be macrophages, a possible T cell involvement in the release of TNF has been suggested by studies performed in animals primed with Propionibacterium acnes (19, 20). In nude Balb/c mice primed with MDP or derivatives, the potentiating effect was quite similar and LPS-induced TNF production was often higher than in nu/+ controls treated with MDP and LPS. The discrepancy with results previously reported with P. acnes is likely to be related to differences in the priming agent since in BCG-infected mice the response to various doses of LPS was similar in nu/+ and in nu/nu mice (18). In our assays the participation of T cell activity was not required for the priming effect of MDP or MDP-GDP. In both normal Swiss mice and Balb/c nude mice, gram-negative bacterial vaccines (typhoid or Bordetella pertussis vaccines) were very potent as eliciting agents at dosage levels which are less toxic than the effective dose LPS as evaluated in adrenalectomized mice or in mice primed with MDP.

<u>Absence of Correlation Between Circulating TNF Level Induced after Priming with MDP and Toxicity of the Combined Treatment</u>

In comparing several adjuvant-active MDP derivatives for their priming effect on TNF production, it was found that only some of them were active, i.e., those that have already been shown to stimulate resistance to infec-

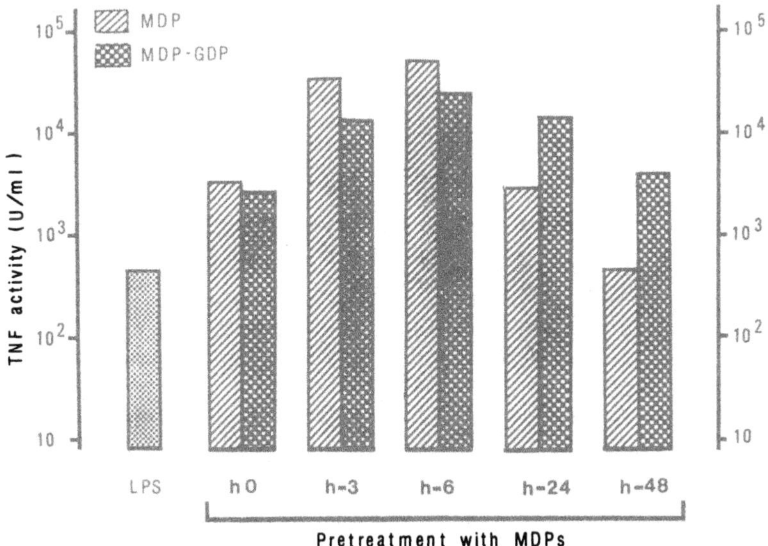

Fig 1. Priming effect of MDP or MDP-GDP on TNF production in mice subsequently treated with LPS at various time intervals. All mice received 25 μg of LPS intravenously and were bled 2 hr later. MDP or MDP-GDP was given by the same route.

Table 5. Comparative effect of some MDPs on TNF production and toxicity displayed by LPS

Priming agent*	Priming effect on TNF production	Toxicity
-	+	-
MDP	+ + +	+ + +
MDP (D,D)	+	-
Murabutide	+ + +	+

*300 μg by the intravenous route 3 hr before 25 μg LPS by the same route.

tions. Further comparative assays on toxic synergism with LPS have then demonstrated that there was no correlation between toxicity and level of circulating TNF. An example has been provided with murabutide as summarized in Table 5. The non-pyrogenic MDP analog is as potent as MDP in priming animals challenged with LPS to produce circulating TNF. MDP (D,D), an inactive analog of MDP used as a control, did not prime mice for TNF release and did not increase LPS toxicity. A similar pattern of response was observed with lipophilic derivatives. Thus, MDP-GDP enhanced the lethal effect of LPS and primed animals to produce TNF (see Fig 1), whereas MDP (D,D)-GDP, a stereoisomer which displayed comparable immunostimulating properties and was as effective in priming mice, did not decrease resistance to LPS toxicity. Several other examples have also been observed.

DISCUSSION

Many deleterious effects of LPS have been reproduced by injecting large amounts of recombinant human or mouse TNF to various animal species (1, 32). The prominent role of TNF in mediating the lethal effect of LPS in mice has been established by experiments showing that antibody to recombinant TNF could prevent the development of endotoxic shock (2). It has then been reported that sensitization to the lethal effect of LPS by various methods caused a high sensitivity to the toxicity of TNF, such as treatment with galactosamine (16), adrenalectomy, infections, etc. However, interactions with other cytokines cannot be excluded yet in the sensitizing effect to LPS toxicity.

Mechanisms involved in the toxic synergism produced by prior administration of MDP in LPS-treated mice are still unknown. The fact that MDP could prime mice for an increased production of circulating TNF when challenged with LPS indicated a possible relation between toxic effects and TNF level in the blood. However, comparative assays with several MDP derivatives were inconsistent with this hypothesis since, depending on the chemical structure, dissociation between the effects have been observed. Some MDP derivatives, particularly among the lipophilic ones, caused the production of large yields of circulating TNF without increasing the susceptibility of mice to LPS toxicity. All the cytotoxic activity found in sera was inhibited by rabbit antibodies raised to rMuTNF. Studies are being pursued to evaluate the capacity of the muramyl peptides to sensitize - or the opposite, i.e., to desensitize - animals to the toxic effect of exogenous TNF. MDP preparations are not contaminated by LPS but a synergy between TNF and other bacterial products has been reported to cause lethal shock (30).

The potentiation of LPS-induced tumor necrosis is likely to be related to an increased production of circulating TNF obtained with MDP and very small doses of LPS. After such treatment, which induced tumor necrosis, the level of TNF in the blood was rather low, confirming observations reported by Bloksma et al (3, 4). Obviously, the amount of exogenous TNF that induced tumor necrosis factor is higher than the circulating level recovered in the blood 2 hr after the LPS injection. This level may correspond to a continuous production and to an endogenous factor with a longer half-life than the single injection of exogenous factor. A possible role of vasoamine release should be considered (4), amplifying the vascular effects of TNF (21).

The priming effect of MDP and derivatives on the subsequent production of TNF elicited by a larger dose of LPS or a gram-negative bacterial preparation which could be demonstrated within a few hr induced the same pattern of response as priming with BCG organisms, i.e., the peak of cytotoxic activity found in the blood was reached within 2 hr and then declined, returning to the baseline 4 hr after LPS injection. Our working hypothesis is that the priming effect of MDPs which display an anti-infectious effect is related to the protection against a bacterial challenge. The bacterial inoculum may induce a rapid and transient production of TNF, sufficient to ensure an increased resistance. A marked enhancement of nonspecific resistance has been demonstrated against various gram-negative or gram-positive organisms (23, 27). The importance of TNF release at the early beginning of a bacterial challenge has been shown by the effect of anti-rTNF antibodies injected in mice that converted a non-lethal Listeria infection into a lethal one (11).

REFERENCES

1. Bauss, F., Dröge, W. and Männel, D. N., 1985, Tumor necrosis factor mediates endotoxic effects in mice. Infect. Immun. 55: 1622.

2. Beutler, B., Milsark, I. W. and Cerami, A. C., 1985, Passive immunization against cachectin/tumor necrosis factor protects mice from lethal effect of endotoxin. Science 229: 869.

3. Bloksma, N., Hofhuis, F. M. and Willers, J. M., 1984, Endotoxin-induced antitumor activity in the mouse is highly potentiated by muramyl dipeptide. Cancer Letters 23: 159.

4. Bloksma, N., Hofhuis, F. M. and Willers, J. M., 1984, Muramyl dipeptide is a powerful potentiator of the antitumor action of various tumor necrotizing agents. Cancer Immunol. Immunother. 17: 154.

5. Carswell, E. A., Old, L. J., Kassel, R. L., Green, S., Fiore, N. and Williamson, B., 1975, An endotoxin-induced serum factor that causes necrosis of tumors. Proc. Natl. Acad. Sci. USA 72: 3666.

6. Chedid, L., 1983, Muramyl peptides as possible endogenous immunopharmacological mediators. Microbiol. Immun. 27: 723.

7. Chedid, L., Audibert, F., Bona, C., Damais, C., Parant, F. and Parant, M., 1975, Biological activities of endotoxin detoxified by alkylation. Infect. Immun. 12: 714.

8. Chedid, L., Parant, M., Audibert, F., Riveau, G., Parant, F., Lederer, E., Choay, J. and Lefrancier, P., 1982, Biological activity of a new synthetic muramyl peptide adjuvant devoid of pyrogenicity. Infect. Immun. 35: 417.

9. Chedid, L., Parant, M., Parant, F., Lefrancier, P., Choay, J. and Lederer, E.,, 1977, Enhancement of non-specific immunity to Klebsiella

pneumoniae infection by a synthetic immunoadjuvant (N-acetyl-muramyl-L-alanyl-D-isoglutamine) and several analogs. Proc. Natl. Acad. Sci. USA 74: 2089.

10. Chedid, L., Parant, M., Parant, F., Audibert, F., Lefrancier, P., Choay, J. and Sela, M., 1979, Enhancement of certain biological activities of muramyl dipeptide derivatives after conjugation to a multi-poly(DL-alanyl)--poly(L-lysine) carrier. Proc. Natl. Acad. Sci. USA 76: 6557.

11. Havell, E. A., 1987, Production of tumor necrosis factor during murine Listeriosis. J. Immunol. 139: 4225.

12. Kotani, S., Takeda, H., Tsujimoto, M., Ogawa, T., Mori, Y., Koga, T., Iribe, H., Tanaka, A., Nagao, S., McGhee, J. R., Michalek, S. M., Kawata, S., Shiba, T. and Kusumoto, S., 1983, Lipophilic muramyl peptides and synthetic lipid A analogs as immunomodulators, in: "Progress in Immunology V," Y. Yamamura and T. Tada, eds., Academic Press, Japan.

13. Lederer, E., 1980, Syntheric immunostimulants derived from the bacterial cell wall. J. Med. Chem. 23: 819.

14. Lefrancier, P., Derrien, M., Jamet, X., Choay, J., Lederer, E., Audibert, F., Parant, F., Parant, M. and Chedid, L., 1982, Apyrogenic adjuvant-active N-acetylmuramyl dipeptides. J. Med. Chem. 25: 87.

15. Lefrancier, P. and Lederer, E., 1981, Chemistry of synthetic immunomodulant muramyl peptides. Prog. Chem. Org. Nat. Prod. 40: 1.

16. Lehmann, V., Freudenberg, M. A. and Galanos, C., 1987, Lethal toxicity of lipopolysaccharide and tumor necrosis factor in normal and D-galactosamine-treated mice. J. Exp. Med. 165: 657.

17. Level, M., Bernard, J. M., Lefrancier, P. and Phillips, N., 1984, New lipophilic muramyl dipeptide derivatives: synthesis and biological activity of their liposome encapsulated formulation, in: "Forum Peptides," B. Castro and J. Martinez, eds., Centre de Pharmacologie, Montpellier, France, p. 250.

18. Männel, D., Meltzer, M. S. and Mergenhagen, S. E., 1980, Generation and characterization of a lipopolysaccharide-induced and serum-derived factor for tumor cells. Infect. Immun. 28: 204.

19. Niitsu, Y., Watanabe, N., Sone, H., Neda, H. and Urushizaki, I., 1985, T cell involvement in production of tumor necrosis factor: reconstitution experiment with nude mice. Japanese J. Cancer Res. 76: 395.

20. Old. L. J., 1976, Tumor necrosis factor. Clin. Bull. 6: 118.

21. Palladino, M. A., Shalaby, M. R., Kramer, S. M., Ferraiolo, B. L., Baughman, R. A., Deleo, A. B., Crase, D., Marafino, B., Aggarwal, B. B., Figari, I. S., Liggitt, D. and Patton, J. S., 1987, Characterization of the antitumor activities of human tumor necrosis factor-α and the comparison with other cytokines: induction of tumor specific immunity. J. Immunol. 138: 4023.

22. Parant, M., 1983, Effect of LPS on nonspecific resistance to bacterial infections, in: "Beneficial Effects of Endotoxins," A. Nowotny, ed., Plenum Press, New York, p. 179.

23. Parant, M., 1988, Role of tumor necrosis factor in nonspecific stimulation of the mouse resistance to infections, in: "Tumor Necrosis

Factor/Cachectin, Lymphotoxins and Related Cytokines," H. Kirchner and B. Bonavida, eds., Karger, Basel, p. 234.

24. Parant, M. and Chedid, L., 1984, Stimulation of nonspecific resistance to infections by synthetic immunoregulatory agents. Infection 12: 230.

25. Parant, M. and Chedid, L., 1987, Muramyl dipeptides, host immunity and enhancement, in: "Antibiosis and Host Immunity," A. Szentivanyi, H. Friedman and G. Gillissen, eds., Plenum Press, New York, p. 291.

26. Parant, M., Parant, F. and Chedid, L., 1978, Enhancement of the neonate's non specific immunity to Klebsiella infection by muramyl dipeptide, a synthetic immunoadjuvant. Proc. Natl. Acad. Sci. USA 75: 3395.

27. Parant, M., Parant, F., Vinit, M. A. and Chedid, L., 1987, Action protectrice du tumor necrosis factor (TNF) obtenu par recombinaison génétique contre l'infection expérimentale bactérienne et fongique. C. R. Acad. Sci. Paris 304: 1.

28. Ribi, E. E., Cantrell, J. L., VonEschen, K. B. and Schwartzman, S. M., 1979, Enhancement of endotoxic shock by N-acetyl-L-alanyl-(L- seryl)-D-isoglutamine (muramyl dipeptide), Cancer Res. 39: 4756.

29. Ribi, E., Parker, R., Strain, S. M., Mizuno, Y., Nowotny, A., VonEschen, K. B., Cantrell, J. L., McLaughlin, C. A., Hwang, K. M. and Goren, M. B., 1979, Peptides as requirement for immunotherapy of the guinea-pig line-10 tumor with endotoxins. Cancer Immunol. Immunother. 7: 43.

30. Rothstein, J. L. and Schreiber, H., 1988, Synergy between tumor necrosis factor and bacterial products causes hemorrhagic necrosis and lethal shock in normal mice. Proc. Natl. Acad. Sci. USA 85: 607.

31. Ruff, M. R. and Gifford, G. E., 1981, Tumor necrosis factor, in: "Lymphokines Vol. 2," E. Pick, ed., Academic Press, New York, p. 235.

32. Tracey, K. J., Beutler, B., Lowry, S. F., Merryweather, J., Wolpe, S., Milsark, I. W., Hariri, R. J., Fahey, T. J., Zentella, A., Albert, J. D., Shires, G. T, and Cerami, A., 1986, Shock and tissue injury induced by recombinant human cachectin. Science 234: 470.

THE MEDIATION OF ENDOTOXIN-INDUCED BENEFICIAL EFFECTS BY CYTOKINES

R. Urbaschek and B. Urbaschek

Department of Immunology and Serology, Institute of Medical Microbiology and Hygiene, Klinikum Mannheim, University of Heidelberg, D6, 5; 6800 Mannheim; FRG

INTRODUCTION

Endotoxins, when entering the circulation in sufficient amounts, elicit multiple effects that can lead to shock and death. Besides these detrimental effects, endotoxins in minute concentrations may nonspecifically contribute to regulate the steady state of host defense. Moreover, various experimental approaches have shown, already in the early years of endotoxin research, that injection of small amounts of extracted endotoxins can induce beneficial effects, such as tolerance to the pyrogenic and lethal effects of endotoxin, nonspecific resistance to microbial infections and irradiation disease, stimulation of hematopoiesis, as well as tumor regression. These beneficial effects of endotoxins have been reviewed recently (13).

It is well established that the major target cell of endotoxin is the macrophage and that cytokines are involved in the mediation of endotoxic effects. Our interest was to study in several experimental models whether tumor necrosis factor (TNF) or interleukin-1 (IL-1) are involved in mediating endotoxin-induced beneficial effects. These two cytokines were chosen because TNF and IL-1 were detected in those serum fractions from mediator-rich tumor necrosis serum (TNS) that transferred radioprotection, nonspecific resistance to gut-derived infection and stimulation of hematopoiesis (18, 19, 20).

The results of the experiments presented here, 1) emphasize that ng amounts of endotoxins are sufficient to induce potent protection to the lethal effects of endotoxin and that dose-dependent timing of pretreatment is crucial, 2) demonstrate that IL-1 and TNF differ in their mediation of beneficial effects in the experimental models used.

MATERIALS AND METHODS

Female NMRI mice (Zentralinstitut fur Versuchstierzucht, Hannover, FRG) or C3H/HeJ mice (Jackson Laboratory, Bar Harbor, Maine) were used. Endotoxin was extracted from E. coli 0119. Recombinant human TNF α (specific activity 2 x 10^7 U/mg) was supplied by Knoll/BASF (Ludwigshafen, FRG). The Limulus-Amebocyte-Lysate (LAL) activity measured with a kinetic LAL microtiter test (6) was < 0.4 ng/μg rHuTNF. Recombinant mouse and human IL-1 α (specific activity 2 x 10^8 U/mg and 1 x 10^8 U/mg respectively) were a kind gift of Dr. P. Lomedico (Hoffmann-La Roche, Nutley, New Jersey). The LAL activity was 1.7 ng/2000 U and 15 pg/2000 U respectively.

Table 1. Endotoxin tolerance. NMRI mice were challenged i.v. with different concentrations of endotoxin without or with i.v. pretreatment (-3 days) of 1 ug of endotoxin. n = 10

Endotoxin ug/mouse	% Lethality	
	Pretreated	Control*
250	0	
225	0	
200	0	100
175	0	70
150		60
125		40

*LD_{50} = 144 μg; f = 2.4

Endotoxin Tolerance

Three days or 24 hr before a lethal i.v. challenge with endotoxin mice were injected i.v. with either endotoxin, rHuTNF or rMuIL-1, or rHuIL-1. In order to provide the means to compare the potency of endotoxin tolerance inducing substances with other laboratories in addition to the shift in LD_{50} we describe an index taking into account the steepness of endotoxin lethality curves. Thus, a potency factor is calculated:

$$f = \frac{\text{Dosis } (LD_{50})}{\text{Dosis } (LD_{75}) - \text{Dosis } (LD_{25})}$$

The endotoxin used resulted in f = 2.4 (Table 1).

Irradiation

Mice were exposed in plexiglass containers to 650, 725 or 850 cGy whole body irradiation with a ^{60}Cobalt source (72 cGy/min) at the German Cancer Research Center, Heidelberg, FRG. They were pretreated i.v. with rHuTNF (5 μg) or rHuIL-1 (2000 U) at 24 hr before irradiation exposure.

Septicemia

In ether anesthesia, septicemia was induced by cecal ligation and puncture in mice (17). They were treated i.v. with rHuIL-1, rMuIL-1 or rHuTNF. Lethality rates following endotoxin challenge, irradiation or septicemia were recorded.

GM-CFC Assay

Colony formation by GM-CFC's (granulocyte macrophage colony forming cells) was measured by a semi-solid agar assay in 35 mm culture dishes. To 1.0 ml enriched McCoy medium and 0.3% agar containing 1 x 10^5 nucleated murine bone marrow cells 25 μl of standard GM-CSF (obtained from mice 2 hr after 5 μg of endotoxin) was added as well as different concentrations of rHuIL-1, rMuIL-1, rHuTNF, or endotoxin in a volume of 25 μl. After incubation at 37°C for 7 days in a humidified atmosphere of 7.5% CO_2, colonies of more than 50 cells were counted. They were compared to the number of colonies stimulated by 25 μl CSF plus 25 μl saline.

Statistics

Statistical comparisons were carried out using Chi square and student's tests.

RESULTS AND DISCUSSION

The results in Table 1 represent an example of the characteristic potency of one single injection of endotoxin (1 μg) to induce tolerance to the lethal effects of endotoxin. After pretreatment with 1 μg at day 7 before the lethal challenge the induction of tolerance is lost (data not shown). The significance of the time of pretreatment and the concentration of endotoxin used to elicit tolerance (9) is supported by the results shown in Table 2. Moreover, the fact that a concentration of as low as 1 ng of endotoxin has a protective effect is demonstrated. Complete protection is achieved with 10 ng of endotoxin in this experiment when injected 3 days before the lethal challenge. This tolerance is lost when this amount is injected at -24 hr. At this time 100 ng of endotoxin are sufficient to cause complete tolerance to the 100% lethal challenge. These results emphasize the need to consider the potential effect of ng amounts of endotoxin when testing activities of substances that may be contaminated with endotoxins; especially when synergistic effects with endotoxin are expected, for example with cytokines such as TNF (16).

The complex phenomenon of tolerance to endotoxin lethality has been discussed in detail by Greisman (10) who pointed to the role of RES macrophages, in particular the Kupffer cells, as a major endotoxin target. Vital microscopic observations of responses of Kupffer cells and the hepatic microvasculature to endotoxin revealed the impairment of Kupffer cell function and integrity, which is reversed during endotoxin tolerance (11). The results obtained from studies of different endotoxin mediators - CSF, IL-1, TNF, and IFN - measured individually in the same samples of serum from endotoxin-tolerant and nontolerant BCG-infected mice, respectively, further support the central role of macrophages in the mechanisms of endotoxin tolerance. The refractory status of the macrophage that is established by the tolerance-inducing injection (10) was indicated in our experiments by the absence of TNF - a macrophage product - in tolerant BCG-infected mice after a lethal challenge with endotoxin (20). Macrophages also had been found to be refractory to endotoxin-induced prostaglandin production in the state of endotoxin tolerance (15). Further studies of the changes in the production or release of different mediators in endotoxin tolerance may give more insight into the

Table 2. Endotoxin tolerance. NMRI mice were challenged with 200 μg of endotoxin after i.v. pretreatment with endotoxin or rMuIL-1. Control 100% lethality; 10/10 mice.

Substances	Pretreatment -4 days		Pretreatment -24 hr	
	dead/total	% lethality	dead/total	%lethality
Endotoxin 1 ng	6/10	60*	9/10	90
Endotoxin 10 ng	0/10	0***	9/10	90
Endotoxin 100 ng	0/10	0***	6/10	60*
rMuIL-1 2000U			3/8	37.5**

* $p \leq 0.05$
** $p \leq 0.01$
*** $P \leq 0.001$

underlying mechanisms. This may also explain why the time of expression of tolerance to endotoxin is inversely related to tolerance to endotoxin-induced responses of the thermoregulatory center (9). Mice tolerating the lethal challenge did not produce TNF, however, IL-1 and IFN, both fever inducing substances (5), still were detectable in these mice (20).

Whereas IL-1 significantly reduced endotoxin-related lethality (Table 2). TNF failed to induce endotoxin tolerance in these experiments also when injected 3 days before lethal doses of endotoxin (data not shown). When the endotoxin challenge resulted in 63% lethality in control mice, pretreatment with 5 µg of TNF at -24 hr did induce tolerance ($p \leq 0.05$). By repeated pretreatment with TNF tolerance was achieved to the lethal effects of endotoxin as well as to TNF toxicity in rats (7).

IL-1 has been described to induce nonspecific resistance to Listeria, Pseudomonas or Klebsiella infection (3, 14). In the cecal ligation and puncture model used - simulating clinical situations after severe peritonitis-IL-1 significantly reduced the lethality, whereas TNF did not (Table 3).

On the other hand, IL-1 failed to elicit a radioprotective effect in endotoxin low responder C3H/HeJ mice, while TNF was capable of significantly reducing radiation caused lethality (Table 4). TNF induced radioprotection was first reported in 1986 (22). This radioprotection correlates with the stimulation of hematopoiesis as evidenced by an increase of GM-CFC and CSF by TNF (21, 24). Both IL-1 preparations did not show an elevation of GM-CFC in our experiments (22). The fact that rHuIL-1 and also rMuIL-1 (tested in several experiments, data not shown) failed to elicit in C3H/HeJ mice the reported potent IL-1 induced radioprotection (12) is still unexplained. When IL-1 and TNF were compared in their effects on GM-CFC in culture in the presence of postendotoxin serum as source of CSF, only TNF induced an increase in the number of GM-CFC (Table 5). Suppressive effects on the development of GM-CFC by TNF in culture was observed when murine cell-conditioned media were used as sources of GM-CSF (2). Thus, the enhancing effects of TNF on GM-CSF used in our experiments are due to factors present in postendotoxin serum. Endotoxin per se did not influence the activity of CSF (Table 5).

Table 3. Gut-derived septicemia induced by cecal ligation and puncture in NMRI mice without or with i.v. treatment of endotoxin rHuIL-1, rMuIL-1, or rHuTNF. n = 10

Substances	Time of Treatment	% Lethality
Control		80
Endotoxin 1 µg	- 24 hr	20**
rHuIL-1 2000U	- 24 hr	30*
rMuIL-1 2000U	- 24 hr	30*
rHuTNF 5 µg	- 24 hr	50

* $p \leq 0.05$
** $p \leq 0.01$

Table 4. Radioprotection. C3H/HeJ mice were exposed to different doses of ^{60}Cobalt whole body irradiation without or with i.v. pretreatment (-24hr) of rHuTNF (5 µg) or rHuIL-1 (2000 U). n = 9

Pretreatment	Doses cGy	Cumulative Lethality in % Days after Irradiation 12	16	20	24	30
Control	700	0	22	33	33	33
	775	11	66	100		
	850	11	100			
rHuTNF	700	0	0	0	11	11
	775	0	0	0	0	0**
	850	22	55	55	55	55*
rHuIL-1	700	0	0	0	0	0
	775	11	33	77	77	77
	850	11	88	100		

* $p \leq 0.05$
** $p \leq 0.001$

It can be concluded that both TNF and IL-1 mediate endotoxin-induced beneficial effects. Whereas TNF is capable of stimulating granulopoiesis and of inducing radioprotection in our experiments, IL-1 was more potent in eliciting protective effects to lethal doses of endotoxin and to gut-derived septicemia. The cytokines have been described to share many biological activities in common, however, it becomes more apparent that they differ in some of their activities (4).

Considering these beneficial effects of IL-1 and TNF it is evident that in all models tested, the mediator-rich TNS is more potent (18, 19, 20) than these cytokines per se. This points to the potential synergistic effect of several cytokines present in TNS. Synergisms of cytokines in the induction of resistance to infection has been described (1). Moreover, small amounts of endotoxin are more effective than IL-1 or TNF alone. In regard to the potential therapeutic use, however, endotoxin is not suitable because of its toxicity. In this respect preparations that have beneficial effects such as a nontoxic native protoplasmic polysaccharide, NPP, from E. coli (23) or an endotoxin-derived polysaccharide (8) are of special interest. It was observed for instance that the nontoxic White polysaccharide preparation induces the release of IL-1 (8). The endogenous release of cytokines by injecting nontoxic substances mediating beneficial effects may be more efficient than the administration of cytokines. In this case several mediators would be released in their physiological sequence, they may be available more continuously at their site of action, and their physiological synergism may occur.

ACKNOWLEDGEMENT

We wish to thank Dr. K.-H. Höver, German Cancer Research Center, Heidelberg, for his interest, and his advice in the performance of irradiation. We are grateful to Bettina Sieburg and Birgit Gropp for excellent technical assistance.

Table 5. Number of colonies stimulated in the presence of CSF

rHuTNF pro ml	Colonies[1]	rHuIL-1 U/ml	Colonies[1]	rMuIL-1 U/ml	Colonies[1]	Endotoxin pro ml	Colonies[1]
0.1 ng	93±6	0.2	115±12	0.02	77±11	1.0 pg	103±10
1.0 ng	100±4	2.0	111±14	0.2	91±6	10.0 pg	99±10
10.0 ng	118±8	20.0	122±5	2.0	100±15	0.1 ng	95±18
0.1 ug	145±12***	200.0	116±4	20.0	85±9	1.0 ng	101±22
1.0 ug	150±8***	2000.0	107±14	200.0	98±9	10.0 ng	91±16
10.0 ug	145±9***					1.0 ug	93±8

[1]In % of control (100% = 74 ± 12 colonies/25 ul CSF/1 x 10^5 bone marrow cells/ml; ± sd

***$p \leq 0.001$

REFERENCES

1. Belosevic, M., Davis, C. E., Meltzer, M. S., and Nacy, C. A., 1988, Regulation of activated macrophage antimicrobial activities, Identification of lymphokines that cooperate with IFN-γ for induction of resistance to infection. J. Immunol. 141: 890.

2. Broxmeyer, H. E., Williams, D. E., Lu, L., Cooper, S., Anderson, S. L., Beyer, G. S., Hoffman, R., and Rubin, B. Y., 1986, The suppressive influences of human tumor necrosis factors on bone marrow hematopoietic progenitor cells from normal donors and patients with leukemia: synergism of tumor necrosis factor and interferon-γ, J. Immunol. 136: 4487.

3. Czuprynski, C. J., and Brown, J. F., 1987, Recombinant murine interleukin-1 enhancement of nonspecific antibacterial resistance. Infect. Immun. 55: 2061.

4. Dinarello, C. A., 1987, The biology of interleukin 1 and comparison to tumor necrosis factor. Immunol. Letters 16: 227.

5. Dinarello, C. A., Cannon, J. G., and Wolff, S. M., 1988, New concepts on the pathogenesis of fever, in: "Perspectives on Bacterial Pathogenesis and Host Defense," B. Urbaschek, ed., The University of Chicago Press, Chicago.

6. Ditter, B., Becker, K.-P., Urbaschek, R., and Urbaschek, B., 1983, Quantitativer Endotoxinnachweis. Automatisierter, kinetischer Limulus-Amobozyten-Lysat Mikrotiter-Test mit Messung probenabhängiger Interferenzen. ArzneimittelForsch/Drug Res. 33: 681.

7. Fraker, D. L., Stovroff, M. C., Merino, M. J., and Norton, J. A., 1988, Tolerance to tumor necrosis factor in rats and the relationship to endotoxin tolerance and toxicity. J. Exp. Med. 168: 95.

8. Friedman, H., Blanchard, D. K., Newton, C., Klein, T., Stewart, II, W., Keler, T., and Nowotny, A., 1987, Distinctive immunomodulatory effects of endotoxin and nontoxic lipopolysaccharide derivatives in lymphoid cell cultures. J. Biol. Resp. Modif. 6: 664.

9. Greer, G. G., and Rietschel, E. Th., 1978, Inverse relationship between the susceptibility of lipoplysaccharide (lipid A)-pretreated mice to the hypothermic and lethal effect of lipopolysaccharide. Infect. Immun. 20: 366.

10. Greisman, S. E., 1983, Induction of endotoxin tolerance, in: "Beneficial Effects of Endotoxins," A. Nowotny, ed., Plenum Press, New York.

11. McCuskey, R. S., Urbaschek, R., McCuskey, P. A., and Urbaschek, B., 1983, In vivo microscopic observations of the responses of Kupffer cells and the hepatic microcirculation to Mycobacterium bovis BCG alone and in combination with endotoxin. Infect. Immun. 42: 362.

12. Neta, R., Douches, S. D., and Oppenheim, J. J., 1986, Interleukin-1 is a radioprotector. J. Immunol. 136: 2483.

13. Nowotny, A., 1983, "Beneficial Effects of Endotoxins," Plenum Press, New York

14. Ozaki, Y., Ohashi, T., Minami, A., and Nakamura, S.-I., 1987, Enhanced resistance of mice to bacterial infection induced by recombinant human interleukin-1α, Infect. Immun. 55: 1436.

15. Rietschel, E. Th., Schade, U., Jensen, M., Wollenweber, H. W., Lüderitz, O., and Greisman, S. E., 1982, Bacterial endotoxins: Chemical structure, biological activity and role in septicaemia. Scand. J. Infect. Dis. 31 (Suppl.): 8.

16. Rothstein, J. L., and Schreiber, H., 1988, Synergy between tumor necrosis factor and bacterial products causes hemorrhagic necrosis and lethal shock in normal mice. Proc. Natl. Acad. Sci. (USA) 85: 607.

17. Urbaschek, B., Ditter, B., Becker, K.-P., and Urbaschek, R., 1984, Protective effects and role of endotoxin in experimental septicemia. Circ. Shock 14: 209.

18. Urbaschek, R., and Urbaschek, B., 1982, Aspects of beneficial endotoxin-mediated effects. Klin. Wochenschr. 60: 746.

19. Urbaschek, R., and Urbaschek, B., 1983, Ability of post-endotoxin serum from BCG-infected mice to induce nonspecific resistance and stimulation of granulopoiesis. Infect. Immun. 39: 1488.

20. Urbaschek, R., Männel, D. N., Mergenhagen, S. E., and Urbaschek, B., 1986, The role of post-endotoxin serum components from BCG infected mice in the protection of compromised hosts, in: "Immunobiology and Immunopharmacology of Bacterial Endotoxins," A. Szentivanyi, H. Friedman, and A. Nowotny, eds. Plenum Press, New York.

21. Urbaschek, R., Männel, D. N., and Urbaschek, B., 1987, Tumor necrosis factor induced stimulation of granulopoiesis and radioprotection. Lymph. Res. 6: 179.

22. Urbaschek, R., and Urbaschek, B., 1987, Tumor necrosis factor and interleukin 1 as mediators of endotoxin-induced beneficial effects. Rev. Infect. Dis. 9: S607.

23. Urbaschek, R., Urbaschek, B., and Ribi, E., 1985, Induction of nonspecific resistance, endotoxin tolerance and colony-stimulating activity (CSA) by nontoxic LPS components. Fed. Proc. 44: 1490.

24. Vogel, S. N., Douches, S. D., Kaufman, E. N., Neta, R., 1987, Induction of colony stimulating factor in vivo by recombinant interleukin 1 α and recombinant tumor necrosis factor α . J. Immunol. 138: 2143.

THE MECHANISM OF ADJUVANT ACTION OF BACTERIAL LIPOPOLYSACCHARIDE (LPS) IN SUBCUTANEOUS IMMUNIZATION

Y. Inoue and T. Yokochi

Department of Microbiology, Fukui Medical School
Fukui 910-11, Japan

Bacterial lipopolysaccharide (LPS) exhibits an adjuvant action on antibody response to various antigens in mice. The adjuvant action induced by subcutaneous (s.c.) injection of LPS with antigen is different from that by intraperitoneal (i.p.) or intravenous (i.v.) injection (2). In the present study, we investigated histological changes at the regional s.c. tissues after injection with LPS and the tissue distribution of the LPS. It was suggested that there were two distinct mechanisms of adjuvant action which operated at the early and late stages after s.c. immunization, respectively.

Klebsiella LPS (KO3 LPS) and Escherichia coli LPS (EO9 LPS) were prepared from Klebsiella sp. strain LEN-1 (O3:K1-), and E. coli O9 strain B993 (O9:K-:H-), respectively, by the phenol water method (4). LPS from Salmonella typhosa (Stph LPS), S. enteritidis (Sent LPS), E. coli O128 (EO128 LPS) and E. coli O111 (EO111 LPS) prepared by the Westphal method were purchased from Difco Laboratories, Detroit, Mich., U.S.A. The rough form of LPS (R-LPS) was prepared from the rough mutant of strain LEN-1. The lipid A was isolated from the KO3 LPS by hydrolysis with acetic acid. LPS was injected s.c. at the inguinal region of the SMA strain of mice and the regional skin tissues were removed various days after injection, fixed and stained with hematoxylin and eosin. LPS was radiolabeled with ^{125}I or ^{51}Cr (1, 3), and the radioactivity in various organs was determined by a gamma scintillation counter.

Histology

The histological examinations were made in the regional skin tissues of mice injected s.c. with 100 μg of LPS. At one day after injection with KO3 LPS, a number of polymorphonuclear leukocytes (PMN) infiltrated in the dermis and fatty tissue, and the number of PMN increased markedly up to 5 days. The cells infiltrated even into the s.c. muscular tissue. At 10 days, a large number of endothelial cells and fibroblasts proliferated in the lesions induced by KO3 LPS. At 14 days, the s.c. fatty tissue was virtually occupied by granulation tissues, and the formation of several lymphoid follicles was observed in those tissues. The mitosis of lymphocytes was seen at the center of the follicles and many plasma cells were detected in the periphery of the follicles. Injection with Styp LPS also induced the accumulation of PMN, although the number of PMN was much less. On the other hand, Sent LPS, EO9 LPS, EO128 LPS and EO111 LPS exclusively induced the infiltration of mononuclear (MN) cells in the dermis. The order of intensity to promote cell infiltration was K03 LPS (3:1)> > Styp LPS (2:1) > Sent LPS (1:2), E09 LPS (1:2), E0128 LPS (1:2) > E0111 LPS (1:2). The proportion in parenthesis indicates the ratio of PMN to MN cells, infiltrating at the regional site. All LPSs tested except K03 LPS, caused no significant histological changes at the regional site throughout the course of experiment. R-LPS and lipid A derived from K03 LPS mainly induced the accumulation of MN cells at the dermis with neither significant tissue damages nor proliferation of endothelial cells and the formation of lymphoid follicles.

Tissue Distribution of LPS

The tissue distribution of ^{51}Cr- or ^{125}I-labeled K03 LPS after s.c. and i.p. injection was examined. A large amount of K03 LPS remained for a long period at the regional site when injected s.c.. About half of the injected LPS still remained even after 14 days, while there was no such retention of LPS in the case of i.p. injection. There was no marked difference in the level of retention at the regional site among various LPS tested. R-LPS and lipid A remained at the regional site for a longer time than K03 LPS.

Adjuvant Action

The 20% suspension of the syngeneic eyeball extract (0.1 ml) and LPS (100 μg) was injected s.c., and the intensity of the adjuvant action of LPS on the primary antibody response to the eyeball antigen was measured. The titer of antibody was estimated by an indirect solid phase radioimmunoassay using ^{125}I-labeled protein A. The antibody production to the syngeneic eye extract was strongly augmented by K03 LPS and Styp LPS, although the adjuvant action of K03 LPS was the strongest. The order of strength of adjuvant action was K03 LPS > Styp LPS > E09 LPS > Sent LPS > E0128 LPS > E0111 LPS.

The intensity of adjuvant action of various LPSs on antibody response to otherwise nonimmunogenic autoantigen paralleled the activity to induce the infiltration of inflammatory cells. The infiltration of PMN seemed to play an important role for triggering helper T cells, because K03 LPS and Styp LPS which preferentially induced the accumulation of PMN at the regional site exhibited the strong adjuvant action. It is conceivable that the lysozomal enzymes released by PMN promote antigen processing in the regional s.c. microenvironment, resulting in enhanced activation of antigen-specific helper T cells.

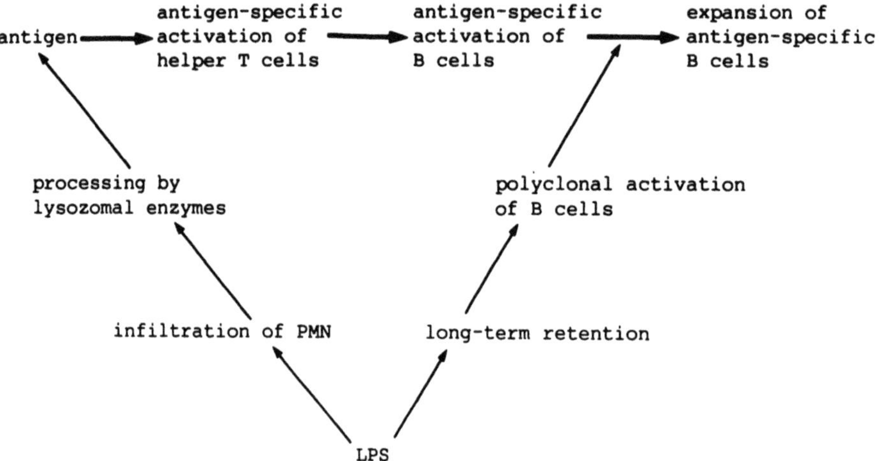

Fig 1. A proposed scheme of the mechanism of adjuvant action of LPS.

All LPSs remained at the regional site for a long period. The remaining LPS could persistently stimulate polyclonal activation of antigen-specific B cells which were initially triggered by helper T cell at the early stage. This idea was supported by the histological findings that B lymphocytes proliferated in the lymphoid follicles in the s.c. tissues at the late stage. Finally, we provide the possible scheme of two mechanisms which consecutively operate at the early and late stages in the adjuvant action of s.c. injected LPS (Fig 1).

REFERENCES

1. Braun, D. G., Hild, K. and Ziegler, A., 1979, Resolution of immunoglobulin patterns by analytical isoelectrofocusing, in: "Immunological Methods," I. Lefkovits and B. Permis, eds., Academic Press, New York.

2. Nakashima, I., Nagase, F., Matsuura, A., Yokochi, T. and Kato, N., 1980, Adjuvant actions of polyclonal lymphocyte activators. III. Two distinct types of T-initiating adjuvant action demonstrated under different experimental conditions. Cell Immunol. 52: 429.

3. Noyes, H. E., McInturf, C. R. and Blahuta, G. J., 1959, Studies on distribution of Escherichia coli endotoxin in mice. Pro. Soc. Exp. Biol. and Med. 100: 65.

4. Westphal, O., 1975, Bacterial endotoxins. Int. Rev. Allergy Appl. Immunol. 49: 1.

LIPID A, THE IMMUNOSTIMULATORY PRINCIPLE OF LIPOPOLYSACCHARIDES ?

H. Loppnow**, I. Dürrbaum*, H. Brade*, C. A. Dinarello**, S. Kusumoto***, E. Th. Rietschel* and H.-D. Flad*

*Forschungsinstitut Borstel, D-2061 Borstel, FRG;
**Tufts University School of Medicine, Boston, USA; and
***University of Osaka, Osaka, Japan

INTRODUCTION

Lipopolysaccharide (LPS) is an inducer of toxic and immunostimulatory or immunoregulatory responses (2). The lipid A moiety was shown to be the endotoxic principle of LPS (3, 9). Data about immunostimulatory properties like induction of interleukin 1 (IL-1) by LPS and lipid A are still conflicting. In this report LPS and partial structures thereof were used to define the structural element of LPS which is responsible for IL-1 induction. Evidence is given that lipid A is not only the endotoxic but also the major immunostimulatory and immunoregulatory principle of LPS.

MATERIAL AND METHODS

The substances used for induction experiments are S- and R-form LPS, synthetic lipid A or synthetic lipid A partial structures (Fig 1), and core-oligosaccharides of LPS (Fig 2; see also Ref. 1, 4, 8). For induction experiments 5 x 10^6 mononuclear cells per ml (MNC/ml) isolated on Percoll or two types of adherent cells were used. Briefly, cells adherent to culture flasks (ADH) were isolated and adjusted to 2 x 10^6 ADH/ml. Furthermore, cells adherent to wells of 24 well culture plates (C-ADH) were used. All induction experiments were performed at serum free conditions. IL-1 activities were detected in thymocyte comitogenic and/or fibroblast proliferation assays as described (6). Intracellular IL-1 (icIL-1) was detected after disrupting the cells by freezing.

RESULTS

Numerous dose response experiments with LPS and partial structures thereof are summarized in Fig 3, where the minimal concentrations necessary for IL-1 induction are listed. The results varied within two or three orders of magnitude because different donors were used in the various experiments. It is obvious that lipid A (506) like LPS is a strong inducer of IL-1. Synthetic monodephosphorylated lipid A compounds (505, 504) are weaker inducers. Pentaacylated partial structures like LA20PH are very weak inducers or not active. The tetraacylated synthetic precursor of lipid A failed to induce release of IL-1, bisacylated oligoacyl structures also failed to induce IL-1 release. Core-oligosaccharides are very weak inducers of IL-1 or not active. Dose response experiments were also performed with MNC and two types of adherent cells (ADH and C-ADH). Comparable minimal doses were detected when

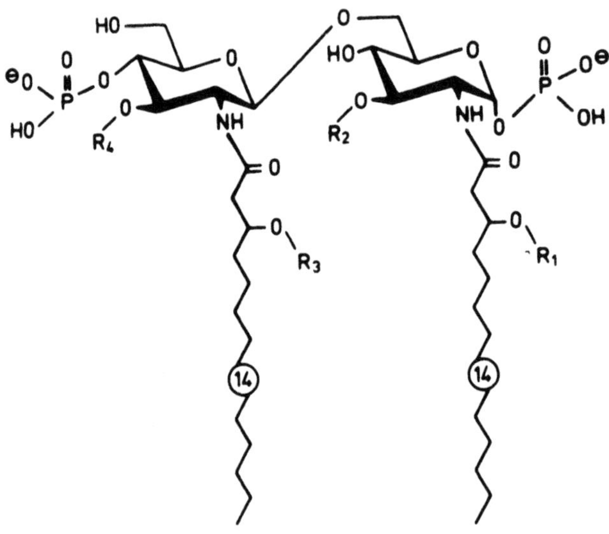

Synthetic compound		Nature of R4	R3	R2	R1	Number of fatty acids
516 (LA 16-PP)	(Heptaacyl S.minnesota Lipid A)	14:0 (3-0 14:0)[1]	12:0[2]	14:0 (3-OH)[3]	16:0[4]	7
506 (LA 15-PP)	(E.coli Lipid A)	14:0 (3-0 14:0)	12:0	14:0 (3-OH)	H	6
LA 22-PP	(C.violaceum-type Lipid A	14:0 (3-OH)	14:0[5]	14:0 (3-OH)	14:0	6
LA 21-PP	(Isomer of precursor Ib)	14:0 (3-OH)	16:0	14:0 (3-OH)	H	5
LA 20-PP	(Precursor Ib)	14:0 (3-OH)	H	14:0 (3-OH)	16:0	5
406 (LA 14-PP)	(Precursor Ia)	14:0 (3-OH)	H	14:0 (3-OH)	H	4
606 (LA 19-PP)	(De-O-acyl-Lipid A)	H	H	H	H	2

1) (R)-3-(tetradecanoyloxy)tetradecanoyl 2) dodecanoyl
3) (R)-3-Hydroxytetradecanoyl 4) hexadecanoyl
5) tetradecanoyl

Fig 1. Chemical structures of synthetic lipid A and synthetic partial structures of lipid A.

The structures of the bisphosphorylated compounds are shown. The monophosphorylated structures can be derived from this figure by using the code as shown in the example below:

506/LA15-PP = Bisphosphorylated compound
505/LA15-HP = 4'-monodephospho partial structure
504/LA15-PH = 1-monodephospho partial structure

I

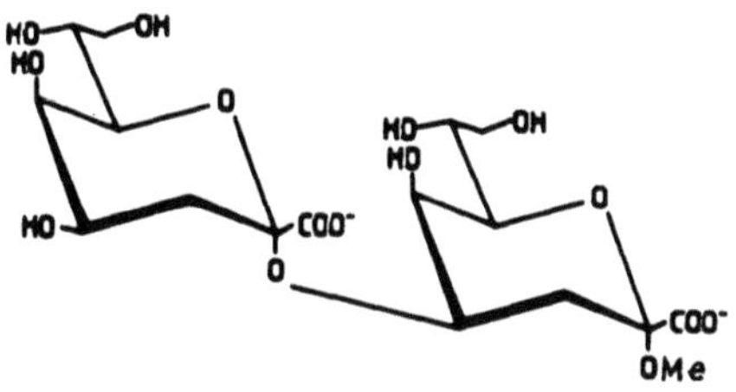

II

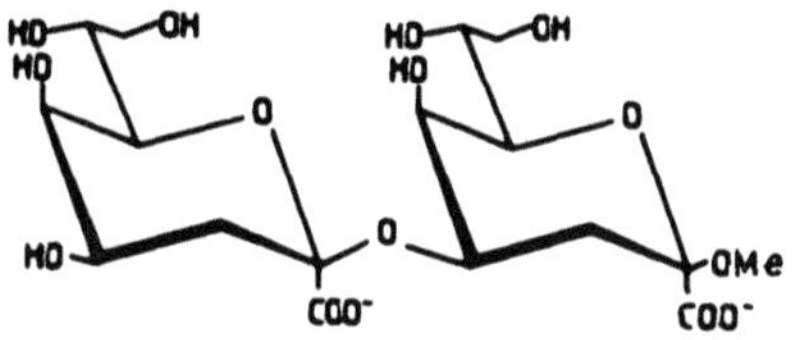

III

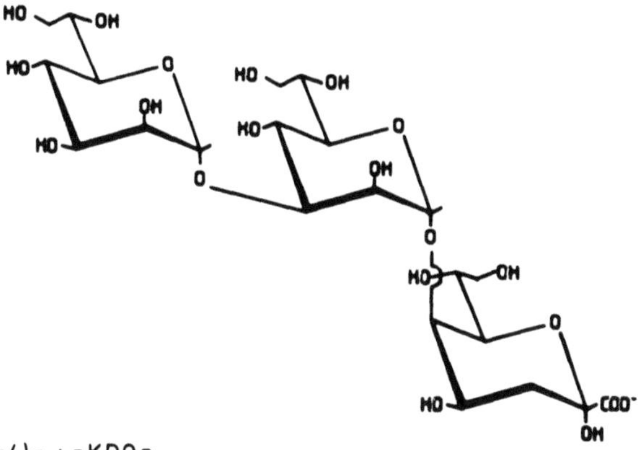

I - α-KDOp-(2-4)-α-KDOp

II - β-KDOp-(2-4)-α-KDOp

III - α-Hep-(1-3)-α-Hep-(1-5)-KDO (isolated from *S minnesota*)

Fig 2. Structures of synthetic and natural core oligosaccharides. Compounds I and II are synthetic disaccharides (see ref. 8). Compound III is a natural core oligosaccharide isolated from **S. minnesota.**

	-----α-helix----- ---Ca^{2+} binding loop--- ----α-helix----	Score
TEST	E L - - L L - - L O - O - O G - L O - - O L - - L L - - L	
(a)	Ⓔ H S V R N F V G Ⓠ A K S Ⓢ Ⓖ L Ⓘ Ⓣ Q R Ⓠ A E Q Ⓕ Ⓘ S Q Y	9
(b)	Ⓔ H S V R D F V S Ⓠ A K S Ⓢ Ⓖ L Ⓘ Ⓣ E K Ⓔ A Q T Ⓕ Ⓘ S Q Y	9
(c)	Q A K S S G L I T Ⓠ R Ⓠ A Ⓔ Q F Ⓘ Ⓢ Q Y Ⓝ	6
(d)	Q A K S S G L I T Ⓔ K Ⓔ A Ⓠ T F Ⓘ Ⓢ Q Y Ⓠ/Ⓔ	6

Fig 3. Minimal concentrations necessary for induction of IL-1 as detected in numerous experiments, determined in thymocyte comitogenic and/or fibroblast proliferation assay (Reproduced from 11; courtesy of J. Immunol.).

a) - synthetic **S. minnesota** lipid A
b) - synthetic **E. coli** lipid A
c) - synthetic **E. coli** monodephospho lipid A
d) - synthetic **C. violaceum** lipid A
e, f, g) - core-oligosaccharides

Table 1. Comparison of two differently isolated types of adherent cells in IL-1 induction experiments

Interleukin 1 inducer	Minimal concentration (pg/ml) necessary for IL-1[a] induction with two types of adherent cells			
	Experiment A		Experiment B	
	MNC	ADH[b]	MNC	C-ADH[c]
S-form LPS	10^1	10^2	1	1
Re LPS	10^1	10^2	1	10^7
Synthetic lipid A (506)	10^2	10^3	10^2	10^7
Synthetic lipid A precursor Ia (406)	0	0	0	0

[a] determined in fibroblast proliferation assay
[b] cells isolated by adherence on culture flasks
[c] cells adherent to wells of 24 well culture plates

MNC and ADH were analyzed (Table 1); in contrast ill defined C-ADH were stimulated by S-form LPS over a wide dose range, whereas R-form LPS and lipid A were only weak inducers of IL-1 (Table 1). The synthetic precursor Ia (compound 406) of lipid A did not induce release of IL-1 activity in any of these experiments. To ascertain that indeed IL-1 is not induced by the synthetic precursor Ia, MNC were analyzed for icIL-1. Table 2 shows that LPS and synthetic lipid A induce icIL-1, while the precursor was completely inactive.

Table 2. Comparison of released and intracellular IL-1 activity induced with synthetic lipid A precursor Ia

Stimuli	Concentration (pg/ml)	IL-1 activity (U/ml)[a]	
		Released to supernatant	Intracellular
Medium	-	2	1
LPS	10	156	103
Synthetic lipid A (506)	10	55	48
Synthetic lipid A precursor Ia (406)	10	< 1	< 1

[a] determined in fibroblast proliferation assay

DISCUSSION

Lipid A was postulated to be the endotoxic principle of LPS (9), a hypothesis which has been proven to be correct (7). Besides the endotoxic activities, the beneficial activities of LPS are important. IL-1 induction was used here as an immunostimulatory model for beneficial activities. We could show in this report that synthetic lipid A is a potent inducer of IL-1, comparable to LPS in terms of minimal doses necessary for IL-1 induction. Induction experiments with defined ADH (2×10^6/ml) showed that in contrast to C-ADH, these 90-95% nonspecific-esterase positive cells induced IL-1 activity as found with MNC. If cell concentration of ADH was lowered to correspond to the cell concentration of C-ADH, no IL-1 could be detected. These results showed that cell concentration and also the composition of the cell population are of importance for IL-1 induction. The failure of synthetic precursor Ia of lipid A was detected in all induction systems described here. Subsequent determination of icIL-1 showed that synthetic precursor Ia of lipid A was completely inactive in IL-1 induction as proposed (6, 7). This holds true also for some endotoxic activities (3). These findings indicate structure function relationship with regard to biological activity. It is thought that LPS and lipid A insert into the membrane (5), but the present results and competition experiments (data not shown) support the evidence that specific binding of LPS and lipid A to cells is required for IL-1 induction. Possibly this occurs by binding to receptor proteins as described recently (10). Probably endotoxic and immunostimulatory or immunoregulatory functions are initiated by binding of LPS or lipid A to the same membrane structures. The structural requirements for induction of tumor necrosis factor, a mediator of endotoxic activities of LPS, are identical to those of IL-1 (11). A further aspect of dose response experiments for induction of IL-1 is the analysis of absolute amounts of IL-1 activity. In most experiments more IL-1 activity was detected in cultures stimulated by LPS than in cultures stimulated by lipid A or core-oligosaccharides. This suggests that oligosaccharides may be modulators of lipid A mediated induction of IL-1.

SUMMARY AND CONCLUSION

Lipid A has been found to be an inducer of IL-1 with similar potency as LPS. Partial structures of lipid A or core oligosaccharides are less active or not active at all. We propose that lipid A is the structure responsible for induction of immunostimulatory or immunoregulatory properties of LPS.

REFERENCES

1. Brade, L., Brandenburg, K., Kuhn, H.-M., Kusumoto, Sh., Macher, I., Rietschel, E. Th. and Brade, H., 1987, The immunogenicity and antigenicity of lipid A are influenced by its physicochemical state and environment. Inf. Immun. 55: 2636.

2. Dinarello, C. A., 1984, Interleukin 1. Rev. Inf. Dis. 6: 51.

3. Galanos, C., Lüderitz, O., Rietschel, E. Th., Westphal, O., Brade, H., Brade, L., Freudenberg, M., Schade, U., Imoto, M., Yoshimura, H., Kusumoto, S. and Shiba, T., 1985, Synthetic and natural **E. coli** free lipid A express identical endotoxic activities. Eur. J. Biochem. 148: 1.

4. Imoto, M., Yoshimura, H., Shimamoto, T., Sakaguchi, N., Kusumoto, S. and Shiba, T., 1987, Total synthesis of **E. coli** lipid A, the endotoxically active principle of cell surface LPS. Bull. Chem. Soc. Jpn. 60: 2205.

5. Larsen, N. E. and Sullivan, R., 1984, Interaction between endotoxin and human monocytes. Proc. Natl. Acad. Sci. USA 81: 3491.

6. Loppnow, H., Brade, L., Brade, H., Rietschel, E. Th., Kusumoto, S., Shiba, T. and Flad, H.-D., 1986, Induction of human IL-1 by bacterial and synthetic lipid A. Eur. J. Immunol. 16: 1263.

7. Rietschel, E. Th., Brade, L., Loppnow, H., Flad, H.-D., Schade, U., Zähringer, U., Kuhn, H.-M., Holst, O., Helander, I., Kondo, S. and Brade, H., 1988, Chemical structure and biological activity of the lipid A component of bacterial endotoxin. Adv. Biosc. 68: 143.

8. Waldstätten, P., Christian, R., Schulz, G., Unger, F. M., Kosma, P., Kratzky, C. and Paulsen, H., 1983, Synthesis of oligosaccharides containing KDO residues, in: "Bacterial LPS. Structure, Synthesis and Biological Activities," L. M. Anderson and F. M. Unger, eds., Am. Chem. Soc., p. 121.

9. Westphal, O. and Lüderitz, O., 1954, Chemische Erforschung von LPS Gram-negativer Bakterien. Angew. Chem. 66: 407.

10. Wright, S. O. and Jong, M. T. C., 1986, Adhesion-promoting receptors on human macrophages recognize **E. coli** by binding to LPS. J. Exp. Med. 164: 1876.

11. Loppnow, H., Brade, H., Dürrbaum, I., Dinarello, C. A., Kusumoto, Sh., Rietschel, E. Th., and Flad, H. D., 1989, IL-1 induction-capacity of defined lipopolysaccharide partial structures. J. Immunol. 142: 3229.

A STUDY OF THE CELLULAR AND MOLECULAR MEDIATORS OF THE ADJUVANT ACTION OF A NONTOXIC MONOPHOSPHORYL LIPID A

A. G. Johnson and M. A. Tomai

Department of Microbiology/Immunology, School of Medicine
University of Minnesota, Duluth, 55812

INTRODUCTION

With the current resurgence of efforts to improve and expand human vaccines, attention is again being focused on the development of safe and effective adjuvants (17). In particular, the utilization of synthetic antigenic determinants or ligands of low molecular weight, which are inherently weak antigenically, necessitates the use of adjuvant carriers for optimum efficiency.

The potent adjuvant action on antibody formation in animals of endotoxic lipopolysaccharides (LPS) marks these compounds as worthy candidates for study in this respect. Although their extraordinary activities on the immune response have been known for over thirty years, their profound toxicity in minute amounts for man has prevented their inclusion in human vaccines (11, 23). Identification of the lipid A fraction of the lipopolysaccharide as responsible for most of the adjuvant action of the molecule was accompanied by the knowledge that this fraction also was responsible for its toxicity (23). Early efforts to detoxify these compounds achieved only partial success, insufficient to permit their serious usage in human beings (4, 12, 20).

A significant breakthrough, however, was achieved in 1981 when Takayama, et al., reported the isolation of a nontoxic lipid A fraction which retained the ability of the parent endotoxin to cause the regression of certain established tumors (31). The loss in toxicity, typified by a 1000 fold drop in lethality, a 2000 fold drop in pyrogenicity, and absence of local Shwartzman activity, was achieved by exposure to mild acid of LPS isolated from cell walls of various deep rough mutants of Salmonella species (27). A year later its structure was reported, and the loss in toxicity was linked to the loss of a phosphate group at the 1 position of the reducing sugar of the parent molecule, a D glucosamine disaccharide with ester and amide linked fatty acids (25, 30). Accordingly it was termed monophosphoryl lipid A (MPL, Ribi), and further characterization established its retention of mitogenic activity, ability to increase antibody formation, nonspecific resistance and phagocytosis as well as to protect against radiation damage (28, 29).

In earlier studies we described the suprising efficacy of MPL in stimulating antibody formation and mitogenicity in mice normally hyporesponsive to native LPS (32, 33). This was attributed to the lack of oligosaccharide residues on MPL, which, as postulated previously by Vukajlovich and Morrison

(36) and Vogel, et al., (34) may mask the ability of intact lipid A to transmit an appropriate stimulatory signal. Recently, we have extended characterization of the adjuvant properties of MPL to a model of immunodeficiency, the aging mouse. Inclusion of microgram amounts of MPL together with antigen resulted in restoration of the usual 60-70% drop in antibody forming cells in aging mice to the normal levels seen in young adult mice (32). Accordingly, we summarize herein the results of our current efforts to define the cell type(s) affected by MPL as well as the cytokines mediating the action of this nontoxic glycolipid in restoring the immunocompetence of aging mice.

MATERIALS AND METHODS

Mice

Balb/c mice originally purchased from the Charles River Laboratory, Wilmington, MA were bred in our animal facilities by brother and sister matings. The young adult mice used were males between 1 1/2 and 5 months of age and aging mice were males between 17 and 24 months of age.

Monophosphoryl Lipid A

MPL from S. minnesota, strain R595 was prepared at Ribi Immunochem Research Inc., Hamilton, MT using the Galanos extraction method (6). Isolation and characterization of MPL have been described previously (25, 26, 31). MPL was essentially nontoxic and non-pyrogenic, and retained several of the beneficial activities ascribed to the parent molecule. Stock solutions of MPL were prepared by dissolving 2 mg quantities in 1 or 2 ml volumes of pyrogen-free water containing 0.05-0.1% triethylamine. The solutions were clarified to slight opalescence after brief warming in a 50-60°C water bath and sonication. These stock solutions were further diluted in phosphate buffered saline (PBS), pH 7.2 for in vivo experiments, or in Click's medium containing 10% fetal bovine serum (FBS) for in vitro experiments.

Antigen

Defibrinated sheep red blood cells (SRBC), Kroy Medical, Stillwater, MN were used as antigen. SRBC were first washed 3X in Hank's balanced salt solution (HBSS) before use. For in vitro studies 1 x 10^7 SRBC were added to each culture dish in a 0.025 ml volume of Click's medium.

In Vitro Culture of Spleen Cells

Spleen cells were cultured using a modified Mishell and Dutton system (21). Briefly, mice were sacrificed by cervical dislocation, their spleens removed and single cell suspensions made. Debris was allowed to settle for 4 min after which the supernatant was removed and centrifuged for 10 min at 1200 rpm. After cells were water shocked to remove red blood cells, if desired, they were washed 2X in HBSS, and counted and diluted in Click's medium containing 10% FBS to 1 x 10^7 cells/ml. The cells were then added to 35 x 10 mm plastic tissue culture dishes, Corning, Corning, N.Y. (2 wells/ experimental group) and were incubated in the presence of antigen for 4 days in a 37°C humidified incubator containing 5% CO_2. On day 4 of culture, suspensions were harvested from the wells and antibody producing cells were measured.

Hemolytic Plaque Assay

Antibody production was measured using a modified hemolytic plaque assay (13). Briefly, 60 x 15 mm Nunc plastic tissue culture dishes, Nunclon Intermed, Roskilde, Denmark were coated with 2.0 ml of poly-L-lysine (50 μg/ml). After 15 min the plates were washed with PBS and 2.0 ml of washed

SRBC's (diluted 1:20) were added. After 15 min the plates were swirled and allowed to settle for an additional 15 min and rinsed with PBS. Finally, 1.5 ml PBS (pH 7.2) were added to each plate. For in vitro experiments 1 x 10^6 cells were added to plates (3 plates/experimental group). The plates were subsequently incubated in the presence of guinea pig complement, Texas Biological Labs, Fort Worth, Texas, for one hr at 37°C, and plaques were counted. Results were expressed as mean PFC $\pm$ standard error of the mean (S.E.M.).

Isolation of Adherent and Non-adherent Cell Populations

Adherent cells, primarily macrophages, were isolated from spleen cell populations by the method of Ackerman and Douglas (1). Briefly, spleens were removed and a suspension prepared as described in the section on in vitro culture. Cell numbers were adjusted to 2.5 x 10^7 cells/ml in HBSS and 5% FBS. 10.0 ml of the suspension were added to baby hamster kidney cell (BHK) microexudate coated tissue culture flasks, Corning, Corning, NY. The flasks were then incubated for 2 hr at 37°C in a humidified atmosphere of 5% CO_2. After incubation, non-adherent cells were further purified by passage of this population over Sephadex G-10 columns according to the protocol of Ly and Mishell (15). Briefly, a 25 ml syringe barrel containing a glass wool plug was packed with 15 ml of hydrated Sephadex G-10. The column was washed with warm HBSS + 5% FBS and incubated for 10 min at 37°C. After incubation, 5 x 10^8 cells in 5 ml HBSS + 5% FBS were added dropwise and allowed to incorporate into the column for 10 min. The non-adherent cells were then eluted with 30 ml of warm HBSS + 5% FBS. Adherent cells, which were still stuck to the BHK flasks, were washed 3X with HBSS and removed from the flask by incubating at 37°C for 10 min with 10 mM EDTA. The flasks were subsequently tapped to detach the cells, which were collected and washed to remove the EDTA. Non-adherent populations contained less than 1% Mac 1^+ cells.

Isolation of T and B Lymphocytes

The procedure was used as described by Mage et al., (16) and Wysocki et al. (38). It involved separating B and T lymphocytes using plastic petri dishes that were coated with rabbit anti-mouse immunoglobulin (RAMig), Accurate Chemical Co., Hicksville, NY. The RaMig was diluted 1:5 with a solution of normal rabbit immunoglobulin (NRig), Accurate Chemical Co., Hicksville, NY. Both the RaMig and the NRig were diluted to 5 μg/ml in 0.05 M Tris buffer, pH 9.5, Sigma Chemical, St. Louis, MO. 10.0 ml of the 1:5 dilution of RaMig and NRig were added to sterile plastic petri dishes. After 40 min at room temperature, the plates were washed with PBS, pH 7.2, 4X and 1X with PBS + 1% FBS. Spleen cells prepared as described previously were diluted in PBS + 5% FBS to 6.7 x 10^6 cells/ml, and 3.0 ml of this suspension were added to each plate. Plates were incubated an additional 30 min at 4°C. Subsequently, unattached cells were removed by swirling the dishes and decanting the effluent into a sterile centrifuge tube. Plates were washed 3X with PBS containing 1% FBS, and the supernatant decanted into the same centrifuge tube. Plates were washed 2 more times and the fluid discarded. B lymphocytes were recovered by adding 10.0 ml PBS + 1% FBS, flushing the plates with a Pasteur pipette, and decanting the liquid into a sterile centrifuge tube. The tubes were then centrifuged at 1200 rpm for 10 min, after which cells were suspended to appropriate concentrations in Click's medium containing 10% FBS.

Interleukin-1 Assay

Interleukin 1 (IL-1) was assessed using the standard mouse thymocyte assay as described by Mizel et al. (22). Briefly, thymocytes were obtained from 4 wk old C3H/HeJ male mice, counted and diluted to 1.5 x 10^7 cells/ml in RPMI complete medium containing 5% FCS. 0.1 ml of the cell suspension was then added to flat bottom 96 well microtiter plates, Corning, Corning, NY that contained medium or dilutions of test supernatants. In addition, concanavalin A (Con A), Sigma Chemical, St. Louis, MO was added to each well (0.1 μg/well). Cultures were incubated at 37°C in a humidified environment of 5% CC_2 for 72 hr. During the last 18 hr of incubation, each well was pulsed with 1 uCi of ^{3}HTdR (specific activity 40Ci/nmol, Amersham, Arlington Heights, IL). After incubation cultures were harvested and radioactivity counted as described in the mitogenicity section. Results were expressed in units of IL-1. Arbitrarily, 10 units of IL-1 were assigned to that amount of IL-1 that induced half the maximal proliferation induced by the standard, supernatant from LPS stimulated P388D1 cells.

Interleukin 2 Assay

Interleukin 2 (IL-2) activity was measured as described by Gillis, et al., (7) using the IL-2 dependent CTL-2 cell line which proliferates only in response to IL-2. Briefly, CTL's were washed 2X in HBSS and diluted in Click's medium containing 10% FBS to 1 x 10^5 cells/ml. 0.1 ml of the cell suspension was added to round bottom 96 well microtiter plates, Corning, Corning, NY that contained dilutions of the test supernatants or medium. Volumes were adjusted to 0.2 ml and plates were incubated for 24 hr at 37°C in a humidified environnment of 5% CO_2. During the final 6 hr of incubation cells were pulsed with 1 uCi ^{3}HTdR as described in the IL-1 assay section. Cultures were harvested as previously described. Results were expressed in units of IL-2 where 10 units of IL-2 were arbitrarily assigned as that amount of IL-2 that induced half of the maximal proliferation induced by the standard, a supernatant from PMA-stimulated E1-4 cells (5).

Isolation of Macrophages from the Peritoneal Cavity

Peritoneal exudate cells (PEC) were obtained by washing with 6.0 ml HBSS, Gibco, Grand Island, NY, the peritoneal cavity of mice injected three days previously with 3.0 ml of 1M thioglycollate broth, Difco, Detroit, MI. Cells were centrifuged at 800 rpm for 10 min after which they were counted and diluted to appropriate concentrations in RPMI + 1% FBS. Cells were about 90% positive for Mac 1 antigen (10).

IL-1 Generation

Splenic adherent cells or thioglycollate induced PEC were diluted in RPMI + 1% FBS to 1 or 2 x 10^6 cells/ml and subsequently 1 ml was added to 6 well tissue culture dishes, Corning, Corning, NY. The cells were incubated for 48 hr ± MPL unless otherwise specified. After incubation, supernatants were collected by centrifugation for 15 min at 2200 rpm. Supernatants were frozen until they were assayed for IL-1 activity as described above.

IL-2 Generation

Spleen cells from young or aging mice were diluted in Click's medium containing 10% FBS to 1 x 10^7 cells/ml. The cells were then added to 12 well tissue cultures dishes, Corning, Corning, NY and incubated with the various stimulating agents at 37°C and 5% CO_2 for various times. Supernatants were aspirated from the cultures after incubation and centrifuged at 2200 rpm for 15 min. The fluid was then added to a sterile tube and frozen until assayed for IL-2 activity as described above.

Generation of Supernatant Fluids from MPL and Medium Stimulated Cells

Purified populations of B cells, T cells and macrophages (1-2 x 10^6 cells/ml) were incubated in Click's medium + 10% FCS + 1 μg/ml of MPL for two hr at 37°C in an atmosphere of 5% CO_2. After incubation, the cultures were washed three times in HBSS and resuspended in fresh Click's medium containing 10% FCS. The cultures were allowed to incubate for an additional 48 hr at 37°C in a humidified environment containing 5% CO_2. After incubation the supernatant fluids were collected and centrifuged for 15 min at 2200 rpm to remove cellular debris. 0.4 ml of the various supernatant fluids were added to 6 well plates containing 1×10^7 spleen cells from aging mice. The volume was adjusted to 1.0 ml and 10^7 SRBC were added and PFC measured 4 days later. Results from MPL stimulated populations were always compared to their respective unstimulated populations.

Inhibition of the Adjuvant Action of MPL by Anti-interferon Antisera

Two preparations of anti-interferon antisera were generously provided by Dr. Sidney Grossberg, University of Wisconsin, Madison. The first was an anti-type 1 mouse interferon (IFN) with viral plaque inhibition titers of anti-IFN vs. 10 units of murine IFN alpha and beta of 1:4,000 and 1:36,000 respectively. The second preparation was an anti-mouse IFN beta preparation from Lee Biomolecular, San Diego, CA, Lot #84042, which however, contained antibody against all three IFN, alpha, beta and gamma. The titers vs. 10 units of murine IFN alpha, beta, and gamma were 1:1,600, 1:137,000 and 1:560 respectively. The anti-alpha/beta preparation and the anti-alpha/beta/gamma preparation were diluted in Click's medium 1:160 and 1:17 respectively. The ability of these antisera to inhibit the enhancement of antibody production by splenic cultures from aging mice induced by supernatants from MPL stimulated T cells was tested by addition of 0.1 ml of the antibody diluted 1:16 to 0.4 ml of the various supernatants. These mixtures were incubated for 1 hr at 4°C and subsequently tested for the ability to enhance antibody production in a modified Mishell-Dutton system.

Statistical Analysis

Data were analyzed by a BMDP statistical program for a one-sample t test after taking the log 10 of each pair of groups to be compared. A P-value less than 0.05 was considered a statistically significant difference.

RESULTS

The ability of MPL to restore antibody formation when injected into aging mice of the Balb and C3H strains is documented in Table 1. However, to facilitate definition of the cell target for MPL, an in vitro culture system was adopted as described in Materials and Methods. Enhancement of antibody forming cells in both young and aging Balb mice was readily achieved in this in vitro system as well, as is evident in Table 2.

Subsequent separation of aging Balb spleen cells into adherent, T and B cell compartments, and their exposure in vitro to MPL for two hr followed by antigen and co-culture with unexposed splenocytes at a 1:10 ratio for four days, revealed the T cell as the most likely candidate for receipt of an adjuvant signal from MPL (Fig 1). Exposure of the adherent or B cell populations to MPL did not result in any increase in PFC when mixed and co-cultured with unexposed splenocytes from 22 month old mice.

To determine whether the stimulatory action of the T cell population was exerted through secretion of a lymphokine mediator, T and B and adherent cells from aging mice were again isolated and each exposed to MPL for 2 hr, washed and incubated for 48 hr. The supernatant fluids were collected and added to cultures of unexposed spleen cells from aging mice together with antigen, and PFC enumerated 4 days later. The results are depicted in Fig 2 and indicate the adjuvant action of the MPL treated T cell compartment was mediated by a lymphokine secreted into the supernatant fluids. Also apparent was a slight but statistically insignificant effect of supernatant fluids

Table 1. Adjuvant action of MPL in vivo

MPL	Mouse Strain	
	Balb	C3H
-	116 ± 38	14 ± 4
+	562 ± 214	152 ± 78

Data modified from (13). PFC/2 x 10^5 spleen cells

Table 2. Adjuvant action of MPL in vitro

	Average PFC/culture*		
Mice	SRBC	SRBC + MPL	p
3-5 months	590 ± 188	1790 ± 790	0.02
18-22 months	252 ± 148	1300 ± 460	0.01

*1μg MPL was added along with 10^6 SRBC to splenic cultures and PFC were assayed on day 4. The results are expressed as the mean PFC culture ± SEM of 3 experiments in which 3 mice were assayed individually/experiment.

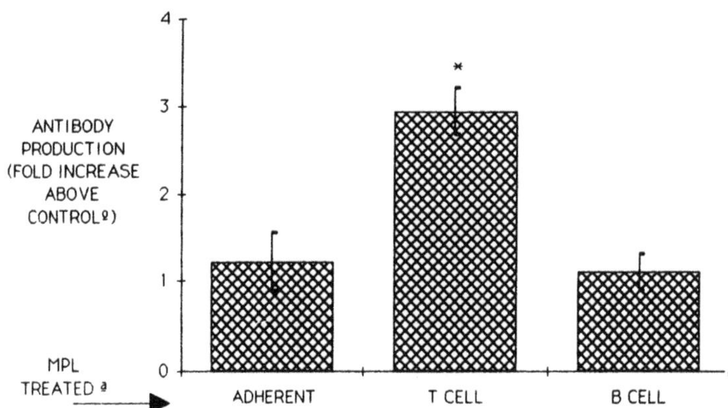

Fig 1. [a]Cell populations were stimulated in vitro with 1 μg/ml of MPL. Populations were then washed and 1 x 10^6 cells were added to 9 x 10^6 whole spleen cells from 22 month old male Balb/c mice. Cultures were incubated for 4 days with 10^7 SRBC and PFC were measured on day 4. Results were expressed as the mean of 4 experiments ± SEM.

[o]Control cultures contained 10^6 untreated cells along with the whole spleen cells.

*indicates a statistically significant difference ($p<0.05$) when compared to the control.

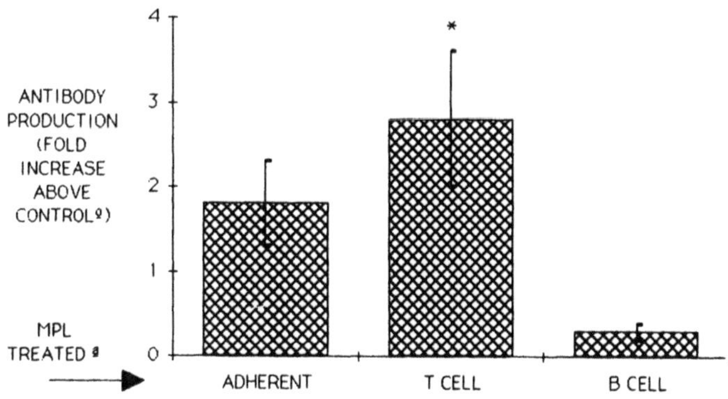

Fig 2. [a]Cell populations (10^6 cells/ml) were treated with 1 μg/ml of MPL. Populations were washed and incubated an additional 48 hr after which cell-free supernatant fluids were collected. 0.4 ml of this fluid was added to 10^7 spleen cells from 22 month old male Balb/c mice (3 mice pooled/exp) and cultures were incubated for 4 days with 10^7 SRBC. Results were expressed as the mean of 3-5 experiments ± SEM.

[b]Control cultures contained supernatants from unstimulated cell populations.

*indicates a statistically significant difference ($p<0.05$) when compared to supernatants from unstimulated populations.

from the adherent cell population exposed to MPL. On the other hand, the B cell population appeared inhibitory.

Identification of the active factor in the T cell supernatant fluids initially involved testing for increased interleukin-2 secretion following exposure to MPL. However MPL was ineffective in stimulating IL-2 production directly in cells from either young or aging mice (data not shown). In addition, MPL was also incapable of augmenting concanavalin A inducible IL-2 production in splenic cultures from young adult or aging mice. The amount of IL-2 released by control Con-A stimulated young adult spleen cells was 10-fold higher than levels observed in spleen cells from aging mice, as expected.

Evidence suggesting that the lymphokine responsible for the enhanced numbers of antibody forming cells induced by MPL exposed T cells was interferon gamma is seen in Fig 3. An antiserum to alpha and beta interferon, which was devoid of interferon gamma activity, did not inhibit significantly the adjuvant action of MPL in either the aging or young adult mice, although the numbers of PFC were lowered in both age groups. On the other hand, an antiserum containing activity against gamma interferon abolished the enhancing action. This latter antiserum also totally abrogated the enhancement of PFC numbers induced by supernatant fluids from MPL stimulated T cells (Table 3).

Since one of the major attributes of interferon gamma is the capacity of this lymphokine to promote the secretion of IL-1 by the macrophage, our T cell supernatant fluids were evaluated for their ability to augment IL-1 production by splenic macrophages. As may be seen in Figure 4, supernatant fluids from MPL stimulated T cells enhanced IL-1 secretion by macrophages significantly in comparison to MPL alone. This activity was also inhibitable by an anti-gamma interferon antiserum.

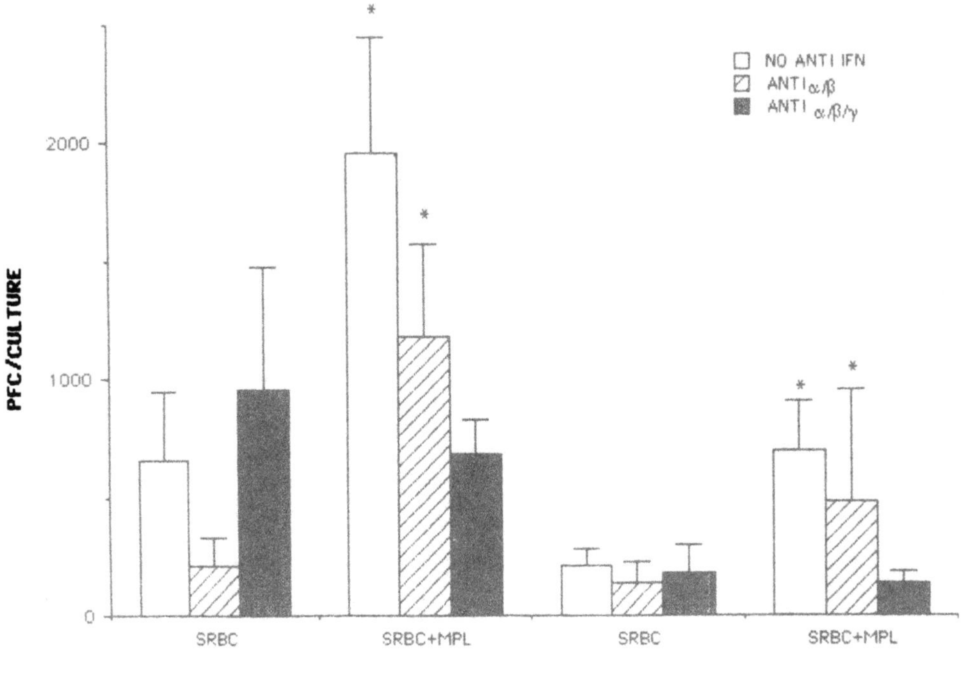

Fig 3. [a]10^7 spleen cells from either 8 week or 22 month male Balb/c mice were cultured with 10^7 SRBC + 1μg/ml MPL for 4 days. In addition, certain cultures received antiserum to either α/β IFN or αβ and γ. After culture PFC were measured. The white bars received no antibody, the hatched bars received anti-α/β IFN, and the dark bars received anti-α/β/γ IFN. Results were expressed as the mean of 3 experiments ± SEM.

*indicates $p<0.05$ when compared to appropriate control.

Table 3. Abrogation of the adjuvant action of MPL induced supernatant fluids by anti-gamma interferon serum

Mice	Average PFC/Culture			
	Untreated		Antiserum Treated	
	Control	Experimental	Control	Experimental
22-24 months	149 ± 20	794 ± 64	321 ± 76	158 ± 8

*Control cultures received 10^6 SRBC and experimental cultures received 1 μg MPL in addition to SRBC. PFC were measured on day 4 and are expressed as the mean PFC/culture + SEM of three experiments in which 3 male Balb mouse spleens were pooled per experiment. Supernatant fluids were treated with anti-gamma IFN for 1 hr before addition to spleen cells.

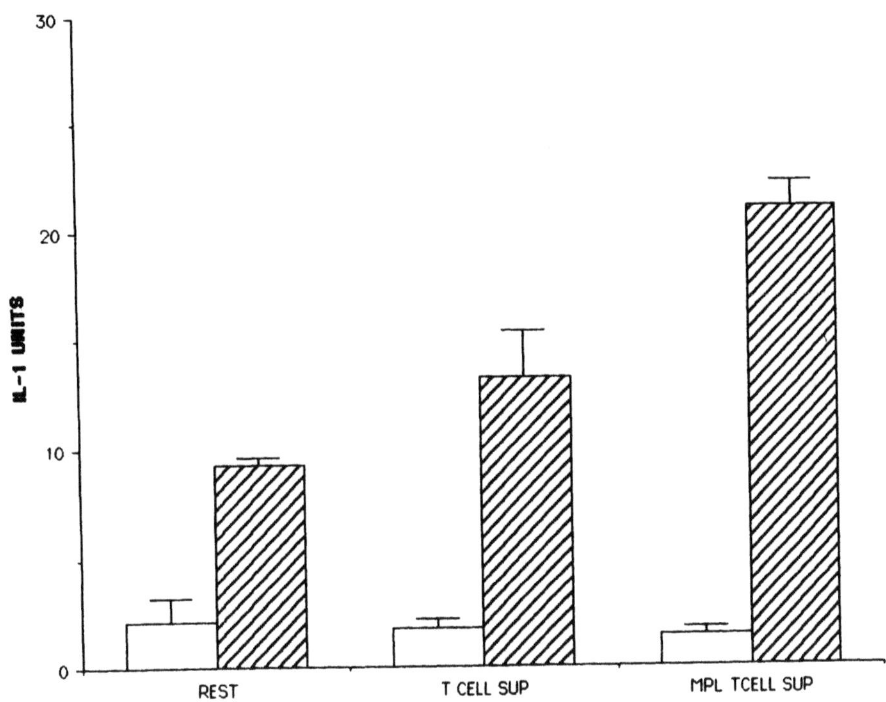

Fig 4. [a]0.1 ml of the supernatant fluids from MPL and unstimulated T cells was added along with 0.9 ml of medium to splenic adherent cells from aging mice. In addition, MPL at 10 µg/ml was added to some of the cultures and all were incubated for 48 hr. Supernatant fluids were collected and assayed for IL-1. Results were expressed as the mean of 2 experiments ± SEM.

DISCUSSION

Although aging mice exhibit a dramatic decrease in the ability to produce antibody on antigen challenge both in vivo and in vitro (18), Han and Johnson (23) showed that the adjuvant poly adenylic:poly uridylic acid complexes was capable of restoring antibody production in aging mice. Thus, the potential for adequate responsiveness is inherent in such animals. Later studies indicated, however, that intact LPS was ineffective in enhancing antibody production in splenic cultures from aging mice (8, 14, 37). The activity of MPL in aging mice shown in our previous study (32) as well as herein, however, contrasts with these reports of the inability of the native LPS to function in this model. An explanation for this may lie in our rather surprising previous finding that MPL was also capable of enhancing antibody formation as well as stimulating proliferation of splenic cultures form LPS hyporesponsive mouse strains (32, 33). The structural difference between LPS and MPL preparations may explain this paradox since evidence has accumulated recently that increasing the polysaccharide content of the LPS molecule may in some instances inhibit the functional activity of these glycolipids (34, 36). Thus, the polysaccharide portion of LPS may have to be removed enzymatically to allow triggering to occur in both the aging and LPS hyporesponsive mice. This putative enzyme may be defective in cells from both of these models.

Our experiments favor the T cell as the initial target for the adjuvant action of MPL. Although we cannot rule out contamination of our T cell preparations with minute numbers of macrophages, macrophages isolated from the spleen as well as thioglycollate stimulated PEC, when stimulated with MPL showed no greater enhancement of antibody production in splenic cultures from aging mice than unstimulated PEC. Other evidence also is supportive of LPS action on the T cell. The studies of Allison and Davies (2) demonstrated that mice depleted of T cells by adult thymectomy or treatment with anti-lymphocyte serum and reconstituted with bone marrow cells were not able to respond to the antigen, even in the presence of endotoxin unless these mice received syngeneic thymus cells. Nakano, et al., (24) reported that LPS acted primarily on a non-adherent, Ig negative cell population in enhancing both 7S and 19S PFC to SRBC. Some of the most compelling data that support a T dependent mode of action for LPS was described in the elegant studies performed by McGhee et al. (19). These investigators showed that LPS was capable of enhancing antibody production in vitro only if T cells and macrophages were from LPS responsive mice. Baker, et al., (3) have found that MPL enhanced antibody production to pneumococcal polysaccharide type 3 and did so by decreasing T suppressor activity.

Most of these studies did not however, distinguish between a direct or indirect effect of LPS on T lymphocytes. Vogel et al, however, recently (35) demonstrated that LPS acted directly on T lymphocytes. They observed that a cytotoxic T lymphocyte CTL line as well as a highly purified subpopulation of splenic T cells were capable of proliferating in response to LPS.

The ability of antisera containing antibody to gamma interferon to abrogate the enhanced PFC numbers induced by MPL implicates this T cell lymphokine as a prime mediator. Together with the evidence discussed above and the additional finding that MPL induced T cell supernatant fluids containing gamma interferon, stimulated macrophages to secrete increased amounts of interleukin 1 suggests the following hypothesis to describe the adjuvant action of MPL in aging mice: MPL acts initially on the T helper lymphocyte stimulating the secretion of gamma interferon. The latter in turn causes increased expression of Ia antigen on the macrophage and secretion of higher than normal levels of IL-1, which in turn increase the well-described sequence of cell activations and further cytokine release associated with antibody synthesis.

SUMMARY

A detoxified endotoxin, termed monophosphoryl lipid A (MPL, Ribi), has been shown to increase antibody forming cell numbers in aging Balb mice both in vivo and in vitro. Separation of splenocytes from aging mice into purified T, B and adherent cell populations and subsequent incubation of each with MPL and admixture with their cellular counterparts and antigen, revealed only the T cell compartment capable of transferring the adjuvant action. Incubation of purified T cells from aging mice with MPL for 2 hr, followed by washing and culture for 48 hr, resulted in a supernatant fluid which enhanced antibody formation in cultures of aging spleen cells. This enhancing action was eliminated by an antiserum containing anti-alpha/beta/gamma interferon, but not by an anti-alpha/beta interferon antiserum. These data, as well as evidence gained by others as discussed, suggests the hypothesis wherein MPL increases antibody formation in aging mice by inducing the helper T cell population to secrete interferon gamma. The latter activates the macrophage to secrete increased levels of interleukin 1, thereby resulting in increased responsiveness throughout the ensuing sequence of cellular and molecular events leading to antibody synthesis.

ACKNOWLEDGEMENTS

This research was supported by USPHS Grant AI 25810. We thank the National Institute of Aging for numbers of aging mice.

REFERENCES

1. Ackerman, S. K. and Douglas, S. D., 1978, Purification of human monocytes on microexudate coated surfaces. J. Immunol. 120: 1372.

2. Allison, A. C. and Davies, A. J. S., 1971, Requirement of thymus dependent lymphocytes for potentiation by adjuvants of antibody formation. Nature 233: 330.

3. Baker, P. J., Hiernaux, J. R., Faunterloy, M. B., Prescott, B., Cantrell, J. L. and Rudbach, J. A., 1988, Inactivation of suppressor T cell activity by non-toxic monophosphoryl lipid A. Infect. Immun. 56: 1076.

4. Chedid, L., Audibert, F. and Bona, C., 1975, Adjuvant and mitogenic effects of detoxified lipopolysaccharides. CR. Acad. Sci. (Paris) 280: 1197.

5. Farrar, J. J., Fuller-Farrar, J., Simon, P. L., Hilfiker, M. L., Stadler, B. M. and Farrar, W. L., 1980, Thymoma production of T cell growth factor (interleukin 2). J. Immunol. 126: 1120.

6. Galanos, C., Luderitz, O. and Westphal, O., 1969, A new method for the extraction of R lipopolysaccharides. Eur. J. Immunol. 9: 245.

7. Gillis, S., Ferm, M. M., Ou, W. and Smith, K. A., 1978, T cell growth factor: parameters of production and a quantitative microassay for activity. J. Immunol. 120: 2027.

8. Goodman, M. G. and Weigle, W. O., 1985, Restoration of humoral immunity in vitro in immunodeficient aging mice by C8-derivatized guanine ribonucleosides. J. Immunol. 134: 3808.

9. Han, I. and Johnson, A., 1976, Regulation of the immune system by synthetic polynucleotides. VI. Amplification of the immune response in young and aging mice. J. Immunol. 117: 423.

10. Ho, M. K. and Springer, T. A., 1982, Mac-1 antigen: quantitative expression in macrophage populations and tissues and immunofluorescent localization in the spleen. J. Immunol. 128: 2281.

11. Johnson, A. G., Gaines, S. and Landy, M., 1956, Studies on the O-antigen of Salmonella typhosa. V. Enhancement of the antibody response to protein antigens by the purified lipopolysaccharide. J. Exp. Med. 103: 225.

12. Johnson, A. G. and Nowotny, A., 1964, Relationship of structure to function in bacterial O antigens. III. Biological properties of endotoxoids. J. Bacteriol. 87: 809.

13. Kennedy, J. and Axelrad, M., 1971, An improved assay for hemolytic plaque forming cells. Immunology 20: 253.

14. Kishimoto, S., Takahama, T. and Mizumachi, H., 1976, In vitro immune response to the 2,4,6 trinitrophenyl determinant in aged C57 Bl/6J mice: Changes in the humoral immune response to avidity for the TNP determinant and responsiveness to LPS effect with aging. J. Immunol. 116: 294.

15. Ly, I. A. and Mishell, R. I., 1974, Separation of mouse spleen cells by passage through columns of Sephadex G-10. J. Immunol. Methods 5: 239.

16. Mage, M. G., McHugh, L. L. and Rothstein, T. L., 1977, Mouse lymphocytes with and without surface immunoglobulin: Preparative scale separation in polystyrene tissue culture dishes coated with specifically purified anti-immunoglobulin. J. Immunol. Methods 15: 47.

17. Majde, J. A., 1987, Immunopharmacology of Infectious Diseases: Vaccine adjuvants and Modulators of Non-specific Resistance. Progess in Leukocyte Biology, Alan R. Liss Publishing, New York. (Whole text cited).

18. Makinodan, T. and Peterson, W. J., 1962, Relative antibody forming capacity of spleen cells as a function of age. Proc. Natl. Acad. Sci. USA 48: 234.

19. McGhee, J. R., Farrar, J. J., Michalek, S. M., Mergenhagen, S. E. and Rosenstreich, D. L., 1979, Cellular requirements for lipopolysaccharide adjuvanticity. J. Exp. Med. 149: 793.

20. McIntire, F., Hargie, M., Schend, J., et al., 1976, Biological properties of non-toxic derivatives of a lipopolysaccharide from E. coli K235. J. Immunol. 117: 674.

21. Mishell, R. and Dutton, R., 1967, Immunization of dissociated spleen cell cultures in normal mice. J. Exp. Med. 126: 423.

22. Mizel, S. B., Rosenstreich, D. L. and Oppenheim, J. J., 1978, Phorbol myristicacetate stimulates LAF production by the macrophage cell line P388D1. Cell Immunol. 40: 230.

23. Morrison, D. and Ryan, J., 1979, Bacterial endotoxins and host immune responses. Adv. Immunol. 23: 293.

24. Nakano, M., Uchiyama, T. and Saito, K., 1973, Adjuvant effect of endotoxin: Antibody to sheep erythrocytes in mice after transfer of syngeneic lymhoid cells treated with bacterial lipopolysaccharide in vitro. J. Immunol. 110: 408.

25. Qureshi, N. and Takayama, K., 1982, Purification and structural determination of non-toxic lipid A obtained from the lipopolysaccharide of Salmonella typhimurium. J. Biol. Chem. 257: 11,808.

26. Qureshi, N., Mascagni, P., Ribi, E. and Takayama, K., 1985, Monophosphoryl lipid A obtained from lipopolysacharides of Salmonella minnesota R595. Purification of the dimethyl derivative by high performance lipid chromatography and complete structural determination. J. Biol. Chem. 260: 5271.

27. Ribi, E., Cantrell, J. L., Takayama, K., Quereshi, N., Peterson, J. and Ribi, H. O., 1984, Lipid A and Immunotherapy. Rev. Infect. Dis. 6: 567.

28. Ribi, E., Ulrich, J. T. and Masihi, K. N., in: "Immunopharmacology of Infectious Diseases," J. A. Majde, ed., Alan R. Liss Publishing, New York, p. 101.

29. Ribi, E., Cantrell, J., Feldner, T., Myers, K. and Peterson, J., 1986, Biological activities of monophosphoryl lipid A, in: "Microbiology, 1986," L. Levine, P. F. Bonventre, J. A. Morello, F. D. Silver and H. C. Wu, eds., Amer. Soc. for Microbiol., Washington, D.C.

30. Rietschel, E. H., Brade, L., Schade, U., Zahringer, U. and Brade, H., 1987, Bacterial Endotoxins: Relation of Chemical Structure to Biologi-

cal Activity, in: "Immunopharmacology of Infectious Diseases," J. A. Majde, ed., Alan R. Liss Publishing, New York, p. 79.

31. Takayama, K., Ribi, E. and Cantrell, J. L., 1981, Isolation of a non-toxic lipid A fraction containing tumor regression activity. Cancer Res. 41: 2654.

32. Tomai, M. A., Solem, L. E., Johnson, A. G. and Ribi, E., 1987, The adjuvant properties of a non-toxic monophosphoryl lipid A in hyporesponsive and aging mice. J. Biol. Resp. Modifiers 6: 99.

33. Tomai, M. A., Johnson, A. G. and Ribi, E., 1988, Glycolipid induced proliferation of lipopolysaccharide hyporesponsive splenocytes. J. Leuk. Biol. 43: 11.

34. Vogel, S., Madonna, G., Wahl, L. and Rick, P., 1984, In vitro stimulation of C3H/HeJ spleen cells and macrophages by a lipid A precursor molecule derived from Salmonella typhimurium. J. Immunol. 132: 347.

35. Vogel, S. N., Hilfiker, M. L. and Caulfield, M. J., 1983, Endotoxin-induced T lymphocyte proliferation. J. Immunol. 130: 1774.

36. Vukajlovich, S. and Morrison, D., 1983, Conversion of lipopolysaccharides to molecular aggregates with reduced subunit heterogeneity - demonstration of LPS responsiveness in "endotoxin unresponsive" C3H/HeJ splenocytes. J. Immunol. 130: 2804.

37. Winchurch, R. A., Birminghan, W., Hilberg, C. and Munster, A., 1982, Effects of endotoxin on immunity in aging mice. Cell. Immunol. 67: 384.

38. Wysocki, L. J. and Sato, Y. L., 1978, Panning for lymphocytes: A method for cell selection. Proc. Natl. Acad. Sci. 75: 2844.

ANTI-LPS REGION ANTIBODY RESPONSES AND CELLULAR IMMUNE RESPONSIVENESS IN TYPHOID PATIENTS

C. M. Mastroianni, A. Misefari*, E. Jirillo**, C. De Simone***
V. Vullo and S. Delia

Malattie Infettive III, Universitá "La Sapienza" Roma, Italy
*Cattedra di Immunologia, Universitá di Messina, Messina, Italy, **Cattedra di Immunologia, Universitá di Bari, Bari, Italy, ***Malattie Infettive, Universitá dell Aquila degli Abruzzi, L'Aquila, Italy

INTRODUCTION

In recent years, several reports have provided evidence for an involvement of the immune system during typhoid fever (3). In particular, a reduction of several immunological parameters such as leukocyte inhibiting factor (LIF) release, plaque-forming cell (PFC) production and natural killer (NK) cell activity have been demonstrated (1). In addition, Salmonella typhi organisms possess on their outermembrane the lipopolysaccharide (LPS) which is a powerful immunomodulating agent (4). Therefore, to better investigate the relationship between immune function and typhoid fever, we analyzed humoral and cell-mediated responses in typhoid patients towards LPS or whole bacteria.

Antibody responses to O-polysaccharide chain and lipid A regions of S. typhi LPS have been evaluated by using a new developed enzyme immunoassay, the Dot immunobinding (DIB) (2, 6). On the other hand, the cellular response to S. typhi has been determined with the anti-bacterial antibody-dependent cellular cytotoxicity (ADCC) which represents a novel mechanism of host protection against enteric pathogens (5).

METHODS, RESULTS AND DISCUSSION

Blood samples were collected from 9 children with typhoid fever at the first, second and third wk after the onset of fever.

The DIB assay was performed on nitrocellulose paper as previously described (6). Positive reactions appeared as well-defined blue dots on a white background. Antibody titers were determined by testing two-fold dilutions of serum samples. Anti-bacterial activity exerted by typhoid peripheral mononuclear cells has been determined according to the method of Tagliabue et al. (5). ADCC was evaluated during the course of infection at Effector/Target (E/T) ratios of 50, 25, and 12.

Results show that anti-O polysaccharide chain antibody titers are lower (mean=53; range=20-160) at the first wk and progressively augment with the time (mean=728; range=160-1280). On the other hand, anti-lipid A antibody titers are already higher (mean=302; range=80-160) at the onset of the

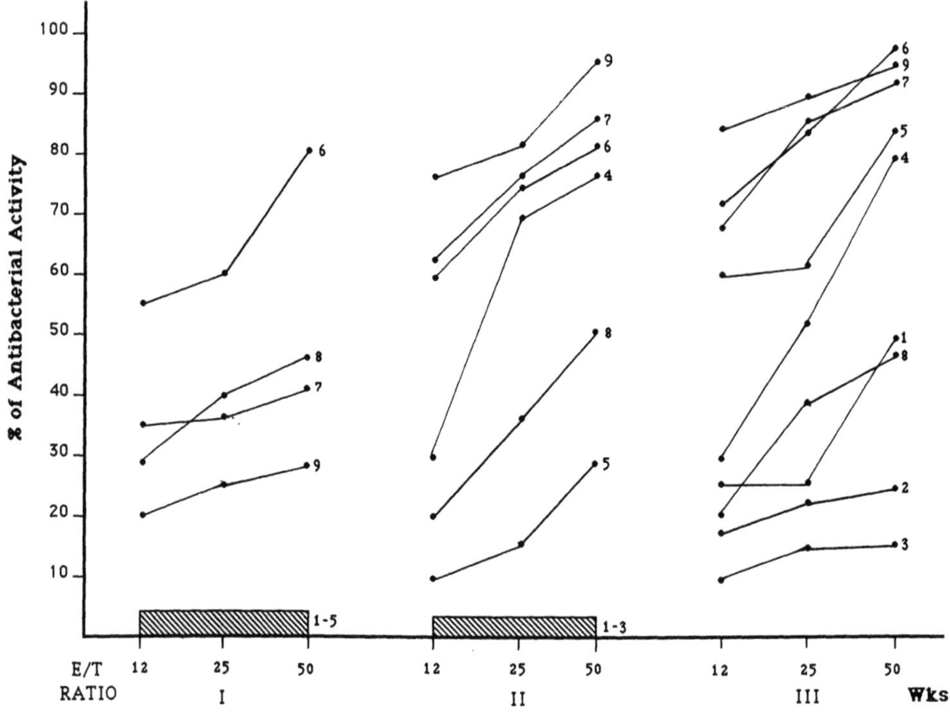

Fig 1. Antibacterial activity against S. typhi by PBMC in typhoid patients. Numbers indicate the patients studied.

disease and slightly increase in the following two wks (mean=577; range = 80-1280).

The pattern of anti-bacterial activity against S. typhi is expressed in Figure 1. ADCC anti-S. typhi is in general depressed at the first wk and is almost recovered at the third wk of the disease.

Our data indicate that immune responsiveness in the course of typhoid fever undergoes a biphasic pattern. Either humoral or cellular responses are initially depressed and recover in the later stage. Several factors may be responsible for this impaired immune responsiveness such as prostaglandins and macrophage products, e.g., arachidonic acid metabolites or free oxygens radicals (3). However, also release of suppressive substances should be taken into consideration following massive ingestion of organisms by macrophages (3). Taken together, all these data bring new insight in the comprehension of Salmonellosis pathogenesis and will facilitate the development of more sophisticated methods and therapeutical strategies, even including vaccines.

ACKNOWLEDGEMENTS

Paper supported by a Grant from regione Puglia, Italy.

REFERENCES

1. Antonaci, S., Garofalo, A. R., Stasi, D., Caretto, G., Jirilli, E. and Bonomo, L., 1987, Cell-mediated immunity in typhoid fever patients. Microbios Letters 35: 19.

2. Delia, S., Vullo, V., Mastroianni, C. M., Contini, C., Massetti, A. P., Cignarella, L. and Sorice, F., 1987, Use of dot immunobinding assay (DIB) for the rapid diagnosis of human brucellosis. J. Infection 14: 88.

3. Edelman, R. and Levine, M. M., 1986, Summary of an International Workshop of Typhoid Fever. Rev. Infect. Dis. 8: 329.

4. Galanos, C., Lüderitz, O., Rietschel, E. T. and Westphal, O., 1977, Newer aspects of the chemistry and biology of bacterial lipopolysaccharides, with special reference to their lipid A component, in: "International Review of Biochemistry. Biochemistry of lipids. II. Vol. 14," T. W. Goodwin, ed., Baltimore, p. 239.

5. Tagliabue, A., Villa, L., Boraschi, D., Peri, G., De Gori, V. and Nencioni, L., 1985, Natural anti-bacterial activity against Salmonella typhi by human T4+ lymphocytes armed with IgA antibodies. J. Immunol. 135: 4178.

6. Vullo, V., Contini, C., Mastroianni, C. M., Massetti, A. P., Cignarella, L. and Delia, S., 1987, Evaluation of Dot Immunobinding Assay (DIB) for the Detection of Antibodies Against Brucella Melitensis, EOS Riv. Immunol. Immunopharmacol. 7: 147.

LIPOPOLYSACCHARIDE, BUT NOT LETHAL INFECTION, RELEASES TUMOR NECROSIS FACTOR IN MICE

R. D. Cornwell, D. T. Golenbock and R. A. Proctor

University of Wisconsin, Departments of Medicine and Medical Microbiology, Madison, WI 53706

An endogenously produced cytokine, tumor necrosis factor (TNF), is thought to be an important mediator in the pathophysiology of gram-negative sepsis (10). Infusions of TNF in animals reproduce the metabolic, hormonal, hemodynamic, and histopathologic finding seen in lethal gram-negative infection (7, 11). Pretreatment with polyclonal anti-TNF antibodies was shown to reduce endotoxin (LPS) lethality in mice (1). Passive immunization with monoclonal antibodies against recombinant human TNF conferred complete protection against shock and death in baboons challenged with an otherwise lethal infusion of E. coli (9). Measurable circulating levels of TNF have been found in animals following a lethal bolus infusion of LPS (2, 8) or live gram-negative bacteria (6, 9), while little has been reported concerning TNF production in other models of lethal gram-negative infection.

In this study, we measured serum TNF levels in response to a mouse thigh infection using both cyclophosphomide-induced neutropenic and normopenic mice. This model provides reproducible sepsis and 100% mortality within 24-36 hr using E. coli (5) or K. pneumoniae (Dr. B. Vogelman, University of Wisconsin, personal communication). Serum TNF levels in cyclophosphamide-treated and untreated mice were measured following a lethal intraperitoneal dose of LPS.

For these experiments, male C57BL/10 mice, weighing 20-25 g each, were obtained from Jackson Laboratory, Bar Harbor, ME. Cyclophosphamide-treated mice received intraperitoneal injections of cyclophosphamide at 150 mg/kg 5 days prior and 100 mg/kg 2 days prior to experimentation, a regimen which has been shown to reliably produce profound neutropenia in mice for days after the last injection (5). At various time points following LPS challenge or bacterial thigh muscle inoculation, blood was collected from ether-anesthetized mice by axillary artery exsanguination, allowed to clot at room temperature, and serum stored at -70°C until assayed for TNF. The assay used for TNF was a standard L929 cell cytotoxicity bioassay using a final antinomycin D concentration of 1 μg/ml and a target cell seeding density of 3.0 x 10^4 cells/well on 96 well microtiter plate, as previously described (4). After exposure of target cells to serial dilutions of serum samples at 37°C for 20 hr, cytotoxicity was quantified using a colorimetric assay with a tetrazolium salt, MTT. One unit of TNF activity was defined as the amount required to lyse 50% L929 target cells.

The sensitivity of this assay was comparable to the bioassay used at

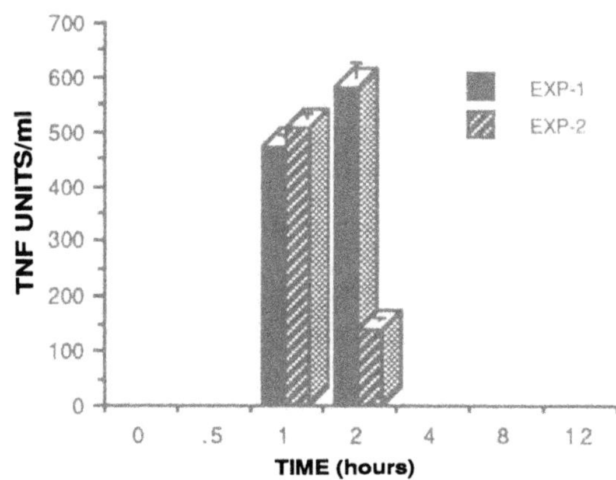

Fig 1. Circulating TNF in normopenic mice following lethal (500 μg) intraperitoneal LPS challenge. TNF activity was determined in a actinomycin D sensitized L929 cell cytotoxicity assay by measuring MTT reduction. Each experiment represents one mouse per time point, with measurable activity at 1 and 2 hr. No activity was found at 0, 0.5, 4, 8 and 12 hr.

Genentech to standardize recombinant human TNF (rhTNF) as determined by the activity of a rhTNF (Genentech, Inc., San Francisco, CA), and specificity was shown by using a polyclonal antibody against recombinant murine TNF (Genzyme Corp., Boston, MA).

Following intraperitoneal injection of 500 μg of endotoxin, prepared from E. coli 0111:B4 by the Westphal method (Difco, Detroit, MI), measurable circulating levels of TNF were seen in the untreated and cyclophosphamide-treated mice as shown in Figs 1 and 2. The rapid rise at 1-2 hr followed by a fall to undetectable levels at 4 hr are consistent with previous reports of circulating TNF following LPS challenge in animals and humans (2, 6, 8). Although the numbers of animals for comparison are small, cyclophosphamide-pretreatment enhanced TNF release following LPS challenge, which is consistent with reports of cyclophosphamide sensitization of mice to LPS challenge (3).

In another experiment designed to measure circulating TNF in a model of gram-negative infection, mice were given a bilateral thigh muscle inoculation with live bacteria. In cyclophosphamide-treated C57BL/10 mice, a 10^6 CFU/mouse inoculum of E. coli (ATCC 25922) resulted in overt signs of sepsis within 4-6 hr; i.e., hair ruffling, decreased spontaneous activity, shivering, and increased respiratory rate. Noncyclophosphamide-treated mice received an inoculum 10^6 CFU/mouse of a highly virulent K. pneumoniae. No measurable circulating serum TNF was found in either model (Fig 2).

In this study, deep seated lethal gram-negative infection failed to produce detectable circulating levels of TNF, in contrast to what has been seen with bolus infusion of LPS and bacteria (2, 6, 8, 9). While endotoxin infusion and bacteremia produce a rapid peak and disappearance of circulating TNF, localized infection may release TNF locally or systemically in amounts that fail to produce detectable circulating LPS needed to produce circulating levels of TNF may be greater for mice, a less LPS-responsive species, than primates. As suggested by others, undetectable levels of TNF may synergize with other mediators such as gamma interferon and interleukin-1 to mediate the lethal host response to sepsis (6). Alternatively, other virulence factors, such as α-hemolysin, may predominate in these strains which lead to death without endotoxemia.

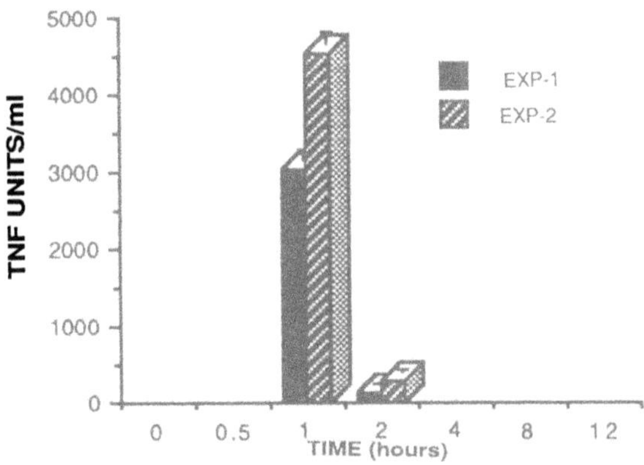

Fig 2. Circulating TNF in cyclophosphamide-induced neutropenic mice following 500 μg LPS challenge. As in Fig 1, each experiment represents one mouse per time point. Measurable TNF activity was found at 1 and 2 hr, with no activity at 0, 0.5, 4, 8 and 12 hr.

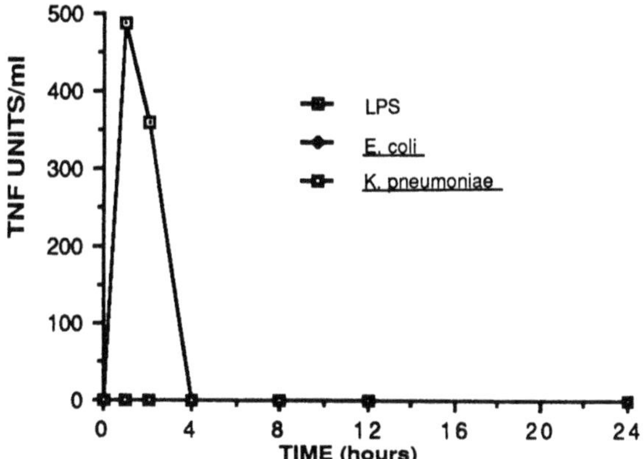

Fig 3. Serum TNF activity following LPS challenge vs. lethal thigh infection with 10^6 CFU E. coli (cyclophosphamide-induced neutropenic mice) and 10^6 CFU K. pneumoniae (normopenic mice). No measurable activity was found with either bacterial challenges.

REFERENCES

1. Beutler, B. A., Milsack, I. W. and Cerami, A., 1985, Passive immunization against cachectin tumor necrosis factor protects mice from lethal effects of endotoxin. Science 229: 869-871.

2. Beutler, B. A., Milsack, I. W. and Cerami, A., 1985, Cachectin/tumor necrosis factor: production, distribution and metabolic fate in vivo. J. Immunol. 135: 3972-3977.

3. Bradley, S. G., 1985, Interactions between endotoxin and protein synthesis, in: "Handbook of Endotoxin," Vol. 3, Cellular Biology of Endotoxin, L. J. Berry, ed., Elsevier, Amsterdam, New York, p. 340-371.

4. Flick, D. A. and Gifford, G. E., 1983, Comparison of in vitro cytotoxic assays for tumor necrosis factor. J. Immunol. Methods 68: 167-175.

5. Golenbock, D. T., Leggett, J. E., Rasmussen, P., Craig, W. A., Raetz, C.

R. H. and Proctor, R. A., 1988, Lipid X protects mice against fatal gram-negative infection. Infect. Immun. 56: 779-784.

6. Hesse, D. G., Tracey, K. J., Fong, Y., et al., 1988, Cytokine appearance in human endotoxemia and primate bacteremia. Surg. Gynecol. Obstet. 166: 147-153.

7. Mannel, D. N., Northoff, H., Bauss, F. and Felk, W., 1987, Tumor necrosis factor: cytokine involved in toxic effects of endotoxin. Rev. Infect. Dis. 9: S602-S606.

8. Rothstein, J. L. and Schreiber, H., 1987, Relationship of tumor necrosis factor and endotoxin to macrophage cytotoxicity, hemorrhagic necrosis and lethal shock, in: "Tumor necrosis factor and related cytotoxins," J. Wiley, ed., London, England (Ciba Found. Symp. 131), p. 124-135.

9. Tracey, K. J., Fong, Y., Hesse, A. G., et al., 1987, Anti-cachectin/ TNF monoclonal antibodies prevent septic shock during lethal bacteremia. Nature 330: 662-664.

10. Tracey, K. J., Lowry, S. F. and Cerami, A., 1988, Cachectin: a hormone that triggers acute shock and chronic cachexia. J. Infect. Dis. 157: 413-420.

11. Tracey, K. J., Lowry, S. F., Fahey, T. J., et al., 1987, Cachectin/ tumor necrosis factor induces lethal shock and stress hormone responses in the dog. Surg. Gynecol. Obstet. 164: 415-422.

BIOLOGICAL PROPERTIES OF LIPOPOLYSACCHARIDES ISOLATED FROM BORDETELLA

M. Watanabe, H. Takimoto, Y. Kumazawa* and K. Amano**

The Kitasato Institute and *School of Pharmaceutical Sciences, Kitasato University, 5-9-1 Shirokane, Minato-ku Tokyo 108 and **Hirosaki University School of Medicine Hirosaki 036, Japan

ABSTRACT

Biological activity of lipopolysaccharides (LPSs) separated from Bordetella, i.e., **B. pertussis** (Bp), **B. parapertussis** (Bpp) and **B. bronchiseptica** (Bbs), was determined and compared with that of an **Escherichia coli** LPS as a control. Two Bp-LPS preparations showed marked biological activities comparable to those of **E. coli** LPS in terms of lethal toxicity in galactosamine-sensitized mice, pyrogenicity in rabbits, mitogenicity in C3H/He spleen cell cultures, macrophage activation and tumor necrosis factor-inducing activity. All the activities except mitogenicity of two Bpp-LPS preparations were lower than or comparable to those of E. coli LPS. Activities stronger than or comparable to those of E. coli LPS were observed in two Bbs-LPS preparations. Among six LPS preparations from Bordetella tested, a Bbs-LPS from L3 strain exhibited the most intensive activities.

INTRODUCTION

There is little information on LPS of **B. parapertussis** and **B. bronchiseptica**, though a nontoxic and Shwartzman-negative lipid A possessing high adjuvant activities was isolated from **B. pertussis** LPS (1). Accordingly, it was attempted to determine biological activities, i.e., lethal toxicity in galactosamine-sensitized mice, pyrogenicity, mitogenicity, macrophage activation and tumor necrosis factor (TNF)-inducing activity, of six LPS preparations from three **Bordetella** species and to compare with those of a LPS preparation from **E. coli** 055:B5 strain (Difco Laboratories).

RESULTS AND DISCUSSION

All LPS preparations separated from the **Bordetella** contained glucosamine, xylose, heptose, KDO, uronic acid, phosphate and fatty acids. Protein contents differed in each LPS preparation. KDO contents of the LPSs were very low as compared with heptose contents. Myristic, palmitic, isopalmitic and β-hydroxymiristic acids were the major fatty acid composition in the LPSs, suggesting that the lipid A moiety of the **Bordetella** LPSs is similar to that of an enterobacterial lipid A.

Lethality in galactosamine-sensitized mice was tested using male 10-wk-old C57BL/6 mice according to the method of Galanos (2). Among LPSs tested, a Bbs-LPS (L3) preparation exhibited the most intensive activity (100%

lethality at 1 ng/mouse). The activity of two Bp-LPS preparations (Tohama and AK-168) was almost comparable to that of **E. coli** LPS showing 100% lethality at a dose of 10 ng/mouse. Another Bbs-LPS preparation (H-214) exhibited somewhat stronger lethality than the Bp-LPSs (1 ng/mouse), but the activity of two Bpp-LPS preparations (21815 and AK-167) was weaker than the Bp-LPS (100 ng/mouse).

Pyrogenicity was assessed by determining mean fever response of three Japanese white rabbits each of which was administered intravenously (i.v.) a test sample dose (3). The smallest dose that consistently evoked rise in rabbit body temperature (at least a 0.6°C) was found to be 10 ng/kg for Bp-LPS (Tohama) and Bbs-LPSs (L3 and H-214). Pyrogenicity of the Bpp-LPSs was detected at a dose of 100 ng/kg, while Bp-LPS (AK-168) did not show detectable activity at a dose of 100 ng/kg.

Macrophage activation by **Bordetella** LPSs was judged by measuring phagocytic, cellular lysosomal enzyme (acid phosphatase) and cytostatic activities of macrophages obtained from the peritoneal cavity of mice which had been injected intraperitoneally with 1 µg of test sample 4 days earlier, as described previously (3). All of the **Bordetella** LPSs tested induced significant macrophage activation at a dose of 1 µg/mouse. The ability of both Bbs-LPSs was almost comparable to or somewhat weaker than that of a control E. coli LPS. Macrophage activation by Bp-LPSs (Tohama and AK-168) was almost equivalent to that by a Bbs-LPS (H-214), while the activity of Bpp-LPSs was much weaker than that of **E. coli** LPS.

TNF-inducing activity was assessed by determining whether or not samples induced detectable TNF into sera of **P. acnes**-primed mice when they were injected i.v. at varying doses (3). The activity of TNF in the sera was determined by the cytolytic assay using L929 cells. All preparations showed significant TNF-inducing activity at a dose of 1 µg/mouse. The activity of Bp-LPSs and Bbs-LPSs was almost comparable to or somewhat stronger than that of **E. coli** LPS, while Bpp-LPSs was less active in TNF-induction than **E. coli** LPS.

Mitogenic activity was assessed by estimating tritiated thymidine uptake into C3H/He and C3H/HeJ spleen cells which were incubated with test samples (3). All LPS preparations tested showed significant mitogenic activity in C3H/He spleen cell cultures at a concentration of more than 10 ng/0.1 ml/well. The activity of Bp- and Bbs-LPSs was almost equivalent to or higher than that of **E. coli** LPS. Both Bpp-LPS preparations showed much stronger mitogenicity than **E. coli** LPS, though other biological activities were weaker than those of **E. coli** LPS. Both LPS preparations (Tohama and 21815) containing trace amounts of protein did not show detectable mitogenicity even at the high concentration of 10 µg/0.1 ml/well.

These results indicate that six LPS preparations from three species of **Bordetella** were stronger or weaker in the biological activities tested than an **E. coli** LPS preparation and that there is significant difference in the expression of activities among them.

REFERENCES

1. Ayme, G., Caroff, M., Chaby, R., H-Cavaillon, N., Dur, A. D., Moreau, M., Muset, M., Mynard, M. C., Roumiantzeff, M., Schulz, D. and Szabo, L., 1980, Biological activities of fragments derived from **Bordetella pertussis** endotoxin: isolation of a nontoxic, Shwartzman negative lipid A possessing high adjuvant properties. Infect. Immun. 27: 739.

2. Galanos, C., Freudenberg, M. A. and Reutter, W., 1979, Galactosamine-

induced sensitization to the lethal effects of endotoxin. Proc. Natl. Acad. Sci. USA 76: 5939.

3. Kumazawa, Y., Nakatsuka, M., Takimoto, H., Furuya, T., Nagumo, T., Yamamoto, A., Homma, J. Y., Inada, K., Yoshida, M., Kiso, M. and Hasegawa, A., 1988, Importance of fatty acid substituents of chemically synthesized lipid A-subunit analogs in the expression of immunopharmacological activity. Infect. Immun. 56: 149.

ALTERATIONS OF RESPONSES TO BACTERIAL ENDOTOXIN BY BACTEROIDES FRAGILIS IN VIVO AND IN VITRO

A. C. Rodloff, S. Ehlers, D. K. Blanchard* and H. Hahn

Institute for Medical Microbiology and Immunology, Free University of Berlin, Federal Republic of Germany and *Department of Medical Microbiology and Immunology University of South Florida, Tampa, USA

INTRODUCTION

Gram negative obligately anaerobic bacteria constitute a major part of the normal indigenous bacterial flora of humans, however, they also have to be considered to be important opportunistic pathogens, e.g., infections with Bacteroidaceae may arise, when the function of the mucous membranes as anatomic barrier for microorganisms is compromised and bacteria are introduced into otherwise sterile tissues. In such instances, the resulting infection is often of polymicrobial etiology and Bacteroidaceae are found especially in association with Enterobacteriaceae. It is clinical experience that these mixed aerobic/anaerobic infections create significant therapeutical problems even if the individual causative microorganisms display a high in-vitro-susceptibility to antimicrobial agents employed. Therefore, efforts were made to study the interaction of aerobes and anaerobes in mixed infections with a number of different animal models.

Altemeier (1) showed as early as in 1942, that bacterial mixtures isolated from several cases of human peritonitis had higher pathogenic potential in experimental animals than pure cultures of any of the microorganisms involved. A more precise evaluation of synergistic effects of mixed inocula was given by Hite et al., (3) and later by Socransky and Gibbons (12), who emphasized the role of the Bacteroidaceae in augmenting the virulence of the bacterial associations. Weinstein, Onderdonk and co-workers (8, 13) reported on syngergistic effects in a model of peritonitis (intra-abdominal sepsis) in Wistar rats, while Kelly (6) described synergy for the same bacteria in experimental wound infections.

Our studies were aimed at developing a simple and reproducible experimental model of synergistic infection with Escherichia coli and Bacteroides species and at investigating the mechanisms responsible for the synergistic action of these bacteria.

MATERIALS AND METHODS

Experimental Animals

Female (C57Bl/6 x DBA/2)F1 hybrid mice at the age of approximately 10 wk were used throughout the experiments. The animals were raised at our own breeding facilities and kept under specific pathogen free conditions.

Bacteria

Bacteroides fragilis ATCC 25285 (BF) was grown in Schaedler-broth (BBL Microbiology Systems, Cockeysville, MD, USA; supplemented with 0.1 mg/1 Vitamin K1) under anaerobic conditions for 24 hr at 37°C and appropriate bacterial concentrations were established by adding fresh medium. BF was either passaged repeatedly through animals to ensure maximal encapsulation (BFa) or was subcultured in broth media until part of the capsular material was lost (BFl). Furthermore, Bacteroides thetaiotaomicron ATCC 29741 and Bacteroides distasonis B 24 were included in some studies. Escherichia coli ATCC 25922 (EC) was used as aerobic organism in mixed infections. When called for, Listeria monocytogenes EGD (LM) and Streptococcus pneumoniae ATCC 6303 (SP) were employed to evaluate unrelated organisms. All aerobes were either grown in nutrient broth or in brain-heart infusion broth (Oxoid, Basingstoke, Hampshire, GB).

Experimental Infections

Infective organisms were introduced into experimental animals by intravenous injections (tail vein) of 0.2 ml fresh broth culture. Mixed infections were established with separate successive injections of pure cultures, monoinfected controls received an additional 0.2 ml of sterile broth. EC was given at a dose of 1×10^7 cfu per animal, which caused death of approx. 10% of the mice challenged within 4 days. Bacteroides species were always injected at 1×10^8 cfu/mouse. This inoculum by itself usually was not lethal. If called for, Escherichia coli 0111:B4-derived lipopolysaccharide (LPS; Sigma Chemical Co., St. Louis, MO, USA) was suspended in phosphate buffered salt solution (PBS) at a concentration of 0.5 g/1 and mice received 0.2 ml of this solution i.v. Experimental animals were observed for 9 days post infection (p.i.) and lethality was recorded. At day 9 p.i., survivors were killed, livers and kidneys recovered, homogenized in PBS, and aliquots appropriately cultivated to establish bacterial organ content.

Proliferation of Spleen Cells from Infected Animals

Spleens were obtained from infected mice at indicated times after injection of the bacteria and disrupted into single cell suspensions. Red blood cells were lysed, remaining cells washed three times and resuspended in RPMI 1640 (Biochrom KG, Berlin, Germany; supplemented with per liter 3.7 g $NaHCO_3$, 100 ml fetal bovine serum, 100,000 I.E. penicillin, and 10 mg streptomycin) at a concentration of 2×10^6/ml. When called for, RPMI was further supplemented with 5 mg/1 indomethacin (Sigma). Wells of microtitration plates were filled with 0.2 ml of spleen cell suspension and 0.01 mg of LPS were added to each culture to induce proliferation. After incubation for 24 hr at 37°C in 5% CO_2, 0.001 mCi of ^{3}H-thymidine was added to each well. After additional incubation for 24 hr, cells were harvested on filter paper and radioactivity of the cells was counted with a liquid scintillation spectrometer (Packard Instrument Co., Rockville, MD, USA).

Proliferation of Spleen Cells Treated with Bacteroides fragilis In Vitro

Spleens were obtained from healthy mice and cells were taken into culture as described above. Various amounts of appropriate heat killed bacteria were placed into each well and cultures were then incubated for 6 hr before LPS was added and the above mentioned procedure was followed again.

Effect of Bacteroides fragilis on Interferon Production by Spleen Cells

Spleen cells were taken into culture as described above and incubated in the presence of 1×10^8 heat killed bacteria/ml (BFa, EC, LM, or SP), 10 mg/1 LPS, 5 mg/1 Concanavalin A (Con A; Sigma), or 2 mg/1 phytohemagglutinin (PHA,

Burroughs Wellcome Corp., Research Triangle, NC, USA). Supernatants were collected after 24 hr of incubation and assayed for interferon (IFN) activity. For this purpose, 0.05 ml of serial half-log dilutions were placed into wells of microtitration plates together with 2 x 10^4 L929 cells and incubated for 24 hr. Then, 4000 plaque forming units of vesicular stomatitis virus were added to each culture and after further incubation (24 hr), virus-induced cytopathogenic effects and protection afforded by the supernatants were evaluated. Results were expressed in units calibrated against a reference mouse IFN obtained from the National Institute of Allergy and Infectious Diseases, USA.

RESULTS

Experimental Infections

Mice were infected with selected doses of bacteria that were either shown to cause no lethality (1 x 10^8 Bacteroides species) or that inflicted death on approx. 10% of the animals challenged (LD_{10}; 1 x 10^7 EC). Table 1 shows that when mixed inocula were used, a significant increase in lethality of experimental animals was observed (LD_{50} to LD_{80}). The synergistic effects were not exclusive for encapsulated or less encapsulated BF and EC, but could also be produced by combining EC with other pathogenic Bacteroides species (BT, BD). Interestingly, when viable BFa were replaced by heat-killed organisms, the synergy was still operative. The latter fact prompted us to determine, whether the vitality of EC was a prerequisite for synergy.

Effect of Bacteroides fragilis on Lipopolysaccharide Toxicity in Experimental Animals

The lipopolysaccharide of gram negative bacteria such as EC are of major importance in the pathogenicity of these microorganisms. Therefore, in additional experiments, the viable EC were replaced by a dose of 0.1 mg of LPS per mouse. This inoculum proved to be equivalent to the bacteria in terms of lethality induced in experimental animals (Table 2). When combined with an injection of BFa, the synergistic effects observed for the viable bacteria did not recur. However, when animals were pretreated with Bacter-

Table 1.

Lethality of mice infected with different bacteria either alone or in combination. In addition, the yield of infecting organisms in liver and kidneys of animals surviving at day 9 post infection are given.

bacteria injected	lethality[1]	yield of Bacteroides in[2] liver		kidneys		yield of Escherichia coli in[3] liver			kidneys		
		$<10^2$	10^2-10^5	$<10^2$	10^2-10^5	$<10^2$	10^2-10^5	$>10^5$	$<10^2$	10^2-10^5	$>10^5$
BFa	0/20	19x	1x	20x	no	does not apply					
BFl	0/20	20x	no	20x	no	does not apply					
BT	0/20	14x	6x	20x	no	does not apply					
BD	0/20	15x	5x	18x	2x	does not apply					
EC	2/20	does not apply				17x	1x	no	17x	1x	no
BFa+EC	11/20	6x	3x	8x	1x	3x	6x	no	3x	4x	2x
BFl+EC	10/20	10x	no	10x	no	8x	2x	no	4x	6x	no
BT+EC	16/20	4x	no	4x	no	3x	1x	no	3x	1x	no
BD+EC	12/20	6x	2x	7x	1x	5x	2x	1x	6x	2x	no
BFa[4]+EC	8/20	does not apply				9x	3x	no	6x	4x	2x

[1]Lethality: Number of animals dead 9 days post infection/ total number of animals infected
[2]Number of surviving animals yielding Bacteroides species in liver and/or kidneys 9 days post infection. Detection limit: 10^2 cfu/organ
[3]Number of surviving animals yielding Escherichia coli in liver and/or kidneys 9 days post infection. Detection limit: 10^2 cfu/organ
[4]Heat - killed encapsulates Bacteroides fragilis

Table 2. LPS-susceptibility of mice pretreated with Bacteroides species at different times

bacteria injected	time between injections	LPS injected	lethality[1)]
1×10^8 BFA	0 hr	0.1 mg	2/20
1×10^8 BFA	3 hr	0.1 mg	1/20
1×10^8 BFA	6 hr	0.1 mg	11/20
1×10^8 BFA	12 hr	0.1 mg	7/20
1×10^8 BFA	24 hr	0.1 mg	4/20
1×10^8 BFA	48 hr	0.1 mg	0/20
1×10^8 BT	6 hr	0.1 mg	17/20
1×10^8 BD	6 hr	0.1 mg	8/20
1×10^8 BFA[2)]	6 hr	0.1 mg	9/20

1) Lethality: Number of animals dead by day 9 post infection/total number of animals infected

2) Heat-killed encapsulated Bacteroides fragilis

oides species and later challenged with LPS, the synergy was restored. This effect was time dependent and maximal lethality was observed, when BFa was given 6 hr prior to the LPS dose (Table 2). Finally, heat killed BFa and LPS together also displayed synergy.

Lipopolysaccharide-stimulated Proliferation of Spleen Cells from Bacteroides fragilis-Infected Mice

Among the wide variety of biologic effects of LPS, perhaps the best studied phenomenon is the polyclonal expansion of B lymphocytes. Moreover, lymphocytes seem to be essential in mediating the toxic effects of LPS. We therefore addressed the question, whether the injection of BFa into experimental animals alters the proliferative response to LPS of their spleen cells.

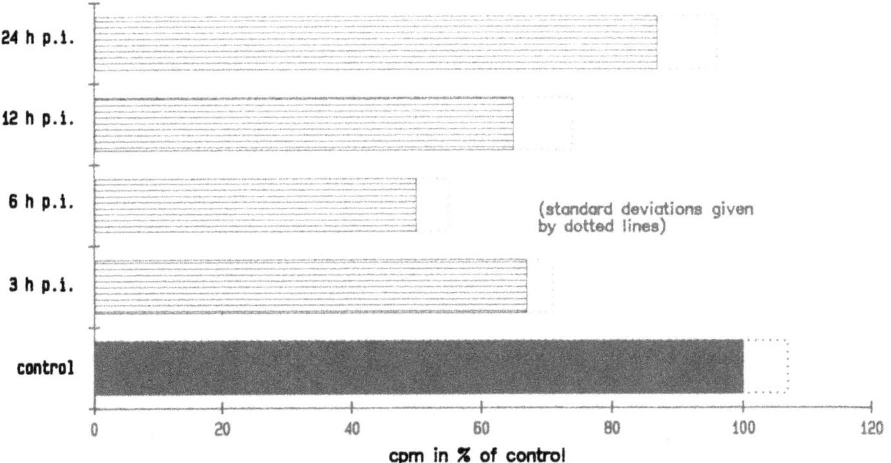

Fig 1. Incorporation of ^{3}H-labeled thymidine by spleen cells harvested from mice at different times post infection (p.i.) with Bacteroides fragilis and stimulated in vitro with LPS.

Splenocytes of BFa infected mice were harvested at different times after introduction of the bacteria into the animals and then tested in vitro for their capacity to proliferate upon stimulation with LPS. The results clearly demonstrate that--if compared to normal splenocytes--cells from infected animals are inhibited in their mitogenic response (Fig 1). The degree of inhibition was time dependent and followed the same pattern as observed for the augmented animal susceptibility to LPS toxicity.

Lipopolysaccharide-stimulated Proliferation of Spleen Cells Treated with Bacteroides fragilis In Vitro

The inhibition of the mitogenic response of splenocytes to LPS was further analyzed with an in vitro system. Spleen cells were incubated together with heat killed BFa and then stimulated with LPS. Again a dose dependent suppression of the proliferation became evident (Fig 2). To test the specificity of this effect, other bacteria were also included in this study (EC, LM, SP). Although there was some inhibition of the LPS induced proliferation with EC and LM, only SP caused similarly extensive suppression as BFa (Fig 3). When the experiment were repeated with 5 mg/l indomethacin present in the culture medium, essentially the same results were obtained (data not shown).

Effect of Bacteroides fragilis on Lipopolysaccharide-induced Interferon Production

Upon stimulation with bacteria, capsular polysaccharides, or lipopolysaccharide, leukocytes are known to produce immunomodulators such as interferons. We therefore became interested to evaluate the effect BFa might have on IFN production. When equal amounts of different heat killed bacteria were tested for their ability to induce IFN in spleen cell cultures, BFa proved to be less effective than EC, LM or SP (Table 3). Neutralization experiments with antibodies against IFN alpha/beta showed that all organisms and LPS induced both, IFN alpha/beta and IFN gamma, while Con A and PHA only induced IFN gamma. When splenocytes of infected mice were investigated, those from animals injected with either LM or SP showed a spontaneous IFN alpha/beta release in vitro (Table 4). Addition of LPS to these cultures resulted in IFN levels well above the values of control cultures with cells from uninfected animals. On the other hand, splenocytes from BFa or EC infected mice

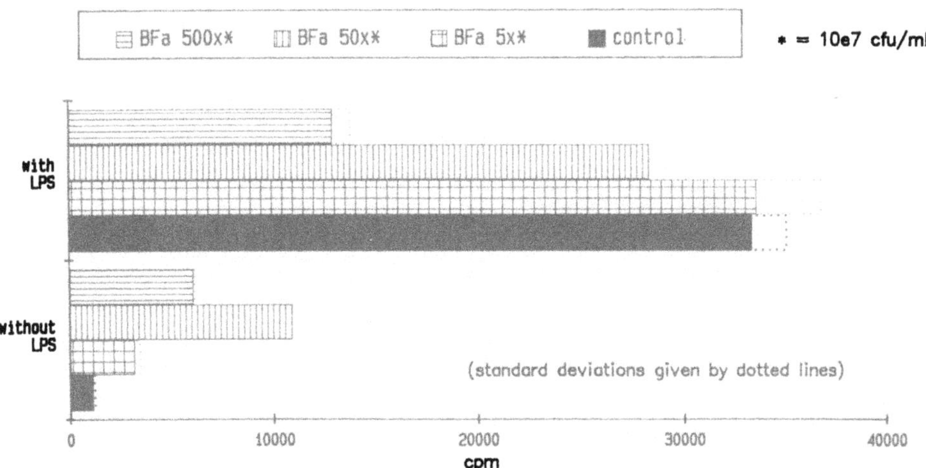

Fig 2. Incorporation of ^{3}H-labeled thymidine by mouse spleen cells treated in vitro with varying amounts of heat killed encapsulated Bacteroides fragilis (BFa) and then stimulated with LPS.

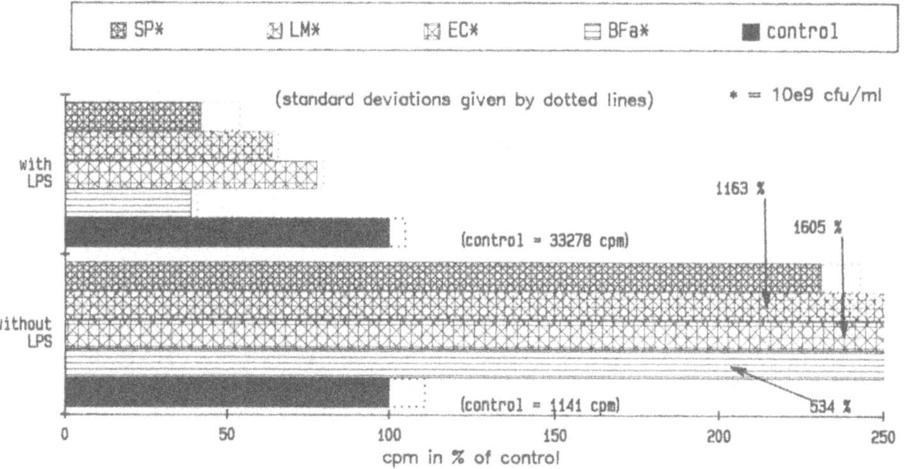

Fig 3. Incorporation of ^{3}H-labeled thymidine by mouse spleen cells treated in vitro with different heat killed bacteria (Bacteroides fragilis, Escherichia coli, Listeria monocytogenes, Streptococcus pneumoniae) and then stimulated with LPS.

did not release IFN spontaneously in vitro, and moreover, were hyporesponsive to stimulation with LPS.

DISCUSSION

Numerous investigators have provided evidence for synergistic effects of Bacteriodaceae and Enterobacteriaceae in experimental infections (3, 6, 8, 10, 12, 13). However, in many of these studies immunologically active substances (8, 13) or alterations of the host's integrity (6) have been used to establish reproducible infections. Accordingly, it was difficult to evaluate the actual contribution of the individual bacterial strains to the disease process. Employing intravenous injections of bacteria, we have developed an experimental model not necessitating such adjuvants for initiating the infec-

Table 3. In vitro production of interferons after induction of spleen cell cultures with heat killed bacteria, LPS, or plant lectins

Induction with	IFN (U/ml) in supernatant
none	<10[1)]
BFa	85(20)[2)]
EC	450(300)
LM	250(100)
SP	300(100)
LPS	100(30)
Con A	1000(1000)
PHA	300(300)

[1)] Levels are the average of three separate experiments
[2)] Remaining IFN activity after treatment of supernatants with sheep anti-mouse-IFN-alpha/beta-antibodies

Table 4. In vitro production of interferons by spleen cells that were harvested from mice 6 hr after injection of different bacteria and either were or were not stimulated by the addition of LPS to the culture media in vitro

Mice infected with	IFN (U/ml) in supernatants	
	no LPS stimulation	LPS stimulated[1)]
control	<10	100(30)[2)]
1 x 10^8	<10	30(<10)
1 x 10^8	<10	30(<10)
1 x 10^8	50(<10)	400(150)
1 x 10^8	50(<10)	500(500)

1) 10 mg/1 LPS
2) Remaining IFN activity after treatment of supernatants with sheep anti-mouse-IFN-alpha/beta-antibodies.

tious process. Again, in this model, Bacteroides species and EC proved to be synergistic in terms of animal lethality (Table 1).

The mechanisms of this bacterial synergy seem to be quite complex. Mayrand and McBride (7) showed that a metabolic product of Klebsiella pneumonia (succinate) enhanced the growth of Bacteroides asaccharolyticus. With our studies it became clear that even heat killed (metabolically inactive) bacteria and/or bacterial components (LPS) can be sufficient to cause synergistic effects in an animal host (Tables 1 and 2). Therefore, it seemed likely that alterations of the host's immune response by Bacteroides species were responsible for the described effects.

Ingham et al., (4) reported in 1977 that anaerobes interfere with the phagocytosis of aerobic bacteria by polymorphonuclear leukocytes in vitro. These results were later confirmed and extended by a number of other authors (2, 5, 11) and competition of the bacteria for serum opsonins was held responsible for the described effects (2, 5). Furthermore, it was shown that BF is capable of inhibiting the phagocytic activity of macrophages in vitro and in vivo (9). This suppression of phagocytic systems might be one explanation of enhanced bacterial concentrations in organs of animals suffering from mixed infections (Table 1), subsequently resulting in augmented organ failure rates and higher lethality.

With the present study, we addressed the question whether Bacteroides fragilis is capable of altering biologic effects of Escherichia coli-derived LPS in experimental animals or in in vitro assay systems, respectively. First, it became evident that BF-infected mice displayed an increased susceptibility to LPS toxicity (Fig 1). This effect was not present immediately after the injection of BF but affected the animal over a certain period of time. The time course followed the pattern established earlier for other in vivo effects of the anaerobe (9).

In an attempt to further characterize the alterations of the LPS-response in BF-infected animals, we concentrated on spleen cell functions. Fig 1 shows that -in vitro- splenocytes from infected mice are inhibited in their LPS-induced mitogenicity. Again, the effect follows the above-mentioned time pattern with maximal inhibition present 6 hr post infection. In vitro, the suppression of LPS-primed proliferation by BF was demonstrated to be directly dose related (Fig 2). Subsequent studies showed that the effect was not specific for BF, since other organisms (EC, LM) were also suppressive; however, the inhibition was significantly less pronounced. Only SP, an organism possessing a polysaccharide capsule like BF, exerted a similarly effective impairment of the LPS-induced spleen cell proliferation. Very preliminary data from our laboratory (data not shown) suggest that isolated capsular polysaccharide of BFa is equally suppressive as the whole organism. Hence, the capsule might be the common denominator for the similar effects of BF and SP described here.

Since BF disturbed the induction of spleen cells proliferation in response to LPS, the capacity of interleukin production of the cells was evaluated employing IFN synthesis as an example. Table 3 shows that BFa itself is not a potent inducer of IFN synthesis in splenocytes. However, BFa is a very effective inducer of IFN production in liver leukocytes (data not shown). Spleen cells from BFa-infected mice are hyporesponsive to IFN induction by LPS. This property is shared by cells from EC- but not from LM- or SP-infected animals. The consequence of the suppression of IFN production at present remains unsettled.

In conclusion, BFa has been demonstrated to significantly inhibit host defense mechanisms. Especially, biologic responses to bacterial LPS seem to be disrupted. At the same time, experimental animals are found to be hypersensitive to the toxic properties of LPS. The latter fact may contribute to the synergistic effects of mixed aerobic/anaerobic infections.

REFERENCES

1. Altemeier, W.A., 1942, The pathogenicity of the bacteria of appendicitis peritonitis. Surgery 11: 374-384.

2. Dijkmans, B. A. C., Leijh, P. C. J., Braat, A. G. P. and van Furth, R., 1985, Effect of bacterial competition on the opsonisation, phagocytosis, and intracellular killing of microorganisms by granulocytes. Infect. Immun. 49: 219-224.

3. Hite, K. E., Locke, M. and Hesseltine, H. C., 1949, Synergism in experimental infections with nonsporulating anaerobic bacteria. J. Infect. Dis. 84: 1-9.

4. Ingham, H. R., Sissons, P. R., Thargonnet, D., Selkon, J. B. and Codd, A. A., 1977, Inhibition of phagocytosis in vitro by obligate anaerobes. Lancet II 1252-1254.

5. Jones, G. R. and Gemmel, C. G., 1982, Impairment by Bacteroides species of opsonisation and phagocytosis of enterobacteria. J. Med. Microbiol. 15: 351-361.

6. Kelly, M. J., 1978, The quantative and histological demonstration of pathogenic synergy between Escherichia coli and Bacteroides fragilis in guinea pig wounds. J. Med. Microbiol. 11: 513-523.

7. Mayrand, D. and McBride, B. C., 1980, Ecological relationship of bacteria involved in a simple, mixed anaerobic infection. Infect. Immun. 27: 44-50.

8. Onderdonk, A. B., Bartlett, J. G., Louie, T., Sullivan-Seigler, N. and Gorbach, S. L., 1976, Microbial synergy in experimental intra-abdominal abscess. Infect. Immun. 13: 22-26.

9. Rodloff, A. C., Becker, J., Blanchard, D. K., Klein, T. W., Hahn, H.

and Friedman, H., 1986, Inhibition of macrophage phagocytosis by Bacteroides fragilis in vivo and in vitro. Infect. Immun. 52: 488-492.

10. Rodloff, A. C. and Hahn, H., 1984, Synergistic lethality in experimental infections with Escherichia coli and Bacteroides fragilis. Zentralbl. Bakteriol. Mikrobiol. Hyg. A 258: 112-119.

11. Rodloff, A. C., Hilliger, F., Friedman, H. and Hahn, H., 1986, Effects of anti-Bacteroides-antibodies on Escherichia coli and different Bacteroides species in vitro and vivo. Zentralbl. Bakteriol. Mikrobiol. Hyg. A 262: 483-491.

12. Socransky, S. S. and Gibbons, R. J., 1965, Required role of Bacteroides melaninogenicus in mixed anaerobic infections. J. Infect. Dis. 115: 247-253.

13. Weinstein, W. M., Onderdonk, A. B., Bartlett, J. G. and Gorbach, S. L., 1974, Experimental intra-abdominal abscesses in rats: development of an experimental model. Infect. Immun. 10: 1250-1255.

MECHANISMS OF THE LETHAL ACTION OF ENDOTOXIN AND ENDOTOXIN HYPERSENSITIVITY

C. Galanos, M. A. Freudenberg, and M. Matsuura

Max-Planck-Institut für Immunbiologie, Stübeweg 51, 7800 Freiburg, FRG

MECHANISMS OF HOST-RESPONSE TO ENDOTOXIN

Endotoxins (lipopolysaccharides, LPS) are endowed with a vast spectrum of biological activities that are both harmful and beneficiary for the host-organism. Many of these activities, e.g., mitogenic and polyclonal stimulation of antibody-producing cells, adjuvance activity or induction of prostaglandin and leucotriene synthesis in macrophages are not exclusively properties of endotoxin. They are also expressed by a number of other substances like zymosan (1, 22) or muramyl dipeptide (MDP) (9, 25, 26, 27) which are in some cases even more powerful inducers than endotoxin itself. Conversely, however, neither zymosan nor MDP elicit acute, hazardous effects that are in any way comparable to those seen in experimental endotoxin shock. Many activities of endotoxins are not necessarily side-effects of their toxic action as believed earlier but are induced independently by discrete structures in the lipid A. Evidence for this has been obtained in recent years by studying partial structures of natural and synthetic lipid A. We could thus show that a natural lipid A precursor structure containing 4 unsubstituted 3-hydroxy-tetradecanoid acid residues (2 amide- and 2 ester linked) expresses significant lethal toxicity. This molecule was incapable of inducing the local Shwartzman reaction, the induction of which requires the additional substitution of at least one of the amide-linked 3-OH-tetradecanoic acids with hexadecanoic acid (12). Similarly a number of synthetic analogues and partial structures of lipid A, despite their low toxicity were potent in inducing proliferation and polyclonal antibody synthesis in mouse B-cells (16, 28, 29, 30). It thus becomes evident that many activities of endotoxin proceed independently and are based on self-contained mechanisms. For this reason, the elucidation of, for example, the mechanism of B-cell activation by endotoxin, although extremely important for the understanding of the effect of LPS on the immune system, and the mechanisms by which LPS interacts and triggers these cells, it will not necessarily disclose the mechanism of endotoxin induced lethality.

The object pursued in our studies has been the identification of the cells and endogenous mediator(s) involved in the lethal toxicity of LPS. Today it is generally agreed upon that the pathophysiological activities of endotoxin are not direct LPS effects, but are induced indirectly through the action of endogenous mediators that are formed after interaction of LPS with humoral and cellular targets. In the past, lymphoreticular cells were shown to mediate endotoxin activity (18, 19, 20, 21); however, the precise identity

Table 1. Lethal toxicity of LPS in normal and D-galactosamine-treated C3H/HeN mice

Mouse strain	Lethality (LD_{50}) in untreated	D-GalN-treated
	(μg LPS)	
C3H/HeN	270	0.0068
C3H/HeJ	> 5,000	1,760

of the cell-type involved was not established. More recently indirect evidence was obtained that tumor-necrosis factor (TNF) (7) represents a primary mediator of the toxicity of LPS (4, 5, 6). In the following chapters direct evidence will be presented that macrophages are the effectors of the lethal activity of LPS. In direct lethality tests it will be shown that TNF is a mediator of lethal toxicity and can replace endotoxin in different LPS-dependent toxicity models.

The Lethal Activity of Endotoxin is Mediated by Macrophages (11)

The role of macrophages in endotoxin-induced lethality was studied in mice made hypersensitive to endotoxin by D-galactosamine. Treatment of different animals with D-galactosamine increases their sensitivity to endotoxin more than 100,000-fold (13). D-galactosamine induces an early depletion of UTP in hepatocytes which leads to inhibition of RNA synthesis (8). These early biochemical alterations are prerequisite for the development of sensitization to endotoxin because their inhibition by uridine also inhibits sensitization (13).

Induction of hypersensitivity to endotoxin by D-galactosamine was found to proceed in rabbits, rats, guinea pigs and in all endotoxin-responder mouse strains tested so far. Treatment of endotoxin-resistant mice (C3H/HeJ or C57Bl/10 SccR) with D-galactosamine had no apparent effect on their high resistance to endotoxin (Table 1). Measurement of UTP levels in the liver of D-galactosamine treated C3H/HeJ mice showed a strong UTP depletion identical to that seen in endotoxin-sensitive C3H/HeN mice (Table 2). This shows that endotoxin-resistant mice are in principle sensitized to endotoxin by D-

Table 2. D-galactosamine-induced changes in liver UTP in C3H/HeN and C3H/HeJ mice

Mouse strain	Treatment	UTP (mmol/kg liver)
C3H/HeN	PBS	0.22 ± 0.02
	D-GalN	0.02 ± 0.002
C3H/HeJ	PBS	0.21 ± 0.04
	D-GalN	0.02 ± 0.003

Table 3. Lethal toxicity of LPS in D-galactosamine treated C3H/HeJ mice administered C3H/HeN macrophages

C3H/HeN macrophages	D-galactosamine (mg)	LPS (μg)	Lethality %
2×10^7	20	100	100
2×10^7	20	10	90
2×10^7	20	1	74
2×10^7	20	0.1	0
none	20	500	0
2×10^7	20	none	0

C3H/HeJ mice received 2×10^7 bone marrow-derived C3H/HeN macrophages (i.v.) and 2 hr later D-galactosamine and different amounts of LPS as a mixture (i.v.).

galactosamine; the sensitization, however, is not evident because the animals lack the mechanism or response to endotoxin. The sensitization of endotoxin-resistant mice by D-galactosamine became evident after transfer of endotoxin-sensitive macrophages in these animals. 2×10^7 pure, cultured macrophages (from histocompatible C3H/HeN mice), administered to C3H/HeJ mice, rendered them sensitive to the lethal activity of sub-microgram amounts of LPS after D-galactosamine treatment, showing that macrophages are the effector cells of the lethal toxicity of LPS (Table 3).

Induction of Lethality by Macrophages may be Triggered With LPS In Vitro (10)

Induction of lethality in D-galactosamine treated C3H/HeJ mice is also achieved by macrophages stimulated with LPS in vitro. Thus C3H/HeN cultured macrophages incubated with LPS, washed and transferred (2×10^7/mouse) into D-galactosamine-treated C3H/HeJ mice, induced lethality without further treatment of the animals with LPS. As seen in Table 4 the amounts of LPS causing lethality in these highly resistant mice are very small. These are given by the values in parenthesis which represent the quantities of LPS associated with the macrophages and which are actually effecting lethality.

The above results lead to the following conclusions. Macrophages mediate the lethal activity of endotoxin. The direct interaction of LPS with macrophages is the first step in the triggering of endotoxin lethality. In the galactosamine-model, sensitization to LPS and induction of lethal toxicity develop independently and are based on different mechanisms. Thus GalN exerts its sensitizing effects by increasing the susceptibility of the host to the lethal action of toxic macrophage products, without increasing susceptibility to LPS itself.

There exist several substances, including zymosan, which are known to be potent activators of macrophages, inducing formation of prostaglandins and leucotrienes, mediators which are also formed upon activation of macrophages with endotoxin (15, 22). It is interesting that none of these substances show toxic effects in normal or D-galactosamine-treated mice. They are equally without toxic activity when we used them to stimulate macrophages in vitro which were subsequently transferred into D-galactosamine treated animals. In this context it may be said that the induction of "lethal" macro-

Table 4. Lethal toxicity of C3H/HeN macrophages treated with LPS in vitro in D-galactosamine sensitized C3H/HeJ mice

LPS/2 x 10^7 macrophages µg	Lethality %
0.5(0.05)	100
0.1(°)	80
0.02(°)	60
0.004	0
control macrophages	0

Pure cultured macrophages derived from bone-marrow precursors of C3H/HeN mice were incubated with different amounts of S. abortus equi LPS at 37°C/90 min. The cells were washed and 2 x 10^7 macrophages transferred into D-galactosamine-treated (20 mg/mouse) C3H/HeJ mice, i.v. Animals receiving 2 x 10^7 macrophages treated under identical conditions but without LPS served as controls.

Values in parenthesis are µg of LPS actually associated with macrophages after incubation and washing. This was measured using ^{14}C LPS.

° = not detectable.

phages is a property unique for LPS. It also becomes evident that those LPS-mediators which are also stimulated in macrophages by nontoxic activators, may be excluded as being directly responsible for endotoxin lethality. Therefore the macrophage-dependent lethal activity of endotoxin must be related to the induction of unique mediators.

TNF a Mediator of the Lethal Activity of LPS (17)

In the above chapter it was shown that D-galactosamine sensitization is a model by which the treated host is sensitized to mediators of LPS rather than to the LPS itself. In the search for the endogenous mediators of LPS lethality we looked therefore for mediators that are released from macrophages and whose toxicity would be enhanceable by D-galactosamine. A number of mediators of macrophage and non-macrophage origin such as prostaglandins, leucotrienes, histamine, serotonin, adrenalin, and platelet activating factor were found to be either nontoxic or, where toxic, their toxicity was not increased after D-galactosamine treatment.

A clue as to be the possible nature of the relevant mediator involved in endotoxin lethality was obtained when TNF-rich sera obtained from P. acnes-treated mice (7) after challenge with LPS were investigated for their toxicity in D-galactosamine-treated mice. In order to exclude that any possible toxic effects of the sera were due to endotoxin contamination, the lethality tests were carried out in D-galactosamine-treated endotoxin resistant C3H/HeJ mice. Such sera, depending on the time of their collection after LPS challenge were highly toxic, approximately 12 µl of the 2 hr serum sufficing to cause lethality (Coumbos, Freudenberg and Galanos, unpublished). These results were suggesting a possible role for TNF in endotoxin lethality.

Evidence for the toxicity of TNF was obtained using human recombinant TNF in normal and D-galactosamine-sensitized mice. The results of these experiments depicted in Table 5, show that TNF is lethal in normal mice in

Table 5. Lethal toxicity of TNF or LPS in D-galactosamine-treated endotoxin-sensitive C57Bl/6 and -resistant C3H/HeJ mice.

D-GalN (mg)	TNF or LPS (μg)	Lethality (dead/total) C56Bl/6	C3H/HeJ
18	TNF: 1.0	6/6	6/6
18	0.1	3/6	4/6
18	0.01	0/6	1/6
18	-	0/6	0/6
-	150	0/6	0/6
-	250	3/6	1/4
-	500	6/6	3/4
18	LPS: 0.01	6/6	0/6
18	500.0	ND	0/6
-	100.0	3/6	0/6

Groups of mice received D-galactosamine and TNF or LPS as mixture intraperitoneally in 0.5 ml PBS. Controls received, D-galactosamine, TNF, or LPS alone.

ND = not determined.

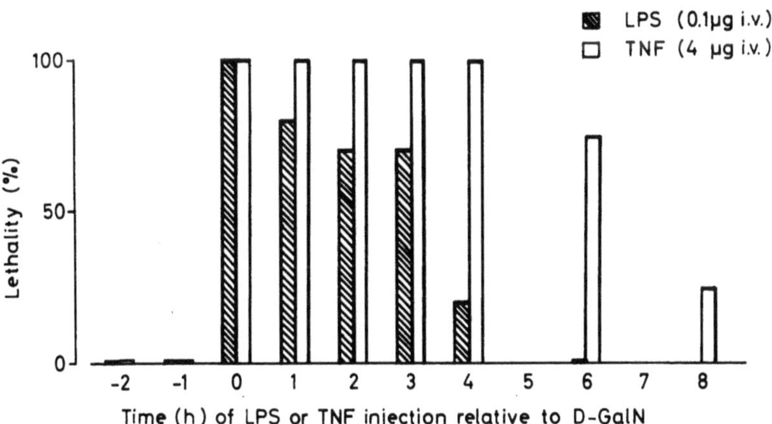

Fig 1. Effect of time interval between D-galactosamine and LPS or TNF administration on sensitization (C57BL/6 mice).

Table 6. Protection to the lethal activity of TNF by specific antiserum

Antiserum (μl)	Lethality (%)
none	100
25	83
50	50
100	0
200	0
normal serum (200 μl)	100

Mice received different amounts of antiserum i.v. Fifteen min later they were challenged with 18 mg D-galactosamine (i.p.) and 1μg TNF (i.v.). Mice receiving normal rabbit serum or no serum and the same amounts of D-galactosamine and TNF served as controls.

a dose of 250-500 μg and that its toxicity is very strongly enhanced by D-galactosamine (LD_{50} = 0,1μg). Unlike LPS, TNF is equally toxic for endotoxin-sensitive and -resistant mice (17).

Administration of uridine which inhibits the D-galactosamine sensitization to LPS also inhibits sensitization to TNF.

The duration of sensitization to TNF by D-galactosamine is shown in Fig 1 and compared to that towards LPS. It may be seen that sensitization to TNF lasts longer than to LPS. This probably reflects the induction time for TNF formation after LPS treatment, which results in the appearance of this mediator at a time when the galactosamine sensitization has already subsided.

It should be noted that neither LPS nor TNF induce lethality when administered before D-galactosamine, an important phenomenon investigated in detail below.

Protective Effect of Anti-TNF Anti-Serum to TNF Lethality

Antiserum to human recombinant TNF raised in rabbits, was found to afford complete protection to the lethal activity of TNF in D-galactosamine-treated mice (Galanos and Freudenberg, unpublished). Table 6 shows that a partial or total protection is obtained with 25 to 100 μl of antiserum. Normal rabbit serum serving as control showed no protective activity.

Induction of Tolerance to LPS/D-galactosamine by Pretreatment with LPS (10)

In Fig 1 it was shown that administration of LPS 1 or 2 hr before D-galactosamine does not cause lethality. Absence of lethality was seen also when amounts of LPS 10,000 times in excess of a lethal dose (10 μg) were administered 1 or 2 hr before D-galactosamine. This result was unexpected because in blood clearance studies it was found that the LPS used (S. abortus equi), has a long time of blood-clearance, so that over 80% of the injected LPS still circulates at the time of D-galactosamine injection (1-2 hr later). The above absence of lethality was found to be due to an induction of tolerance to LPS. Minute amounts of LPS administered in mice rendered them tolerant to a subsequent challenge with D-galactosamine and a second lethal dose of LPS, carried out 1 to 56 hr later (Table 7).

Table 7. Effect of LPS pretreatment on the lethal toxicity of LPS in D-galactosamine-treated mice

Pretreatment (LPS in μg)	Lethality after LPS/D-galactosamine challenge (dead total)
0.1	0/8
0.01	0/8
0.001	4/8
0.0001	8/8
none	8/8

C3H/Tif F mice were injected with different amounts of LPS (in 0.1 ml) intravenously and 90 min later received a mixture of 0.1 μg LPS and 18 mg D-galactosamine (in 0.2 ml) i.v.

Macrophages Mediate the Tolerance Induced by LPS Pretreatment (10)

As shown above, C3H/HeJ mice become highly sensitive to LPS and D-galactosamine when administered endotoxin-sensitive macrophages. Endotoxin-resistant mice receiving LPS-responder macrophages, remain sensitive to LPS for more than 1 week. This model is therefore very useful because it allows a large flexibility with respect to, the time of LPS-pretreatment, LPS/D-galactosamine challenge, or of a second macrophage application. Pretreatment of C3H/HeJ mice with LPS, before administration of D-galactosamine and macrophages, did not protect them of lethality. Complete protection was obtained however, when at the time of LPS pretreatment, endotoxin-sensitive macrophages were administered. In this way the animals were tolerant to a lethal challenge with D-galactosamine and LPS (Table 8). The tolerance could not be broken by a second administration of sensitive macrophages given at the time

Table 8. Induction of tolerance in C3H/HeJ mice by LPS-pretreatment requires LPS-sensitive macrophages

Pretreatment		Challenge			Lethality
Macrophages (C3H/HeN)	LPS (μg)	D-GalN (mg)	Macrophages (C3H/HeN)	LPS (μg)	%
-	-	18	2.10^7	20	100
-	20	18	2.10^7	20	100
2.10^7	-	18	-	20	100
2.10^7	20	18	-	20	0
2.10^7	20	18	2.10^7	20	0

For pretreatment macrophages were injected i.v., followed by LPS i.p. For challenge, D-galactosamine was injected i.p., followed 30 min later by macrophages i.v. and LPS i.p. The interval between pretreatment and challenge may be any time between 90 min and 24 hr.

Table 9. Induction of tolerance to LPS-D-galactosamine by macrophages pretreated with LPS in vitro.

Pretreatment in vitro LPS/2 x 10^7 macrophages μg	Lethality after challenge in vivo with LPS/D-galactosamine
0.5	0
0.1	0
0.02	20
control macrophages	100

Macrophages (C3H/HeN) were incubated with different amounts of LPS at 37°C/1h, washed and 2 x 10^7 cells transferred to C3H/HeJ mice. 2 hr later the animals were challenged with D-galactosamine 18 mg and a lethal dose (1 μg) of LPS i.p. Mice receiving untreated macrophages and challenged with LPS/D-galactosamine served as control.

of challenge. Thus the mice remain tolerant in the presence of macrophages that are capable of being triggered the LPS to cause lethality. This indicates that the tolerance is not necessarily due to a tolerance of the macrophages which were induced by the LPS pretreatment. From these results it is concluded that endotoxin-sensitive macrophages mediate the tolerance-inducing activity of LPS.

Induction of Tolerance by Macrophages Treated with LPS In Vitro (10)

Induction of tolerance by LPS in C3H/HeJ mice in the presence of C3H/HeN macrophages, is also achieved by carrying the LPS-pretreatment directly on macrophages in vitro.

C3H/HeN macrophages incubated with LPS in vitro, washed and transferred (2 x 10^7 cells) into C3H/HeJ mice induce tolerance to a subsequent challenge with LPS/D-galactosamine (Table 9).

From this result it is concluded that the direct interaction of LPS with macrophages is the first step in the induction of tolerance to endotoxin.

TNF - a Mediator of LPS-Induced Tolerance (Galanos and Freudenberg, in press)

Endotoxin-responder mice made tolerant to LPS/D-galactosamine by pretreatment with LPS are also found to be tolerant to the lethal activity of TNF.

Conversely pretreatment of the animals with TNF renders them tolerant to both TNF and LPS (Table 10). The tolerance-inducing property of TNF may be demonstrated directly also in D-galactosamine-treated C3H/HeJ mice. Pretreatment of these animals with TNF makes them tolerant to a subsequent challenge with D-galactosamine and lethal amounts of TNF.

Summary and General Conclusions

The property of endotoxin to induce lethality and tolerance to its own toxic action is mediated by macrophages. Induction of both activities may be carried out extracorporally by treating macrophages with LPS in vitro. Such

Table 10. Induction of tolerance by TNF to the enhanced lethal toxicity of TNF and LPS in D-galactosamine-treated C3H/HeN mice.

Pretreatment (TNF μg)	Lethality after challenge with D-galactosamine (18mg) and TNF (1 μg)	LPS (0.1 μg)
	dead/total	
4	0/6	0/6
1	2/20	8/20
0.1	10/16	6/9
0.01	5/6	6/6
none	6/6	6/6

TNF pretreatment was carried out intravenously, 4 hr before challenge. Challenge with D-galactosamine and TNF or LPS was carried out intraperitoneally.

"triggered" macrophages induce lethality when administered into mice together with or after D-galactosamine, and tolerance when administered before D-galactosamine. Therefore the direct interaction of LPS with macrophages is the first step in the initiation of both activities. The sensitization to LPS of endotoxin resistant mice by D-galactosamine, which becomes apparent after LPS-responsive macrophages are administered to the animals, makes it evident that sensitization to endotoxin and development of LPS toxicity proceed independently and are based on different mechanisms. D-galactosamine does not increase the sensitivity of the host to the LPS itself but to the lethal activity of toxic mediators.

TNF is a mediator of the lethal activity of LPS, and sensitization by D-galactosamine represents also a sensitization to this mediator. Induction of tolerance by LPS is mediated by TNF. LPS and TNF are cross-reacting in their tolerance-inducing property.

HYPERSENSITIVITY TO ENDOTOXIN

Sensitivity to the lethal activity of endotoxin is genetically determined and differs considerably among different species of animals. Apart from genetic factors, endotoxin sensitivity may be influenced by environmental conditions to which the animals are exposed. In a long-term study carried out in rabbits several years ago (Galanos, unpublished) it was found that when the animals were kept under SPF-equivalent conditions about 4% of the animals were naturally hypersensitive to endotoxin. In contrast, in a population kept under less favourable conditions of hygiene, as many as 20% of the animals were hypersensitive. Such hypersensitive rabbits appeared always normal with no obvious signs of illness.

The phenomenon of natural sensitization to endotoxin has been known for many years, yet the underlying mechanisms remained unknown. The experimental evidence obtained during the last six years suggests strongly that endotoxin hypersensitivity may be a frequent cause of lethal outcome in gram-negative infection. We believe that gram-negative septic shock probably always proceeds in a state of hypersensitivity to endotoxin which is acquired by the host during the infection.

Table 11. Models of sensitization to endotoxin developed in recent years

Sensitizing agent	Sensitization factor
Gram-negative infection:	
Coxiella burnetii (phase I)	100
Klebsiella pneumoniae	> 500
Salmonella typhimurium	> 500
Bacterial products:	
Muramyl dipeptide (MDP), (early phase toxicity)	100
Bacterial proteins	50
Hepatoxic agents	
D-galactosamine	100,000
Growing Tumours	
Lewis lung carcinoma	> 10,000
EMT6 sarcoma	200

Experimental models of sensitization may help to understand the mechanisms leading to endotoxin hypersensitivity. A number of sensitization models which we believe to be relevant to natural sensitization have been developed in our laboratory. These are listed in Table 11 and are discussed in the following chapters.

Sensitization by Muramyldipeptide (MDP) (24)

Treatment of mice with MDP (e.g., 100 μg) and subsequent challenge with endotoxin 4 hr later was found to increase the sensitivity of mice to the lethal effects of endotoxin. MDP-hypersensitivity is expressed as two timely distinct toxic manifestations, an early-phase toxicity developing 10 to 20 min after LPS injection and a late-phase toxicity developing 15 hr to 72 hr after LPS administration (Table 12).

Late phase toxicity is a true hypersensitivity to the lethal activity of LPS. It is inducible only in endotoxin-responder mice strains by small amounts (1 to 10 μg) of endotoxically active S- and R-form LPS and free lipid A. Late-phase toxicity is characterized by a slow deterioration in the health of the animals comparable to that seen in nonsensitized animals receiving lethal amounts of LPS.

Late-phase toxicity is a TNF dependent activity. Mice made hypersensitive to LPS by MDP are also hypersensitive to the lethal activity of TNF (Galanos and Freudenberg, unpublished). Thus C57Bl/6 mice treated with MDP (100 μg) were sensitive to as little as 5 μg human recombinant TNF administered 4 hr later, compared to several hundred microgram that are necessary to cause lethality in non-treated animals.

Table 12. Induction of early- and late-phase toxicity by S- and R-form LPS in MDP-treated C57Bl/6 and C3H/HeJ mice

		C57Bl/6		C3H/HeJ	
		deaths/total in phase:		deaths/total in phase:	
MDP (μg)	LPS (μg)	early	late	early	late
100	S-form 100	6/6	-*	6/6	-*
100	10	0/6	6/6	1/6	0/6
100	R-form 100	0/6	6/6	0/6	0/6
100	10	0/6	1/6	0/6	0/6

S-form LPS = S. abortus equi; R-form LPS = S. minnesota R595. The LD_{50} of the LPS of S. abortus equi in normal C57Bl/6 mice is approx. 150 μg that of the R595 approx. 600 μg.

*No survivals from early-phase toxicity.

Early phase toxicity is an anaphylactic-like reaction and may be accompanied by severe convulsions and unconsciousness. It is inducible only by some S-form LPS in amounts of 100 μg but cannot be elicited by R-form LPS of free lipid A even in much higher amounts (Table 12).

Early-phase toxicity is seen also with nontoxic LPS such as that of **Bacteroides gingivalis.** Further a strong early phase toxicity with lethal outcome proceeded also in endotoxin-resistant C3H/HeJ mice. Unlike late phase toxicity it is not a true endotoxic activity. Mice surviving the early-phase toxicity after challenge with toxic LPS usually recover or partly recover during the following 2 or 3 hr. The condition of such animals however slowly deteriorates again and they always die 15 to 75 hr later as a result of the late-phase toxicity.

An analysis of data then leads to the following conclusions. Late-phase toxicity is a lipid A-dependent activity. This is evident from the fact that late-phase toxicity proceeds only in LPS-responder mice with endotoxically active LPS and lipid A. A strong argument for this is also the fact that late-phase toxicity is a TNF-induced activity, because we believe that the classical lethal toxicity of LPS is mediated through TNF. In contrast, early phase toxicity is not obligatorily an activity of toxic lipid A and therefore not mediated through TNF as shown here. It is not known at present which part of the LPS molecule is responsible for this activity.

The present data make it evident that, under certain circumstances, LPS may induce lethal effects which are not related to their classical endotoxic activity.

Protein-Dependent Sensitization (14)

A mixture of proteins isolated from different S- and R-form bacteria in an LPS-free form was found to express no intrinsic toxicity in mice or rabbits even in high concentrations (several mg/animal). Two injections of small amounts (10-50 μg) of such proteins carried out 7 to 14 days apart, was found to increase the sensitivity of mice and rabbits to the lethal activity of endotoxin. The reaction is anaphylactic-like, the animals dying within 10 to 20 min of injection of a low amount (5-10 μg) of LPS. The result in mice is shown in Table 13. The protein sensitization to endotoxin proceeds in

Table 13. Lethal toxicity of LPS/bacterial protein in protein-sensitized NMRI/mice.

Sensitization	LPS + Protein (μg, i.v.) on day 0		Lethality %
	25	100	100
100 μg Protein subcutaneously on day -7	12.5	100	80
	none	100	0
	25	none	0
none	25	100	0

different mice-strains including the endotoxin-resistant C3H/HeJ mice. Similar sensitizing effects were seen also with non-bacterial proteins e.g., with bovine-serum albumin. The sensitization is seen only when the same protein is used for both injections. Anti-protein antiserum may substitute for the first priming protein injection, however there is no direct correlation between anti-protein antibody titers and sensitizing activity. It seems therefore that the above protein sensitization is related to a particular class of anti-protein antibody or to other serum factors, which however, are specific for the protein.

Sensitization by Growing Tumours (2)

Certain tumors were found to exert strong sensitizing effects to the lethal activity of endotoxin, during growth in syngeneic mice. Two such tumors are, a metastatic Lewis lung carcinoma (LLC) growing in C57Bl/6 mice and a EMT6 sarcoma growing in BALB/C mice (Fig 2). With both tumors sensitization becomes detectable on day 3 after tumor inoculation and reaches maximum approximately 2 weeks later. At the height of sensitization the LLC-bearing animals are found to be susceptible to less than 0.1 μg LPS, those

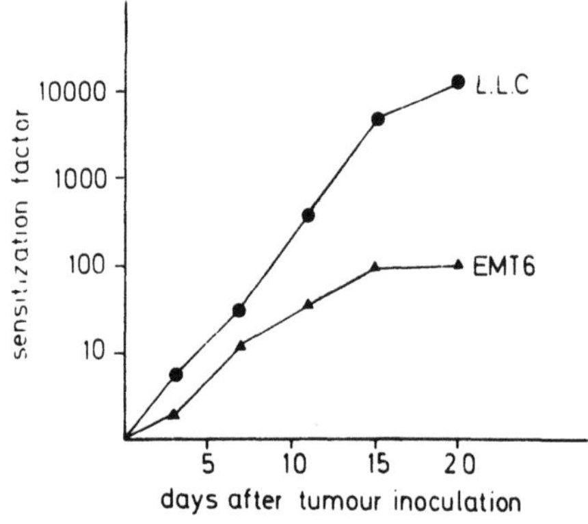

Fig 2. Sensitization to the lethal effects of LPS by growing tumours.

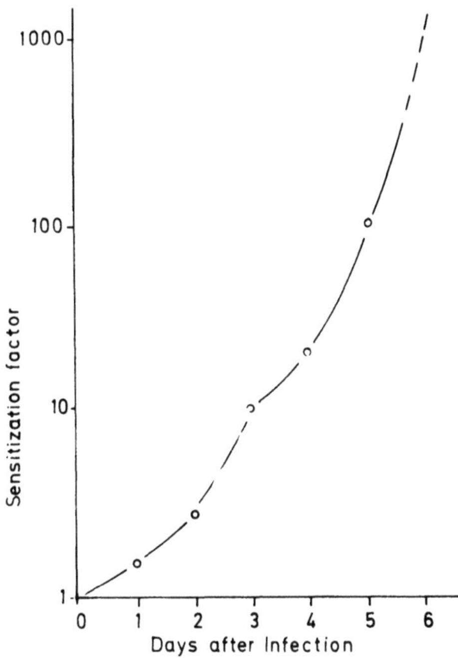

Fig 3. Sensitization of mice to Endotoxin by **S. typhimurium** infection. (Krajewska and Galanos, 1986)

bearing the sarcoma to 1-2 μg. The property to sensitize to endotoxin is not shared by all tumours since a number of other tumours (EL4 lympho-sarcoma growing in C57B1/6 and a methylcholanthrene-induced fibrosarcoma growing in BALB/C mice) showed no comparable sensitization.

In the sensitization to LPS by tumors, TNF represents the likely mediator of endotoxin lethality since very low amounts (0.1-5) μg) of exogenous TNF administered at the height of sensitization, suffices to cause lethality in the above tumor-bearing mice.

It is likely that a tumour-induced hypersensitivity to endotoxin such as the one shown to proceed here in mice, may also occur in naturally occurring tumors. Infection is a very frequent cause of mortality in patients with malignant carcinoma (3). Two thirds of such cases are due to gram-negative infections. It could be possible that this high mortality may be at least partly be related to a higher sensitivity to endotoxin, induced in patients by the growing tumors.

Sensitization by Infection

Mice (C57B1/6) infected with **S. typhimurium** develop a hypersensitivity to the lethal activity of endotoxin. Hypersensitivity is detectable already 1 day after infection at which time significantly lower amounts of LPS are sufficient to cause lethality (Fig 3). Hypersensitivity continues to increase steadily up to the time (day 5 to 6) when the animals would normally die as a result of infection. Consequently the extent of maximum sensitization to LPS caused by a lethal infection cannot be determined because at the later stages of infection the lethality caused by a challenge with endotoxin overlaps with the lethality due to the infection. Although a sensitization factor of approximately 1000 has been calculated on day 5 after infection, the actual value may be much higher.

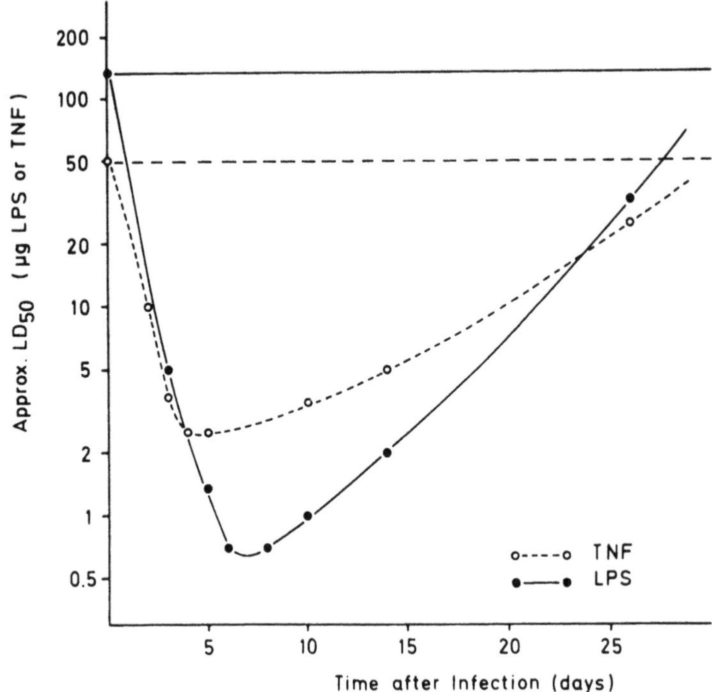

Fig 4. Sensitivity of C3H/Tif mice to LPS- or TNF- lethality during infection with **S. typhimurium.**

Sensitization to endotoxin also develops as a result of sublethal infection. This could be demonstrated with S. typhimurium infection in C3H/Tif mice, which are more resistant to this pathogen and consequently survive infections with up to 10^5 cells. Fig 4 shows the time-course of sensitization of C3H/Tif mice to endotoxin, after infection with 2 x 10^4 cells. An increase in sensitivity was detectable on day 2, and was maximum on day 6 to 8. Thereafter sensitivity decreased reaching pre-infection values 3 weeks after infection.

As seen in the previous chapters, in a number of models sensitizing to endotoxin, the sensitization was paralleled by a sensitization to TNF. A similar situation was found to exist during infection. As seen in Fig 4 the sensitization to LPS by sublethal infection is paralleled by an increased sensitivity to the lethal effects of TNF, indicating the important role of this mediator in endotoxin-dependent activities during gram-negative infection. In addition to **S. typhimurium,** a number of other gram-negative bacteria were demonstrated to increase endotoxin sensitivity (see Table 11). Thus infection of mice with **K. pneumoniae** (14) or **Coxiella burnetii** (23) (in the latter case also by treatment with killed microorganisms), were found to increase endotoxin susceptibility, indicating that induction of hypersensitivity to endotoxin may be a property of infectious gram-negative bacteria in general.

Frequently experimental animals (mice, and especially rabbits) that are apparently healthy are found to succumb to very low, otherwise nonlethal amounts of endotoxin. The reason for this enhanced sensitivity is not known. In the present report we showed that sublethal infection with gram negative bacteria increases endotoxin sensitivity. We therefore propose that latent gram-negative infection, proceeding without apparent symptoms, represents an underlying mechanism of natural sensitization to endotoxin.

ACKNOWLEDGEMENTS

The authors are indebted to M.-L. Gundelach, H. Stübig, I. Minner, C. Strohmeier and C. Steidle for expert technical assistance. The work was supported in part by the Deutsche Forschungsgemeinschaft through SFB 154.

REFERENCES

1. Aderem, A. A., Keum, M. M., Pure, E., and Cohn, Z. A., 1986, Bacterial lipopolysaccharides, phorbol myristate acetate, and zymosan induce the myristoylation of specific macrophage proteins. Proc. Natl. Acad. Sci. 83: 5817-5821.

2. Bartoleyns, J., Freudenberg, M. A., and Galanos, C., 1987, Growing tumors induce hypersensitivity to endotoxin and tumor necrosis factor. Infect. Immun. 55: 2230-2233.

3. Berger, H. and Freudenberg, N., 1983, Todesursachen by Malignompatienten. Med. Welt 34: 112-118.

4. Beutler, B., Greenwald, D., Hulmes, J. D., Chang, M., Pan, A.-C. E., Mathison, J., Ulevitch, R. J., and Cerami, A., 1985, Identity of tumour necrosis factor and the macrophage-secreted factor cachectin. Nature 316: 562.

5. Beutler, B., Mahoney, J., Le Trang, N., Pekala, P., and Cerami, A., 1985, Purification of cachectin, a lipoprotein lipase-suppressing hormone secreted by endotoxin-induced raw 264.7 cells. J. Exp. Med. 161: 984.

6. Beutler, B., Milsark, I. W., and Cerami, A. C., 1985, Passive immunization against Cachectin/Tumor necrosis factor protects mice from lethal effect of endotoxin. Science 229: 869.

7. Carswell, E., Old, L., Kassel, R., Green, S., Fiore, N., and Williamson, B., 1975, An endotoxin-induced serum factor that causes necrosis of tumors. Proc. Nat. Acad. Sci. USA 72: 3666-3670.

8. Decker, K. and Keppler, D., 1974, Galactosamine hepatitis. Key role of the nucleotide deficiency period in the pathogenesis of cell injury and cell death. Rev. Physiol. Biochem. Pharmacol. 71: 77-106.

9. Dinarello, C. A., Elin, R. J., Chedid, L., Wolff, M., 1978, The pyrogenicity of the synthetic adjuvant muramyl dipeptide and two structural analogues. J. Infect. Dis 138: 760.

10. Freudenberg, M. A. and Galanos, C., 1988, Induction of tolerance to LPS/D-galactosamine lethality by pretreatment with LPS is mediated by macrophages. Infect. Immun. (in press).

11. Freudenberg, M., Keppler, D., and Galanos, C., 1986, Requirement for lipopolysaccharide-responsive macrophages in D-galactosamine-induced sensitization to endotoxin. Infect. Immun. 51: 891-895.

12. Galanos, C., Hansen-Hagge, T., Lehmann, V., and Lüderitz, O., 1985, Comparison of the capacity of two lipid A precursor molecules to express the local Shwartzman reaction. Infect. Immun. 48: 355-358.

13. Galanos, C., Freudenberg, M. A., and Reutter, W., Galactosamine-induced

sensitization to the lethal effects of endotoxin. Proc. Natl. Acad. Sci. USA 76: 5939-5943.

14. Galanos, C., Freudenberg, M. A., Krajewska, D., Takada, H. Georgier, G., and Bartoleyns, J., 1986, Hypersensitivity to endotoxin, in: "Endotoxin: Structural aspects and immunobiology of host Responses," E. Jivillo, G. Miragliotta, C. Galanos, E. Th. Rietschel, S. M. Michalek, J. R. McGhee, eds., EOS 6.

15. Keppler, D., Hagman, W., Rapp, S., Denzlinger, C., and Koch, K., 1985, The relation of leucotrienes to liver injury. Hepatology 5: 883-891.

16. Kotani, S., Takada, H., Tsujimoto, M., Ogawa, T., Mori, Y., Sakuta, N., Kawasaki, A., Inage, M., Kusumoto, S., Shiba, T., and Kasai, N., 1983, Immunobiological activities of synthetic lipid A analogs and related compounds as compared with those of bacterial lipopolysaccharide, Re-glycolipid, lipid A, and muramyl dipeptide. Infect. Immun. 41: 758.

17. Lehman, V., Freudenberg, M. A., and Galanos, C., 1987, Lipopolysaccharide and TNF express similar lethal toxicity in D-galactosamine-treated mice. J. Exp. Med.

18. Michalek, S. M., Moore, R. N., McGhee, J. R., Rosenstreich, D. L., and Mergenhagen, S. E., 1980, The primary role of lymphoreticular cells in the mediation of host responses to bacterial endotoxin. J. Infect. Dis. 141: 55-63.

19. Morrison, D. C. and Ryan, J. F., 1979, Bacterial endotoxins and host immune responses. Adv. Immunol. 28: 294-431.

20. Rosenstreich, D. L., Glode, L. M., Wahl, L. M., Sandberg, A. L., and Mergenhagen, S. E., 1977, Analysis of the cellular defects of endotoxin-unresponsive C3H/HeJ mice, in: "Microbiology," D. Schlesinger, ed., Am. Soc. Microbiol., Washington, DC, pp. 314-320.

21. Rosenstreich, D. L. and Vogel, S. N., 1980, Central role of macrophages in the host response to endotoxin, in: "Microbiology," D. Schlesinger, ed., Am. Soc. Microbiol., Washington, DC, pp. 11-15.

22. Schade, V., Lüderitz, O., Rietschel, E. Th., 1986, Arachidonic acid metabolism in LPS activated macrophages, in: "Endotoxin: Structural aspects and immunobiology of host-responses," EOS VI.

23. Schramek, S., Kazar, J., Sekeyova, Z., Freudenberg, M. A., and Galanos, C., 1984, Induction of hyperreactivity to endotoxin in mice by Coxiella burnetii. Infect. Immun. 45: 713-717.

24. Takada, H. and Galanos, C., 1987, Enhancement of endotoxin lethality and generation of anaphylactoid reactions by LPS in MDP-treated mice. Infect. Immun. 55: 409-413.

25. Takada, H., Kotani, S., Kusumoto, S., Tarumi, Y., Ikenada, K., and Shiba, T., 1977, Mitogenic activity of adjuvant-active N-acetylmuramyl-L-alanyl-D-isoglutamine and its analogues. Biken J. 20: 81-85.

26. Tanaka, A., Saito, R., Sugiyama, K., Morisaki, I., Kotani, S., Kusumoto, S., and Shiba, T., 1977, Adjuvant activity of synthetic N-acetylmuramyl peptides in rats. Infect. Immun. 15: 332-334.

27. Tanaka, A., Nagao, S., Saito, R., Kotani, S., Kusumoto, S., and Shiba, T., 1977, Correlation of stereochemically specific structure in muramyl

dipeptide between macrophage activation and adjuvant activity. Biochem. Biophys. Res. Comm. 77: 621.

28. Tanamoto, K., Galanos, C., Lüderitz, O., Kusumoto, S., Shiba, T., 1984, Mitogenic activities of synthetic lipid A analogs and suppression of mitogenicity of lipid A. Infect. Immun. 44: 427.

29. Tanamoto, K., Zähringer, U., McKenzie, G. R., Galanos, C., Rietschel, E. Th., Lüderitz, O., Kusumoto, S., and Shiba, T., 1984, Biological activities of synthetic lipid A analogs: Pyrogenicity, lethal toxicity, anticomplement activity, and induction of gelation of Limulus amoebocyte lysate. Infect. Immun. 44: 421.

30. Vogel, S. N., Madonna, G. S., Wahl, L. M., and Rich, P. D., 1983, in vitro stimulation of C3H/HeJ spleen cells and macrophages by a precursor molecule derived from Salmonella typhimurium. J. Immunol. 132: 347.

SEPTIC SHOCK IN THE ELDERLY

A. Shibusawa and H. Ogata

Dept. of Anesthesiology, Dokkyo University, School of Medicine
Kitakobayashi, Mibumachi, Shimotsugagun, Tochigi 321-02, Japan

INTRODUCTION

In septicemia, it is well-known in animal experiments that endotoxin activates coagulation, fibrinolysis (1), kallikrein systems (4, 10, 15, 17, 19) and the complement cascade (2, 16). This study was performed to investigate retrospectively how sudden and simultaneous activations of the blood coagulation, fibrinolysis, complement and kinin systems occur in septic elderly patients from the time of their admission until shock in order to ascertain the etiology of death in such patients.

MATERIAL AND METHODS

The subjects of the study were 19 patients who were studied randomly after admission. Their clinical examinations were analyzed retrospectively for 16 wk since shock for deceased patients, and for 12 wk for survivors. Comparisons were made between those who died in shock and non-shocked survivors. These patients received ordinary nursing care, antibiotics, electrolyte solution for their treatments and blood transfusion, corticosteroid, albumin, dopamine drip infusion, etc., during this time. Laboratory findings were the following: red blood cell and white blood cell counts, hemoglobin, total protein, fibrin degradation product, fibrinogen, platelet, erythrocyte sedimentation rate, complement (C_3) (C_4), CH_{50}, plasminogen, $\alpha_1$antitrypsin, $\alpha_2$macroglobulin, antithrombin III, prekallikrein, and total kininogen levels.

Laboratory assays were prepared for fibrin degradation products, fibrinogen, plasminogen, α_1Macroglobulin, α_2Antitrypsin and Antithrombin III, Complement C_3, C_4 and CH_{50}, Prekallikrein (13), Kininogen (18) and endotoxin. Each examination value was expressed after correction for plasma protein content. Serum endotoxin was measured only one time in the clinical course. The laboratory findings of the nineteen patients were divided into two groups for analysis: 15 deceased patients after shock and 4 survivors without shock. The laboratory data in the deceased group was rearranged retrospectively for time in weeks before shock. The data was analyzed by paired t test statistically.

RESULTS

Fifteen deceased patients were 6 males and 9 females. The average age was 74 $\pm$ 9. There were four survivors, one male and three females. The

Table 1. Diseases and death causes in 19 patients

Name	Sex	Age	Disease	Death cause
S.I.	M	50	Herpetic meningoencephalitis	sepsis intestinal bleeding
M.F.	M	66	Cerebral infarction	acute bronchopneumonia
S.K.	M	82	Multiple cerebral infarction	sepsis
T.S.	F	71	Cerebral infarction	sepsis acute bronchopneumonia
G.S.	F	82	Cerebral infarction	sepsis urethral infection
Y.K.	M	67	Cerebral infarction	uremia
I.I.	F	82	Multiple cerebral infarction	sepsis
T.I.	F	77	Cerebral infarction	sepsis
F.K.	F	68	Cerebral infarction	sepsis
F.K.	F	75	Subarachnoid hemorrhage	sepsis
K.M.	M	75	Cerebral hemorrhage	sepsis acute bronchopneumonia
T.F.	F	81	Cerebral hemorrhage	sepsis acute bronchopneumonia
N.I.	F	71	Multiple cerebral infarction	sepsis
S.K.	F	83	Multiple cerebral infarction	cerebral hemorrhage
T.T.	M	83	Cerebral infarction	pneumothorax
Y.Y.	F	66	Cerebral infarction	lived
K.S.	F	88	Cerebral infarction	lived
Y.A.	F	57	Cerebral infarction	lived
R.Y.	M	74	Cerebral hemorrhage	lived

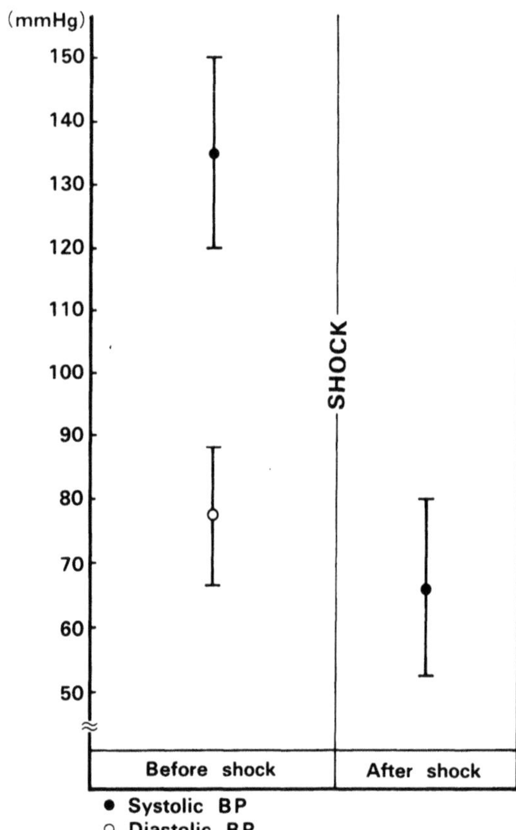

Fig 1. Systolic and diastolic blood pressure before and after shock in 15 deceased patients

average age was 71 + 11. Their main disease was cerebral infarction and main causes of death were sepsis due to infections (Table 1).

In the deceased group, the average systolic and diastolic blood pressure immediately before shock were 135 + 15 mmHg and 75 + 10 mmHg, respectively, but after shock the average systolic blood pressure was 65 + 15 mmHg, and the diastolic blood pressure was unmeasurable. The average survival after the onset of shock was 4.8 + 4.9 days (Fig 1). The data for red blood cell (RBC) count, hemoglobin (Hb) level and white blood cell (WBC) count are given in Tables 2 and 3 and in Fig 2 and 3. In the deceased patients, the RBC decreased from 357 x $10^4/mm^3$ to 260 x $10^4/mm^3$ for 16 wk. Hb decreased from 11.3 g/dl to 7.7 g/dl at 16 wk WBC increased from 7,750/mm^3 to 15.700/mm^3. On the other hand, in the survivors, the values remained almost the same for 12 wk.

The results of the fibrin degradation products (FDP), Fibrinogen (Fbg), platelet, erythrocyte and sedimentation rate (ESR) are given in Tables 2 and 3 and in Fig 4 and 5. In the deceased patients, FDP increased from 30 μg/ml, a threefold increase from normal with statistic significance. Fibrinogen gradually decreased from 495 mg/dl to 250 mg/dl. Platelets remained almost within the normal range, and ESR was more than 35 mm/hr. On the other hand, in the survivors, FDP decreased from 30 μg/ml to a normal range. Fibrinogen decreased from 333 mg/dl to 165 mg/Dl. Platelets remained almost within normal range, and ESR decreased from 40 mm/h to normal values.

Table 2. Results of clinical from 16 wks to one wk before shock in 15 deceased patients

	16w before	12w	8w	4w	3w	2w	1w
Number of patients	4	4	11	11	12	15	15
R.B.C. (10^4 mm^3)	357 ±67	363 ±31	326 ±41	305 ±49	264 ±52*	276 ±49*	259 ±85*
Hb(g/dl)	11.3±1.3	10.4±0.9	10.2±1.2	9.5 ±1.2	9.0 ±1.5*	8.8 ±1.6*	7.7 ±2.8*
W.B.C. (/mm^3)	7750±2650	6450±1650	6600±1500	10100 ±3500	11700 ±2500	17300 ±2220*	15700 ±2300*
F.D.P. (μg/ml)	30±12	30±14	39±40	60±18*	70±14*	50±22*	60±24*
Fbg(mg/dl)	495 ±17	270 ±23*	335 ±57.1*	465 ±35	380 ±40*	362 ±110*	256 ±142*
Platelet (10^4 mm^3)	14±3.5	20±7	21±7.8	23±1.8*	26±6.2*	19±5.7	20±14
E.S.R. (mm/hr)	32±7	57±34.5*	35±21.5	66±33*	82±45*	61±49	39±32
Total-protein(g/dl)	7.0 ±1.4	7.2 ±0.8	5.9 ±0.7	5.62±0.3	5.6 ±0.2	5.6 ±0.4*	5.5 ±1.3*
Plasminogen(mg/dl)	11.9±6.7	20±4*	9.66±5.08	10.2±3	12.4±4.5	12.5±5.3	13.2±5.6
α_2-MG(mg/dl)	107 ±91	25±21*	161 ±76	196 ±43	86±20	20±10*	188 ±76
α_1- AT(mg/dl)	299 ±191	127 ±30	367 ±145	437 ±110	241 ±75	60±30	428 ±117
AT- III(mg/dl)	16±9	10±1	23±11	19±6	12±1	11±5	25±7
C_3 (mg/dl)	132 ±144	102 ±231	96±14.4	83±17*	82±20*	87±22*	61±15*
C_4 (mg/dl)	43±2.3	36±11.5	30±6.2	30±7.5*	24±6.8*	24±6.6*	22±7.6*
CH_{50} (U/ ml)	33±5.8	20±6	28±7.3	31±6	26±5	24±10.4	20±7.6*
Prekallikrein (AMC10^{-2}=100)	20±15	24±20	23±19	46±16	17±15	15±10	19±16
Total kininogen μg/dl (N=3.66)	1.32±0.43	0.76±0.44	1.24±0.48	32±0.4	1.18±0.46	1.06±0.44	39±0.39
H.M.W. kininogen μg/dl (N=0.82)	0.37±0.32	0.12±0.02	0.33±0.22	0.26±0.19	0.18±0.13	0.17±0.09	27±0.23
L.M.W. kininogen μg/dl (N=2.77)	1.07±0.45	0.59±0.43	0.91±0.31	1.06±0.25	0.98±0.29	0.87±0.31	08±0.27

*P<0.05 compared with the values in 16 wks before shock

Table 3. Results of clinical examinations in 4 survived patients for 12 wks

	1st time	4wk later	12wk later
R.B.C. ($10^4/mm^3$)	398±35.5	429±11	402±17
Hb (g/dl)	13±1.0	13.3±1.5	11.7±1.7
W.B.C. ($/mm^3$)	8200±30.3	6000±1700	7650±1250
F.D.P. (ug/ml)	25±17	12.5±5	10±5
Fbg (mg/dl)	333±143	210±120	165±100*
Platelet ($10^4/mm^3$)	19±4.7	17±5	20±5
E.S.R. (mm/hr)	41±10	28±12	20±5
Total-protein (g/dl)	6.5±0.5	6.7±0.3	6.6±0.2
Plasminogen (mg/dl)	15.2±5.8	9.2±4.8	13.2±1.9
α_2-MG(mg/dl)	188±115	145±135	164±124
α_1-AT(mg/dl)	316±155	339±7	380±165
AT-III (mg/dl)	23±5	29.5±1.5	28.4±5.5
C_3(mg/dl)	101±9.0	89±3.5	87±9.8
C_4(mg/dl)	32±9.0	25±1.2	29±4.6
CH_{50}(U/ml)	23±7.0	29±3.5	35±8.7
Prekallikrein (AMC10^{-7}=100)	21.3±14.7	18.4±12.1	14.1±13.9
Total kininogen μg/dl (N=3.66)	1.77±0.4	1.65±0.35	1.11±0.21
H.M.W. kininogen μg/dl (N=0.82)	0.36±0.32	0.55±0.1	0.17±0.16
L.M.W. kininogen μg/dl (N=2.77)	1.39±0.11	1.13±0.08	0.95±0.05

*$P<0.05$ compared with the value at the first time

Total protein levels are given in Tables 2 and 3. In the deceased patients the total protein decreased from 7 g/dl to 5.5 g/dl. In the survivors, these values remained at 6.5 g/dl, its normal values, for 12 wk. The lack of plasminogen, $\alpha_2$macroglobulin (α_2MG), $\alpha_1$antitrypsin (α_1AT) and antithrombin III (AT III) are presented in Tables 2 and 3 and in Fig 6 and 7. In the case of the deceased patients, plasminogen showed a lower level than normal. This correlates with a strong activation of the plasminogen and release of plasmin prior to shock. Both antiplasmin α_2MG and antiprotease α_1AT were activated and removed in parallel with each other. For 16 wk, AT III

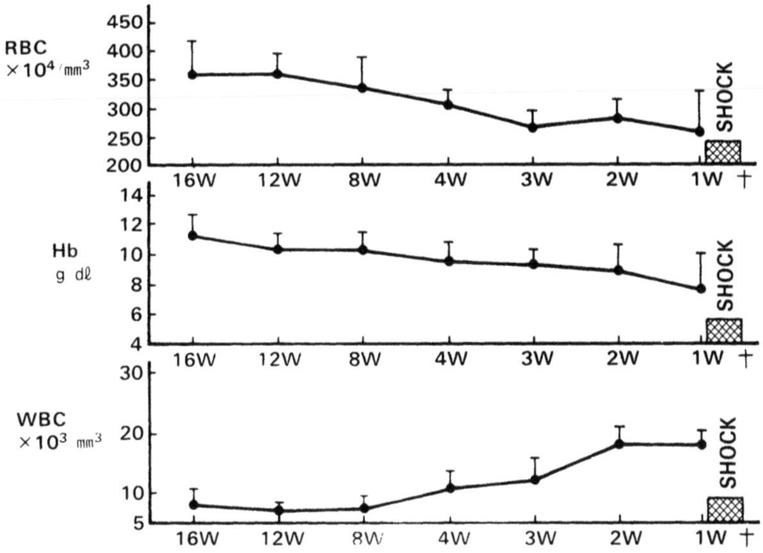

Fig 2. Changes of RBC, Hb, WBC in dead case

remained almost within the lower level normal limit. On the other hand, in survivors, the levels of plasminogen, α_2MG, α_1AT and AT III remained almost within normal limits for 12 wk.

The levels of C_3, C_4, and CH_{50} are given in Tables 2 and 3 and in Fig 8 and 9. In deceased patients, complement (C_3) decreased from 132 mg/dl to 61 mg/dl. Complement (C_4) decreased from 43 mg/dl to 22 mg/dl gradually. Their rate of decrease was 50% and 49% respectively. CH_{50} decreased from 33 U/ml

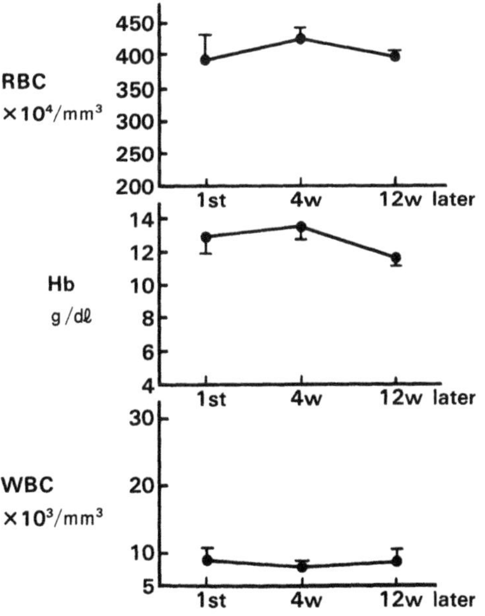

Fig 3. Changes of RBC, Hb, WBC in survived case

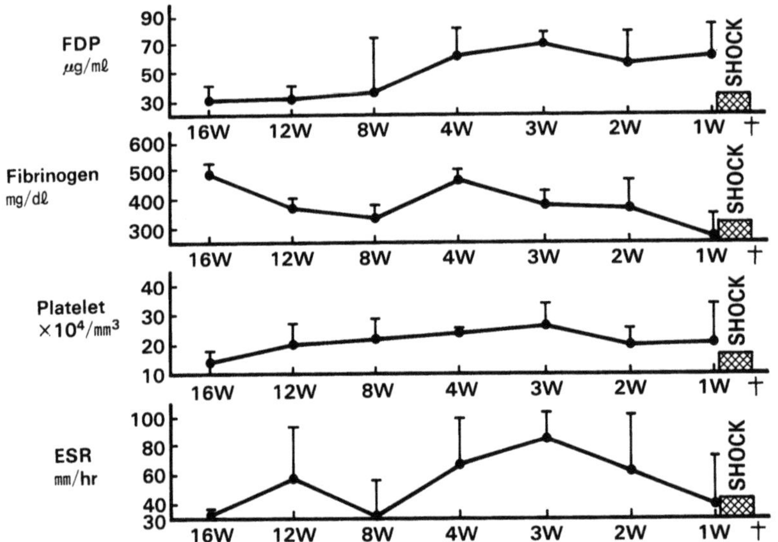

Fig 4. Changes of FDP, Fibrinogen, Platelet, ESR in dead case

to 20 U/ml with a 39% decreasing rate. Thus an activation of the complement system was recognized in the fatal cases.

The levels of prekallikrein and kinin are given in Tables 2 and 3. In the fatal cases, prekallikrein was lower (20 units) prior to shock and a minimum level of 15 units two wk prior to shock. This suggests a strong activation of prekallikrein and release of kallikrein. Total kininogen remained about 1.2 μg/dl. The level of high molecular weight kininogen was approximately 0.24 μg/dl. Low molecular weight kininogen was at approxi-

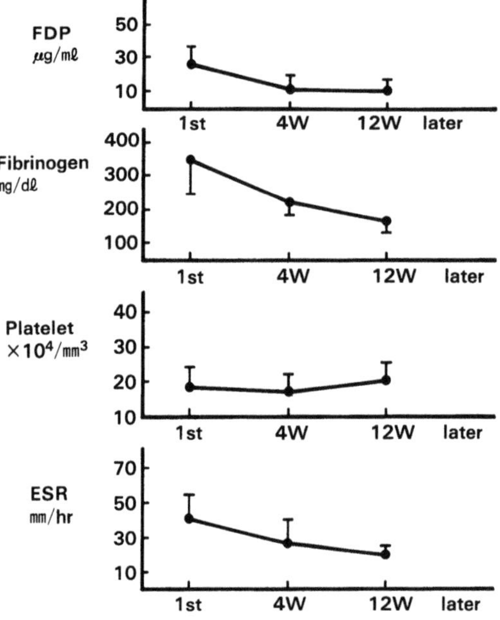

Fig 5. Changes of FDP, Fibrinogen, Platelet, ESR in survived case

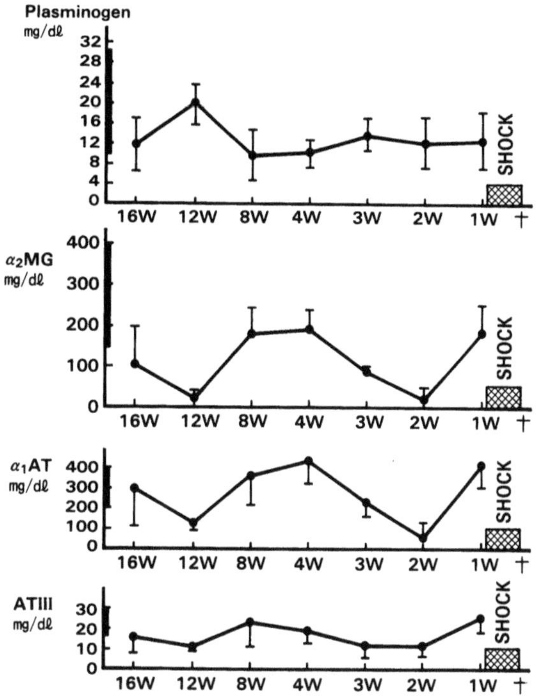

Fig 6. Changes of plasminogen, α_2MG, α_1AT, ATIII in dead cases

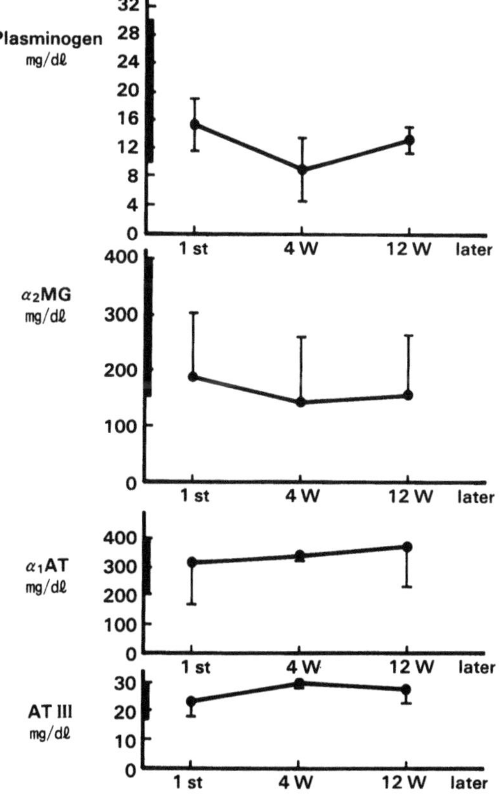

Fig 7. Changes of plasminogen, α_2MG, α_1AT, ATIII in survived case

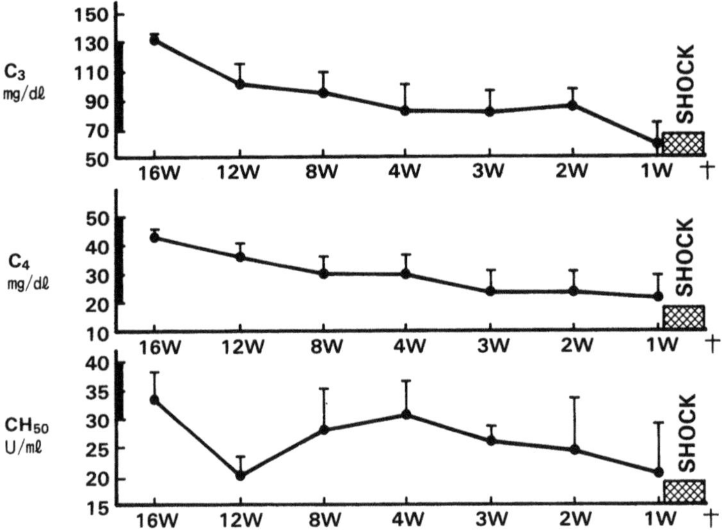

Fig 8. Changes of C_3, C_4, CH_{50} in dead case

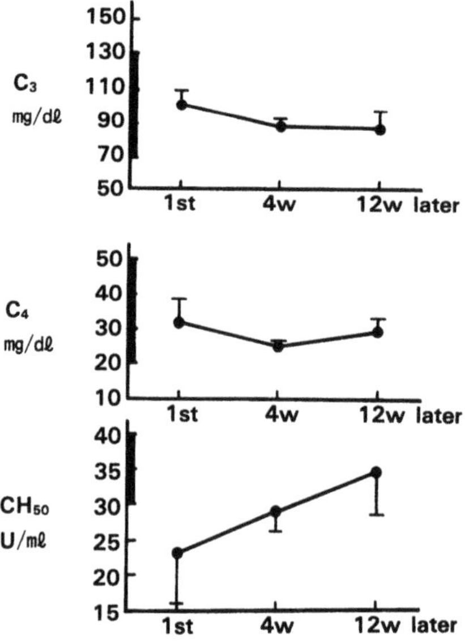

Fig 9. Changes of C_3, C_4, CH_{50} in survived case

mately 0.9 μg/dl. In the survivors, prekallikrein remained at as low as 21-14 units. Total kininogen changed from 1.8 μg/dl to 1.2 μg/dl. High molecular weight kininogen decreased from a level of 0.36 μg/dl to 0.17 μg/dl. Low molecular weight kininogen changed from 1.39 μg/dl to 0.95 μg/dl.

An average concentration of serum endotoxin measured by pyrodic method in the 15 deceased patients was 2.45 $\pm$ 0.93 ng/ml, while it was 1.55 $\pm$ 0.67 ng/ml in the four subjects who survived. However, there was no statistically significant difference between the two groups.

The results of the above-mentioned laboratory data are summarized in Table 4. Marked differences between both deceased and survival groups were observed for RBC, Hb, WBC, FDP, ESR, serum protein, C_3, C_4 and CH_{50} levels. The deceased group tended to show a decrease of RBC, Hb, serum protein, complement (C_3), (C_4), CH_{50} and an increase in WBC, FDP and ESR. On the contrary, the survival group did not show remarkable decreases in RBC, Hb, serum protein, complement (C_3), (C_4), or CH_{50} but a remarkable increase in WBC, FDP and ESR levels. These differences seemed thought to be good indexes for prognosis.

DISCUSSION

A decrease in red blood cell or hemoglobin counts compatible with anemia and hypoprotenemia in the deceased subjects appeared to be an effective and simple clinical indicator to ascertain prognosis of the subjects. The causes of leukocytosis was considered due to bacterial infection originating from

Table 4. Comparison of clinical examinations between dead and survived patients

Clinical examinations	Dead 15	Survived 4
• Red Blood Cell	↓	—
• Haemoglobin	↓	—
• White Blood Cell	↑	—
• FDP	↑	↓
Fibrinogen	↓	↓
Platelet	—	—
• Erythrocyate Sedimentation Rate	↑	↓
Serum protein	↓	—
Plasminogen	↓	↓
α_2Macroglobulin	↓	↓
α_1Antitrypsin	↓	↓
Antithrombin III	↓	↓
• Complement C_3	↓	—
• C_4	↓	—
• CH_{50}	↓	↑
Prekallikrein	↓	↓
HMW Kininogen	↓	↓
LMW Kininogen	↓	↓
Total Kininogen	↓	↓
Endotoxin	↑	↑

↑ Increase ↓ Decrease
- No remarkable changes
• Effective test to determine the prognosis

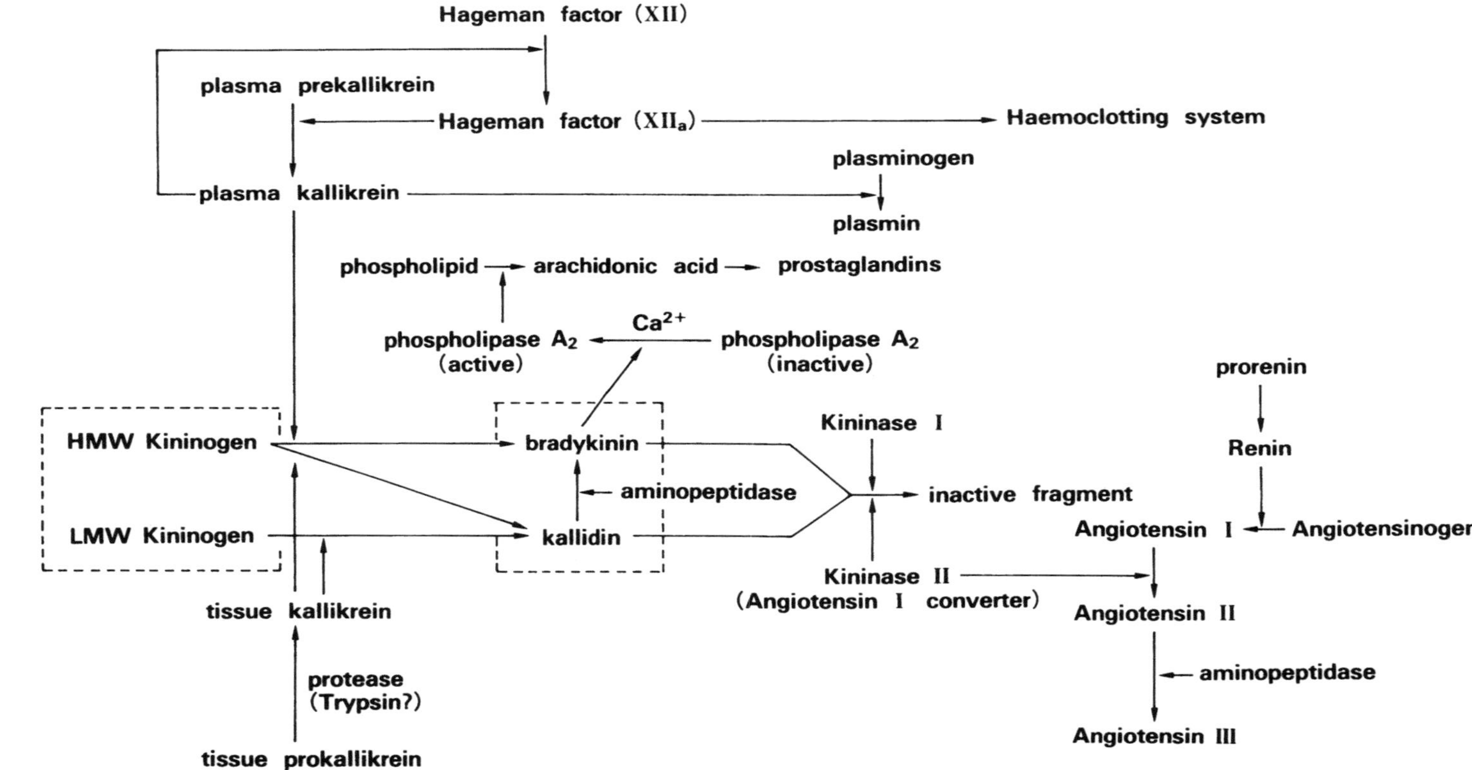

Fig 10. Relationships of Kallikrein-Kinin and other Systems.

the respiratory airway, decubituses and/or urinary tract indwelling catheter. We did not observe leukopenia in the subjects as predicted by Jacob (7).

DIC is well known in septic shock, but we could not diagnose DIC in these deceased patients because of a lack of extreme thrombocytopenia. According to McCabe (9), 10% to 20% of patients with gram negative sepsis will exhibit alterations in hemostasis and Hale (5) states that DIC may also, in part, be secondary to endothelial damage induced by vasoactive substances. Therefore, there might be some relationships between the absences of leukopenia and DIC seen in our data. However, it appeared that an activation of the coagulation system in the deceased subjects occurred because of decreased fibrinogen and AT III as well as increased FDP. An increase of FDP may be due to either primary or secondary fibrinolysis. It also seemed that because of a decrease of plasminogen endotoxin-activated Hageman factor stimulated plasmin release is followed by prekallikrein activation. It is likely that plasmin would have caused a decrease in the fourth complement component followed by activation of the classical pathway of the complement system. Our data also showed that plasmin inhibitor α_1AT or α_2MG may antagonize activation of plasminogen.

Marked differences in the complement system was evident between both groups. In the deceased subjects, the decreasing rate of C_3, C_4, and CH_{50} was 50%, 49%, 39%, respectively, but in the survivors the decreasing rate of C_3 or C_4 was 14%, 9%, respectively. Thus it appears to be important to measure C_3, C_4, and CH_{50} levels to determine prognosis. The cause of diminished C_3 or C_4 may be due to direct action of endotoxin into the alternative pathway as well as direct involvement of plasmin in that classical pathway (2, 3, 16).

It is known that C_5a activates polymorphoneutrophils followed by pulmonary endothelial cell damage due to involvement of free radicals of oxygen, proteolytic enzymes, and products of arachidonic acid metabolism (6, 14). Therefore it seems important to suppress activation of the complement cascade in such patients.

A depletion of prekallikrein is considered the result of activation of Hageman factor due to endotoxin (11). Gallimore (4) and Ogata (12) revealed diminished levels of prekallikrein and/or kininogen in endotoxin shock in dogs. Lower values of prekallikrein, total kininogen, HMW kininogen, and LMW kininogen were observed in both groups. The reasons of these lower values could not be explained. As suggested by Vliet (1981) (19), there might be a diminished production of prekallikrein or kininogen in the liver due to sepsis. It is thought that kallikrein stimulates high molecular wt kininogen, which releases bradykinin. Low molecular weight kininogen may release kallidin through activation of trypsin. Both bradykinin and kallidin are thought to activate phospholipase A2 and then phospholipid results in arachidonic acid and prostaglandin production (Fig 10) (8).

CONCLUSION AND SUMMARY

Fifteen patients suffered from severe cerebral vascular infarction and immobilized for long period died and with four survivors. Their laboratory findings were analyzed retrospectively in regard to shock. 1) Hypoprotenemia, anemia and leukocytosis were markedly recognized in the deceased, 2) there was no tendency for DIC, although patients manifested septic shock and high levels of FDP, 3) activation of plasmin, complement and kallikrein-kinin systems were observed, probably because of endotoxin, 4) survivors had no remarkable decrease in RBC, Hb, serum protein, complement (C_3) (C_4) or CH_{50} levels and no remarkable increase in WBC, FDP or ESR levels. These laboratory findings seemed to be effective indexes of prognosis.

ACKNOWLEDGMENTS

The authors deeply express sorrow and thankfulness for the fifteen patients who died in the midst of this study, and also our appreciation to Mrs. H. Hosaka for analyzing prekallikrein and endotoxin levels and Miss N. Yamaguchi for her typing.

REFERENCES

1. Barreno, P. G., Balibrea, J. L. and Aparicio, P., 1978, Blood coagulation changes in shock. Surg., Gyn. & Obs. 147: 6.

2. Corbeil, L. B., 1978, Role of the complement system in immunity and immunopathology. Vet. clin. of N. America 8: 585.

3. Cristmen, J. K., Silverstein, S. C. and Acs, G., 1977, Plasminogen activators, in: "Proteinases in Mammalian Cells and Tissues," Barrett, ed., Elsevier/North-Holl and Biomedical Press, North-Hollan Publishing Company 91.

4. Gallimore, M. J., Aasen, A. O., Lyngaas, K. H. N., Larsbraaten, M. and Amundsen, E., 1978, Falls in plasma levels of prekallikrein, high molecular weight kininogen and kallikrein inhibitors during lethal endotoxin shock in dogs. Thromb. Res. 12: 307.

5. Hale, D. J., Robinson, J. A., Gunnar, L. R., 1986, Pathophysiology of endotoxin shock in man, in: "Handbook of Endotoxin," R. A. Proctor, ed., Elsevier 4: 1.

6. Hammerschmidt, L. H., Weaver, L. J., Hudson, L. D., Craddock, P. R. and Jacob, H. S., 1980, Associated of complement activation and elevated plasma-C5a with adult respiratory distress syndrome. Lancet 1: 947.

7. Jacob, H. S., Craddock, P. R., Hammerschmidt, D. E. and Moldw, C. F., 1980, Complement-induced granulocyte aggregation: An unsuspected mechanism of disease. N. Engl. J. Med. 302: 789.

8. Kizaki, K., Moriya, H., 1986, Biochemistry of kinin system. Japanese J. of Inflammation 6: 221.

9. McCabe, W. R., 1973, Serum complement levels in bacteremia due to gram negative organisms. N. Engl. J. Med. 288: 21.

10. Morrison, D. C. and Cochrane, C. G., 1974, Direct evidence for Hageman factor (Factor XII) activation by bacterial lipopolysaccharides (endotoxin). The J. of Exper. Med. 140: 797.

11. Nies, A. S., Forsyth, R. P., Williams. H. E. and Melmon, K. L., 1968, Contribution of kinins to endotoxin shock in unanesthetized rhesus monkeys. Circ. Res. 22: 155.

12. Ogata, H., Kim, S., Fukasawa, T., Midorikawa, Y. and Yamashiro, C., 1983, The effects of aprotinin on the phagocytic activity of the RES and plasma prekallikrein levels during endotoxin shock, in: "Molecular and cellular aspects of shock and trauma," Allan M. Lefer and William Schumer, eds., Alan R. Liss, Inc., N. Y. 309.

13. Oh-ishi, S. and Katori, M., 1979, Fluorometric assay for plasma prekallikrein using peptidylmethylcoumarinylamide as a substrate. Thromb. Res. 14: 559.

14. Rinald, J. E. and Rogers, R. M., 1986, Adult respiratory distress syndrome. The New England J. of Med. : 578.

15. Sardesai, V. M. and Rosenberg, J. C., 1974, Proteolysis and bradykinin turnover in endotoxin shock. The J. of Trauma 14: 945.

16. Seelig, R. and Seelig H. P., 1975, The possible role of serum complement system in the formal pathogenesis of acute pancreatitis. Acta Hepato-Gastroenterol. 22: 263.

17. Sumida, S., 1979, Experimental studies on the effect of prophylactic endotoxin shock, in: "Kinins-II systemic proteases and cellular function," S. Fuji, H. Moriya, and T. Suzuki, eds., Plenum Press, N. Y. p. 395.

18. Ueno, A., Oh-ishi, S., Kitagawa, T. and Katori, M., 1981, Enzyme immunoassay of bradykinin using B-D-Galactosidase as a labeling enzyme. Biochem. Pharmacol. 30: 1659.

19. Vliet, A. C. M., Vliet, H. H. D. M., Danilovic, G. D. and Wilson, J. H. P., 1981, Plasma prekallikrein and endotoxin in liver cirrhosis. Thromb. Haemostasis 45: 65.

ENDOTOXIN-INDUCED CYTOKINES IN HUMAN SEPTICEMIA

I. de Vries[1], S. J. H. van Deventer[2], J. Debets[3], H. R. Buller[2], J. W. ten Cate[2], W. Pauw[4], L. W. Statius van Eps[1] and A. Sturk[2]

Department of Internal Medicine[1] and Bacteriology[4] Slotervaart Hospital Amsterdam, Department of Hemostasis and Thrombosis Academical Medical Center Amsterdam[2], and Department of Surgery, Biomedical Center, University of Limburg, Maastricht, The Netherlands[3]

The Gram-negative septic syndrome is characterized by hypotension, intravascular coagulation and multiple organ failure (1). A large body of clinical and experimental evidence indicates that lipopolysaccharides present in the Gram-negative bacterial outer membrane -endotoxins- play a pivotal role in the pathogenesis of septicemia (2). In fact, we have recently reported that endotoxemia (as detected by the Limulus assay) is a better predictor of septicemia than Gram-negative bacteremia (3). Interestingly, the majority of patients with Gram-negative bacteremia who did not develop septicemia as defined by clinical criteria had a negative endotoxin test, whereas patients with endotoxemia had a high probability of developing septicemia. Therefore, we concluded that Gram-negative bacteremia and endotoxemia should be considered separate clinical entities, the latter being associated with the Gram-negative septic syndrome (3, 4).

Bacterial lipopolysaccharides have myriads of biological effects (5), including coagulation (6) and complement activation (7). In the recent past it has become clear that endotoxin-induced macrophage activation (6), resulting in the release of inflammatory mediators (prostaglandins (9), leukotrienes (10), platelet-activating factor (11)) and lymphokines (interleukins (12), tumor necrosis factor (13)) is a crucial mechanism in the pathogenesis of the Gram-negative septic syndrome. In particular, the induction of tumor necrosis factor (TNF, also called cachectin) is thought to be of importance in the development of septicemia, because many of the clinical and laboratory features of Gram-negative septicemia can be evoked by intravenous administration of recombinant TNF (14, 15). Furthermore, immunological intervention directed at TNF reduces the mortality due to experimental Gram-negative septicemia (16).

A possible explanation for the high positive and negative predictive values of the Limulus assay for septicemia is that a positive test detects a concentration of biologically active endotoxins in blood capable of induction of tumor necrosis factor. We present here preliminary results of a study that was designed to prospectively investigate the kinetics of endotoxemia and the release of TNF in blood during the development of the Gram-negative septic syndrome in febrile patients with Gram-negative bacteremia.

METHODS

The study was performed at the Slotervaart Hospital, a general teaching hospital in Amsterdam, The Netherlands. Febrile patients (temp >38°C) who were suspected of a serious Gram-negative bacterial infection (e.g., pyelonephritis, cholangitis, diverticulitis) were enrolled in the study. Patients already having criteria for Gram-negative septicemia were excluded. All patients were prospectively followed for 48 hr during which period blood samples were obtained every six hours for blood culture and determination of endotoxins and TNF. In addition biochemical (creatinine, alkaline phosphatase, bilirubin, plasma bicarbonate) and hematological parameters (white cell count, platelet count, hematocrit) were assessed. Blood pressure was recorded every six hours by sphygmomanometer, and the urine output was measured. Septicemia was defined as the occurrence of one or more of the following criteria: 1) hypotension (systolic blood pressure <90 mm Hg). 2) thrombocytopenia (blood platelets $<100 \times 10^9$/ L). 3) oliguria (urine output < 20 ml/hr). 4) metabolic acidosis (plasma bicarbonate <15 mMol/L). The study was approved by the hospital ethics committee.

In this report we will describe the kinetics of endotoxemia and TNF release in two patients who developed the Gram-negative septic syndrome.

Blood Cultures, Limulus Test and Determination of TNF

Blood for bacterial culture was processed by routine bacterial techniques. Blood for the Limulus assay was collected in two polystyrene tubes (Falcon 2063, Oxnard, Ca., USA) which were immediately placed in melting ice, and platelet-rich plasma was prepared by centrifugation at 190 g at 4°C for 10 min. Duplicate aliquots were frozen at -70°C, and the Limulus assay was performed batchwise as has been described (17, 18). This chromogenic method can detect endotoxins in blood at a concentration of 5 ng/L. TNF was determined in serum with a sensitive ELISA as has been described (19). The detection limit of this assay in blood is 5 ng/L.

Case 1

This 44-year old woman known to have multiple sclerosis for twenty years was admitted because of chills, fever and hematuria. A history of recurrent urinary tract infections was obtained. Physical examination revealed mild tenderness in the left and right lower quadrant and the right costovertebral angle. A severe decubitus ulcer on the right hip was noted. Microscopical examination of a stained urinary specimen showed many Gram-negative rods. A presumptive diagnosis of pyelonephritis was made and antibiotics and intravenous fluids were administered. Despite these measurements septic shock developed 12 hr after admission, complicated by thrombocytopenia and metabolic acidosis. Blood cultures revealed growth of Proteus mirabilis (as did the urine cultures), Streptococcus milleri and Staphylococcus aureus.

Case 2

A 93-year old woman was admitted to the hospital because of obstructive jaundice. An endoscopic retrograde cholangiopancreaticographic (ERCP) examination showed a dilated choledochal duct due to an impacted gallstone. A papillotomy was performed. Twelve hours after the procedure fever (39°C) developed and a diagnosis of cholangitis was made. Despite administration of antibiotics and intravenous fluids, septic shock ensued. Blood cultures revealed growth of Pseudomonas aeruginosa. Although the patient initially recovered from septic shock, after many hours on vasopressors, she died five days later because of heart failure.

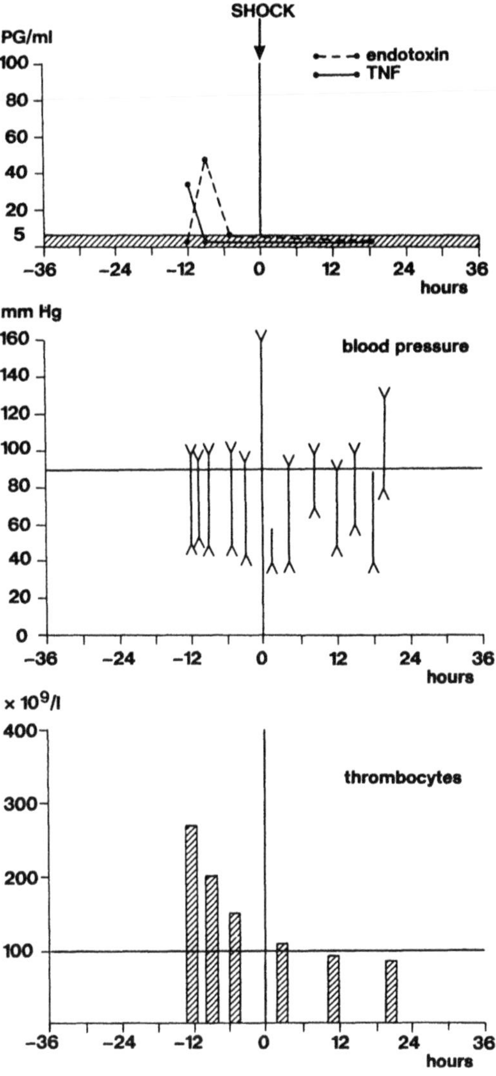

Fig 1. Changes in endotoxin and TNF serum levels, blood pressure and thrombocytes in a patient with shock.

RESULTS

In both patients septic shock ensued, characterized by hypotension, severe thrombocytopenia and metabolic acidosis, requiring vasopressor support and fluid challenge. In the first patient blood pressure dropped below 90 mm Hg twelve hours after TNF became detectable. In fact, in this patient TNF was detectable three hours prior to the first positive endotoxin assay (Fig 1). Furthermore, in this case, both TNF and endotoxin were detectable only in the period preceding the onset of septic shock. The second patient had continuous endotoxemia, starting 18 hr before septic shock established (Fig 2). In this patient TNF became detectable during the period of hypotension. In contrast to endotoxemia, TNF release was pulsatile, as only three of the six subsequent samples obtained during septic shock contained TNF.

In three patients with Gram-negative bacteremia not complicated by septicemia who were studied in the same period, neither endotoxins nor TNF were detectable in blood.

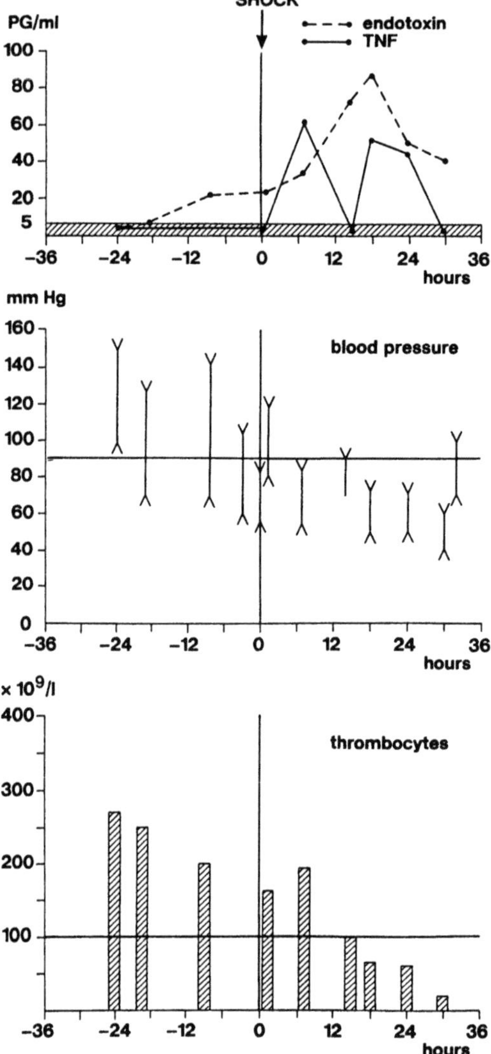

Fig 2. Changes in endotoxin and TNF serum levels, blood pressure and thrombocytes in a patient with shock.

DISCUSSION

In both patients with septicemia endotoxin and TNF were detectable in blood. However, the kinetics of endotoxemia and TNF release differed substantially in the two patients. In the first patient TNF was detectable before the onset of endotoxemia. One possible explanation is that transient endotoxemia was present before this patient entered the study protocol, and therefore remained undetected. On the other hand, this patient also had Gram-positive bacteremia, and it is possible that Gram-positive bacterial products activate macrophages to synthesize and release TNF. In addition, in this patient both endotoxemia and TNF release were detected only before the onset of septic shock. This finding stresses the importance of a prospective study design in the investigation of septicemia, as pivotal factors in the development of septicemia may sometimes be detectable only in the period preceding septic shock. The most significant observation in the second patient was the distinctive behavior of the release of TNF in blood, despite persisting endotoxemia. Although the half-life of recombinant TNF after intravenous administration in humans is known to be approximately 20 min (20), this cannot be the sole explanation for this phenomenon, as macrophage activation by endotoxins was continuous in this patient.

Despite the limited amount of data, several conclusions can be drawn from the results of this study. Firstly, endotoxemia and TNF release were exclusively detected in patients with bacteremia complicated by septic shock. These results confirm our previous study, in which endotoxemia was found to be a reliable indicator of septicemia in febrile patients (3, 4), and are compatible with the hypothesis that the presence of biologically active endotoxin in blood induces release of TNF. Secondly, endotoxin levels in blood may range widely over a short period of time. Therefore a single test result does not accurately reflect the endotoxin burden of the patient, although a positive endotoxin test result has a high predictive value for the development of septicemia (3). In summary, we observed different patterns of endotoxemia and TNF release in human septicemia. More detailed knowledge of the kinetics of endotoxins and cytokines during the development of Gram-negative septicemia will rationalize immunological intervention directed at endotoxin (21, 22) or its endogenous mediators (16).

REFERENCES

1. Hale, D. J., Robinson, J. A., Loeb, H. S., Gunnar, R. M., 1986, Pathophysiology of endotoxin shock in man, in: "Handbook of Endotoxin," Vol. 4, R. A. Proctor, ed., Elsevier, Amsterdam, p. 1-15.

2. Ryan, J. L., 1985, Microbial factors in pathogenesis: Lipopolysaccharides, in: "Septic Shock," R. K. Root and M. A. Sande, eds., New York, Churchill Livingstone, p. 13-25.

3. Van Deventer, S. J. H., Buller, H. R., ten Cate, J. W., et al., 1988, Endotoxemia: an early predictor of septicemia in febrile patients. Lancet i: 605-609.

4. Van Deventer, S. J. H., de Vries, I., Statius van Eps, L. W., et al., 1988, Endotoxemia, bacteremia and urosepsis. Prog. Clin. Biol. Res. 272: 213-24.

5. Morrison, D. C. and Ryan, J. C., 1987, Endotoxin and disease mechanisms. Ann. Rev. Med. 38: 417-432.

6. Maier, R. V., Hahnel, G. B., 1984, Microthrombosis during endotoxemia: Potential role of hepatic versus alveolar macrophages. J. Surg. Res. 36: 362-370.

7. Demling, R. H., Wenger, H., Lalonde, C. C., 1986, Endotoxin-induced prostanoid production by the burn wound can cause distant lung dysfunction. Surgery 99: 421-430.

8. Johnston, R. B., Jr., 1988, Current Concepts - Immunology: Monocytes and macrophages. New Engl. J. Med. 318: 747-752.

9. Kurland, J. I. and Bockman, R. J., 1978, Prostaglandin E2 production by human blood monocytes and mouse peritoneal macrophages. J. Exp. Med. 147: 952.

10. Luderitz, T., Schade, U. F. and Rietschel, E. T., 1986, Formation and metabolism of leukotriene C4 in macrophages exposed to bacterial lipopolysaccharide. Eur. J. Biochem. 15: 377.

11. Doebber, T. W., Wu, M. S. and Robbins, J. C., 1985, Platelet activating factor (PAF) involvement in endotoxin-induced hypotension in rats. Studies with PAF-receptor antagonist Kadsurone. Biochem. Biophys. Res. Comm. 127: 799-808.

12. Dinarello, C. A., 1984, Interleukin-1. Rev. Infect. Dis. 6: 51-95.

13. Beutler, B. and Cerami, A., 1987, The endogenous mediator of endotoxin shock. Clin. Res. 35: 192-197.

14. Tracey, K. J., Beutler, B., Lowry, S. F., et al., 1986, Shock and tissue injury induced by recombinant human chachectin. Science 234: 470-474.

15. Hesse, D. G., Tracey, K. J., Fong, Y., et al., Cytokine appearance in human endotoxemia and non-human primate bacteremia.

16. Tracey, K. J., Fong, Y., Hesse, D. G., et al., 1987, Anti-cachectin/TNF monoclonal antibodies prevent septic shock during lethal bacteremia. Nature 330: 662-664.

17. Sturk, A., Joop, K., ten Cate, J. W., and Thomas, L. L. M., 1985, Optimalization of a chromogenic assay for endotoxin in blood. Prog. Clin. Biol. Res. 189: 117-136.

18. Sturk, A., Janssen, M. E., Muylaert, F. R., Joop, K., Thomas, L. L. M. and ten Cate, J. W., 1987, Endotoxin testing in blood. Prog. Clin. Biol. Res. 231: 371-385.

19. Debets, J. M. H., Van der Linden, C. J., Spronken, I. E. M., and Buurman, W. A., 1988, T-cell mediated TNF-alpha production by monocytes. Scand. J. Immunol. in press.

20. Blick, M., Sherwin, S. A., Rosenblum, M. and Gutterman, J., 1987, Phase I study of recombinant tumor necrosis factor in cancer patients. Cancer Res. 47: 2986-2989.

21. Ziegler, E. J., McCutchan, J. A., Fierer, J.; Glauser, M. P., Sadoff, J. C., Douglas, H. and Braude, A. I., 1982, Treatment of Gram negative bacteremia and shock with human antiserum to a mutant Escherichia coli. New Engl. J. Med. 307: 1225-1230.

22. Baumgartner, J. D., Glauser, M. P., McCutchan, J. A., et al., 1985, Prevention of Gram negative shock and death in surgical patients by antibody to endotoxin core glycolipid. Lancet ii: 59-63.

LIPID A PRECURSORS PROTECT AGAINST ENDOTOXIN CHALLENGE

R. A. Proctor

Department of Medical Microbiology and Department of Medicine, University of Wisconsin Medical School, Madison, Wisconsin 53706

INTRODUCTION

Gram-negative bacteremia, when accompanied by shock, carried a 20-75 percent mortality (4, 23, 26). The advent of more active antibiotics and improved supportive therapy such as fluids, respirators and pressors have benefitted many patients, but the mortality rate remains high in spite of the best therapy (4, 23, 26). This has led to the search for further therapies such as high dose glucocorticoids (19, 20, 42, 43), narcotic antagonists (18, 21) and prostacycline infusion (11, 14). Although these approaches proved exciting in animal models, they have not come into widespread clinical use (13, 42, 43).

Because much of the pathogenecity of serious gram-negative septic shock can be reproduced by bacterial lipopolysaccharide (LPS, endotoxin), anti-endotoxin antibodies, which recognize the common core antigens of LPS, have been developed to neutralize the circulating LPS (1, 50-52). Both monoclonal and polyclonal antibodies have been reported as effective against a broad range of gram-negative pathogens (1, 50-52). However, several studies have failed to demonstrate efficacy of these antibodies and none are as effective as antibodies directed against specific serotypes when the same serotype is used as the challenge organism (reviewed by Dr. M. Pollack in this volume). This remains an area of active clinical and basic research.

Another approach to therapy has involved the use of lipid A biosynthetic precursors or derivatives of these molecules. The concept behind this approach is that endotoxin subunits might compete for a common mammalian receptor with endotoxin, while being less toxic than the complete molecule. The recent information demonstrating the biosynthetic pathway and structure of lipid A, the portion of endotoxin imparting most of its toxicity, has made this approach possible (3, 5, 30, 31, 35-38, 44-46).

Structure and Biosynthesis of Lipid A

Lipid A biosynthesis begins with UDP-n-acetylglucosamine and is then acylated at the second and third positions with β-hydroxymyristates in a reaction that using acyl carrier protein (3) (see Fig 1). The uridine monophosphate group is then removed to give 2,3-diacyl-glucosamine phosphate, lipid X. Lipid X then combines with UDP-diacylglucosamine to form a tetra-acyldisaccharide (5, 37). The enzyme controlling this interaction, lipid A

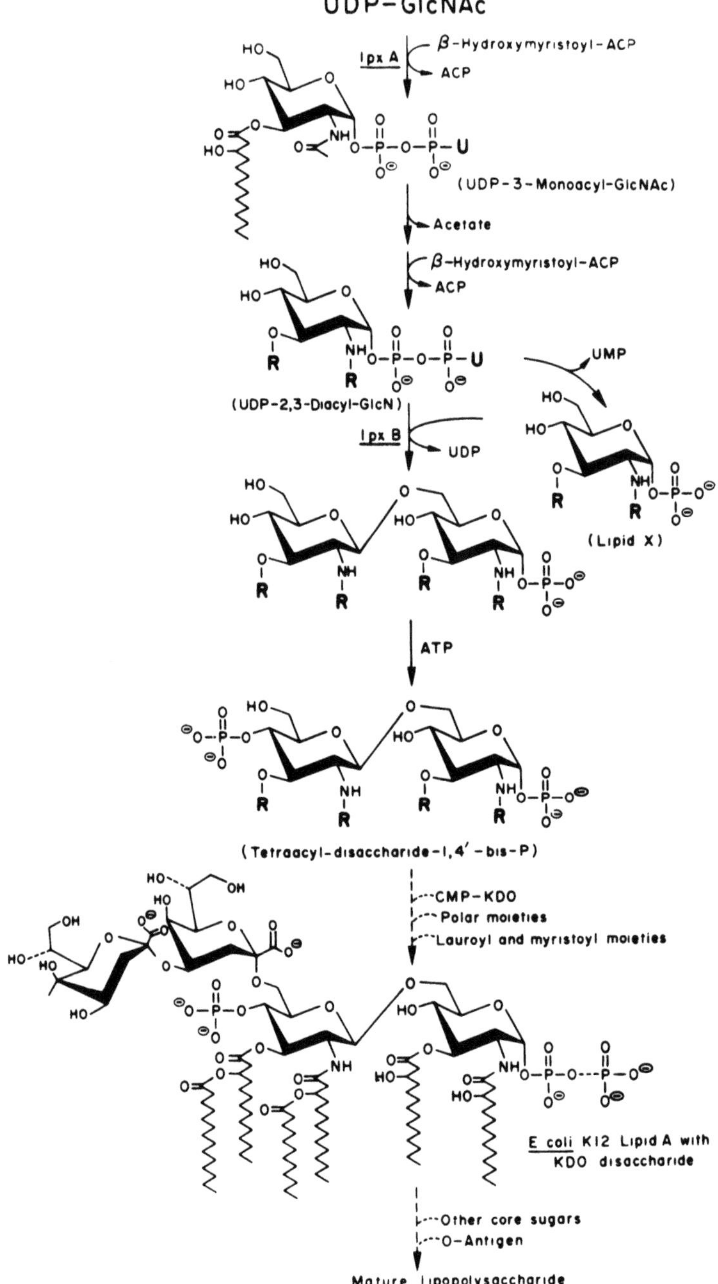
UDP–GlcNAc
lpx A
β-Hydroxymyristoyl-ACP
ACP
(UDP-3-Monoacyl-GlcNAc)
Acetate
β-Hydroxymyristoyl-ACP
ACP
(UDP-2,3-Diacyl-GlcN)
UMP
lpx B
UDP
(Lipid X)
ATP
(Tetraacyl-disaccharide-1,4′-bis-P)
CMP-KDO
Polar moieties
Lauroyl and myristoyl moieties
E coli K12 Lipid A with KDO disaccharide
Other core sugars
O-Antigen
Mature lipopolysaccharide

Fig 1. Biosynthesis of lipid A (from Ref 38). R designates a β-hydroxymyristoyl moiety and U designates uridine. Evidence for the fatty acylation of UDP-GlcNAc and for the precursor-product relationship between UDP-2,3-diacyl-GlcN and lipid X has been presented by Anderson et al. (3). The tetraacyldisaccharide-1-phosphate synthase is the product of the **lpxB** (**pgsB**) gene. The tetraacyldisaccharide 1,4'-bisphosphate is generated by the 4'-kinase (38) and is also the predominant acidic lipid A precursor (termed polar lipid IVA) that accumulates in temperature-sensitive mutants of **S. typhimurium** defective in KDO biosynthesis. The transfer of two KDO moieties from two molecules of CMP-KDO to this precursor by membranes of wild-type cells has been suggested. In a portion of the lipid A molecules, additional polar moieties are present, and these may be added at the same time as, or shortly after, KDO. Specifically, a portion of the lipid A molecules of **E. coli** bear a pyrophosphate residue at the reducing and (as indicated by the dashed bond), while in **S. typhimurium** additional polar substitutes, including 4-amino-4-deoxy-L-arabinose and/or phosphoethanolamine, may be attached to lipid A. The "late acylations" by which the lauroyl and myristoyl residues are incorporated have not been studied. The final structure shown is the minimal unit thought to be required for cell growth and outer membrane biogenesis **E. coli** (35).

disaccharide synthase (35), is temperature sensitive in the MN7 mutant strain of **E. coli** (30, 31) and the gene controlling its production has recently been characterized (12, 49) along with several other genes in the lipid A biosynthesis operon (10). When grown at 42°C, this strain accumulates lipid X and a related triacyl monosaccharide, lipid Y (30, 31). The MN7 strain was crucial to understanding both the structure of lipid A and its biosynthesis (35). As can be seen from Fig 1, lipid X is at a central point in the biosynthetic pathway. Knowing the structure of lipid X immediately provided an important clue to the lipid A structure in **E. coli**.

Once the disaccharide is formed, it is phosphorylated at the 4' position by a membrane bound kinase (38). The KDO groups are added at the 6' position, further fatty acids are added at the β-hydroxy position (this varies as to species of bacteria), and aminoarabinose and ethanolamine added to the phosphate groups at the 1 and 4' positions, respectively (44). The precise details of these later steps are not yet available.

Biological Activities

Because several other papers in this volume review structure-biological responses (see reviews by Drs. Homma, Kotani, and Rietschel et al.), only a brief synopsis will be provided here so as to place the efficacy of lipid A precursors in perspective with their toxicity and biologic responsibility. Enough studies of lipid A subunits have now been performed to begin to make some generalizations about structure-function relationships of lipid A subunits and derivatives, but the comparisons are somewhat difficult because of differences between methods and experimental design. Disaccharide tetraacyl lipid A derivatives tend to be more toxic than monosaccharide precursors. Removal of the phosphate from the 1-position of disaccharide compounds re-

Table 1. Mortality as a function of dose and time of lipid X administration (33)

Dose of lipid X (μg/mouse)[a]	No. of mice alive or dead at time (h)[b] after lipopolysaccharide administration (250 μg)							
	0		2		4		6	
	Alive	Dead	Alive	Dead	Alive	Dead	Alive	Dead
0	1	11	0	4	0	6	0	12
100	3	3	1	5	1	5	2	4
200	3	3	1	5	2	4	1	5
400	5	1	4	2	2	4	1	5
800	5	0	4	2	4	2	2	4
1,200	5	1	5	0	4	2	3	3
1,600	5	0	5	0	4	2	3	3

[a]Both lipid X and endotoxin were given via the tail vein to C57BL/10 mice weighing 20 to 25 g.
[b]Times in hours are relative to time of endotoxin challenge. There was approximately 30 to 60 s between the endotoxin challenge and the administration of lipid X for time zero.

duces its toxicity (24). Addition of fatty acid groups at the β-hydroxy moiety to both monosaccharides (lipid X vs. lipid Y) and disaccharides enhances the toxic activity. Similarly, removal of the β-hydroxy-linked fatty acids from endotoxin by enzymes found in phagocytes reduces the toxicity of endotoxin (28).

All of the toxic responses may not always be disadvantageous. For example, the disaccharides are more pyrogenic than the monosaccharides and the disaccharides also show greater mitogenic activity. Indeed, pyrogenicity also seems to correlate with the immunoprotective activity of the compounds. Perhaps mediators such as interferons, interleukin-1, and tumor necrosis factor must be released in order to stimulate phagocytes and T-cells to protect the host from subsequent challenge. More detailed structure-function profiles are contained in other portions of this volume.

PROTECTIVE EFFICACY OF ENDOTOXIN SUBUNITS

Protection Against Endotoxin Challenge

As the structure of lipid A became more clearly defined, we began to study a number of lipid A precursors and derivatives for activity to define structure-function relationships. In the course of these studies, the low toxicity of lipid X was noted for sheep (6, 7) and mice (33). Because lipid X was a subunit of lipid A, its ability to block the toxic actions of LPS was tested (33). C57B1/10 mice were challenged with and LD_{100} or LD_{200}. Both pre- and post-LPS challenge treatment with lipid X demonstrated protection (see Ref. 33 and Table 1). As the time between LPS challenge and lipid X therapy increased, larger doses were needed and the effectiveness decreased. Of note, the protective efficacy of lipid X could be overcome by giving higher doses of LPS, whereas increasing the lipid X dose did not overcome the higher LPS doses (Proctor, unpublished data). This suggests that lipid X has a protective "window" wherein it can antagonize the toxic effects of LPS. Similarly, galactosamine-sensitized mice were also protected from LPS by lipid X pretreatment (J. K. Chia et al., Clin Res. 35:470A, 1987). The failure of lipid X to protect galactosamine-sensitized mice, when given after LPS challenge (J. K. Chia et al., Clin Res. 35:470A, 1987), might be due to the steep LPS dose response mortality curve such that the window of protection was so narrow that it was missed.

Sheep can also be protected by lipid X given 1 hr before LPS challenge (see Table 2) (16). The sheep received either 100 or 200 μg of lipid X per kg body weight and then challenged with 20 μg **E. coli** 0111:B4 endotoxin per kg body weight (an LD_{40}). Animals pretreated with 100 μg of lipid X per kg demonstrated significantly lower pulmonary artery pressures during both early and late phase responses to endotoxin challenge. The higher dose of lipid X, 200 μg/kg, produced some pulmonary hypertension, but it still showed protective efficacy. Of interest, lipid X did not prevent endotoxin-induced neutropenia nor did it block the systemic hypotensive response to endotoxin. The one animal that was not protected by lipid X received material that was contaminated by lipid Y, which is toxic to sheep (7). Thus, lipid X protected both sheep and mice from the lethal effects of endotoxin.

A monophosphoryl derivative of lipid A has also been found to protect mice against endotoxin challenge (24). This compound is **Salmonella minnesota** Re-lipid A with the phosphate group removed from the 1-position, hence monophosphoryl lipid A (MPLA) (39-41). When given 1 day prior to LPS challenge, the LD_{50} of LPS increased approximately five-fold (24).

Intact LPS in low doses (4 ng/kg) can protect mice from a subsequent LD_{100} of LPS (9). The mechanism of this "tolerance" to endotoxin challenge

Table 2. Mortality of adult sheep pretreated with lipid X (100 or 200 μg/kg) 1 hr before **E. coli** (0111:B4) endotoxin challenge (16)

Outcome	No. (%) of sheep in the following groups[b]		
	Control	100 μg/kg[c]	200
Survival	12 (63)	13 (100)	5 (83)
Death	7 (37)	0	1 (17)[d]

[a]Lipid X concentration, 100 or 200 μg/kg; endotoxin concentration, 20 μg/kg.
[b]$P<0.05$ for combined mortality of pretreated groups versus the control group. $P<0.05$ for the control group versus the 100 μg/kg group. $P<0.1$ for the control group versus the 200 μg/kg group.
[c]One animal was deleted from the data because of death due to catheter-induced pulmonary infection. Inclusion of this animal would still allow statistical significance at $P<0.05$.
[d]This animal received contaminated lipid X (approximately 10% lipid Y; see the text).

is unknown, but it appears to be mediated through macrophages (15, 22, 27). Macrophages from tolerant animals may release fewer mediators in response to LPS such as tumor necrosis factor and interleukin-1 as compared to normal animals.

Protection Against Bacterial Challenge

Lipid X also reduces the mortality of **E. coli** challenged mice (17) (Fig 2). Lipid X alone slightly increased the time to death (17). However, lipid X in combination with ticarcillin was significantly better than ticarcillin alone. Treatment with lipid X and ticarcillin improved survival two to four-fold over a broad range of antibiotic doses. This efficacy continued for 3 days after ticarcillin was stopped. Lipid X enabled the dose of ticarcillin necessary to protect 50% of mice from death to be reduced by two to five-fold. Pretreatment with lipid X was not necessary to improve survival: 16 of 17 (94%) infected and toxic mice that received lipid X and ticarcillin 6 hr after challenge survived versus 30 of 44 (68%) control animals treated with ticarcillin alone ($P<0.0001$) (17). These data suggest that lipid X may be inhibitting some of the actions of endotoxin released by ticarcillin therapy. An alternative explanation is that lipid X might be stimulating host defenses. However, this second explanation seems less likely because highly purified lipid X alone did show some early protective activity which would be a rapid response for activity host cells (17) and because biologic and synthetic lipid X are very weak mitogens and releasers of cytokines (47; Proctor, unpublished data); whereas less purified lipid X has greater macrophage-activating activity (2, 29).

How lipid X may exert anti-endotoxic activity is not known. Although the original concept was that lipid X might compete for a membrane receptor for LPS was the impetus for testing lipid X for protective efficacy, further data make this possibility less likely. First, lipid X does not compete with LPS in a simple antagonist-agonist pattern. The ratio between agonist and antagonist should be constant. However, lipid X is not able to compete with LPS, or lipid A, over a broad range of concentrations, but only through a specific window. (Of note, the effective range of lipid X protection seems to coincide with levels of LPS expected with gram-negative sepsis.) Second, lipid X does not compete with LPS or lipid IVA for a membrane receptor on

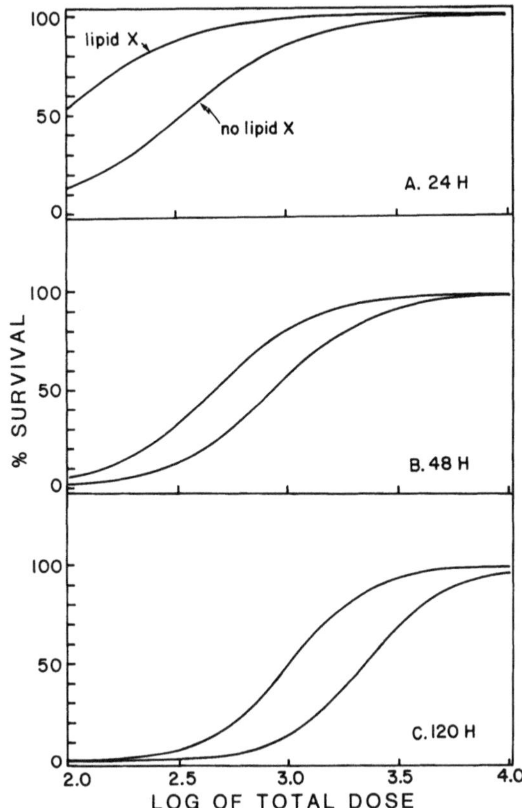

0130u

Fig 2. Percent survival of lipid X-treated and untreated mice versus dose of ticarcillin (17). Using a logistic regression model, survival curves were constructed for neutropenic mice given a lethal **E. coli** thigh infection. Animals were treated with a range of doses of ticarcillin so that this variable could be analyzed separately from the lipid X effect. Mice received lipid 6 hr prior to and 6 hr after **E. coli** challenge. Ticarcillin therapy started at 6 hr and continued through 48 hr. Survival curves are shown for 24, 48 and 120 hr.

macrophages (Drs. Hampton, Golenbock, Raetz, in press, J. Biol. Chem.). Hence, lipid X probably acts on post-receptor binding signal transduction or secretory systems. In support of this concept, we have preliminary data both **in vivo** (see Corwell et al., in this volume) and **in vitro** (RAW 264.7 cells, unpublished data) that lipid X reduces LPS-induced tumor necrosis factor production, which is consistent with data presented by Chia et al., (Clin. Res. 35: 470A, 1987) where they showed reduced TNF production from lipid X-treated, LPS-challenged mouse peritoneal macrophages.

At the cellular level, neither lipid X nor monophosphoryl lipid A were able to inhibit LPS-mediated neutrophil adherence to human umbilical veins, whereas the diphosphoryl tetraacyl lipid A precursor could inhibit their adherence (32). This suggests that these lipids do not mediate protective efficacy by inhibiting neutrophil adherence. Lipid X does inhibit LPS-induced macrophage procoagulant activity both directly at the level of the macrophages and indirectly via the T-cell (B. S. Schwartz and M. C. Monroe, Circulation II, 74: 370, 1986). Finally, lipid X inhibits the Re-LPS-induced mitogenic response of mouse splenocytes (47). Thus, lipid X exerts anti-endotoxin effects in monocytes, T-cells, peritoneal macrophages, RAW 264.7 macrophages, and meutrophils, but most likely not at the level of the cellular receptor.

In contrast to lipid X, monophosphoryl lipid A exhibits many immunostimulating properties and may protect the host from bacterial invasion by activating host defenses. Monophosphoryl lipid A derived from Salmonella minnesota R595 when injected into mice 1 day prior to through 2 days after challenge with **E. coli** or **Staphylococcus epidermidis** (LD_{65} to LD_{100} doses) reduces mortality (8). Also, MPLA enhances the macrophage activity both in vitro and in vivo for tumor lysis, antibody production, and anti-viral activity (25, 39-41, 47). Although the precise mechanisms for these activities are unknown, macrophage activation (39-41) and cytokine release (24) do occur when cells are treated with MPLA.

SUMMARY

These studies provide exciting prospects for the future treatment of gram-negative infections. The anti-endotoxin activity of lipid X, a monosaccharide precursor of lipid A, may be a prototypic compound for agents that can block the toxic effects of endotoxin that is being actively released. In contrast, monophosphoryl lipid A, a disaccharide derivative of lipid A, stimulates host defenses against infections and tumors. With further understanding of the mechanisms by which these compounds exert these effects, we can anticipate that new and more active compounds will be developed and that further activities of existing compounds will be found.

REFERENCES

1. Appelmelk, B. J., 1987, "Antibodies to the LPS core region and their protective role in gram-negative sepsis," Free Univ. Press, Amsterdam.

2. Amano, F., Nishijima, M., and Akamatsu, Y., 1986, A monosaccharide precursor of **Escherichia coli** lipid A has the ability to induce tumor-cytotoxic factor production by a murine macrophage-like cell line, J774.1. J. Immunol. 136: 4122.

3. Anderson, M. S., Bulawa, C. E., and Raetz, C. R. H., 1985, The biosynthesis of gram-negative endotoxin. Formation of lipid A precursors from UDP-GLcNAc in extracts of **Escherichia coli**. J. Biol. Chem. 260: 15536.

4. Bryan, C. S., Reynolds, K. L., and Brenner, E. R., 1983, Analysis of 1,186 episodes of gram-negative bacteremia in non-university hospitals: the effects of antimicrobial therapy. Rev. Infect. Dis. 5: 629.

5. Bulawa, C. E. and Raetz, C. R. H., 1984, The biosynthesis of gram-negative endotoxin and function of UDP-2,3-diacylglucosomine in **Escherichia coli.** J. Biol. Chem. 259: 4846.

6. Burhop, K. E., Proctor, R. A., Helegerson, R. B., Raetz, C. R. H., Starling, J. R., and Will, J. A., 1985, Pulmonary pathophysiological changes in sheep caused by endotoxin precursors, lipid X. J. Appl. Physiol. 59: 1726.

7. Burhop, K. E., Proctor, R. A., Raetz, C. R. H., and Will, J. A., 1987, Pulmonary pressor responses in sheep to chemically-defined precursors of **Escherichia coli** endotoxin. J. Appl. Physiol. 62: 1141.

8. Chase, J. J., Kubey, W., Dulek, M. H., Holmes, C. J., Salit, M. G., Pearson III, F. C., and Ribi, E., 1986, Effect of monophosphoryl lipid A on host resistance to bacterial infection. Infect. Immun. 53: 711.

9. Chong, K.-T. and Huston, M., 1987, Implications of endotoxin contamination in the evaluation of antibodies to lipopolysaccharides in a murine model of gram-negative sepsis. J. Infect. Dis. 156: 713.

10. Coleman, J. and Raetz, C. R. H., 1988, First committed step of lipid A biosynthesis in **Escherichia coli**: sequence of the lpxA gene, J. Bacteriol. 170: 1268.

11. Cook, J. A., Wise, W. C., and Habushka, P. V., 1980, Elevated thromboxane levels in rats during endotoxic shock. Protective effects of imidazole, 13-azaprostanoic acid, or essential fatty acid deficiency. J. Clin. Invest. 65: 227.

12. Crowell, D. N., Reznikoff, W. S., and Raetz, C. R. H., 1987, Nucleotide sequence of **Escherichia coli** gene for lipid A disaccharide synthase. J. Bacteriol. 169: 5727.

13. DeMaria, A., Heffernan, J. J., Grindlinger, G. A., Craven, D. E., McIntosh, T. K., McCabe, W. R., 1985, Naloxone versus placebo in treatment of septic shock. Lancet i: 1363.

14. Flynn, J. T., 1985, The role of arachidonic acid metabolites in endotoxin shock. II. Involvement of prostanoids and thromboxanes. Ch 10, in: "Handbook of Endotoxins, Vol. 2: Pathophysiology of Endotoxin," R. A. Proctor, L. B. Hinshaw, eds., Elsevier, Amsterdam, New York, Oxford, p. 237.

15. Freudenberg, M. A., Keppler, D., and Galanos, C., 1986, Requirements for lipopolysaccharide-responsive macrophages in galactosamine-induced sensitization to endotoxin, Infect. Immun. 51: 891.

16. Golenbock, D. T., Will, J. A., Raetz, C. R. H., and Proctor, R. A., 1987, Lipid X ameliorates pulmonary hypertension and protects sheep from death due to endotoxin. Infect. Immun. 55: 2471.

17. Golenbock, D. T., Leggett, J. E., Craig, W. A., Raetz, C. R. H., and Proctor, R. A., 1988, Lipid X protects mice against fatal **Escherichia coli** infection. Infect. Immun. 56: 779.

18. Gurll, N. J., 1985, Endorphins in endotoxin shock, in: "Handbook of Endotoxins, Vol. 2: Pathophysiology of Endotoxin, Chapter 12," R. A. Proctor, L. B. Hinshaw, eds., Elsevier, Amsterdam, New York, Oxford, p. 299.

19. Hinshaw, L. B., Archer, L. T., Beller-Todd, B. K., Benjamin, B., Flourney, D. J., and Passey, R., 1981, Survival of primates in lethal septic shock following delayed treatment with steroid. Circ. Shock 8: 291.

20. Hinshaw, L. B., Beller-Todd, B. K., Archer, L. T., Benjamin, B., Flourney, D. J., Passey, R., and Wilson, M. F., 1981, Effectiveness of steroid/antibiotic treatment in primates administered LD100 **Escherichia coli.** Ann. Surg. 194: 51.

21. Holaday, J. W. and Faden, A. I., 1978, Naloxone reversal of endotoxin hypotension suggests role of endophins in shock. Nature 275: 450.

22. Johnston, C. A. and Greisman, S. E., 1985, Mechanisms of endotoxin tolerance, in: "Handbook of Endotoxins, Vol. 2: Pathophysiology of Endotoxin," L. B. Hinshaw, ed., Elsevier, Amsterdam, New York, Oxford, p. 359.

23. Kreger, B. E., Craven, D. E., and McCabe, W. R., 1980, Gram-negative bacteremia, IV. Reevaluation of clinical features and treatment in 612 patients. Am. J. Med. 68: 344.

24. Madona, G. S., Peterson, J. E., Ribi, E. E., and Vogel, S. N., 1986, Early-phase endotoxin tolerance: induction by a detoxified lipid A derivative monophosphoryl lipid A. Infect. Immun. 52: 6.

25. Masihi, K. N., Lange, W., Brehmer, W., and Ribi, E., 1986, Immunobiological activities of nontoxic lipid A: enhancement of nonspecific resistance in combination with trehalose dimycolate against viral infection and adjuvant effects. J. Immunopharm. 8: 339.

26. McCabe, W. R. and Jackson, G. G., 1962, Gram-negative bacteremia, I. Etiology and ecology. Arch. Intern. Med. 110: 847.

27. Michalek, S. M., Moore, R. N., McGhee, J. R., Rosenstreich, D. L., and Mergenhagen, S. E., 1980, The primary role of lymphoreticular cells in the mediation of host responses to bacterial endotoxin. J. Infect. Dis. 141: 55.

28. Munford, R. S. and Hall, C. L., 1985, Uptake and deacylation of bacterial lipopolysaccharides by macrophages from normal and endotoxin-hyporesponsive mice. Infect. Immun. 48: 464.

29. Nishijima, M., Amano, F., Akamatsu, Y., Akagawa, K., Tokunaga, T., and Raetz, C. R. H., 1985, Macrophage activation by monosaccharide precursors of **Escherichia coli** lipid A. Proc. Natl. Acad. Sci. (USA) 82: 282.

30. Nishijima, M., Bulawa, C., and Raetz, C. R. H., 1981, Two interesting mutations causing temperature-sensitive phosphatidylglcerol synthesis in **Escherichia coli** membranes. J. Bacteriol. 145: 113.

31. Nishijima, M., and Raetz, C. R. H., 1979, Membrane lipid biogenesis in **Escherichia coli**: identification of genetic loci for phosphatidylglycerophosphate synthetase and construction of mutants lacking phosphatidylglcerol. J. Biol. Chem. 254: 7837.

32. Pohlman, T. H., Munford, R. S., and Harlan, J. M., 1987, Deacylated lipopolysaccharide inhibits neutrophil adherence to endothelial induced by lipopolysaccharide in vitro. J. Exp. Med. 165: 1393.

33. Proctor, R. A., Will, J. A., Burhop, K. E., and Raetz, C. R. H., 1986, Protection of mice against lethal endotoxemia by a lipid A precursor. Infect. Immun. 52: 905.

34. Qureshi, N., Takayama, K., and Ribi, E., 1982, Purification and structural determination of nontoxic lipid A obtained from the lipopolysaccharide of **Salmonella typhimurium**. J. Biol. Chem. 25: 11808.

35. Raetz, C. R. H., 1986, Molecular genetics of membrane phosphological synthesis. Annual Rev. Genet. 13: 319.

36. Raetz, C. R. H., Purcell, S., Meyer, M. V., Qureshi, N., and Takayama, K., 1985, Isolation of eight lipid A precursors from a 3-deoxy-d-monno-octylusonic acid-deficient mutant of **Salmonella typhimurium**. J. Biol. Chem. 260: 16080.

37. Ray, B. L., Painter, G., and Raetz, C. R. H., 1984, The biosynthesis of gram-negative endotoxin. Formation of lipid A disaccharides from monosaccharide precursors in extracts of **Escherichia coli**. J. Biol. Chem. 259: 4852.

38. Ray, B. L. and Raetz, C. R. H., 1987, The biosynthesis of gram-negative endotoxin. A novel kinase in **Escherichia coli** membranes that incorporate the 4'-phosphate of lipid A. J. Biol. Chem. 262: 1122.

39. Ribi, E., 1984, "Advances in carriers and adjuvants for veterinary biologics," Iowa State University Press, Ames, IA.

40. Ribi, E., 1984, Beneficial modification of the endotoxin molecule. J. Biol. Response Modif. 3: 1.

41. Ribi, E., Cantrell, J. L., Takayama, K., Qureshi, N., Peterson, J., and Ribi, H. O., 1984, Lipid A and immunotherapy. Rev. Infect. Dis. 6: 567.

42. Sheagren, J. D., 1981, Septic shock and corticosteroids, (editorial), New Engl. J. Med. 305: 456.

43. Sprung, C. L., Caralis, P. V., Marcial, E. H., Pierce, M., Gelbard, M. A., Long, W. M., Duncan, R. C., Tendler, M. D., and Kardf, M., 1984, The effects of high-dose corticosteroids in patients with septic shock. N. Engl. J. Med. 311: 1137.

44. Strain, S. M., Armitage, I. M., Anderson, L., Takayama, K., Qureshi, N., and Raetz, C. R. H., 1985, Location of polar substitutes and fatty acyl chains on lipid A precursors from a 3-deoxy-D-manno-octulosonic acid-deficient mutant of **Salmonella typhimurium**. J. Biol. Chem. 260: 16089.

45. Takayama, K., Qureshi, N., Mascagni, P., Anderson, L., and Raetz, C. R. H., 1983, Glucosamine-derived phospholipids in **Escherichia coli**. Structure and chemical modification of a triacylglucosamine-1-phosphate found in a phosphatidylglycerol-deficient mutant. J. Biol. Chem. 258: 14245.

46. Takayama, K., Qureshi, N., Mascagni, P., Nashed, M. A., Anderson, L., and Raetz, C. R. H., 1983, Fatty acyl derivatives of glucosamine-1-phosphate in **Escherichia coli** and their structural relationship to lipid A. J. Biol. Chem. 258: 7379.

47. Tomai, M. A., Johnson, A. G., and Ribi, E., 1988, Glycolipid induced proliferation of lipopolysaccharide hyporesponsive C3H/HeJ splenocytes. J. Leukocyte Biol. 43: 11.

48. Tomai, M. A., Solem, L. E., Johnson, A. G., and Ribi, E., 1987, The adjuvant properties of a nontoxic monophosphoryl lipid A in hyporesponsive and aging mice. J. Biol. Response Modif. 6: 99.

49. Tomasiewicz, H. G. and McHenry, C. S., 1987, Sequence analysis of the **dna**E gene of **Escherichia coli**. J. Bacteriol. 169: 5735.

50. Ziegler, E. J., Douglas, H., Sherman, J. E., Davis, C. E., and Braude, A. I., 1973, Treatment of **E. coli** and **Klebsiella** bacteremia in agranulocytic animals with antiserum to a UDP-Gal-epimerase-deficient mutant. J. Immunol. 111: 433.

51. Ziegler, E. J., McCutchan, J. A., Douglas, H., and Braude, A. I., 1975, Prevention of lethal Pseudomonas bacteremia with epimerase-deficient **E. coli** antiserum. Trans. Assoc. Am. Physc. 88: 101.

52. Ziegler, E. J., McCutchan, J. A., Fieker, J., Glauser, M. P., Sadoff, J. C., and Braude, A. I., 1982, Treatment of gram-negative bacteremia and shock with human antiserum to a mutant **Escherichia coli**. N. Engl. J. Med. 307: 1225.

NEW THERAPEUTIC METHOD AGAINST SEPTIC SHOCK - REMOVAL OF ENDOTOXIN USING EXTRACORPOREAL CIRCULATION

M. Kodama, K. Hanasawa and T. Tani

Department of Surgery, Shiga University of Medical Science
Seta-Tsukiwacho, Otsu, Shiga 520-21 Japan

INTRODUCTION

Polymyxin B has been shown to prevent endotoxin-induced mortality of mice and rabbits (9, 10), and to decrease the incidence of endotoxin-disseminated intravascular coagulation (1). However, its use is limited only to oral or local administration because of its strong side effect on the central nervous system and the kidneys. Therefore, it cannot be used by intravenous injection for the therapy of endotoxemia. To solve problems, a new method of preparing polymyxin B by fixing it to an insoluble fiber was developed. We previously reported that polymyxin B would be covalently coupled to an insoluble fiber and could not be removed anymore by washing with isotonic saline (1, 3).

In this paper we will report our evaluation of this newly developed immobilized polymyxin-B fiber (obtained by treating the polystyrene fiber with a solution containing formaldehyde, N-methyl-alpha-chloracetamide and sulfuric acid) with polymyxin B sulfate (Pfizer Taito Co. Ltd., Tokyo) at a pH over 7, followed by reacting it with amine. PMX-F (p-17) is produced by treating the succinylated fiber (obtained by aminating the above-mentioned alpha-chloracetamide methylated and cross-linked polystyrene fiber with a mixture of the primary diamine and of the secondary amine and by succinylating it with succinic acid anhydride) with polymyxin B sulfate under a peptide-condensing agent (Fig 1). P-15 is characterized by having a less expensive and shorter manufacturing process than P-17.

Statistical Analysis

The survival rate was examined by x^2 test. Other observed values (of blood pressure, hematological changes, metabolic changes and histamine levels) were compared by Student's t test.

Endotoxin Assay

We used lipopolysaccharide of E. coli 0111(B4), obtained from Difco Laboratories (Detroit, MI, U.S.A.) as endotoxin throughout the experiments. Endotoxin concentration was measured by the synthetic chromogenic substrate Boc-Leu-Gly-Arg-p-nitroanilide (Seikagaku Kogyo Ltd., Tokyo, Japan) with perchloric acid pre-treatment (4).

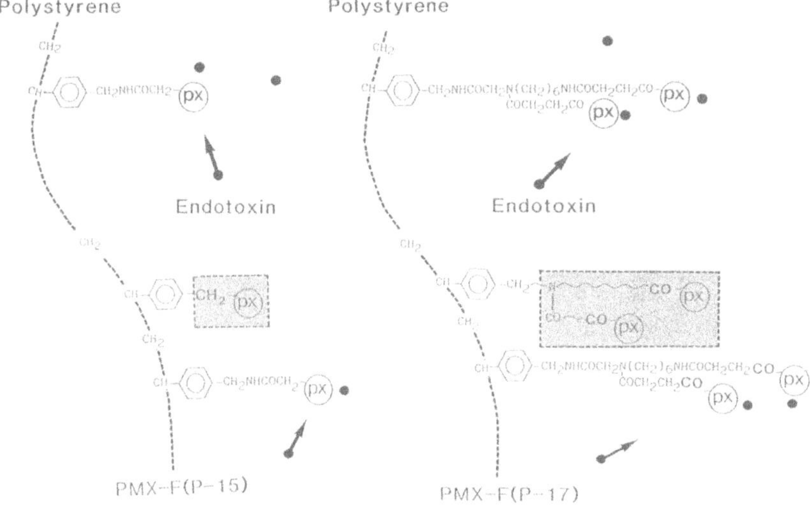

Fig 1. Schema of PMX-F.

Escherichia coli Preparation

E. coli (ATCC 25922) was obtained from American Type Culture. E. coli organisms were incubated overnight in Mueller-Hinton agar (Difco Laboratories) at 37°C., followed by suspension in 0.9% saline. Initial approximation of bacterial numbers was carried out by turbidimetry at a concentration of 10^9 colony forming units per milliliter. Serial dilutions were performed and the final concentration was established by viable colony counting on DHL agar plates (Nissui, Tokyo, Japan).

Determination of the Detoxifying Capacity of PMX-F

Thirty milliliters of endotoxin solution in saline was added to 1 gram of PMX-F (P-15) or PMX-F (P-17) in final endotoxin concentrations of 7.35, 2.0, 0.42 and 0.018 ng/ml. These solutions were incubated for 90 min at 37°C. The residual endotoxin concentrations were examined by the chromogenic limulus amoebocyte assay. The neutralizing capacity per 1 gram of PMX-F was calculated. The neutralizing ability of endotoxin was shown as an isotherm curve.

Effect of PMX-F on Endotoxin Lethality for Mice

The control group of ICR mice was injected with 1 ml of endotoxin solution (0.5 mg/ml) intravenously. The treated group was also injected with 1 ml of endotoxin solution but which had been mixed with 2 grams of PMX-F. Mortality was evaluated 48 hr after injection.

Inhibition of Endotoxin Fever by PMX-F(P-15)

Four groups of 5 rabbits were used to study the inhibition of endotoxin-induced fever by PMX-F. A group was injected with 100 ng/ml endotoxin saline solution per kg body weight. B group was injected with the same solution treated with 4 grams of PMX-F. C group was injected with 5 ng/ml endotoxin solution and D group was given a similar solution treated with 4 grams of PMX-F. Body temperatures were monitored for 3 hr. Rising temperature was calculated as the maximum body temperature minus the temperature before injection.

PMX-F (P-15) Hemoperfusion for the Treatment of Endotoxin Shock

Mongrel adult dogs received saline containing 0.01 percent of E. coli endotoxin (0.5 mg/kg) as a drip infusion for 1 hr in their forepaw, thus producing endotoxin shock (Fig 2). Twenty-four dogs were divided into two groups as follows: 16 dogs underwent direct hemoperfusion (DHP) through a column in which 5 grams of PMX-F were bundled and packed connected with a tube-pump (TR-25, Toray Company, Japan) between the femoral artery and vein at a flow rate of blood of 50 ml/min. This hemoperfusion started 15 min before endotoxin infusion, and was performed for 2 hr with no apparent side effects such as clotting, bursting of the column or blood leakage from the column in the circuit. The other 8 dogs did not receive DHP with PMX-F. All experimental dogs (7-9 kg body wt) were intravenously anesthetized with 15 mg/kg of sodium pentobarbitol. They were not intubated and were allowed to breath room air spontaneously. Measurements of femoral blood pressure, blood pH, histamine level and survival rate were compared between control and treated groups.

Comparative Study between PMX-F and Other Adsorbents (Charcoal and Resin) for Treatment of Endotoxin Shock

For the DHP with adsorbents in dogs with endotoxin shock, 38 adult mongrel dogs of both sexes were anesthetized as mentioned before. The dogs were divided into 4 groups: PMX-F hemoperfusion (n=15), resin (IRA-938) hemoperfusion (n=5), charcoal hemoperfusion (n=5), and carrier fiber hemoperfusion (control) (n=13). The cannulation of the aorta and vena cava inferior was set up through the femoral artery and vein. DHP was performed in the same manner as before. The endotoxic shock model was produced by administering purified endotoxin in an alternative dose of 0.75 mg/kg. The DHP was performed with each adsorbents (resin or charcoal) packed in a 50 ml column. Mean aortic blood pressure, arterial blood gas analysis, white blood cells, platelets, lactic acid, and serum blood sugar were measured. The survival rates of dogs were evaluated at 1 wk after DHP.

Hemoperfusion with PMX-F for Septic Dogs

PMX-F (P-15) of 50 meter length was bundled and packed in a 200 ml column for the hemoperfusion. Mongrel adult dogs weighing 9-15 kg were made septic by intravenous infusion of 1-5 x 10^9 living E. coli organisms (ATCC 25922)/kg body weight over 1 hr. Infusion of the antibiotic gentamicin sulfate (5 mg/kg) was started 30 min after the administration of bacteria (aiming at the increase of endotoxin concentration in the blood stream as a result of breaking down bacteria), and continued for 30 min. Each animal received 10 ml/kg/hr of supplementary saline solution for 1 hr just before the bacteria were administered, and then a 5 ml/kg/hr of saline solution over the following 6 hr as a maintenance dose. DHP was started 30 min just after bacterial administration. This was carried out for 2 hr on the dogs (Table

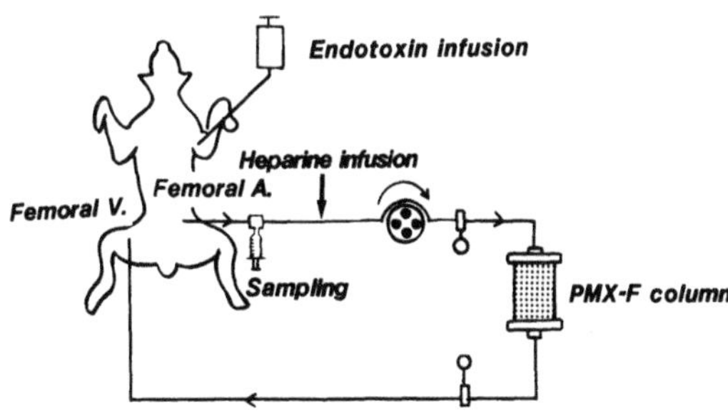

Fig 2. Hemoperfusion for endotoxin shock in canine.

Table 1. Experimental protocol of bacterial sepsis.

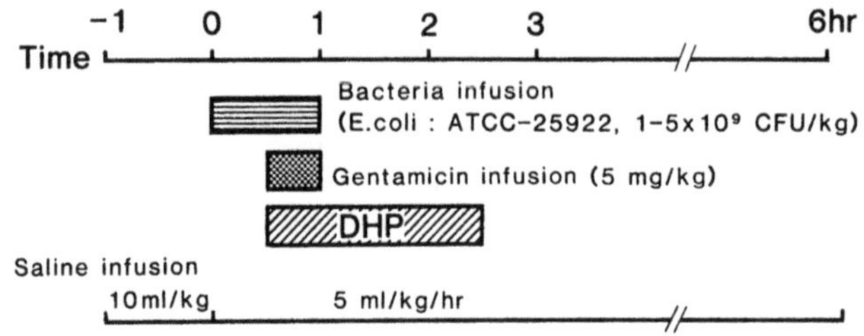

1). Sham-DHP with an empty column (50 ml) was performed as a control in the same manner as the DHP with PMX-F. The anti-coagulant heparin was also infused into the circuit, 3000 units in total for the initial hour. Then for the next hour 1000 units of heparin was infused. Measurements of hematological change, mean aortic blood pressure, plasma glucose, lactate, bacterial counts, and 14-day survival rate were recorded.

RESULTS

Detoxifying Capacity of PMX-F

It was confirmed that both P-15 and P-17 satisfactorily detoxified a very concentrated endotoxin solution. The endotoxin neutralizing capacity is shown as an isotherm curve. P-15 can neutralize a much larger dose of endotoxin than P-17 in the absence of serum. Conversely, in the presence of serum, P-17 can neutralize a much larger amount of endotoxin than P-15 (Fig 3). Therefore, P-17 may theoretically be the more ideal material of the two from the viewpoint of removing a much larger amount of endotoxin in the blood. However, P-17 requires a longer and more expensive manufacturing process than P-15. From a practical point of view we think that P-15 is fully sufficient for the removal of endotoxin from the blood.

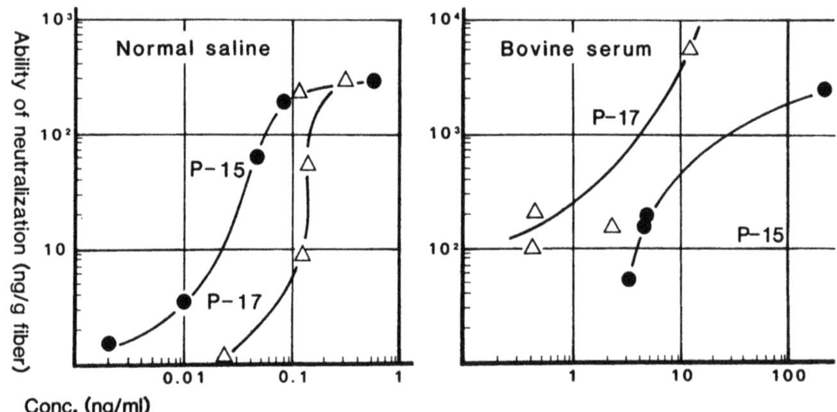

Fig 3. Neutralization of endotoxin by PMX-F in low concentration.

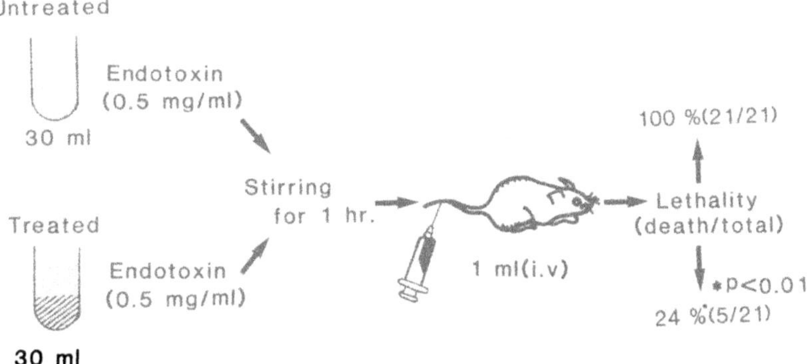

Fig 4. Influence of PMX-F on mice study.

Mice Lethality Study

Untreated mice showed a 100% (21/21) mortality, whereas the group treated with PMX-F experienced a 24% (5/21) mortality. Thus PMX-F treatment significantly decreased the lethality ($p < 0.01$) (Fig 4).

Rabbit Pyrogenicity Test

It is generally recognized that the minimum pyrogenicity of pyrogen is 2 ng/kg and the rising temepratures of 2 ng/kg intravenous administration show more than 0.6°C in rabbits (7). In the rabbits treated with PMX-F, temperatures rose less than 0.6°C. It is evident that PMX-F inactivates the pyrogenicity of endotoxin (Fig 5).

Hemoperfusion in Endotoxin Shock

In the control group of dogs, only one out of 8 (12.5%) was alive after 24 hr. They showed typical symptoms of endotoxin shock, that is, the blood pressure started severely dropping as soon as the endotoxin infusion was begun. This was followed by a gradual but progressive drop in blood pressure

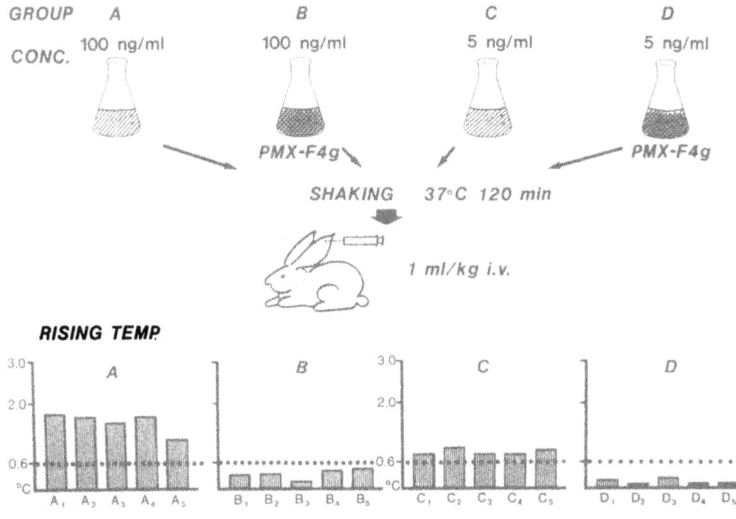

Fig 5. Inhibition of endotoxin fever by PMX-F.

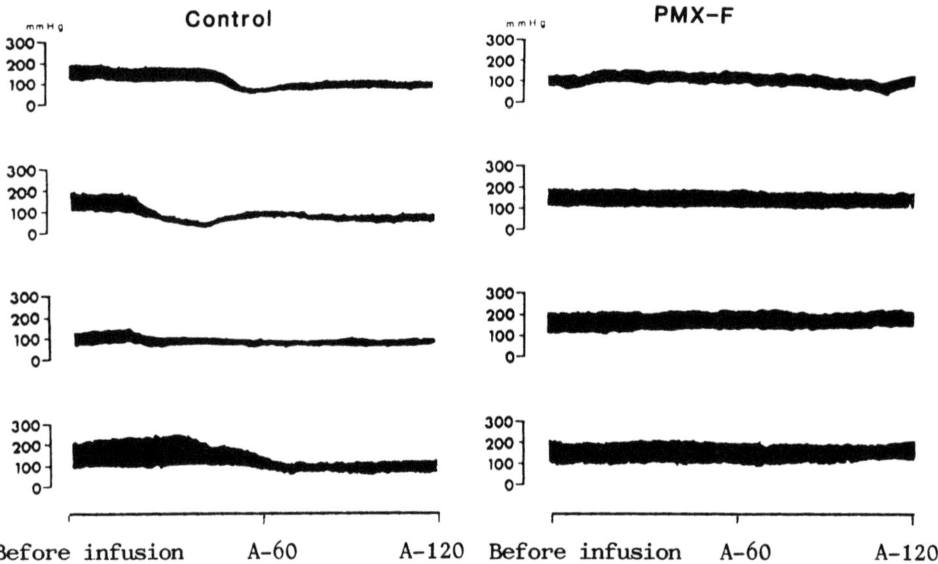

Fig 6. Changes in blood pressure. A60 and A-120 indicate 60 and 120 min after endotoxin infusion. left: blood pressure in the control group; right: blood pressure in the treated group.

with 4-8 hr, until the shocked animals died (Fig 6). The DHP group did not show as high histamine levels as the controls. Significant decreases were observed in the treated group, especially at 30 min post-DHP (P<0.01) (Fig 7). In the blood gas analysis, the blood pH of the treated group exhibited a minimal decrease (pH 7.27 ± 0.04 at a 2 hr post DHP), whereas it exhibited a significant decrease in the control group (pH 7.12 ± 0.06 at 1 hr post-endotoxin administration). Thus direct hemoperfusion with PMX-F was an effective treatment in endotoxin shock.

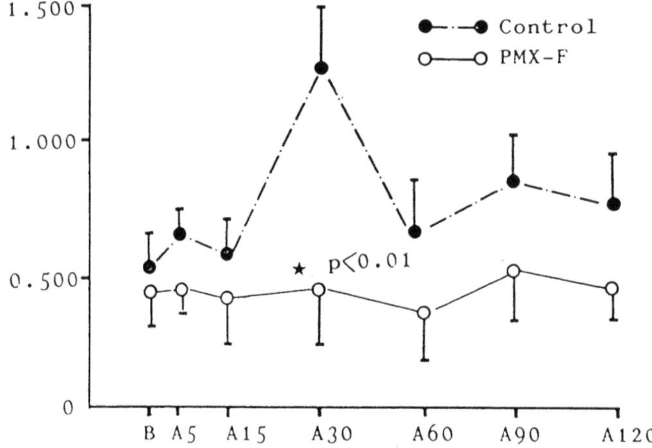

Fig 7. Changes in histamine level. B indicate before endotoxin administration and A15, 30, 60, 90, 120, indicate minutes after endotoxin administration.

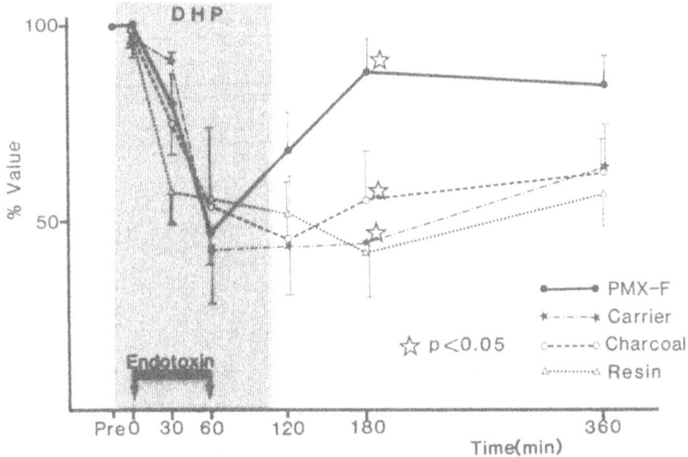

Fig 8. Changes in mean aortic blood pressure.

Comparative Study Using PMX-F, or Resin, or Charcoal

The effectiveness of resin, activated charcoal, and fiber without the attachment of polymyxin B (control) was also studied and compared to that of PMX-F. The blood pressure of all groups immediately dropped following endotoxin infusion. The PMX-F group recovered 80% of the comparative initial value in 3 hr. The differences in blood pressure responses between the PMX-F group and the other three groups 3 hr after administration of endotoxin is shown in Fig 8. All groups showed immediate severe decrease in WBC (Fig 9) and platelet counts (Fig 10) following the administration of endotoxin. However, significant differences in the recovery of WBC counts existed between the PMX-F group and the resin, charcoal and control groups at 6 hr after the administration. All groups showed hyperglycemia just after the administration, but there was a progressive drop in blood glucose until 360 min (Fig 11). All groups showed hyperlacticemia as well, (Fig 12). There were no significant differences at 360 min. The survival rate is shown in Fig 13. The PMX-F group had a much higher rate than the other three groups.

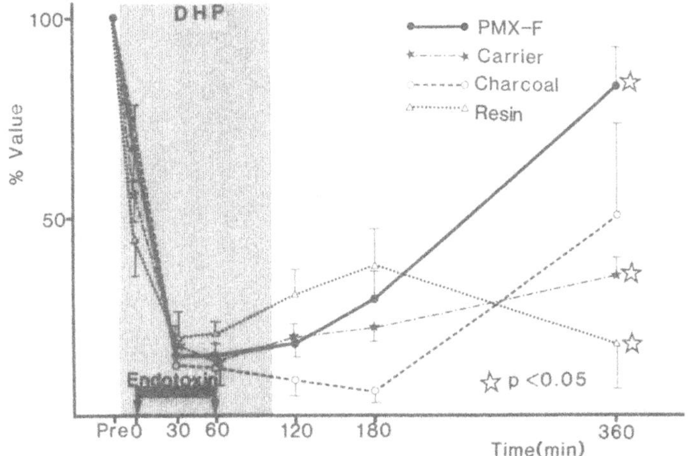

Fig 9. Changes in white blood cell counts.

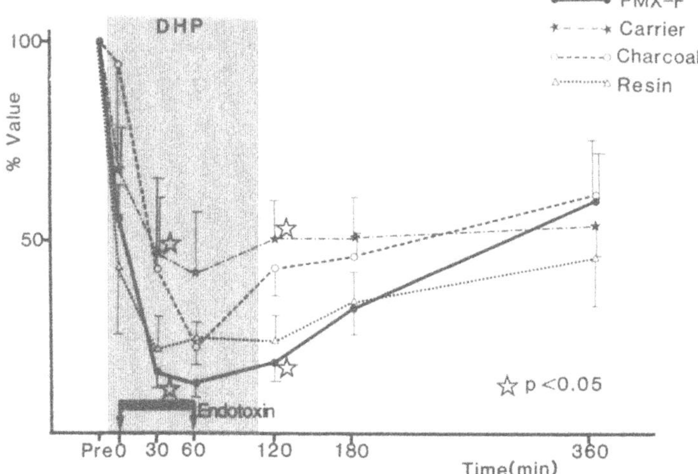

Fig 10. Changes in platelet counts.

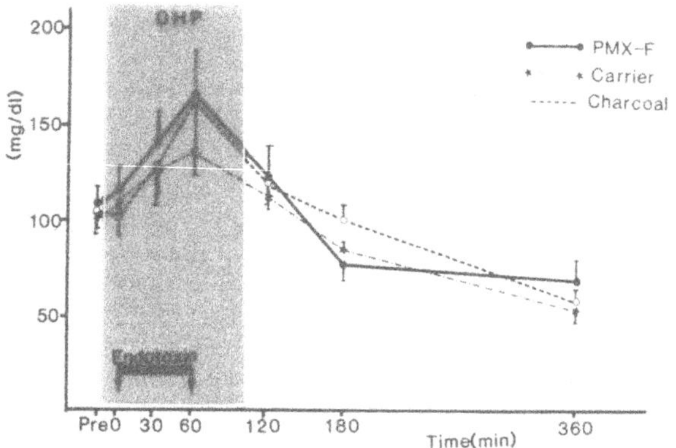

Fig 11. Changes in glucose.

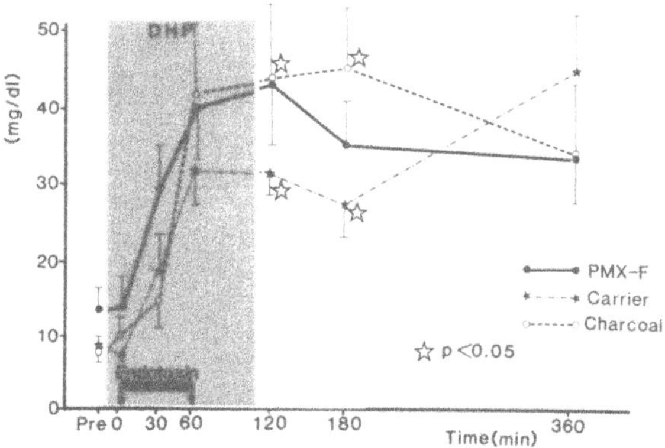

Fig 12. Changes in lactic acid.

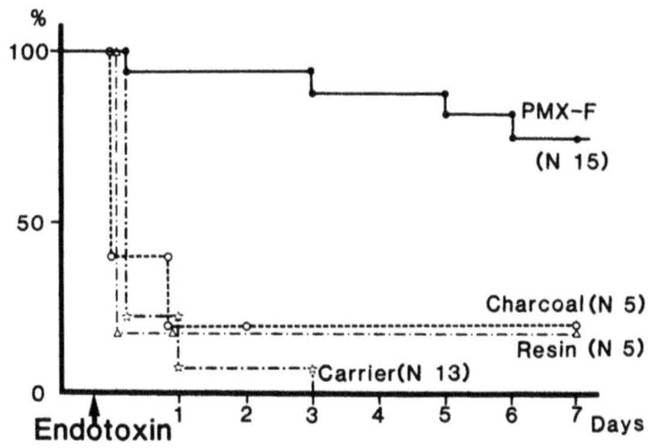

Fig 13. Survival rate of comparative study.

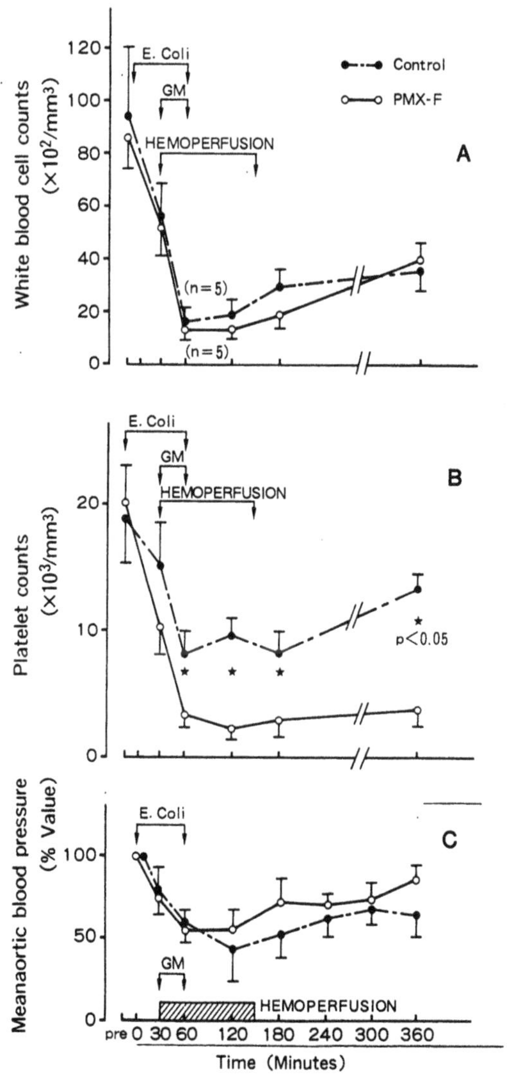

Fig 14. A and B) Hematological changes (white blood cell, platelet).
C) Changes in mean aortic pressure.

Figures 14. A and B show the hematological changes throughout the course of the experiment. White blood cells (WBC) and platelet counts (PLT) declined rapidly during the course of the study in all groups. The decline in the PLT counts in the control group was followed by moderate recovery to 70% of the initial PLT value. Conversely, PMX-F treatment caused a significant fall ($p < 0.05$) in PLT numbers at 60, 120, 180 and 360 min. A search is now being made for the reason why much higher decreases of PLT numbers occur in the group treated with PMX-F. The treated group had higher levels of mean aortic blood pressure than the control group did during the entire period of observation, although the difference was statistically not significant (Fig 14. C).

Plasma glucose and lactate were used during the course of the study to estimate the metabolic changes. All of the dogs in both groups developed transient hyperglycemia 2 hr after bacterial infusion and soon thereafter the glucose levels decreased. The glucose level at 360 min in the treated group was significantly higher than that in the control group ($p < 0.025$). The untreated group fell into severe hypoglycemia (Fig 15. A). The plasma lactate level showed a highly significant decrease in the treated group at 180 and 360 min (Fig 15. B). These observations indicate that PMX-F treatment improves the impaired glucose and lactate metabolism in the septic dog. Table 2 shows the survival time of septic dogs. All of them died within 18 hr in

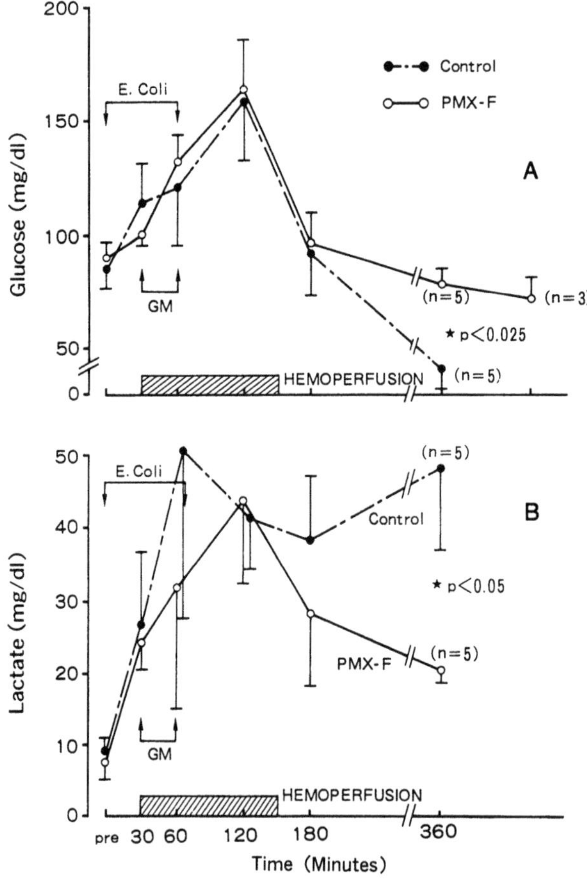

Fig 15. A,B. Metabolic changes (glucose, lactate).

Table 2. Survival rate of septic dogs.

Treatment	Dog No.	Survival
Control group	C-1	<12 hrs
	C-2	<12 hrs
	C-3	<18 hrs
	C-4	<18 hrs
	C-5	10 hrs
Treated group	T-1	permanent
	T-2	permanent
	T-3	14 days
	T-4	7 days
	T-5	3 days

the control group. But all in the treated group survived more than 3 days. Two of the five doges survived permanently. One of the remaining two survived 7 days and the other 14. These results lead us to conclude that PMX-F treatment, namely the selective removal of endotoxin from experimental endotoxemia and septicemia prolongs or increases the chances of survival.

DISCUSSION

Today, plasma exchange has been used to treat various diseases. The primary object of this therapy is to eliminate large molecular substances such as antigens, antibodies, immune complexes, complement split products, protein-bound toxins, toxic drugs, chemical mediators like vasoactive amines and so on. From this viewpoint, plasma or blood exchange appears to be an ideal method of reducing both endotoxins and unspecified protein-bound toxins. However, in such treatments, there is the possibility that a very dangerous infection such as AIDS or hepatitis will be transmitted, as a massive volume of plasma or blood is used. To prevent irreversible damage by post-perfusion complications, another approach is preferable. Many investigators' attention has turned to selective plasma component removal (8).

Currently the authors are developing a new material for the selective removal of endotoxin. The newly developed polymyxin B immobilized on fiber can neutralize a sufficient amount of endotoxin (5). The authors have examined whether polymyxin B is released from PMX-F and have found no leaks from the PMX-F (3). Experiments were also conducted to determine whether PMX-F influences the lethal effect of endotoxin on mice in a batch system. All of the control group died, whereas 76% of the mice treated with PMX-F survived. We then performed DHP with PMX-F after producing shocked dogs by infusing endotoxin. A majority of the dogs survived. Thus the efficacy and safety of PMX-F in vitro and vivo have been confirmed. Subsequently, DHP with PMX-F was performed on septicemic dogs which were given living E. coli organisms. The efficacy of PMX-F treatment for these animals was shown to be equal or better than that for endotoxemic dogs.

There are three conventional therapeutic approaches for the treatment of endotoxemia: the first is blocking the route of the endotoxin source; the second is protecting against endotoxin shock following endotoxemia; the third is improving the function of the organs injured by shock. As for the latest approaches, one is the mechanical removal of endotoxin, and another is the employing of endotoxin-neutralizing properties (2).

Powdered charcoal and certain types of resins are known to be useful for binding endotoxins in vitro (6). We compared the effectiveness of PMX-F with two other adsorbents, resin and coated charcoal, on endotoxin shock dogs in vivo. While resin and coated charcoal hemoperfusion resulted in survival rate lower than expected, PMX-F treatment significantly decreased the mortality rate of endotoxemic dogs.

Finally, it must be emphasized here that the present procedure makes it possible to bring blood in contact with polymyxin B directly and safely, and provides a new endotoxin detoxifying material which can be used as a therapy for endotoxemia or prophylaxis of endotoxemia. The combination of PMX-F treatment with other therapies such as anti-shock drugs, antibiotics, specific immunological approaches or surgical drainage of a septic focus may play an important role in the radical treatment for endotoxemia.

REFERENCES

1. Corrigan, J. J. and Bell, B. M., 1917, Comparison between the polymyxins and gentamicin in preventing endotoxin-induced intravascular coagulation and leukopenia. Infect. Immun. 4: 563.

2. Dunn, D. L. and Ferguson, R. M., 1982, Immunotherapy of gram-negative bacterial sepsis: Enhanced survival in a guinea pig model by use of rabbit antiserum to Escherichia coli J5. Surgery 92: 212.

3. Hanasawa, K., Tani, T., Oka, T., Yoshioka, T., Endo, Y., Horisawa, M., Nakane, Y., Kodama, M., Teramoto, K. and Nishiumi, S., 1984, A new treatment for endotoxemia with direct hemoperfusion by polymyxin immobilized fiber, in: "Therapeutic apheresis: a critical look," Y. Nose, P. S. Malchesky and J. W. Smith, eds., Cleveland: ISAO Press, : 167.

4. Kanoh, S., Yoshida, M., Kobayashi, T. and Ogawa, S., 1966, Studies on pyrogen (I). Jpn. J. Pharmacol. 62: 135.

5. Kodama, M., Oka, T., Tani, T. and Hanasawa, K., 1985, Therapeutic plasmapheresis for hepatic disorder in surgical patients new strategies for dealing with hyperbilirubinemia, endotoxemia and hemorrhagic disorder, in: "Current practice in therapeutic plasmaphoresis," T. Hoshino, ed., Excerpta Medica, Amsterdam, p. 102.

6. Nolan, J. P., Mcdevitt, J. J. and Goldmann, G. S., 1975, Endotoxin binding by charged and uncharged resin. Proc. Soc. Exp. Biol. Med. 149: 766.

7. Obayashi, T., 1984, Addition of perchloric acid to blood samples for colorimetric limulus test using chromogenic substrate: Comparison with conventional procedures and clinical applications. J. Lab. Clin. Med. 104: 321.

8. Pineda, A. A. and Taswell, H. F., 1981, Selective plasma component removal: alternatives to plasma exchange. Artif Organs 5: 234.

9. Rifkind, D., 1967, Prevention by polymyxin B of endotoxin lethality in mice. J. Bacteriol. 93: 1463.

10. Rifkind, D. and Hill, B. J., Rolla, 1967, Neutralization of the Shwartzman reactions by polymyxin B. J. Immunol. 99: 564.

IMMUNOTHERAPY WITH BACTERIAL ENDOTOXINS

J. A. Rudbach*, J. L. Cantrell*, J. T. Ulrich*, and M. S. Mitchell+

*Ribi ImmunoChem Research, Inc., Hamilton, MT, and
+Departments of Medicine and Microbiology, University of Southern California School of Medicine, Los Angeles, CA

INTRODUCTION

Since the recognition that humoral and cellular elements of the body provide protection and are responsible for natural recovery from various diseases (32), attempts have been made to enhance these mechanisms. At first, vaccines specifically targeted to the agent of the disease were employed (18). Subsequently, nonspecific stimulants were tested for their ability to protect man and other animals from infectious diseases and to provide therapeutic benefit in diseased hosts (24, 32). Ultimately, it was only natural that the nonspecific stimulants would be tested for their ability to enhance, or adjuvantize the specific resistance induced by vaccines.

The main source of most of these immunostimulants was microorganisms (16). Initially, either the whole organisms or crude extracts thereform were used. Although these materials displayed potent nonspecific and specific immunostimulatory properties, they also induced severe side effects in the treated animals (5, 16). Therefore, before clinical applications of such immunostimulants could be realized, a separation of biological activities had to be achieved, with isolation and purification of those molecular entities which possessed only the immunostimulatory properties.

Extracts from Gram-negative bacteria are some of the most powerful immunostimulants known (15). The potent immunizing properties of DPT (diptheria toxoid; pertussis bacterin; tetanus toxoid) were attributed to, in part, the potent adjuvant activities elicited by the killed pertussis bacteria in the vaccine (16). Subsequent work over the next several decades ultimately resulted in identification of endotoxin (ET) as the active immunostimulating component of enterobacteria (7). However, bacterial endotoxin could not be used in humans or other animals as a nonspecific immunostimulant or as an adjuvant for vaccines because of its inherent immunogenicity (10) and toxicity (12). Meanwhile, investigations in other laboratories were directed toward elucidating the biochemistry of bacterial endotoxins and relating this to biological function (31). A breakthrough in these studies was the isolation of mutant enterobacteria, which were unable to complete the addition of the oligosaccharide side chains (8). Endotoxins isolated from these bacteria still possessed the stimulatory characteristics of the complete lipopolysaccharides. However, those glycolipids were much simpler to work with and, ultimately, from them came the material known as diphosphoryl lipid A, or

DPL, which is the ultimate biologically active and toxic principle of endotoxin (19, 21, 28).

During the course of purifying and characterizing DPL, other materials, assumed to be related homologues, were observed and isolated (21). Several of these were tested in bioassays routinely used for endotoxins (pyrogenicity and lethality) and were found to be biologically inactive. However, further testing of these homologues showed that they retained the full immunostimulant and adjuvant properties, which were present in the toxic materials (22). Chemical analyses subsequently showed that the nontoxic, immunostimulatory homologue of DPL was a monophosphoryl derivative, which lacked a phosphate on the reducing end of the disaccharide (20). This material is thus referred to as monophosphoryl Lipid A (MPL™) (20).

MPL™ is a chemically defined entity, which has been extensively investigated for uses as an immunotherapetuic, an immunoprophylactic, and as an adjuvant for vaccines (22). In pure form MPL™ is sufficiently low in pyrogenicity and toxicity so that it can be used in human and in veterinary medicine. In the following will be described some of the properties of MPL™ and examples of where it is being employed in preclinical and in clinical investigations. It will be apparent that MPL™ is the "long sought after" utilitarian immunotherapeutic form of endotoxin.

When tumor-bearing animals are injected with endotoxin, the tumors regress in a certain percentage of the animals (12). Also, endotoxin containing products have been reported to induce tumor regression in man (17). However, the regression induced by this immunotherapy was not always quantitatively reproducible and the mechanisms involved were unknown. Whole mycobacteria or fractions thereof, also were shown to have antitumor activities (23, 34, 35). Data in Table 1 typify the results obtained when endotoxin, MPL™, or mycobacterial cell wall skeleton (CWS) were used alone as intralesional immunotherapeutics. Subsequent investigations demonstrated a synergy between the antitumor properties of CWS and endotoxin; this synergy was also demonstrable when nontoxic MPL™ was substituted for the native endotoxin (23) (Table 1).

That the guinea pig-line 10 tumor model is not a unique model for immunotherapy with MPL™-containing materials is shown in Table 2. Therein are shown data from experiments with a mouse ovarian tumor (MOT) model (2). Neither the **Propionibacterium acnes** - pyridine extract (PA-PE) nor MPL™ alone could cure mice previously challenged with MOT cells. However, the combination of PA-PE + MPL™ reproducibly cured over half of the animals carrying this tumor. Thus, nonspecific immunotherapy was curative when given shortly after transplantation with whole tumor cells. This nonspecific protection induced by PA-PE + MPL™ was dose-dependent as shown in Table 3. However, the lower dose of immunostimulant, which by itself would not protect the animals, could act as an adjuvant and enhance specific immunity generated with a co-administered tumor associated antigen (TAA) extracted from MOT; almost 90% of the animals were tumor free 60 days post-transplantation. In this model the TAA by itself was not protective.

The mouse ovarian tumor grows rapidly, and 2 days or more after transplantation it has established a significant tumor burden within the mice. It is one of the paradigms that the success of either specific or nonspecific immunotherapy is inversely related to the tumor burden (27). As shown in Table 4, 4 days after tumor transplantation, specific immunotherapy with TAA from MOT adjuvantized with PA-PE + MPL™ was ineffective in protecting the

Table 1. Direct immunotherapy of line-10 guinea pig tumor with endotoxin and MPL™-containing products[a]

Material injected[b]	Dose (μg)	Animals cured / Total tested	Percent cured
ET	150	3/19	16
MPL™	50	0/18	0
CWS	50	10/48	21
ET + CWS	50 + 50	8/8	100
MPL™ + CWS	50 + 50	50/52	96

[a]Data adapted from (23).
[b]Strain 2 guinea pigs bearing line-10 tumors were inoculated intralesionally with the designated materials on oil droplets. Definitions - ET = endotoxin; MPL™ = monophosphoryl lipid A; CWS = cell wall skeleton.

tumor bearing mice (3). However, if similar groups of mice were treated with the chemotherapeutic mitomycin C to reduce the tumor burden 6 days after tumor transplantation, and this was followed less than 2 days later by specific immunotherapy, 50% of the animals responded (Table 4). It is not surprising that in a complex disease like cancer, a complex therapeutic regimen will be required.

Table 2. Immunotherapy of a murine ovarian tumor with MPL™ and PA-PE[a]

Material Injected[b]	Dose (μg)	Percent Survival at 40 days
None	-	0
MPL™	150	0
PA-PE	700	0
PA-PE + MPL™	700 + 150	60

[a]Data adapted from (2).
[b]All mice injected with murine ovarian tumor cells i.p., and subsequently injected i.p. with the materials indicated. Definitions - MPL™ = monophosphoryl lipid A; PA-PE = Propionibacterium acnes - pyridine extract.

Table 3. Nonspecific and specific immunotherapy in the murine ovarian tumor system[a]

Material injected[b]	Dosage	No. tumor free[c] / Total no. injected	Percent tumor-free
PA-PE + MPL™	1200 + 240	43/49	88
PA-PE + MPL™	350 + 75	0/5	0
TAA	500	0/8	0
TAA + PA-PE + MPL™	500 + 300 + 60	8/8	100

[a]Adapted from (3).
[b]Female C3HeB/FeJ mice inoculated i.p. with 1-2 x 10^4 MOT cells on day 0. Immunostimulants given 24 hr later. Definitions - PA-PE = **Propionibacterium acnes** - pyridine extract; MPL™ = monophosphoyl lipid A; TAA = tumor-associated antigen.
[c]Numbers of tumor-free mice determined 60 days after tumor transplantation.

Pretreatment of experimental animals with bacterial endotoxin is known to induce, nonspecifically, heightened resistance to challenge with a variety of infectious agents (9). Non-toxic MPL™ can have a similar effect (29). The data in Table 5 show that mice pretreated with MPL™ display an increased survival after challenge with 5 LD_{50}'s of a facultative intracellular bacterial parasite. Another microbial immunostimulant, trehalose dimycolate (TDM) also can enhance the resistance of these mice. Furthermore, the effect of a combination of MPL™ plus TDM is shown to be at least additive, if not synergistic (29).

Gram-negative bacterial sepsis is a major cause of morbidity and mortality in hospitalized patients, especially those undergoing certain types of high risk surgery (33). Reduction of incidence and severity of infections might be achieved if patients at high risk could have their immune systems stimulated prior to exposure to the high risk situation. As shown in Table 6, MPL™ can induce resistance to Gram-negative bacterial sepsis. When administered in an aqueous solution, the immunostimulatory window of MPL™ lasts for only several days, which encompass the high risk period. This allows the immunopyrophylaxis to be temporally focused and reduces the potential for side effects which might be induced by a continual high level of immunostimulation. The data do show that injection of MPL™ one or two days before a massive experimental infection with **E. coli** does offer almost complete protection.

One of the main, if not the major cause of death in Gram-negative sepsis is endotoxin shock (14). This can be induced experimentally by injection of purified endotoxin from Gram-negative bacteria. It has been known for decades that a sublethal dose of endotoxin, introduced a day or two before, can induce a state of physiological tolerance to the effects of a biologically toxic challenge dose of an unrelated endotoxin (6). The data in Table 7 show that pretreatment of mice with MPL™ can likewise increase the resistance of mice to a lethal challenge with LPS, as manifested by about a two-fold average increase in the LD_{50}. Thus, resistance to both Gram-negative bacterial sepsis and pathogenic endotoxemia can be increased nonspecifically by pretreatment with the nontoxic MPL™ derivative of endotoxin.

Table 4. Effect of combined chemotherapy and immunotherapy in a mouse ovarian tumor model[a]

Material injected[b]	Dose (μg)	Days after tumor	No. tumor free / No. injected	Percent tumor free
TAA + PA-PE + MPL™	500+300+60	4	0/6	0
Mitomycin C	100	6	0/6	0
Mitomycin C +	100	6		
TAA + PA-PE + MPL™	1000+300+60	7.5	3/6	50

[a]Adapted from (3).
[b]Female C3HeB/FeJ mice inoculated i.p. with 1-2 x 10^4 MOT tumor cells on day 0. Chemotherapy was given on day 6 followed by immunotherapy 1.5 days later. Definitions - TAA = tumor-associated antigen; PA-PE = Propionibacterium acnes - pyridine extract; MPL™ - monophosphoryl lipid A.

Table 5. Induction of nonspecific resistance to Listeria monocytogenes by MPL™ and TDM[a]

Material[b]	Dose (μg)	Alive/Total	Percent survival
Placebo	-	1/10	10
MPL™	100	4/10	40
TDM	100	6/10	60
MPL™ + TDM	100 + 100	10/10	100

[a]Data adapted from (29).
[b]Placebo = 2% squalane; MPL™ = monophosphoryl lipid A; TDM = trehalose dimycolate; these were given in 2% squalane 8 days before challenge with listeria.

Table 6. Prophylaxis by MPL™ of Gram-negative bacterial sepsis[a]

Treatment[b]	Dose (µg)	Alive/Total	Percent survival
MPL™: Day -3	100	5/10	42
MPL™: Day -2	100	9/10	90
MPL™: Day -1	100	10/10	100
MPL™: -8 hr	100	6/10	60
Saline control	-	0/10	0

[a]All groups challenged with 5 x 10^8 CFU (i.p.) of **Escherichia coli** 487 at Day 0. From Ulrich, J. T., unpublished data.
[b]MPL™ (monophosphoryl lipid A) administered as a saline solution,i.p.

In addition to stimulating, nonspecifically, resistance to infections and their toxicological manifestations, MPL™ and the other immunostimulators, when used in conjunction with antigens specific for infectious agents, can provide adjuvant activity to increase these immune responses (7, 22). Three examples of this are shown in Table 8. The first is with an experimental model antigen, ovalbumin (OA). An aqueous solution of MPL™ and a "light" metabolizable oil emulsion, containing a combination of MPL™ and TDM, both significantly enhanced the humoral antibody response of mice to OA. The immune responses to a subunit antigen from **Brucella abortus** and a synthetic polypeptide antigen specific for human hepatitis B virus were likewise enhanced by MPL™-containing adjuvants. These latter two antigens have the potential to protect "production animals" and man against severe infectious diseases.

Table 7. Induction of tolerance to the lethal effects of endotoxin induced by endotoxin or MPL™[a]

Material,[b] pretreatment	Dose (µg)	Injection day[c]	LD50 of endotoxin (µg) challenge
MPL™	100	-3	916
Endotoxin	25	-3	1013
Saline	-	-3	421

[a]From - Ulrich, J.T., unpublished data.
[b]MPL™ = monophosphoryl lipid A.
[c]Challenge with graded doses of endotoxin on day 0.

Vaccines containing purified polysaccharide antigens have suffered from at least two practical drawbacks; they elicit primarily short-lived IgM class antibody responses and they do not stimulate immunological memory. However, recent studies with an MPL™-containing adjuvant have provided hope that a potential exists for overcoming these deficiencies. Table 9 shows the results with two different purified polysaccharide antigen systems. In the first, SSS-III (the protective capsular polysaccharide from the pneumococcus) is shown to stimulate low levels of IgM antibody after one or two injections of optimally immunogenic doses. When this same amount of SSS-III is injected with MPL™ contained in a metabolizable oil vehicle, both the primary and secondary antibody titers are enhanced. Moreover, a significant boost is obtained in the long-lived IgG class of antibody, following the second injection. This is qualitative and quantitative evidence for elicitation and triggering of a memory response to the SSS-III epitope.

Further evidence for enhancement by the MPL™ adjuvant of immunological memory to a polysaccharide antigen is contained in the bottom half of Table 9. Two doses of a polysaccharide-rich LPS from **Escherichia coli** create a secondary antibody response. However, two doses of an antigenically identical native protoplasmic polysaccharide (NPP) do not elicit a secondary antibody response. NPP does not have the lipid A adjuvant component of the LPS (30). It was theorized that this adjuvant component provided a "second signal" which was necessary to trigger a secondary antibody response in a primed animal (30). This is demonstrated by the capacity of LPS to trigger a secondary response in NPP-primed animals (Table 9). The last line in this table demonstrates that MPL™ can provide the second signal, allowing NPP to trigger a secondary antibody response in primed animals. This technology should allow for the creation of more effective polysaccharide vaccines, especially for use in infants and in the geriatric population.

Ultimately, all of the research on immunotherapy with bacterial endotoxins is directed toward enrichment of mankind, through improvement of his own health or that of his companion and production animals. Adjuvants containing the products described herein have been employed successfully in vaccines for several "animal health"-related vaccines. Moreover, in human clinical trials a standardized mixture of allogeneic melanoma cell lysates, potentiated with an MPL™-containing adjuvant (melanoma vaccine) is proving effective (13). In Table 10 are shown the results of one such phase I study. Five of 17 evaluable patients treated with this vaccine had remissions of melanoma (two complete and three partial); three more had minor responses (25-50% regression of disease or greater than 50% regression for less than 4 weeks). The responses were correlated with increases in cytolytic T lymphocytes specifically recognizing melanoma antigens. The only toxicity of this MPL™-containing vaccine was a slight soreness at the sites one day after the injections; there were no systemic toxic or immunological (e.g., anaphylactic) side effects (13). That this vaccine proved immunologically and clinically effective, while other tumor vaccines have not been successful, was attributed by the author to use of the adjuvant (13).

Incorporation of endotoxin into immunotherapeutics has evolved greatly over the past four decades, and this progress has been extremely rapid during the last five or ten years. What has made the difference is the development of molecular engineering techniques by which the toxic properties of the endotoxin molecules can be reduced greatly, with retention of the beneficial immunopotentiating properties (22). These advances were the result of elucidating the precise minimal chemical structure which is responsible for the biological properties of endotoxin, and subsequently modifying this is a very specific fashion.

There are multiple rationales for clinical use of MPL™ as the immunostimulatory portion of endotoxin. The most obvious is that MPL™ has

Table 8. Adjuvant activity of MPL™ or MPL™ + TDM on humoral antibody responses of mice[a]

Antigen[b]	Dose (ug)	Adjuvant[b]	Dose (ug)	EIA titer on day 6-7	14	21-27	Secondary
OA	50	-	-	200	400	400	12,800
OA	50	MPL™	50	1600	3200	6,400	256,000
OA	50	MPL™+TDM	50+50	3200	-	204,800	-
BA	25	-	-	1280	5120	6,400	-
BA	25	MPL™	100	25,460	40,960	25,600	-
BA	25	MPL™+TDM	100+50	10,240	81,900	204,800	-
HBV	40	-	-	-	400	80	-
HBV	40	MPL™	50	-	800	6,400	-
HBV	40	MPL™+TDM	50+50	-	12,800	204,800	-

[a]Adapted from (26).
[b]Abbreviations - OA = ovalbumin; BA = subunit antigen from **Brucella abortus**; HBV = hepatitis B virus synthetic polypeptide; MPL™ = monophosphoryl lipid A; TDM = trehalose dimycolate. The antigens alone or antigens + MPL™ were injected as saline solutions; the antigens + MPL™ + TDM were prepared as 2% squalene emulsions.

greatly diminished toxicity when compared with the native endotoxin molecule (22). Also, MPL™ can be prepared either as an oil-soluble material or as a polar salt. This allows its incorporation into targeting delivery vehicles, such as liposomes or oil droplets, or formulation into aqueous based immunotherapeutics. Furthermore, selection of oil- or aqueous-compatible forms facilitates its combined use with other immunostimulators that have restricted solubilities.

The availability of the precisely defined chemical entity, responsible for immunostimulatory properties of endotoxin, has allowed dissection of the mechanisms of action of this class of materials. One study on such mechanisms has shown that MPL™ inactivates suppressor T cell activity without affecting amplifier or helper T cell functions (1). This selective effect on a cellular subpopulation is a unique phenomenon and has great promise as a rationale for allowing use of MPL™ to advantage in certain clinical situations. When this observation is combined with the safety and efficacy observed in the pragmatic application of an MPL™-containing adjuvant used with a therapeutic cancer vaccine (13), it appears that the dreams and goals of many scientists in the field of endotoxin research may be close to realization.

Table 9. Effect of MPL™ as an adjuvant on antibody responses to polysaccharide antigens[a]

Primary[b]	Secondary	Antibody titer[c] Primary	Secondary
SSS-III (0.75 μg)	SSS-III (0.75 μg)	240 (78)	182(40)
SSS-III (0.75 μg) + MPL™ (100 μg)	SSS-III (0.75 μg) +MPL™ (100 μg)	1472 (232)	1536(736)
LPS (1 μg)	LPS (1 μg)	17	2560
-	LPS (1 μg)	10	61
NPP (1 μg)	NPP (1 μg)	15	21
NPP (1 μg)	LPS (1 μg)	10	1690
NPP (1 μg)	NPP (1 μg) +MPL™ (100 μg)	10	2320

[a]Adapted from (26).
[b]Abbreviations: SSS-III = pneumococcal polysaccharide type III; LPS = lipopolysaccharide from **Escherichia coli** 0113; NPP = native protoplasmic polysaccharide from **E. coli** 0113, MPL™ = monophosphoryl lipid A in a lipid emulsion system (lecithin, peanut oil, and glycerine).
[c]The first number is the total antibody titer and the number in parentheses is the IgG antibody titer.

Table 10. Results of human clinical trials with a melanoma vaccine adjuvantized with MPL™ + CWS[a]

Evaluable patients	Immunological response[b]	Clinical responses Complete	Partial	Minor	None
17	10	2	3	3	9

[a]Adapted from (13): The MPL™ + CWS was prepared in a 2% squalane emulsion (DETOX™).
[b]The immunological response was the elevation in a patient of numbers of cytotoxic T lymphocyte specific for the melanoma antigens.

ACKNOWLEDGEMENT

We thank Ingrid Poole for excellent work and assistance in preparation of this manuscript.

REFERENCES

1. Baker, P. J., Hiernaux, J. R., Fauntleroy, M. B., Prescott, B., Cantrell, J. L., and Rudbach, J. A., 1988, Inactivation of suppressor T cell activity by nontoxic monophosphoryl lipid A (MPL). Infect. Immun. 56:1076.

2. Berek, J. S., Lichtenstein, A. K., Knox, R. M., Jung, T. S., Rose, T. P., Cantrell, J. L., and Zighelboim, J., 1985, Synergistic effects of combination sequential immunotherapies in a murine ovarian cancer model. Cancer Res. 45: 4215.

3. Cantrell, J. L., and Finn, D. J., 1988, Role of novel adjuvants in specific active immunotherapy, in: "Immunity to Cancer II," M. S. Mitchell, ed. Alan R. Liss, New York.

4. Chase, J. J., Kubey, W., Dulek, M. H., Holmes, C. J., Salit, M. G., Pearson, III, F. C., and Ribi, E., 1986, Effect of monophosphoryl lipid A on host resistance to bacterial infection. Infect. Immun. 53: 711.

5. Freund, J., 1956, The mode of action of immunologic adjuvants, in: "Advances in Tuberculosis Research," vol 7, H. Birkhauser and H. Bloch, eds. S. Krager, New York.

6. Greisman, S. E., Wagner, Jr., H. N., Iio, M., Hornick, R. B., Carozza, Jr., F. M., and Woodward, T. E., 1964, Mechanisms of endotoxin tolerance in man, in: "Bacterial Endotoxins," M. Landy and W. Braun, eds. Rutgers University Press, New Brunswick, N.J.

7. Johnson, A. G., Gaines, S., and Landy, M., 1956, Studies on the O-antigen of **Salmonella typhosa**. V. Enhancement of antibody response to protein antigens by the purified lipopolysaccharide. J. Exptl. Med. 103: 225.

8. Kasai, N., and Nowotny, A., 1967, Endotoxic glycolipid from a heptoseless mutant of **Salmonella minnesota**. J. Bacteriol. 94: 1824.

9. Landy, M. and Pillemer, L., 1956, Increased resistance to infection and accompanying alterations in properdin levels following administration of bacterial lipopolysaccharides. J. Exptl. Med. 104: 383.

10. Leong, D. L. Y. and Rudbach, J. A., 1971, Antigenic competition between an endotoxic adjuvant and a protein antigen. Infect. Immun. 3: 308.

11. McLaughlin, C. A., Cantrell, J. L., Ribi, E., and Goldberg, E., 1978, Intratumor chemoimmunotherapy with mitomycin C and components from mycobacteria in regression of line 10 tumors in guinea pigs. Cancer Res. 38: 1311.

12. Milner, K. C., Rudbach, J. A., and Ribi, E., 1971, General Characteristics, in: "Microbial Toxins," vol 4, G. Weinbaum, S. Kadis, and S. J. Ajl, eds. Academic Press, New York.

13. Mitchell, M. S., 1988, Active specific immunotherapy in the treatment of human cancer, in: "Immunity to Cancer II," M. S. Mitchell, ed. Alan R. Liss, New York.

14. Moore, F. D., 1960, Relevance of experimental shock studies to clinical shock problems, in: "Recent Progress and Present Problems in the Field of Shock," S. F. Seeley, and J. R. Weisiger, eds. Fed. Amer. Soc. for Exper. Biol., Wash. D.C.

15. Morrison, D. C. and Ryan, J. L., 1979, Bacterial endotoxins and host immune responses, in: "Advances in Immunology," vol. 28, F. J. Dixon and H. G. Kunkel, eds. Academic Press, NY.

16. Munoz, J., 1964, Effect of bacteria and bacterial products on antibody response, in: "Advances in Immunology," vol 4, F. J. Dixon, Jr., and J. H. Humphrey, eds. Academic Press, New York.

17. Nauts, A. C., Swift, W. E., and Coley, B. L., 1946, Treatment of malignant tumors by bacterial toxins as developed by the late William B. Coley, M. D., reviewed in light of modern research. Cancer Res. 6: 205.

18. Parish, H. J., 1965, "A History of Immunization," E. S. Livingstone, Ltd., London.

19. Qureshi, N., Mascagni, P., Ribi, E., and Takayama, K., 1985, Monophosphoryl lipid A obtained from lipopolysaccharides of **Salmonella minnesota** R 595. Purification of the dimethyl derivative by high performance liquid chromatography and complete structural determination. J. Biol. Chem. 260: 5271.

20. Qureshi, N., Takayama, K., and Ribi, E., 1982, Purification and structural determination of nontoxic lipid A obtained from lipopolysaccharide of **Salmonella typhimurium**. J. Biol. Chem. 257: 11808.

21. Ribi, E., Amano, K., Cantrell, J., Schwartzman, S., Parker, R., and Takayama, K., 1982, Preparation and antitumor activity of nontoxic lipid A. Cancer Immunol. Immunother. 12: 91.

22. Ribi, E., Cantrell, J., Feldner, T., Myers, K., and Peterson, J., 1986, Biological activities of monophosphoryl lipid A, in: "Microbiology 1986," L. Levie, P. F. Bonventre, J. A. Morello, S. D. Silver, and H. C. Wu, eds. Amer. Soc. for Microbiol., Wash. D.C.

23. Ribi, E. E., Cantrell, J., Schwartzman, S., and Parker, R., 1981, BCG cell wall skeleton, P3, MDP and other microbial components - structure activity studies in animal models, in: "Augmenting Agents in Cancer Therapy," E. M. Hersh, M. A. Chirigos, and M. J. Mastrangelo, eds. Raven Press, New York.

24. Rowley, D., 1964, Endotoxin-induced changes in susceptibility to infections, in: "Bacterial Endotoxins", M. Landy and W. Braun, eds. Rutgers University Press, New Brunswick, N.J.

25. Rudbach, J. A., 1971, Molecular immunogenicity of bacterial lipopolysaccharide antigens: establishing a quantitative system. J. Immunol. 4: 993.

26. Rudbach, J. A., Cantrell, J. L., and Ulrich, J. T., 1989, Molecularly engineered microbial immunostimulators, in: "Technological Advances in Vaccine Development," Alan R. Liss, Inc., New York.

27. Simmons, R. L., and Rios, A., 1972, Immunospecific regression of methylcholanthrene fibrosarcoma with the use of neuraminidase II. Intratumor injections of neuraminidase. Surgery 71: 556.

28. Takayama, K., Qureshi, N., Ribi, E., and Cantrell, J. L., 1984, Separation and characterization of toxic and nontoxic forms of lipid A. Rev. Infect. Dis. 6: 439.

29. Ulrich, J. T., Masihi, K. N., and Lange, W., 1988, Mechanisms of nonspecific resistance to microbial infections induced by trehalose dimycolate (TDM) and monophosphoryl lipid A (MPL), in: "Advances in the Biosciences" vol 68, K. N. Masihi and W. Lange, eds. Pergamon Press, New York.

30. Von Eschen, K. B., and Rudbach, J. A., 1974, Immunological responses of mice to native protoplasmic polysaccharide and lipopolysaccharide. J. Exptl. Med. 140: 1604.

31. Westphal, O., and Luderitz, O., 1954, Chemische Erforschung von Lipopolysacchariden gramnegativer Bakterien. Angew. Chem. 66: 407.

32. Wilson, G. S., and Miles, A. A., 1955, "Topley and Wilson's Principles of Bacteriology and Immunity," The Williams & Wilkins Co.

33. Young, L. S., 1985, Gram-negative sepsis, in: "Principles and Practice of Infectious Diseases," G. L. Mandell, R. G. Douglas, Jr., and J. E. Bennett, eds. John Wiley & Sons, New York.

34. Zbar, B., Bernstein, I. D., Bartlett, G. L., Hanna, Jr., M. G., and Rapp, H. J., 1972, Immunotherapy of Cancer: Regression of intradermal tumors and prevention of growth of lymph node metastases after injection of living **Mycobacterium bovis**. J. Natl. Cancer Inst. 49: 119.

35. Zbar, B., Ribi, E., and Rapp, H. J., 1973, An experimental model for immunotherapy of cancer. Natl. Cancer Inst. Monograph 39: 3.

STIMULATION OF NONSPECIFIC RESISTANCE BY RADIO-DETOXIFIED ENDOTOXIN

L. Bertok

"Frederic Joliot-Curie" National Research
Institüte for Radiobiology and Radiohygiene
Budapest, P.O. Box 101, 1775, Hungary

Different immunodeficiency states and infections in immunosuppressed patients are serious problems of medicine. Specific humoral and cellular immune responses are widely investigated, but mechanisms of nonspecific resistance (NSR) gained attention just recently (8). Serious decrease of NSR might be the cause of opportunistic infections in patients receiving radiation therapy, cytotoxic or immunosuppressive drugs, or suffering from certain viral diseases, e.g., AIDS (1-5). Recently some immunomodulators are tested as potential stimulators of NSR. Among them the bacterial endotoxin (LPS) is one of the most active materials. Unfortunately, the parenteral administration of LPS is associated with untolerable side effects, so this compound (in its original form) is not suitable for enhancing of NSR in endotoxin-sensitive mammals or in humans. Various attempts have been made to modify LPS to reduce its toxicity without altering its beneficial immunological activities (15, 17, 18). Perhaps, one of the best detoxification techniques is the use of ionizing radiation (1, 3, 5, 13, 16). As it was demonstrated by many in vitro and in vivo studies irradiation of LPS with ^{60}Co-gamma (150 kGy) decreased its harmful side effects in a dose dependent manner (1-6, 10, 13, 19), but this radiodetoxified LPS preparation (RD-LPS or so-called TOLERIN) preserved the beneficial effects of LPS (1-3, 5, 13). These findings are confirmed by other authors, too (9, 14). Irradiation modifies markedly the chemical structure of LPS, decreases the amount of certain constituents: e.g., glucosamine, KDO, fatty acids, etc. (9, 11, 12).

A single parenteral injection of RD-LPS can prevent the experimental endotoxin shock in all investigated mammals (5). Eighty-four per cent of dogs survived the hemorrhagic shock, and 90% of rats survived the fecal septic peritonitis when they were pretreated with RD-LPS. Such pretreatment may be useful in the preparation of gastrointestinal surgery (cit. 3, 5). The RD-LPS protected 74% of rats with experimental intestinal ischemia induced by superior mesenteric artery occlusion, too (cit. 3, 5) and sixty percent of pretreated rats survived tourniquet shock: experimental limb ischemia (cit. 3, 5). The RD-LPS pretreatment prevented the abortifacient effect of LPS: 90% of the fetuses survived (cit. 1-3, 5). Moreover, the RD-LPS has a membrane-stabilizing effect and hereby can prevent the membrane-damaging effect of LPS and some cytostatics (7, cit. 3, 5). The cardiovascular action of endotoxin is well known in various forms of shock. However, the RD-LPS has barely any hypotensive effect. The RD-LPS pretreatment can prevent practically all hemodynamic changes induced by LPS (cit. 2, 3, 5). LPS plays an important role in the pathogenesis of the so-called intestinal syndrome of radiation disease, too (cit. 3, 5). However, the RD-LPS pretreatment saved 70% of the irradiated rats (1). Moreover the RD-LPS pretreatment can prevent the effect of LPS induced oxydative stress in glutathion redox system and can moderate the level of hypoxic metabolites (lactic and uric acids) and severity of acidosis (Boda et al., unpublished data, 1988). LPS is well known to exert a marked adjuvant activity on the immune response of mammals. The RD-LPS preparation retained this adjuvant activity (5, 10).

Perhaps one of the most important effects of RD-LPS is the influence on regeneration of lymphoreticular-immune system. It is well known that ionizing radiation decreases all immune functions. We have found that the immune response against the sheep red blood cells of sublethally irradiated (7.0 Gy, ^{60}Co-gamma) rats was regenerated by treatment with a single dose of RD-LPS on day 21. The immune response was detected by PFC of spleen and hemolysin titre of sera on day 26. The regeneration of immune system was speedy and significant (10, cit. 4, 5). The relative radioresistant T-helper cell population has an important role in this regenerating effect of RD-LPS (cit. 5). The RD-LPS can evoke the regeneration of immune system in irradiated animals. Decrease of NSR in immune deficient or immunosuppressed patients is the most important cause of the opportunistic infections, sepsis, endotoxemia, pneumonia, etc. It is well known that the majority of the patients after organ transplantation die from common septicemia. Antilymphocyte serum (ALS) is a potent immunosuppressant and it was commonly used in organ transplantation. For this reason, the possibility of augmenting of NSR or induction of endotoxin tolerance after ALS treatment has great importance. If RD-LPS was given to ALS-treated rats they became tolerant against lethal dose of LPS. It is evident that in spite of suppression of T-lymphocytes by ALS, induction of endotoxin tolerance (enhancement of NSR) was normal (6). Moreover, the RD-LPS pretreatment can prevent lethal bacterial (Klebsiella pneumoniae, Proteus vulgaris) infections by elevation of NSR. Facultative pathogen (opportunistic) bacteria may flourish and cause disease when specific and nonspecific resistances are impaired. The lethality of experimental Aujeszky-disease (pseudorabies virus, herpes group) was also reduced by RD-LPS pretreatment from 100% to 30% (1-3, 5). Moreover, the RD-LPS can produce significant proliferation of lymphoreticular-immune system in germ-free (practically immune deficient) animals, too (cit. 5). The proliferation of lymphoreticular-immune system by RD-LPS could also be demonstrated in newborn mice. These animals became sensitive against LCM virus, though, the untreated mice survived the infection because their lymphoreticular system (T-lymphocyte function) was insufficient at this age (cit. 4, 5). The RD-LPS preparation preserve many other beneficial effects such as RES and macrophage activation, antitumor activity, etc. (1-3, 5, 14).

The RD-LPS (TOLERIN) has been tested for innocuity in two trials on volunteers in Hungary under the supervision of the Ministry of Health. The first trial was performed in 5 healthy (31-53 years old) volunteers. Seven μg/kg TOLERIN given subcutaneously caused only a temporary weak febrile and local reaction (weak edema and hyperemia). Clinical and laboratory tests showed practically no changes in the parameters investigated except for the increase of white blood cells and complement C3 fraction at 24 hrs (Bertok et al., unpublished data, 1987).

In the second trial performed on 40 healthy (18-26 years old) volunteers (university students) we had similar results. The subcutaneously given 4 μg/kg TOLERIN caused only a temporary rise of temperature (1 person) and local reaction (weak hyperemia) in 20 per cent (8 persons) of volunteers. The values of clinical and laboratory tests were unchanged except for the number of white blood cells and complement C_3 fraction which were elevated within 24 hrs (Bertok et al., unpublished data, 1987).

On the basis of these results TOLERIN is being tested now in clinical trials in Hungary. If these trials were also successful TOLERIN could be applied for the enhancement of NSR, prevention of endotoxemic shock, regeneration of immune system, complex therapy of cancer and many other aims, too.

REFERENCES

1. Bertók, L., 1980, Radio-detoxified endotoxin as a potent stimulator of nonspecific resistance. Persp. Biol. and Med. 24: 61.

2. Bertók, L., 1983, Stimulation of nonspecific resistance by radiation-detoxified endotoxin, in: "Beneficial effects of endotoxins," A. Nowotny, ed., Plenum Publishing Corporation, New York.

3. Bertók, L., 1983, Bacterial endotoxins and nonspecific resistance, in: "Traumatic Injury: Infection and other immunologic seuquelae," J. L. Ninnemann, ed., University Park Press, Baltimore.

4. Bertók, L., 1986, Possible prevention of immune deficiency by radio-detoxified endotoxin, in: "Abstracts, 6th International Congress of Immunology," K. Charbonneau, ed., Toronto.

5. Bértok, L., 1988, Radio-detoxified endotoxin, a potent stimulator of nonspecific host defense, in: "Immunomodulators and nonspecific host defense mechanisms against microbial infections," K. N. Masihi and W. Lange, eds., Pergamon Press, Oxford-New York.

6. Bertók, L., Elekes, E. and Meretéy, K., 1979, Endotoxin tolerance in rats treated with antilymphocyte serum. Acta Microbiol. Acad. Sci. Hung. 26: 135.

7. Bertók, L., Juhász-Nagy, S. and Sötönyi, P., 1984, Prevention of cardiac damages induced by formyl-leurosine, a potent cytostatic agent, by radio-detoxified endotoxin (TOLERIN) in dogs. Immunopharmacology 8: 13.

8. Chedid, L., 1988, Stimulation of non-specific host defense mechanisms against infections, in: "Immunomodulators and nonspecific host defense mechanisms against microbial infections," K. N. Masihi and W. Lange, eds., Pergamon Press, Oxford-New York.

9. Csakó, Gy., Suba, E. A., Ahlgren, A., Tsai, C. N. and Elin, R. J., 1986, Relation of structure to function for the U. S. reference standard endotoxin after exposure to ^{60}Co radiation. J. Infect. Dis. 153: 98.

10. Elekes, E., Bertók, L. and Meretéy, K., 1978, Adjuvant activity of endotoxin preparations in normal and irradiated rats. Acta Microbiol. Acad. Sci. Hung. 25: 17.

11. Elekes, E., Lüderitz, O., Galanos, C. and Bertók, L., 1986, Chemical analysis of irradiated LPS and lipid A. J. Immunol. Immunopharmacol. 6: 156.

12. ElSabbagh, M., Galanos, C., Bertók, L., Füst, G. and Lüderitz, O., 1982, Effect of ionizing radiation on chemical and biological properties of Salmonella minnesota R595 lipopolysaccharide. Acta Microbiol. Acad. Sci. Hung. 29: 255.

13. Füst, Gy., Bertók, L. and Juhász Nagy, S., 1977, Interactions of the radio-detoxified Escherichia coli endotoxin preparations with the complement system. Infect. Immun. 16: 26.

14. Nerkar, D. P. and Bandekar, J. R., 1986, Stimulation of macrophages and antitumor activity of radiodetoxified endotoxin. Microbiol. Immunol. 30: 893.

15. Nowotny, A., 1964, Chemical detoxification of bacterial endotoxins, in: "Bacterial endotoxins," M. Lady and W. Braun, eds., Rutgers University Press, New Brunswick, N. J.

16. Previte, J. J., Chang, Y. and El-Bisi, H. M., 1967, Detoxification of Salmonella typhimurium lipopolysaccharide by ionizing radiation. J. Bacteriol. 93: 1607.

17. Ribi, E., Cantrell, J. and Takayama, K., 1985, A new immunomodulator with potential clinical applications: Monophosphoryl lipid A, a detoxified endotoxin. Clinical Immunology Newsletter 6: 33.

18. Sultzer, B. M., 1971, Chemical modification of endotoxin and inactivation of its biological properties, in: "Microbial toxins Vol. V," S. Kadis, G. Weinbaum and S. J. Ajl, eds., Academic Press, New York.

19. Walter, R. I., Ledney, G. D. and Bertók, L., 1983, Reduced toxicity of irradiated endotoxin in mice compromised by irradiation, tumor or infection. J. Trauma 23: 225.

MONOCLONAL ANTIBODY TO LIPID A PREVENTS THE DEVELOPMENT OF HAEMODYNAMIC DISORDERS IN ENDOTOXEMIA

A. A. Shnyra, G. F. Kalantarov, T. N. Vlasik, I. N. Trakht, A. Ju. Mayatnikov, A. L. Tabachnik, D.V. Borovikov and V. L. Golubykh

Department of Cellular Biology, Institute of Experimental Cardiology, National Cardiology Research Centre, Academy of Medical Sciences, Moscow, 3-rd Cherepkovskaya str., 15-A USSR

It has been recognized that gram-negative bacteriaemia is the major cause of hospital sepsis. The pathology of gram-negative sepsis is attributed to endotoxin. Endotoxins of all gram-negative bacteria have the same lipid moiety, so called lipid A, which is thought to be responsible for its pathogenic effects (6). Gram-negative endotoxaemia leads to an irreversible cardiovascular collapse (shock), acute pulmonary insufficiency, and disseminated vascular coagulation syndrome that can result in lethality up to 60-80%, despite antibiotic therapy (2). This prompted the search for immunotherapeutic approaches to the protection against gram-negative sepsis (1).

In the present study, we produced a monoclonal antibody to lipid A (IgM) and tested its ability to prevent endotoxic shock in experimental endotoxaemia.

BALB/c mice were immunized with Re LPS isolated form Salmonella minnesota R595 according to (3). The endotoxin was injected intraperitoneally at a dose of 25μg per mouse every other day for 16 days. On the 25th day the mice were boosted with 50μg Re LPS per each animal. Hybridization (5) with certain modifications (4) was performed 3 days after the boost.

Antibody-producing cells were selected by ELISA with the Re LPS antigen. The specificity of the antibody thus obtained was examined in immunoenzyme assay; various mutant strains of Salmonella minnesota, Re LPS, and lipid A were used as antigens. We demonstrated that this antibody bound to lipid A, Re LPS, and Re cells with a high affinity. The affinity decreased as the number of oligosaccharides in the core glycolipid increased. The activity of the monoclonal antibody was estimated by its ability to change the forms of the colonies produced by a specially constructed strain with a Re-chemotype (data not shown).

Degradation and clearance of the antibody from dog bloodstream were

---

Abbreviations used: heart rate (HR), mean arterial pressure (MAP), mean pulmonary pressure (MPP), left ventricular pressure (LVP), contructivity (LVdp/dT/P), cardiac output (CO), total periferal vascular resistance (TPR), pulmonary vascular resistance (PVR).

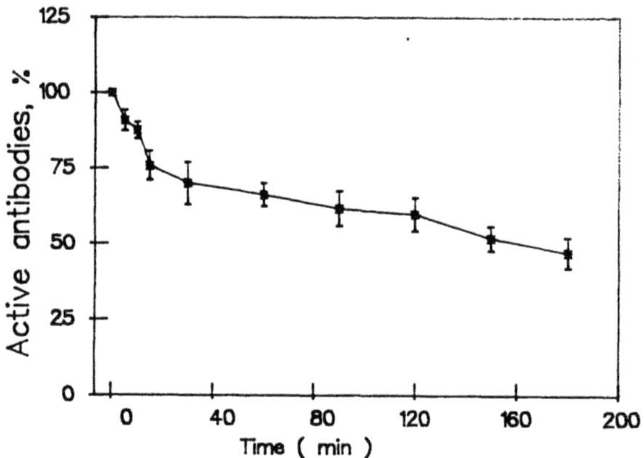

Fig 1. Degradation and clearance of mouse anti-lipid A monoclonal antibody from dog bloodstream (see text for details). The data presented are M±m of five separate experiments. The amount of active antibodies in 1 ml of dog plasma 3 min after the injection of ^{125}I-IgM was taken as 100%.

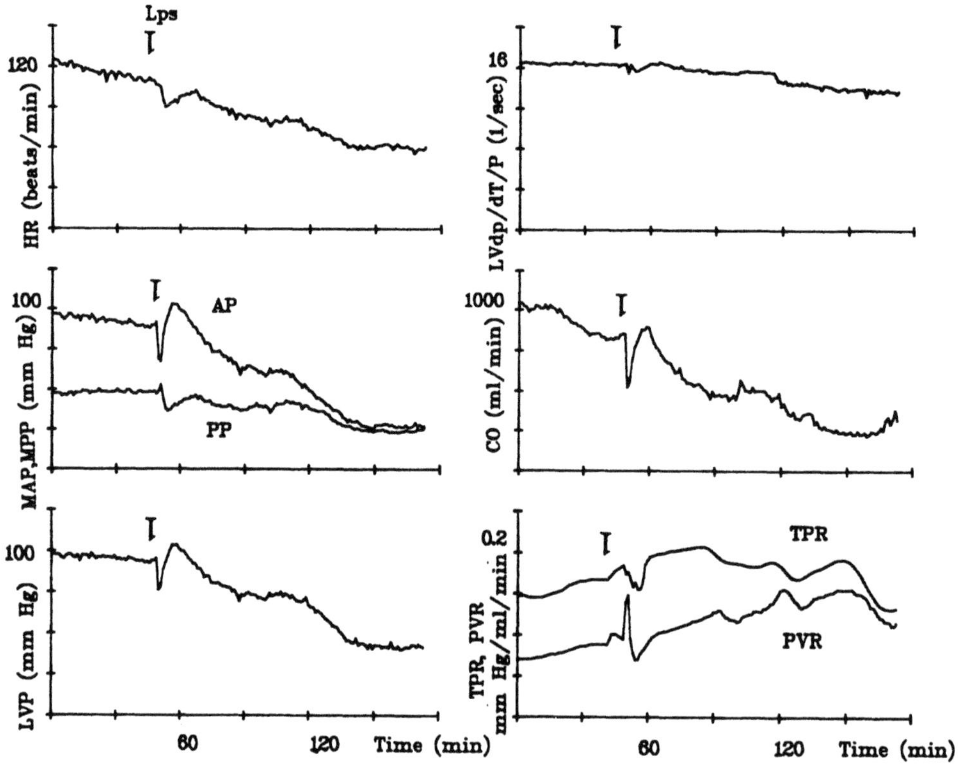

Fig 2. The changes in haemodynamic parameters during experimental endotoxemia. Representative curves for 1 of 4 separate experiments are shown. The arrows indicate the Re LPS injection.

studied with ^{125}I-IgM (2 x 10^7 cpm/kg body weight). At given time periods the amount of active antibodies in dog plasma was determined as the difference between the radioactivity of native plasma and the plasma being applied to a LPS-Sepharose minicolumn (Fig 1). The kinetics of MoAb degradation and clearance in dog bloodstream was of a biphasic character with t1.1/2 = 35 ± 7 min for the first 20 min and t2.1/2= 350 ± 30 min for the further period.

The protective action of the mouse monoclonal anti-lipid A antibody (MoAb) against endotoxic shock was tested in mongrel dogs weighing 10-15 kg. Anaesthetized animals were monitored for blood pressure in the left ventricle, aorta, pulmonary artery, as well as for aortic and pulmonary blood flow. The haemodynamic parameters were recorded in a 7758D System (Hewlett-Packard) and sampled with a Labtam 3015 microcomputer. Endotoxemia was induced by an intravenous administration of Re LPS at a dose of 0.5 mg/kg body weight. Chromatography purified MoAb were injected intravenously at a dose of 1.5-2.0 mg/kg body weight.

25-30 min after the Re LPS injection, the arterial pressure in the dogs dropped, and during 1 h it decreased by 62 ± 8% (Fig 2), which coincided with the decrease in cardiac output and the increase in pulmonary and peripheral resistances. These alterations were irreversible during the first 3 hours.

Based on degradation and clearance experiment, MoAb was administered 30-40 min before the Re LPS injection. This resulted only in minor and transient changes in haemodynamic parameters (Fig 3). In control experi-

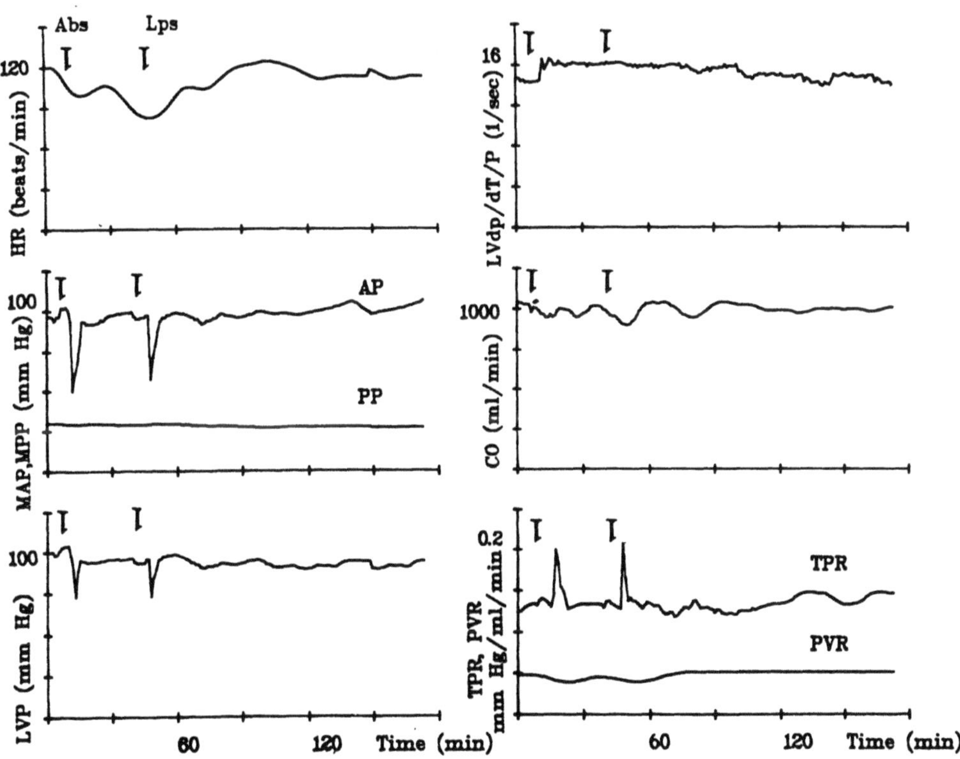

Fig 3. The blocking of the changes in haemodynamic parameters by a passive immunotherapy of experimental endotoxemia. Representative curves for 1 of 4 separate experiments are shown. The arrows indicate the injections of anti-lipid A monoclonal antibody and Re LPS.

ments, anti-fibrin monoclonal IgM had no protective effect against endotoxaemia (data not shown).

Our findings suggest that the interaction of MoAb with the lipid moiety of the endotoxin molecule could block the reactions which are involved in the development of endotoxic shock. According to the literature data, the alterations of haemodynamic parameter may be due to complement activation in endotoxaemia (6). On the other hand, the drop in arterial pressure may be produced by various mediators (for example, tumor necrosis factor) released by macrophages in response to endotoxin (7). The blocking of activation and production of these components upon a passive immunotherapy of experimental endotoxaemia is intensely studied in our laboratory.

REFERENCES

1. Baumgartner, J.-D., McCutchan, J. A., van Melle, G., Vogt, M., Luethy, R., Glauser, M. P., Ziegler, E. J., Klauber, M. R., Muehlen, E., Chiolero, R. and Geroulanos, S., 1985, Prevention of gram-negative shock and death in surgical patients by antibody to endotoxin core glycolipid. Lancet ii: 59.

2. Finland, M., 1980, Changing ecology of bacterial infection as related to antibacterial therapy. J. Infect. Dis. 122: 419.

3. Galanos, G., Luderitz, O. and Westphal, O., 1969, A new method for the extraction of R lipopolysaccharides. Eur. J. Biochem. 9: 245.

4. Galfre, G., Milstein, C. and Wright, B., 1979, Rat x rat hybrid myelomas and a monoclonal anti-Fd portion of mouse IgG. Nature 277: 131.

5. Kohler, G. and Milstein, C., 1975, Continuous culture of fused cells secreting antibody of predetermined specificity. Nature 256: 495.

6. Morrison, D. C. and Ulevitch, R. J., 1978, The effects of Bacterial Endotoxins on Host Mediation Systems. Amer. J. Pathol. 93(2): 526.

7. Tracey, K. J., Fong, Y., Hesse, D. G., Manogue, K. R., Lee, A. T., Kuo, G. C., Lowry, S. F. and Cerami, A., 1987, Anti-cachectin/TNF monoclonal antibodies prevent septic shock during lethal bacteraemia. Nature 300: 662.

ENDOTOXIN SIZE IN HEMODIALYSIS SOLUTIONS: MODIFICATIONS IN PRESENCE OF CONCENTRATED SALT SOLUTIONS AND BACTERIAL PRODUCTS

V. Goury, A. C. Steinmetz, F. Vincent, A. Moufti and J. C. Darbord

Central Pharmacy of Hospitals, Quality Control Laboratory
7 rue du Fer a Moulin, F-75221 Paris Cedex 05

Pyrogenic reactions for which no cause can be found are common in hemodialysis, using non-sterile concentrated salt solutions and membranes which usually retain endotoxins (pore size: 10,000 to 30,000 D). If we admit that endotoxins, the most important pyrogens, might be responsible for these observations, we have to prove that they can cross hemodialysis devices. It is recognized that lipopolysaccharides (LPS) can exist in different forms, aggregated, mono or bi-layer subunits. This has been related to the ionic conditions, the presence of detergent or EDTA (2, 5, 6). In hemodialysis, the extent of the pyrogenic episodes has been shown to depend not only on the presence of gram positive bacteria or, in some cases, Halobacterium species (3). These reactions have only been observed for 40 to 800 $mmol.l^{-1}$ HCO_3^- solutions. We examined the possibility that, under the ionic conditions described above, endotoxins might be the cause of pyrogenic effects associated with hemodialysis. If this were true, we would expect that, after filtration under various conditions, residual endotoxin would be detected in ultra-filtered solutions. Two different procedures were used to meet most of the clinical conditions: filtration experiments were performed with ultrafilters (pore size: 20,000 to 100,000 D), or true hemodialysis devices. Endotoxins were associated with three hemolytic Staphylococcus and two other species commonly isolated in concentrated salt solutions. Moreover, it was known that the effect of toxic shock syndrome toxin (TSS - Staphylococcus) is potentiated by small amount of endotoxin (1), and this unexplained observation supports our Staphylococcus-endotoxin interaction study.

MATERIALS AND METHODS

Endotoxins

Escherichia coli 055B5, provided by SIGMA corp (L 2637) and Chromobacterium violaceum CIP 53.2, endotoxin extracted by the Rudback method (7).

Endotoxin Determination

Limulus amebocyte lysate with chromogenic substrate (LAL-CS), Coatest KABI VITRUM K 82104-1, with microstrips and a Twinreader spectrophotometer (TITERTEK).

Strains

Staphylococcus aureus - Wood - α hemolytic, S. aureus - CIP 5710 - β hemolytic, S. cohnii - DSM 20260 δ hemolytic, Halobacterium halobium - DSM670, Clostridium sporogenes - ATCC 3584.

Culture Conditions and Media

S. aureus (α, β and δ) cultures are obtained with a 2% biotrypcase broth (5364-1 Biomerieux). C. sporogenes cultures are obtained, under an anaerobic atmosphere in a chamber with a TTY medium (biotrypcase, 15 g; Yeast extract, 5 g; NaCl, 2.5 g; Sodium thioglycolate, 0.5 g; distilled water qs 1000 ml) H. halobium cultures are obtained with the DSM broth (NaCl 250 $g.l^{-1}$).

Chemical Reagents

Distilled water for injection (USP XXI), Pyrogen-free isotonic solution (NaCl, $9g.l^{-1}$), concentrated solution for hemodialysis (NaHCO3, 67.2 $g.l^{-1}$; NaCl, 29.2 $g.l^{-1}$).

Ultrafiltrations

1- Ultrasart TM system, cellulose triacetate, ref SARTORIUS 16520C, (size 20,000 D), used with a 30 psi pressure. 2- Minitan system, polysulfone, PTT KOMP 04 (30.000 D) and PTHK OMP 04 (100.000 D) used with 20 psi pressure. 3- Nephross hemodialysis devices, LENTO, Cuprophan^{R}, Organon Teknika corp. In this experiment, the blood compartment of the device was filled with Pyrogen-free isotonic solution.

Acellular Broth Preparations

After a 72-h incubation, each broth was centrifugated (4000 RPM, 15 min) and filtered (0.45 μm). The solutions were kept at -20°C until use. Hemolytic efficiency of these solution were tested on agar plate medium with blood (α and δ rabbit, β sheep). A non-hemolytic "δ-solution", prepared in the same conditions with a non-hemolytic strain obtained by mutation was used.

Electron Microscopy

Endotoxin preparations were examined after negative coloration (2% Potassium phosphotungstate, Philips EM 301).

RESULTS

1- To assay for endotoxin crossing through the two ultrafiltration systems proposed, we thawed the acellular broth preparation and, in the same hour, added 2000 $EU.ml^{-1}$ of E. coli 055B5 or C. violaceum endotoxin before ultrafiltration. The same experiments were done with water and HCO_3^- solutions. Table 1 shows the amount of endotoxin crossing the filter in each case, and demonstrate that the ultrafiltration properties are modified in the presence of HCO_3^-, Halobacterium or δ hemolysin solutions.

Sonification of the ultrafilter after each experiment increased the amount crossing by less than 5%. We couldn't find LAL-CS activity after δ hemolysin confrontation and filtration (Table 1, column*), and in this case we observed liposome-like vesicular forms (Fig 1). This phenomenon was not observed with the δ-hemolysin preparation.

2- To confirm the above results, we performed a simulated hemodialysis with Nephross devices and the same endotoxin - hemolysin - HCO_3- solutions.

Table 1. Ultrafiltration of endotoxin solutions (2000 EU/ml^{-1}) - When two results are given, the upper results were observed with C. violaceum endotoxin, and the lower with E. coli 055B5.

	ULTRASART 20,000 D		MINITAN 30,000 D	MINITAN 100,000 D
	Endotoxin removed (%)	Endotoxin on the filter (%)	Endotoxin removed (%)	Endotoxin removed (%)
Water	< 0.03	65-75	< 0.02	< 0.02
Concentrated solution HCO_3^-	0.03	54-75	< 0.02	< 0.02
S. aureus α hemolysin	0.03	30-60	< 0.02	0.03
S. aureus β hemolysin	< 0.03	25-60	< 0.02	< 0.02
S. cohnii δ hemolysin	0.13	5-10*	< 0.02	0.3-5
S. cohnii δ^-	< 0.03	46-60	< 0.02	< 0.02
H. halobium	0.15	48-60	< 0.02	0.5
C. sporogenes	0.06	65-74	< 0.02	0.2

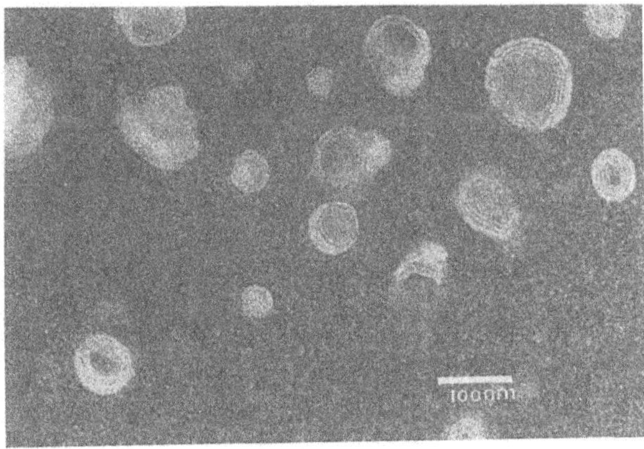

Fig 1. Liposome-like vesicular forms obsrved with δ hemolysin solution and endotoxin.

Table 2. Not removed endotoxin (%) recovered in blood compartment after hemodialysis simulation (E. coli 055B5, Nephross lento)

Water	0.6
HCO_3^-	1.2
S. aureus α hemolysin	0.6
S. aureus β hemolysin	0.6
S. cohnii δ hemolysin	2.05 to 6.6
S. cohnii δ^-	1.2

The results are shown in Table 2 with analogous results for the crossing values but without inactivation after filtration of the LAL-CS reaction by δ hemolysin. Nevertheless, in this case, we observed that endotoxins are recovered after dialysis in an isotonic NaCl solution.

DISCUSSION

We have shown that endotoxin crossing through hemodialysis membranes was increased by δ hemolysin, by unknown Halobacterium products and by HCO_3^-. We observed, simultaneously, the formation of 20-100 nm liposome-like vesicular forms, but the reason of this phenomenon is not known. It is possible that there is chemical hydrolysis of the LPS by δ hemolysin, as it has been shown for the lipoprotein structure in the erythrocyte membrane, with splitting and reorganization in a short time. Therefore there is a modification of the endotoxin structure, and this phenomenon could be of great importance in the pathogenesis of hemodialysis shock.

To conclude, we can say with the procedure tested here, that a strong correlation exists between the presence of bacterial hemolysin in the solution and the endotoxin crossing through a 20,000 D filter. Since both hemolysin and HCO_3^- have been shown to induce a split form of endotoxin, it appears that they are important determinants in the filtration of endotoxins during hemodialysis. These experiments suggest that other bacterial contaminations, yet unknown, and which have presumably no effect, increase the pyrogenic effect of endotoxins released by gram negative bacteria when both are present in concentrated salt solutions. These synergistic activities have led us to introduce new specifications in quality control.

REFERENCES

1. de Azavedo, J. C. S., Hartigan, P. J., de Saxe, M. and Arbuthnott, J. P., 1985, Gram-negative endotoxins and staphylococcal toxic shock syndrome, in: "Bacterial Endotoxins, Structure, Biomedical Significance, and Detection with the Limulus Amebocyte Lysate Test, Alan R. Liss, Inc., p. 419-430.

2. Good, C. M. and Lane, H. E., 1977, The biochemistry of pyrogens. Bull. Parent. Drug. Assoc. 31: 116.

3. Goury, V., Guyomard, S., Mollet, M., Man, N. K., Hamon, M. and Darbord, J. C., 1987, Role des bacteries halophiles ou halotphiles ou halotrophes dans les pathologies chromiques de dialyse au long cours. Bull. Acad. Natle. Med. 171: 561.

4. Guyomard, S., Goury, V. and Darbord, J. C., 1988, Effects of ionizing radiations on bacterial endotoxins: comparison between gamma radiations and accelerated electrons. Radiat. Phys. Chem. 31: 679.

5. Ribi, E., Anacker, R. L., Brown, R., Haskins, W. T., Malhgren, B., Milner, K. C. and Rudback, J. K., 1966, Reaction of endotoxin and surfactants. J. Bact. 92: 1493.

6. Rosen, F. S., Skarnes, R. C., Landy, M. and Shear, M. J., 1958, Inactivation of endotoxin by a humoral component. III. Role of divalent cation and a dialysable component. J. Exp. Med. 108: 701.

7. Rudback, J. K., Akiya, F. I., Elin, R. J., Hochstein, H. D., Luoma, M. K., Milner, E. C. B., Milner, K. C. and Thomas, K. R., 1976, Preparation and properties of a national reference endotoxin. J. of Clinical Microbiol. 13: 21.

8. Sweadner, K. J., Forte, M. and Nelsen, L. L., 1977, Filtration removal of endotoxin (pyrogens) in solutions in different stages of aggregation. Appl. Environ. Microbiol. 34: 382.

PROTECTIVE EFFECT OF SALMONELLA TYPHIMURIUM RE-LPS ANTISERUM

Y. Ching and Y. Shihao

Endotoxin Laboratory, Department of Microbiology
Second Military Medical University, Shanghai,
People's Republic of China

ABSTRACT

There is increasing evidence that antiserum to LPS can reduce the morbidity and mortality of Gram-negative bacterial infections. We reported that antiserum to S. typhimurium SL 1102 (Re mutant strain) has excellent cross-protective activity. Antisera to these bacteria and to its Re-LPS were prepared in rabbits immunized with heat-killed bacterial cells and with Re-LPS preparations. Re-LPS antibody titers were tested by immune hemagglutination (IHA) and by ELISA. These antisera were capable of protecting ICR mice against lethal challenge with S-type S. typhimurium 50014 (100 LD_{50}), E. coli 0111: B4(32 LD_{50}). Pseudomonas aeruginosa (8LD_{50}) and Klebsiella pneumonia (16 LD_{50}). We used gastric mucin (5%) as a virulence enhancing agent for the bacterial challenges in this study. The IHA titer of antibody to the homologous strain was much higher than that of other strains. Protection by the sera was 75-100%, 25% and 0% when injected 24, 48 or 72 hr before the challenge, respectively. Survival rate was more than 50% when the antiserum was injected 5-7 hr after the challenge with a ten-fold or higher lethal dose. No protection was observed against such high challenge if the serum was injected later than this time. According to this report, Re-LPS antiserum provides a better protection than S-type specific antisera.

INTRODUCTION

The first report on the neutralization of endotoxic properties by strain specific hyperimmune anti O-antiserum was published by Nowotny et al in 1965 (14). Lethality, pyrogenicity and Shwartzman skin reactivity of endotoxins could be abolished by in vitro incubation of endotoxin in various dilutions of antisera. The neutralization of toxicity did not effect the non-specific resistance enhancing beneficial effect of the endotoxin against virulent bacterial infections (14, 16).

The involvement of multiple species and serologic types in Gram negative infections prompted the evaluation of the effectiveness of immunization with shared, cross-reactive antigens, such as the core polysaccharide and lipid region of Gram negative endotoxins. It was expected that antisera to these epitopes will cross protect against various Gram negative bacterial infections. Our results using the antiserum to S. typhimurium SL 1102 (Re mutant) strain are reported here.

Table 1a. Antibody titers of different sera to several LPS as determined by IHA

Serum	Titer of antibodies to LPS					
	1102.Re	50014	055B5	41002	0056	lipid A
Anti-re mutant	12800	160	80	40	32	60
Anti-Re LPS	1600	80	80	20	10	80
Anti-50014 bacteria	128	25600	60	16	16	40
Anti-50014 LPS	10	1600	32	10	10	40
Anti-055B5 LPS	60	80	3200	10	10	20
Anti-41002 bacteria	32	8	8	1600	128	16
Anti-Lipid A	80	80	80	160	20	6400
Normal Serum	4	8	4	4	4	10

MATERIALS AND METHODS

Antiserum to the Re mutant of S. typhimurium was produced in New Zealand rabbits with heat-killed bacteria (2×10^9 cell/ml). Rabbits were immunized intravenously receiving 1 ml of above bacterial suspension each time, three times a wk. This was followed by 1 wk rest. Three more injections were given during the third wk. Seven days after the last injection, blood was collected by cardiac puncture and the sera were pooled. Antiserum to isolated Re-LPS was also prepared by intravenous injections of 80, 200, 400, 600 µg of S. typhimurium SL 1102 LPS prepared by the method of Galanos et al (9). One injection was given weekly. The titer of antibodies were determined by ELISA (10) and IHA (5).

Bacterial suspension was mixed with 5% gastric mucin for the intraperitoneal challenge. ICR mice were used in this experiment. The protection was performed by injecting i.p. 0.3 ml antiserum into each mouse 22-24 hr before the viable bacterial challenge or 2 hr before challenging them with LPS. The survival rate was determined 3 or 7 days later.

Table 1b. Antibody titers of sera to several LPS determined by ELISA

Sera	Titer of antibodies to LPS					
	1102.Re	50014	055B5	41002	0056	lipid A
Nonimmune serum	320	100	2000	20	20	3200
Anti-Re mutant	12500	100	10	20	1280	100

NOTE: Titer of the antiserum was based on the titer of nonimmune serum being negative.

Table 2. The capacity of the antiserum to Re mutant in the protection against heterologous bacterial challenge

Challenging bacteria	LD50 (cfu)	Survival rate after one wk (survival/total)		
		Anti-Re serum	Normal serum	Controls
S. typhimurium	2(1.86x10^4)	7/7	6/7	2/7
(50014)	4	7/7	1/7	0/7
	32	6/7	0/7	0/7
	100	4/7	0/7	-
	128	1/7	0/7	-
E. coli	2(3.8x10^6)	7/7	7/7	2/7
(0111:B4)	16	7/7	6/7	1/7
	32	4/7	1/7	0/7
	64	1/7	0/7	0/7
P. aeruginosa	2(3.75x10^6)	7/7	2/7	1/7
	4	6/7	1/7	0/7
	8	3/7	0/7	0/7
K. pneumonia	2(10^7)	7/7	7/7	2/7
	6	6/7	3/7	1/7
	8	6/7	2/7	0/7
	16	2/7	0/7	0/7

Table 3. Passive immunization of mice against several bacteria with antiserum to Re mutant

Bacterial challenge	Sera	LD50 (log10cfu)	Survivors/ Total	P Value
S. typhimurium	Re mutant antiserum	5.63	27/35(77.1%)	
(50014)	Nonimmune serum	4.42	8/35(22.8%)	0.01
E. coli (0111:B4)	Re mutant antiserum	7.89	23/42(76.2%)	
	Nonimmune serum	7.60	23/42(54.7%)	0.05
P. aeruginosa	Re mutant antiserum	7.06	14/21(66.7%)	
	Nonimmune serum	6.46	3/21(14.3%)	0.01
K. pneumoniae	Re mutant antiserum	7.79	27/35(77.1%)	
	Nonimmune serum	7.49	18/35(51.4%)	0.05

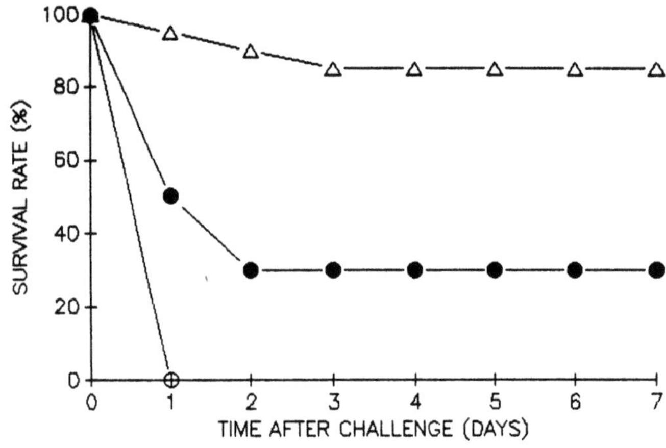

Fig 1. The effect of the antiserum on preventing lethal challenge with bacteria. 16 LD_{50} doses of S. typhimurium (50014) was used after serum injection. - Δ - antiserum to Re mutant, - ● - nonimmune serum, - O - 0.9% saline control.

RESULTS AND DISCUSSION

The results showed that the titer of antiserum to the homologous LPS was the highest. Cross-reactive titer of the Re antiserum to heterologous LPS was also demonstrated but this was found to be low with both IHA and ELISA methods (Table 1a and 1b). In spite of this, Re antisera had good cross-protective effect to heterologous bacteria, particularly within the same genus (Table 2).

Normal serum had slight protective effect against lower dose of bacterial challenge as shown in Tables 2 and 3 and Fig 1. The antibody titer to Re-LPS in mice after injecting them with Re antiserum was determined by exsanguination of randomized mice from different groups. Good correlation between the anti-Re titer and its protective effect against virulent homologous bacterial challenge was observed (Fig 2). Furthermore, the Re antiserum showed a significant protection to lethal challenge with LPS (2-3 LD_{50}) as presented in Table 4.

Analyzing the main component in the protective Re bacterial antiserum, we found that the protective capacity of the antisera to Re-LPS was nearly the same as that of antiserum to Re mutant (Fig 3). The antisera to the O-antigen or to lipid A were not protective against heterologous bacterial challenge. Re antisera and IgG isolated from it showed nearly the same activity (Fig 4). The protective activity of the antiserum was more markedly reduced after absorption with Re-LPS than with smooth LPS (Fig 5 and Table 5).

Very effective protection was observed when the antiserum was administered within 5 hr after the bacterial challenge. This effect could be increased with repeated injections of the antiserum (Fig 6 and 7). The results showed that if Re antiserum was combined with Gentamicine antibiotic or with heparin, it could be more effective than the application of Re antiserum alone (Fig 8 and 9).

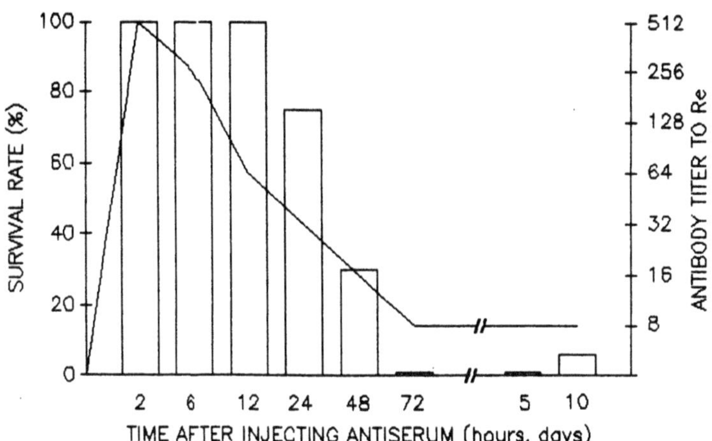

Fig 2. Correlation between protecting activity and titer of antibodies. 32 LD_{50} dose of S. typhimurium was used for challenge. Antiserum (0.3 ml) was administered i.p. Titer of the antiserum in mice was determined by IHA.

Table 4. The protective activity of several sera to LPS

Serum	Survivors/Total (%)	
	50014 LPS	055B5 LPS
0.9% saline	4/28 (14.3)	3/21 (14.3)
Nonimmunol serum	8/28 (28.6)	5/21 (23.8)
Anti-41002 serum	8/28 (28.6)	4/21 (19.0)
Anti-50014 serum	21/28 (75.0)*	5/21 (23.8)
Anti-055B5 serum	7/28 (25.0)	12/21 (57.1)*
Anti-Re serum	19/28 (67.9)*	10/21 (47.6)+

NOTE: Antiserum was compared with nonimmunol serum
* P 0.01; + P 0.05

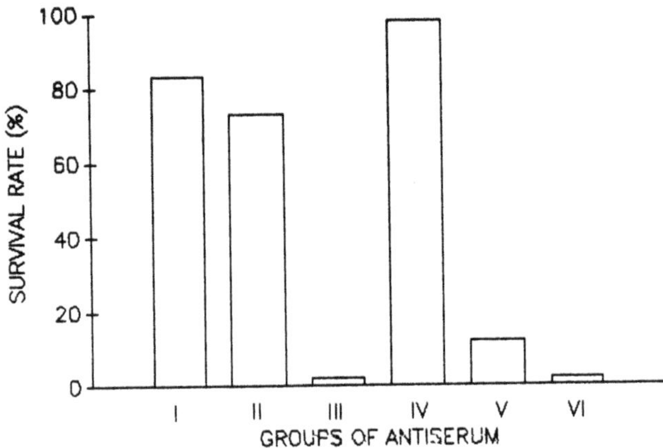

Fig 3. The comparison of different sera for protective effect. Lethal dose of S. typhimurium (50014) bacteria was used for challenge. I: antiserum to Re mutant, II: antiserum to Re-LPS, III: antiserum absorbed with Re-LPS, IV: homologous antiserum, V: antiserum to Lipid A, VI: heterologous antiserum.

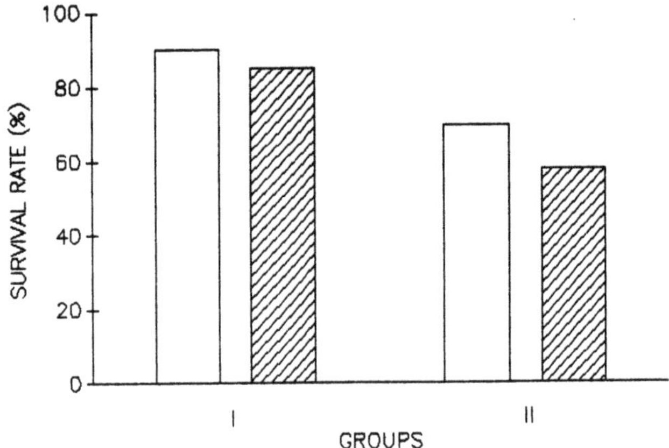

Fig 4. Comparison of the protective effect between antiserum to Re mutant and its immunoglobulin (IgG). IgG (3 mg/0.3 ml) was used by i.p. ▯ : antiserum, ▨ : IgG. I. 32 LD_{50} doses of S. typhimurium, II. 6 LD_{50} doses of P. aeruginosa challenge. Serum or IgG was injected i.p. 22 hr. before challenge.

We used 5% gastric mucin to enhance the virulence of the bacterial challenge. This reduced the challenge dose from 10^7-10^8 to 10^3-10^4 and we obtained reproducible results. This study and our previous work (3) supports the claim of Appelmelk who showed that the most important factor determining the outcome of experiments measuring the protection against infection is the proper choice of the experimental model (1).

The cross-reactive titer of Re antisera was low and it did not reflect the capacity of the antiserum to protect against heterologous bacterial challenge. We assume that organisms growing in logarithmic phase usually lack complete O-specific LPS structure and therefore the core components of the LPS are better exposed to Re antibodies to interact with them (6, 15). Our report shows that after passive immunization the Re antibody titer in the circulation is related to the protective effect of the Re antiserum. That some other components could have contributed to the protection by antiserum has been demonstrated by other laboratories (7, 8, 12, 13, 18). We consider that the antibody to Re-LPS is the main component responsible for the protective activity in such sera. In addition, the non-specific antibodies to the O-antigens which appear in the serum induced by immunization also may have contributed to the cross protection by Re antiserum.

Intravenous injection of Re antiserum during the onset of bacteremia is effective to prevent lethal infection, as has been shown by clinical investigators (4, 11, 19). Though antibiotics are effective in the treatment of bacteremia, one has to realize that free LPS in the blood increases by 10-2000-fold in the initial phase (17). In addition, DIC, glomerular lesions due to complement and to clotting system activation by LPS may also appear (2). Therefore the use of Re antiserum combined with antibiotics and anticoagulants can be very valuable. Clearly, as we are facing more Gram negative bacterial infections, antibiotic resistant strains and an increasing number of severely immunocompromised patients, immunotherapy of the infection becomes increasingly important.

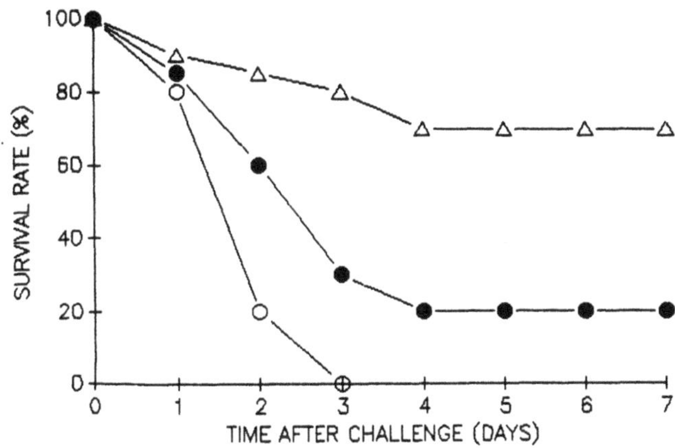

Fig 5. The protective activity of anti-Re serum absorbed with LPS. The absorbed serum was administered i.p. at 22 hr before challenge. Lethal dose of S. typhimurium (50014) was used for challenge. - O -: absorbed with Re-LPS, - ● -: with 40014 LPS, - Δ -: no absorption.

Table 5. Titer of the antisera after absorption with LPS determined by IHA

Antiserum to Re mutant absorbed by	Titer of antibodies to	
	1102 LPS	50014 LPS
No absorption	6400	80
50014 LPS	3200	16
1102 Re-LPS	20	20

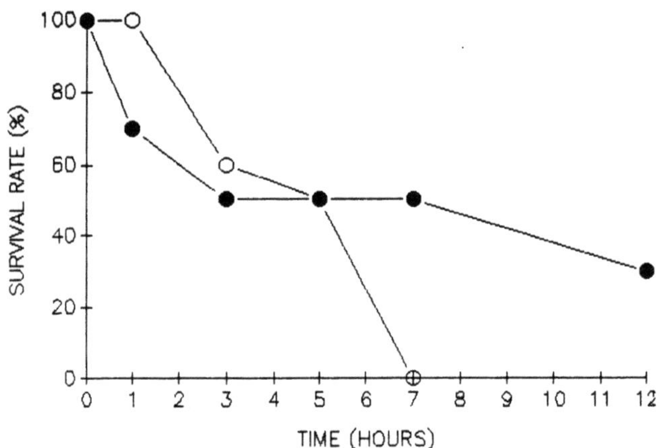

Fig 6. The effect of antiserum on the prevention of lethal bacteremia. Antiserum was administered i.v. at different times after bacterial challenge. - 0 -: 32 LD_{50} doses of S. typhimurium bacteria, - ● -: 4 LD_{50} doses of P. aeruginosa.

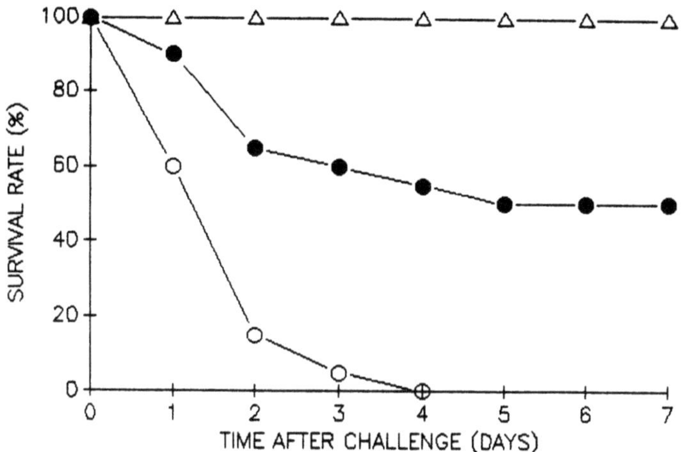

Fig 7. The protective effect of antiserum administered as single-dose or double-dose after i.p. bacterial challenge. 32 LD_{50} doses of S. typhimurium bacteria was used for challenge. Antiserum was administered i.v. - 0 -: serum injected 12 hr after challenge, - ● -: at 3 hr, - Δ-: serum injected twice at 3 and 12 hrs.

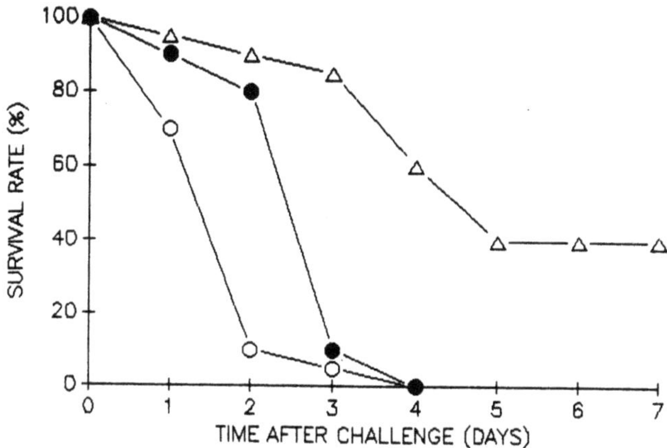

Fig 8. The protective effect of antibiotics combined with antiserum during severe bacteremia. Treatment was performed 12 hr after bacterial challenge. 1000u/mouse of Gentamicin was administered i.m. Serum was administered i.v. - 0 -: antiserum, - ● -: Gentamicin, -Δ -: antiserum and Gentamicin. Challenge with S. typhimurium bacteria.

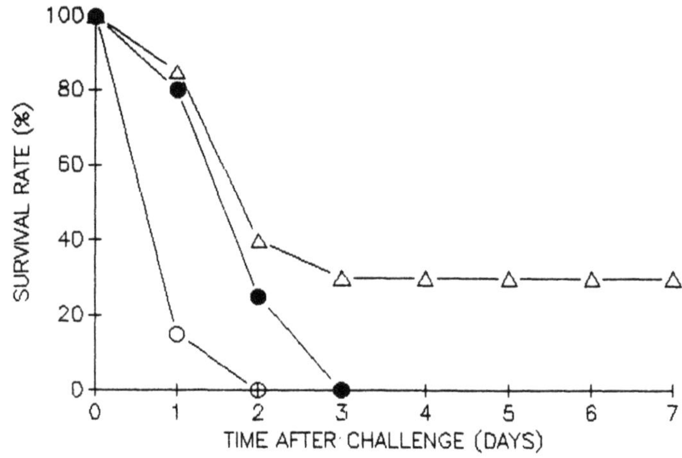

Fig 9. The protective effect of heparin combined with antiserum during severe bacteremia. Treatment was performed 12 hr after bacterial challenge. Heparin (60u/mouse) was administered i.v. at 30-40 min after injecting serum i.v. - O -: normal serum + heparin, - ● -: antiserum + 0.9% saline, - Δ-: antiserum + heparin. Challenge with 32 LD_{50} dose of S. typhimurium.

REFERENCES

1. Appelmelk, B. J., Verwey-van Vught, A. M. J. J., Maaskant, J. J., Schouten, W. F., Thijs, L. G., Maclaren, D. M., 1986, Use of mucin and hemoglobulin in experimental murine Gram-negative bacteremia enhances the immunoprotective action of antibodies reactive with the lipopolysaccharide core region. Antonie van Leeuwenhoek 52: 537.

2. Braude, A. I., Douglas, H. and Davis, C. E., 1973, Treatment and prevention of intravascular coagulation with antiserum to endotoxin. J. Inf. Dis. 128: s157.

3. Ching, Y., Lusen, T., Hsilin, L. and Shihchi, T., 1963, Protective effect of the placental globulin against Pseudomonas aeuginosa infection. Chinese Med. J. 49: 644.

4. Dunn, D. L., Ewald, D. C., Chandan, N. and Cerra, F. B., 1986, Immunotherapy of Gram-negative bacterial sepsis. A single murine monoclonal antibody provides cross-genera protection. Arc. Surg. 121: 58.

5. FanYuh, and Yu Ching, 1986, The immunogenicity and antibody response of endotoxin. Shanghai J. Immunol. 6: 339.

6. Fenwick, B. W., Cullor, J. S., Osburn, B. I. and Olander, H. J., 1986, Mechanisms involved in protection provided by immunization against core lipopolysaccharide of E. coli J5 from lethal Haemophilus pleuromoniae infection in swine. Infect. Immun. 53: 298.

7. Gaffin, S. L., Wells, M. and Jordan, J. P., 1985, Anti-lipopolysaccharide toxin therapy for whole body X-irradiation overdose. The Brit. J. Radiol. 58: 881.

8. Gaffin, S. L., Grinberg, Z., Abraham, C., Birkhan, J. and Shechter, Y., 1981, Protection against hemorrhagic shock in the cat by human plasma containing endotoxin-specific antibodies. J. Surg. Res. 31: 18.

9. Galanos, C., Luderitz, O. and Westphal, O., 1969, A new method for the extraction of R lipopolysaccharides. Eur. J. Biochem. 9: 245.

10. Gigliotti, F. and Shenep, J. L., 1985, Failure of monoclonal antibodies to core glycolipid to bind intact smooth strains of E. coli. J. Inf. Dis. 151: 1105.

11. Lachman, E., Pitsoe, S. B. and Gaffin, S. L., 1984, Anti-lipopolysaccharide immunotherapy in management of septic shock of obstetric and gynecological origin. The Lancet 981.

12. McCabe, W. R., 1972, Immunization with R mutants of S. minnesota. 1. Protection against challenge with heterologous Gram-negative bacilli. J. Immunol. 108: 601.

13. Ng, A. K., Chen, C. L., Chang, C. M. and Nowotny, A., 1976, Relationship of structure to function in bacterial endotoxins: serologically cross-reactive components and their effect on protection of mice against some Gram-negative infection. J. Gen. Microbiol. 94: 107.

14. Nowotny, A. Radvany, R. and Neal, N., 1965, Neutralization of toxic bacterial O-antigens with O-antibodies while maintaining their stimulus on non-specific resistance. Life Sci. 4: 1107.

15. Proctor, R. A., 1986, Role of antibody in the prevention and pathogenesis of endotoxin and Gram-negative septic shock, in: "Handbook of Endotoxin, Vol 4," R. A. Proctor, ed., Elsevier, Amsterdam, p. 161.

16. Radvany, R., Neal, N. and Nowotny, A., 1966, Relation of structure to function in bacterial O-antigens, VI. Neutralization of endotoxic O-antigens by homologous O-antibody. Ann. N.Y. Acad. Sci. 133: 763.

17. Shenep, J. L. and Morgan, K. A., 1984, Kinetic of endotoxin release during antibiotic therapy for experimental Gram-negative bacterial sepsis. J. Inf. Dis. 150: 380.

18. Siber, G. R., Kania, S. A. and Warren, H. S., 1985, Cross-reactivity of rabbit antibodies to LPS of E. coli J5 and other Gram-negative bacteria. J. Inf. Dis. 152: 954.

19. Ziegler, E. J., McCutchan, J. A., Fierer, J., Glauser, M. P., Sadoff, J. C., Douglas, H. and Braude, A. I., 1982, Treatment of Gram-negative bacteremia and shock with human antiserum to a mutant E. coli. N. E. J. Med. 307: 1225.

INDEX

Abequose, 500, 504
Acetylsalicylic acid, 393
Achromobacter lyticus
endopeptidase, 274-278
Acid phosphatase, 102, 590
Acinetobacter calcoaceticus, 84
sp., 82, 228
Actinomycin D, 321, 322, 332 335, 342, 538, 585 585
Acylation, 104, 105
3-Acyloxyacyl hydrolase, 37-38
Adaptation, homeoviscous, 50
Adenocarcinoma cell line
TA-3, 164, 172, 173
Adenosine monophosphate, cyclic 371-373, 378-381, .469, 473-476, 478
Adenylate cyclase, 369, 373 381, 382, 475, 478
Adjuvant activity assay, 102
Adrenal gland
and lipopolysaccharide, 503
Aeromonas salmonicidae, 84
AIDS, **see** Immunodeficiency
Alcaligenes faecalis var.**myxogenes,** 34
Amido black stain, 260
4-Amino-4-deoxy-L-arabinose 46, 49
Amoebocyte and lipopolysaccharide, 225, 257-271
see Limulus, Tachypleus
Anthracene-9-carboxyl chloride
synthesis, 204, 205, 207
Antibody, monoclonal, 320-324, 331-344, 526-527, 530
Antigen, tumor-associated, 668
Anti-lipopolysaccharide factor (ALF), 257-285
function, 273-285
structure, 275-277
Antitumor activity assay, 111-116
Arachidonic acid, 381, 382, 390, 393
Arginine α-amide, 274, 279

Assay, **see** separate compounds
Atherosclerosis, 396-397

Baboon, 585
Bacillus Calmette-Guérin(BCG) 376, 399, 471, 531, 538, 539, 542, 545
Bacillus subtilis, 259, 267
Bacteremia,Gram-negative, 635, 636, 641
Bacteria
-binding, 422
bound concept, 419-422
Gram-negative, 417-425
and T-cell, 417-425
see separate species
Bacteroides asaccharolyticus, 599
B. distasonis, 594
B. fragilis, 593-601
B. gingivalis, 613
B. thetaiotaomicron, 594
B. sp.,, 82, 84, 86
B-cell, 372, 376-378, 571 603
activation, 102, 234
isolation, 569
and lipopolysaccharide, 376

B-cell (continued)
  mitogenicity, 160
  of mouse, 149, 150, 155,156
  polyclonal, 28, 427-443
  proliferation, 378
  stimulation, 28
    assay, 448
BCG, **see** Bacillus Calmette-Guérin
Binding, **see** separate items
Blastogenesis, 514
Blood cell, mononuclear, 447, 455-456
  see B-cell, T-cell, others
B-lymphocyte, **see** B-cell
Bone marrow, 287, 429
Bordetella bronchoseptica, 589-591
  B. parapertussis, 589-591
  B. pertussis, 84, 149-157
  B. sp., 589-591
Bound bacteria concept, **see** Bacteria, bound
Bradyrhizobium sp., 45
Brucella abortus, 672
  B. melitensis, 46, 48
  B. pertussis, 369-374
    toxin, 369-374
Burst, metabolic, 301

Calcium, 247-255, 281, 282 380, 382, 390
  ionophore **A23187**, 347-357
Calmodulin, 349, 352-357
Cancer
  cure, 666-669
  patient, 420
  therapy, **see** Monophosphoryl lipid A
Candida albicans, 221, 259 266-267
  C. quillermondi, 221
CAP, **see** Protein, cationic
CAT, **see** Methyl-30-0-(9-carboxy anthracenyl)tetradecanoate
Cecropin of silkworm, 269
Cell
  adrenocortical, 199
  chrominum release assay, 165 171
  Coulter-counting, 165
  DNA synthesis, 165-166
  glucose uptake, 166
  line:
    Balb/c, 165
    C3HeB/FeJ, 149, 151
    C3H/HeJ, 149-157
    C3H/HeSlc, 160, 161
    C3H/OuJ, 150-152
    L929, 165, 172, 173
Cell (continued)
  line (continued)
    P388D1, 164, 172, 173
    P815, 164
    TA-3, 164-172
  viability assay, 165
Chemiluminescence, 304, 308, 413-415
luminol-dependent, 413-415
Chick embryo, 19-22
Chlorobiaceae, 45
Cholangitis, 636
Cholera toxin, 378
Cholestasis, 482, 491-494
Choline, 381
Chromatiaceae, 45
Chrominum release assay, 165, 171
Chromobacterium violaceum, 15, 16, 19, 71, 85-86, 563, 685
Clostridium sporogenes, 686, 687
Clostripain, 275, 276
Coagulation,disseminated, intravascular(DIC), 389, 653
Coagulation factor C, 31
Cobra venom factor, 391, 392
Cod liver oil, 394
Collagenase, 361, 379
Colony formation by granulocyte
  macrophage, 550
Colony stimulating factor, 102, 377, 379, 467, 468
Complement, 35, 301-317, 389-393
  C1, 301-317
Concanavalin A, 371, 377-379 570, 573, 594, 598
Core disaccharide of lipopolysaccharide, 83-85
Corynebacterium parvum, 471
  and tumor, 376
Coxiella burnetii, 612, 616
Coxsackie virus B, 518-520
Cryptococcus neoformans, 259, 266, 267
Cyclooxygenase, 361, 363, 365, 371, 372, 382
  inhibitor, **see** Indomethacin
Cyclophosphamide, 585-587
  and neutropenia, 585
Cytochalasin E, 32
Cytokine, 516-518, 549-556, 635-640
  and septicemia, human, 635-640
Cytochrome-c, 32
Cytotoxicity assay, 538-539

DCX, **see Serratia marcescens** agent, cytotoxic
2-Deoxy-D-glucose uptake, 178, 179
3-Deoxy-D-manno-2-octulosonic acid(KDO), 3-11, 83-84, 190-193
  synthetic, 3-11
6-Deoxy-L-talose, 132
2,3-Diacylglucosamine phosphate 59
Diacylglycerol, 381, 382
2,3-Diamino-2,3-dideoxy-D-glucose(DAG), 46-48
  in bacteria, 46-47
  isolation, 46
Diamino-glucose type lipid A, 57-63
2,4-Dibromoacetophenone, 393 394
Diethylcarbamazine, 363
Diphenylhexatriene(DPH)
  fluorescence anisotropy, 233-242
Disaccharide, 15
DNA synthesis, 150-153, 165-166, 175, 177
  and polymyxin B, 152, 153
Dog
  and lipid A antibody production, 681-684
  clearance from blood, 682-684
Dot immunobinding assay, 581
DPH, **see** Diphenylhexatriene

Electrodialysis of lipopolysa charide, 248
Electrophoresis, two-dimensional, 447-456
ELISA, 73-77
Endospecy, 216-227
  assay, 217-221, 227
  principle, 216
  specificity, 217, 219
Endocytosis on Kupffer cell, 484, 488, 489
Endotoxemia, 375, 635-636, 681-684
Endotoxin (synonymous with Lipopolysaccharide, **see**)
  absorbents, 655, 659
  and acetylsalicylic acid, 394
  activity, 19-26 **see** function
  antiserum, 691
  assay, 147-229, 391, 653, 685
    new, specific, 215-223

Endotoxin (continued)
  binding, 391-392
    -protein, cationic, 287-299
  challenge, 641-652
    and lipid A precursor as protector, 541-652
  chromogenic test, 225-229
  cod liver oil, 394
  contaminant, 147-229
    lipid as, 163-184
  cytokine, 549-556
  detection, 203-213
    by fluorescence, 203-213
  effects, beneficial, 549-556
  and erythrocyte agglutination, 287-299
  extraction, 163
  fluorescence method, 203-213
  fractionation, 163
  functions, 1-145, 369
  and granulocyte, 287-299
  host response, 497-701
  hypersensitivity, 604, 611-616
  as immunoadjuvant, 525-535
  and immunocyte, 525-535
    leukemic, 525-535
    normal, 525-535
  as immunostimulant, 525
  interactions
    cellular, 245-295
    molecular, 231-344
  and interleukin-1, 369-374
  and Kupffer cell dysfunction 494
  and lethality, 19-21, 226. 603-619
  and liver disease, 228, 481-495
  and **Limulus** amoebocyte lysate assay, 203-204
  lipid contaminant of, 163-184
    biology, 163-184
    chemistry, 163-184
  macrophage as major target cell, **see** Macrophage
  and monocyte, 389-398
  and muramyl dipeptide synergism, 537-547
  neutralization by antiserum, 691
  in plasma in disease, 228
  as probe for immunodeficiency, virus-induced (AIDS), 511-523
  and pyrogenicity, 226
  radiation, ionizing, 677

Endotoxin (continued)
radio-detoxified, 677-680
see Tolerin
and immunostimulation, 677-680
removal by circulation, extracorporeal, 653-644
in rat, 499-509 **see** Rat
and sepsis, 203
and sites, active, 147-229
and size for
hemodialysis, 685-689
ultrafiltration, 686-689
structure, 1-145
synthesis, 1-145
chemical, 3-11
and thromboplastin, 392-394
and tolerance, 551, 552, 609-611, 645-646
induced, 670
and ultrafiltration, 686-689
uptake, 391-392
Endotoxicity, 102-103
and lipid A, 90-91, 102-103
review, 13-43
Erythrocyte
sensitized, 287-299
agglutination, 287-299
and lipopolysaccharide, 287-299
trinitrophenylated, 102
Escherichia coli (E. coli), 3, 15, 71-78, 83-94, 102, 137-145, 361
and lipid A, 563
in macrophage, 407
and sepsis, 668, 670
strains, source of lipopolysaccharide):
ATCC**25922**, 586, 594, 598, 600, 654
D**31m4**, 336
EH**100**, 429
F**515**, 102, 321, 499-509
J**5**, 258, 336, 341, 429
JE**1001**, 247
K**12**, 142, 247-248, 252, 253, 259, 267
K**235**, 429
Re mutant, 3-4
UKTB, 259-260
WF+, 407-412
no.**487**, 668, 670
O**8**:K**42**, 287, 290, 294, 331-340
O**9**:B**993**, 557
O**111**:B**4**, 34, 103, 199-202, 217, 221, 225, 226, 274, 283, 320-326, 391, 399, 403-406, 429, 446, 447, 457, 458, 468, 474, 477

Escherichia coli (continued)
strains (continued)
O**111**:B**4** (continued), 557, 585-587, 594, 643,644, 646, 648, 653, 693
O**113**, 217, 221, 258, 260, 673
O**119**, 549
O**127**:B**8**, 21, 370, 429, 513
O**128**, 557
O**26**:B**6**, 390, 429
O**55**:B**5**, 149, 217, 221, 235, 467, 589-591, 685
Ethyleneimine, 274
Eyeball antigen in mouse, 558
antibody, 558

Factor C, **see Limulus Polyphemus** amidase activity
Fatty acid determination, 204
Ferritin, 305, 3076
Fibroblast
assay, 29, 30, 564
cell lines, 172-179
gingival, human, 165
murine, 165, 174-177
proliferation assay, 564
sensitized, 332, 335
Fibrosarcoma, methylcholanthrene -induced, 538, 541
Flavobacterium sp., 159
flavolipin, 159
lipoamino acid, 159
Flavolipin, 159
Flow cytometry, 332
Fluorescence anisotropy, 235-237
Foam cell, 396
macrophage is, 396
Friend leukemia virus complex
in mouse, 513-518,
lipopolysaccharide, 513-518
and spleen, 513, 515-517
virus, 528-532

D-Galactosamine, 341, 538, 604-612
Gene **rfb**, bacterial, 141-145
rfe, bacterial, 137-139
Gentamicin, 325, 326
G protein, 373, 381, 475, 478, 479
Gi protein, 369, 372, 373, 475, 478, 479
GLA compound, 19, 21, 23-33, 77, 105-112
analog, 103, 104
D-glucan, 215, 217, 219, 222, 257

Glucosamine, 29, 31, 32, 35, 37, 45
1-6-Glucosamine disaccharide, 53-57
Glucosamine phosphate, acylated 23
β-Glucuronidase, 304, 308, 310
Gold, colloidal-protein technique 199-202
Gram-negative septic syndrome, 635-640
  case histories, two, 636-639
Granulocyte, 287-299, 376, 391, 395, 550
G test, 217, 218, 220
Guanosine monophosphate, cyclic 378-381
  and hormone, 378
Guanylate cyclase, 381, 382
Guinea pig, 26, 537-547

Haemophilus influenzae, 84, 86
  H. sp., 82
Halobacterium halobium, 686-688
  and hemodialysis, 685-689
  H. sp., 685
Hamster kidney cell, 569
Handbook of Endotoxins
  volumes **1984-1986**, 82
Hemagglutination, 288-295
Hemocyanin, 341
Hemocyte of horseshoe crab, 273-285
  anti-lipopolysaccharide factor, 273-285
  and tachyplesin peptide, 273-285
Hemodialysis
  and endotoxin, ultrafiltered, 685-689
  and pyrogenicity, 685
    by bacteria, 685
Hemolymph coagulation, 273
β-Hemolysin, 586
Hemolysis, 260-263, 568-569
  plaque assay, 568-569
Hemoperfusion
  and endotoxin shock, 655-656
Heparin, 700
Hepatitis, alcoholic, 481-482 486, 488, 490-492
Hepatitis A, viral, 481-484
Hepatitis B, viral, 672
Hepatocyte, 199, 201, 504
Heptose, 83
Histocompatibility complex, major (MHC), class II,
and Ia molecule, 427-443
Hormone
  action, 378
  thymic, **see** Timostimolina
Horseshoe crab clotting assay, **see Limulus, Tachypleus**
Host and lipopolysaccharide, 497-701
Hydropathy, 281
Hydroperoxyeicosatetranoic acid, 381
Hydroxyeicosatetranoic acid, 381
3-Hydroxy fatty acid, 203-213
  for lipid A detection, new method, 203-213
13-Hydroxylinoleic acid, 361-368
  and macrophage activation, 361-368
13-Hydroxyoctadecadienoic acid, 361-366
3-Hydroxytetradecanoate, 149, 204, 205, 290-211
Hypersensitivity, delayed, 26, 611-616
  to endotoxin, 604, 611, 616

Ia molecule, 427-443
  and lipopolysaccharide, 427-443
  monoclonal antibody, 429 432, 437
Imidazole, 378
Immune response gene **Ir**, 428
Immunization, subcutaneous
  and histology in mouse, 557-558
Immunoadjuvant, **see** Endotoxin
Immunocyte, 525-534
  and endotoxin, 525-535
  leukemic, 525-535
  normal, 525-535
Immunocytochemistry, 200
Immunodeficiency, 511-523
  virus-induced (AIDS), 511-523
    and endotoxin probe of, 511-523
    virus, human (HIV), 511
Immunodot assay, described, 74
Immunoglobulin A (IgA), 422
  in liver disease, 490-492
Immunopharmacology, 102, 105, 375-376
Immunoprecipitation, 174

Immunoprophylaxis
with monophosphoryl lipid A, 668
Immunoreactivity of lipid A, 91-93
Immunostimulation, 36-38, 525, 665
Immunosuppression by virus, 512,
by retrovirus, murine, 513-518
and tumorigenesis, 513
Immunotherapy, 665-676
with endotoxin, bacterial, 665-676
with lipopolysaccharide, 665-676
tumor regression, 376, 666
see BCG, **Corynebacterium parvum, Propionibacterium acnes**
Indomethacin, 369-374, 473-476, 478, 594
Interferon, 102-104, 108, 161
alpha, 377, 379, 571, 574
anti - antiserum, 571
assay, 102, 594
beta, 403-406, 571, 574
gamma, 377, 467-471, 477, 517-518, 571, 573, 574, 576, 594
induction, 24, 25
by lipopolysaccharide, 597-599
production **in vitro**, 598-599
Interleukin-**1**, 29, 30, 150, 161, 303, 308-311, 347-359, 361-365, 369-374, 377, 379, 517, 531, 532 549-556, 561, 564
assay, 370-371, 527, 569-570
and endotoxin, 369-374
inhibition by pertussis toxin, 371
and indomethacin, 369-374
induction by lipid A, 561-566
and lipid A, 561-566, 569
from macrophage, peritoneal, 347-359
from monocyte, 356
and pertussis toxin, 369-374
production, 370-371
and prostaglandin, 371, 372
Interleukin-1β, human, 413-415
Interleukin-**2**, 377, 379, 381, 573
assay, 570
Involution, lymphoid
and coxsackie virus B, 518-520
Ionomycin, 354
Ir gene, 428
Isopeptide antimicrobial, 269

Japanese horseshoe crab, **see Tachypleus tridentatus**
Jaundice, destructive, 493

Kallikrein-kinin in elderly patients, 630
KDO, **see** 3-Deoxy-D-manno-2-octulosonic acid
2-Keto-3-deoxyoctonic acid synthetic, 15
Keyhole limpet hemocyanin, 341
Klebsiella pneumoniae, 71, 141, 552, 585-587, 599, 612, 616, 693
R-form, 247-255
strain LEN-**111**, 247-255, 321-328
and lipopolysaccharide, 247-255, 320, 557
type-**2**, 538, 542
Komuro-Boyse assay, 378
Kupffer cell, 551
and liver disease, 481-495
dysfunction, 481-495
electron micrograph, 483, 487, 488, 493, 494
endocytosis depressed, 484, 488, 489, 494

LA compound, 19-36, 71, 75-77
analog toxicity, lethal, 20
antibody, 25
as immunoadjuvant, 25-26
Limulus activity, 31-36
mitogenicity, 27, 28
pyrogenicity, 20, 22-24
Schwartzman reaction, 20-22
stimulation of
lymphocyte, 27-28
macrophage, 29-33
monokine, 24
toxicity, lethal, 19-21
α-Lactalbumin, 281, 282
LBP, **see** Lipopolysaccharide -binding peptide
Lectin, 381, **see** separate compounds
Legionella pneumophila, 370-372

Lethality, 19-21, 226, 589-590, 595, 596, 603-619, 657
  and lipopolysaccharide, 589-590, 603-619
  and tumor necrosis factor, 606-608
Leukemia
  cell line K562, 264
  see Friend leukemia
Leukotriene, 364, 381
Lewis lung carcinoma, 612, 614-615
Limulus polyphemus amoebocyte lysate
  activity, 31-36, 277, 278
  assay, 103, 105, 204, 210-211, 215, 391, 481, 482, 549
  factor
    C, 215, 273-280
    G, 216, 222
  gelation inhibition, 257, 260
Lipid IV a, 399-402
Lipid A, 21, 54, 82, 91, 94, 160, 356, 375, 419, 429 445, 457, 470, 474, 499 557, 561-566, 603
  activity, biological, 104, 644-645
  antibody, monoclonal, 71, 73 681-684
  assay, 73-74
  bioreactivity, 33-36
  biosynthesis, 641-644
  biphosphorylated, 562
  of **Chromobacterium violaceum** 15-16, 19
  diamino glucose type (DAG), 57-63
  ELISA, 73-75
  endotoxicity, 90-91, 102-103
    endotoxic shock prevention 681-684
  epitope, 71
    analysis, 74-75, 78
  of **Escherichia coli**, 15-16
    type, synthetic, **see** synthetic
  immunochemistry of, 71-79
  immunodot assay, 74
  as immunostimulator, 36-38, 561-566
  and interleukin-1
    induced, 561-566
    not induced, 369
  monophosphoryl, **see** Monophosphoryl lipid A
Lipid A (continued)
  polymorphism, structural, 89
  precursor, 641-652
  state, physical, 87-90
  structure, 90-94, 641-644
    classical, 45
    and function, 90-94, 645-646
  synthetic, **E. coli** type, 3-43, 87-89, 204, 209, 210 561-566
    analog, 101, 119
    activity, 14-18
    endotoxicity, 13-43
      structural requirement for, 13-43
    procedure described, 3-11
    variant, natural, 45-70
    x-ray diffraction, 89
Lipid A synthetase of **E. coli**, 59
Lipid X (2,3-Diacylglucosamine phosphate), 59, 155, 233, 241, 242, 399-402, 641-648
  and mortality of mouse, 644-647
  and ticarcillin, 646-647
Lipoamino acid, bacterial, 159-162
Lipooxygenase, 361-367
  inhibitor, 393, 395
Lipopolysaccharide (LPS, synonymous with endotoxin) 301-317, 399-402
  as adjuvant in immunization, 557-559
  and antibody, 641
    monoclonal, 331-344
  and anti-LPS factor from amoebocyte, 257-271
  and B-cell activation, 378, 428-514
  binding, 201
    assay, 469
    capacity, 422
    to lymphocyte, murine, 234
    peptide, 257-271, **see** Tachyplesin
    protein, 446, 449-456
      80kDa, 449-450, 456-464
    site, 467-480
  bioactivities, listed, 14
  and blastogenesis, 514
  and calcium, 378
  carbohydrate composition 241
  and cell activation, 149-157
  and chemiluminescence by macrophage, 413-415

Lipopolysaccharide (continued)
chemistry, 82-87
clearance, 500-502
and colony stimulating factor, 377
and complement, 301-317
activation, 376
core, inner, 3, 83-85
oligosaccharides of, 561-566
3-deoxy-D-manno-2-octulosonic acid (KDO), 3-11
detection by fluorescence, 233-245
in model membrane, 233-245
detoxification by polymyxin B fiber, 654
effects, deleterious, 544
electrodialysis, 248
endotoxicity, 81-99
erythrocyte agglutination, 287-299
expression of, 467-480
mechanism for, 467-480
and fatty acids, 504-506
and fever, 377, **see** pyrogenicity
and Friend leukemia complex, 513-518
functions, 81-99, 273, 331 603, 635
and host, 375
response, 497-701
hypersensitivity, 611-616
and immunity, 375-376
as immunoadjuvant, 557-559
and immunocyte, 515
and immunopharmacology, 375-376
as immunostimulant, 539
immunotherapy with, 376, 665-676
and inflammation, 389
interaction
cellular, 345-495
molecular, 231-344
and interleukin-1, 376, 413
KDO moiety, 3-11, 85
lattice structure, 247-250
lethality, 322, 589-590, 603-619
and lipid A, **see** Lipid A
and lipoprotein, high-density 500, 502
localization, immunocytochemical, 199-202
and gold, colloidal, 199-202
and macrophage, 361-368, 379-380, 399-406, 580

Lipopolysaccharide (continued)
and membrane, cytoplasmic, 407-412
mitogenicity, 590
and monocyte, 389-398
in mouse
skin, 557-558
tissue, 558
unresponsive, 347-359
neutralization by antibody, 319-330
and nucleotide, cyclic, 375-387
and O-polysaccharides, 504-506
and plasma cell, 377
and polymyxin B, 321
properties, biological, 57
and protothymocyte, 378
pyrogenicity, 267, 590
receptor on lymphoid cell, 445-466
signaling in macrophage, 467-480
specificity, serological, 81-99
state, physical, 87-90
structure, 81-99, 319, 331
synthetic, 3-11, **see** Lipid
and T-cell, 377, 378, 417-425
tests for, 34-35
and thymocyte, 377-379
toxicity, 81, 539-540
transmembrane signal, 380-382
and tumor necrosis factor, 377, 585-588, 590
Lipoprotein, high-density
and LPS-binding, 500, 502
Listeria monocytogenes, 407, 552, 594, 598, 600, 669
Liver
disease, 228, 481-495
and endotoxin, 481-495
and lipopolysaccharide, 502-505
see Hepatocyte
LPS, **see** Lipopolysaccharide
Lung
Lewis carcinoma, 612, 614-615
and lipopolysaccharide excretion, 506
macrophages, 506
Lymphocyte, 150-157, 417-425
and bacteria, 417-425
see B-cell, T-cell, others
Lymphoid cell, murine
and lipopolysaccharide receptor, 445-466

Lymphokine, 377, 428
Lymphosarcoma, 180
Lysozyme test, 266
and **Micrococcus leisodeikticus**, 266
Lysylendopeptidase, 274-278

MAC, **see** Membrane attack complex
Macrophage, 104, 160, 161, 287 301-317, 332, 378-380, 467-480, 549-556, 569
activating factor, 377
activation, 413-415
by BCG, 342
by 13-hydroxylinoleic acid, 361-368
by lipopolysaccharide, 361 -368, 590
adherence to bacteria, 306
alveolar, 506
and lipopolysaccharide excretion, 506
bacteria-infected, 303, 308 309, 407
BCG-activated, 342
C1g, 301-307
membrane-associated, 301-317
calmodulin, soluble, 349
cell lines, 399-406
chemiluminescence, 413-415
colony stimulating factor, 467
cytotoxicity, 163
electron microscopy, 407-412
as foam cell, 396
functions, 377
and β-glucuronidase, 304
γ-interferon, 377, 467
interleukin-1, 347-359, 467
isolation, 570
and lipopolysaccharide, 306 -311, 377, 379-380, 407 -412, 467-480, 515-516 604-605, 609-610
and signaling in, 467-480
lymphokine, 377
peritoneal, murine, 102, 347 -359, 370-373
preparation, 468
production in mouse, 302
prostaglandin, 303, 467
protein kinase C, 349
mRNA, 348-350, 352, 354, 357
stimulation, 27-33
survival of bacteria within 303, 407, **see** bacteria
Macrophage (continued)
tumor necrosis factor, 399-402, 467
uptake of bacteria, **see** bacteria, Phagocytosis
Magnesium, 247-255
Mannopyranosyl groups
in lipid A, 52-53
D-Mannose, 52
in bacteria, 54
Mastocytoma cell line, 164, 171
Measles and tuberculin anergy, 511
Melanoma vaccine, 671, 673
and remission, 671
Mellitin, 270
Membrane
attack complex (MAC), 301
bacterial, 93-94
cellular, 233-245
cytoplasmic, 407-412
and lipopolysaccharide, 407-412
and macrophage stimulation 407-412
Met-enkephalin, 421
Meth A fibrosarcoma, 111-116
antitumor assay, 111-116
healing in mouse, 26
Methylchloranthrene
and fibrosarcoma, 538, 541
Methyl-3-O-(9-carboxy anthracenyl)tetradecanoate (CAT), 205-209
MHC, **see** Histocompatibility complex, major
Micrococcus leisodeikticus, 266
Migration inhibitory factor, 377
Mitogenicity, 104-106, 590, 667, 669
Monocyte, 302, 356, 389-398, 418
and lipopolysaccharide, 389-398
Monokine, **see** Interferon, Tumor necrosis factor
Monophosphoryl lipid A, 233, 242, 567-579, 666-676
and ovarian tumor, murine, 666-669
Morganella sp., 46
Mouse
adrenalectomized, 538
athymic, nude, 27
bone marrow cell, 287
cell lines, 149-157
cyclophosphamide-treated 585-587

Mouse (continued)
endotoxin-resistant strains 550, 551, 604-610
D-galactosamine primed, 19-22, 109, 226, 604-611
infected, experimentally, 109-111, 585
irradiation, 550
lethality, 55-553
meth A fibrosarcoma healing 26
and **Mycobacterium tuberculosis** BCG strain, 24
myeloma cell line, 455
necrosis of tumor, 26
nude, thymic, 27
ovarian tumor model, 666-669
and cancer cure, 666-669
and **Propionibacterium acnes** 24, 25, 102, 667
pyrogenicity, 102, 104
radioprotection, 552-553
Schwartzman reaction, 102, 104
septicemia, induced, 550, 552
skin histology, 557-559
strains:
BALB/c, 379, 413, 447, 526-533, 537-547, 568-576, 681
BDF-1, 370-373
C3H/HeJ, 347-359, 370-373, 379, 418-420, 549-559, 613
C3H/HeSlc, 467
C3H/He, 347-359
C3H/HeN, 604-606, 610
C3H/Tif, 616
C3HeB/FeJ, 446, 448
C3H (normal), 445-446, 572
C57Bl/6, 379, 589-591, 613-616
C57Bl/6xDBA/2 (hybrid) 593-601
C57BL/6, 102, 104
C57BL/10, 585-588
MRL, 413, 415
NMRI, 614
tolerance, 609-611
tumor necrosis, 26
Mucin, gastric, 697
Murabutide, 539, 540, 544
Muramyl peptide, 413, 531 537-547, 612-613
and endotoxin synergism, 537-547
hypersensitivity, 612-613
sensitization, 612-613
Mycobacterium tuberculosis, 399-402, 342, 429
see Bacillus Calmette Guérin
Mycoplasma pneumoniae, 301
Myoglobin, 275

Naja naja kaouthia (cobra) venom, 391
Neisseria gonorrhoeae, 82, 86
Neoplasm, lymphoid, induced, 164 172, 173
Neuraminidase, 420
Neuropeptide, 420-421
Neutropenia, 585, 587
Nitrobacter sp., 45
Nordihydroguaiaretic acid, 393, 395
Nucleotide, cyclic, 375-387
and lipopolysaccharide, 375-387

O-antigen, **see** Lipopolysaccharide
O-specific chain, 82
Ovarian tumor model in mouse 666-669
cured by
mitomycin C, 667
monophosphoryl lipid A, 667
Propionibacterium acnes pyridine extract, 667
tumor-associated antigen, 668
3-Oxomyristic acid, 50
in bacteria, 51
Oxygen intermediate, reactive (ROI), 403-406

Paracoccus denitrificans, 62
Peptide
lipopolysaccharide-binding (LBP), 257-271
from Japanese horseshoe crab, 257-271
see Tachyplesin I
Perchloric acid
and human plasma, 225-229
Peritonitis, bacterial, 593
Pertussis toxin, 369-374, 475-476
and interleukin-1, 369-374
Pertussis vaccine, 543
Phagocyte, mononuclear, 413
Phagocytosis, 102, 104, 301, 306, 308, 361, 364, 365, 417, 422
assay, 303
Phagolysosome, 301, 409
Phagosome, 409, 411

Phenylobacterium immobile, 57-59
Phorbol myristate acetate, 381
Phosphatidylcholine vesicle, 233
Phosphoinositidase, 373
Phosphatidylinositol, 372, 373, 381
Phosphatidylinositol 4, 5-bisphosphate, 356
Phosphodiesterase, 353
Phosphoinositidase, 373
Phospholipase
  A-2, 381, 390, 393
  C, 369, 372, 381, 382, 390
    inhibitor, 393-394
Phospholipid, 235, 381
4-O-Phosphono-D-glucosamine, 103, 107-109
Phosphorylation, 104, 105
Photoaffinity lipopolysaccharide probe, 446-447
Phytohemagglutinin (PHA), 29, 303, 309, 377, 378, 594, 598
Plaque assay, hemolytic, 568-569
Plaque-forming cell, reverse assay, 430
Plaque reduction method, 102
Plasma, human, 225-229, 377
  and perchloric acid, 225-229
Platelet, 390, 391, 396
Plesiomonas shigelloides, 71
Pneumococcus vaccine, 671
Pneumocyte type II, 199, 201
Polymyxin B, 121-126, 152, 153, 293, 297, 321-323 326, 335, 364, 379, 471 653-662
Porin, 185-187, 419
  isolation, 186
Precipitation in gel, 259-260 267, 269
  double diffusion, 259-260
Pronase, 474, 477
Propionibacterium acnes, 24, 25, 26, 102, 590, 606, 666
  -pyridine extract for tumor therapy, 667
Prostacyclin, 381
Prostaglandin
  E1, 372, 373, 378, 379
  E2, 29, 161, 303, 308, 310, 312, 478
Protein
  bacterial, 612
    sensitization, 613-614
  cationic, 287-288
  endotoxin-associated, 149-150
Protein (continued)
  gold, colloidal, technique 199-202
  of lipopolysaccharide, 80kDa 449-450, 456-461
    antiserum, 459-464
    binding to, 293, 295
Protein kinase, 378
  A, 372
  C, 278, 349, 352, 353, 372, 380-382
Proteus mirabilis, 121-130, 636
  P. vulgaris, 127-130
Protothymocyte, 378
Providencia rettgeri, 49
  P. sp., 46
Pseudomonas aeruginosa, 109, 110, 217, 221, 259 267, 337, 537, 552 636, 693
  strain 18S, 320-328
  P. diminuta, 57-60, 71, 72, 75-78
  P. fluorescens, 131-135
  P. sp., 86
  P. vesicularis, 72, 75-78
Purple bacteria dendogram, 63
Pyelonephritis, 636
Pyrogen, 377
Pyrogenicity, 22-24, 102, 104, 226, 268, 250, 645, 655, 685
Pyrogen test, 259, 267

Rabbit, 21, 540
Radiation, ionizing, 677-678
Radiodetoxification of endotoxin, **see** Tolerin
Radioimmunoassay (RIA), 31
Radioprotection, 552-553
Raji cell assay, 481, 484
Rat, 199, 407-412, 499-509
  and endotoxin, 499-509
  fed alcohol chronically, 488-489
  and macrophage, peritoneal, 407-412
Receptor for lipopolysaccharide on lymphoid cell, 445-466
Red blood cell hemolysis, 258-261
Resistance of patient, non-specific, 677-680
Retrovirus, murine, 513-518
  and immunosuppression, 513-518
Rhodobacter capsulatus, 45, 53-56, 60, 61
  R. sphaeroides, 45, 50, 54, 55, 60, 61

Rhodobacter sp., 52
Rhodocyclus gelatinosus, 60
  R. purpureus, 46
  R. tenuis, 46, 53
Rhodomicrobium vannielii, 52-54
Rhodopseudomonas blastica, 62
  R. palustris, 59, 60 87
  R. sphaeroides, 87
  R. viridis, 58-60, 87
RNA, 348
  messenger(mRNA), 350, 352, 354, 357

Salmonella abortus-equi, 22, 204, 210, 217, 221, 361, 499-509, 613
  S. enteritidis, 217, 221, 538, 557
S. minnesota, 15, 16, 19,71-78, 83, 87, 90, 258-260, 264, 267, 331-344 418-425, 429, 457, 613
  strain R595(Re), 150-155 204, 210, 235, 259, 260, 264, 267, 283, 287, 290-292, 307-312 319-330, 418-425, 429 563, 568, 645, 681
S. sp., 46, 50, 53-55, 83,94
S. typhimurium, 37, 38, 137, 144, 149, 217, 221,233 235, 238, 242, 258,264 265, 267, 283, 287 290-294, 302, 308, 348 418-425, 429, 612, 615 616, 643, 691-701
S. typhosa(S. typhi), 150, 151, 154, 155, 217 221, 417, 557, 581-583
Salmonellosis, 581-583
  in Bari, Italy, 418
  see Typhoid patient
Sarcoma EMT-6, 612-615
Sarcophaga peregrina, 283
Sarcotoxin, 283
  of flesh fly, 270
Schwartzman reaction, 20-22, 102, 104
Scorpion toxin, 283
Sepsis,bacterial, 203, 375, 668
Septicemia,human, 389, 550 552, 635-640
Serratia marcescens, 164-181 217, 221, 429, 525
Serum,bactericidal, 301,302 305
Sheep mortality after
  endotoxin challenge, 646
Shigella flexneri, 217, 221
  S. dysenteriae, 144
Shigella sonnei, 125
Shock
  lethal, 544
  Septic, 228, 319, 636-639, 641
    in the elderly, 621-633
    treatment,new, 653-664
  toxic, syndrome
    and **Staphylococcus**, 685
Simian virus-40(SV40), 174-179
Spleen cell, 568, 569, 574 575, 594-598, 600
  and lipopolysaccharide, 597-600
  T-cell depleted, 430-432
Splenocyte, murine, 27, 447-450, 459, 526-532,597
Staphylococcus aureus, 259, 267,407, 636, 686-688
  S. cohnii, 686-688
  S. epidermidis, 228, 259, 267, 648
Streptococcus milleri, 636
  S. pneumoniae, 594, 598, 600
  S. pyogenes, 181
Superoxide anion, 29, 32

Tachyplesin peptide, 273-285
  in hemocyte of horseshoe crab 273-285
    assay, 274
    isolation, 277
    purification, 274
    structure, 257-285
      and function, 258, 273 -285
  see Tachypleus tridentatus
  see Japanese horseshoe crab
Tachypleus tridentatus, 273, 280
  anti-lipopolysaccharide factor, 273-285
T-cell, 155, 377-379, 417-425, 428, 451, 569, 571, 573, 575, 576
  and lipopolysaccharide, 377 -379, 417-425, 451
Tetraacetyl-KDO-glucosamine-4-phosphate,synthetic, 15
Theophylline, 378
Thiobacillus versutus, 62
  T. sp., 45
Thromboplastin, 389-397
  synthesis, 392-397
Thomboxan, 381
Thymidine,radioactive
  uptake, 27, 149-155, 371

Thymocyte, 29, 30, 303,377-379, 527
assay, 303
and lipopolysaccharide,377-379
Ticarcillin, 646-647
and lipid X, 646-647
Timostimolina(thymic hormone), 420
Tissue factor, **see** Thromboplastin
Tissue thromboplastin, 287, 288
Tolerance of mouse, 551, 552, 609-611, 645-646, 670
Tolerin, 677-680
is lipopolysaccharide radio-detoxified, 677-680
functions,beneficial, 677-678
immunostimulation, 677-680
Toxic shock syndrome by **Staphylococcus**, 685
Toxicolor assay, 217-222, 347
Toxin,bacterial,mixed(MBT), 180-181
described in **1895**, 180
and lymphosarcoma, 180
Transmembrane signal, 380-382
Trehalose dimycolate, 668, 669, 672
Tuberculin, 153
anergy in measles, 511
Tuftsin, 379
Tumor
antigen associated with(TAA), 668, 669
assay, 538
cytotoxicity - , 469
cytotoxicity, 470, 475, 476
assay, 469
and endotoxin, 376
immunotherapy, 376, 666
growing, 612-616
and sensitization of mouse, 614-615
model:ovarian tumor in mouse 666-669
necrosis, 541, 545
necrosis factor **see** Tumor necrosis factor
regression, 666
Tumor necrosis factor, 60, 102-106, 160, 332, 335, 336, 377, 399-406, 467, 477-479, 538-545, 549-550, 604, 606, 607, 611, 612, 636-639
assay, 102, 469
and lipopolysaccharide, 377, 399-402,585-588, 590, 606-608
Tumorigenesis
and immunosuppression, 513
Typhoid patient, 581-583
immune system, 581-583
Typhoid vaccine, 543

Vaccinia virus, 110-113
Vasomine, 545
Vesicle, 233-238
Vesicular stomatitis virus, 102, 595
Vibrio anguillarum, 50
V. cholerae, 84
Hakata, 189-197
0-1, 189-197
type Inaba, 189
type Ogawa, 189
V. fluvialis, 189-197
V. non-cholera, 189-197
V. parahaemolyticus, 84
V. sp.,189-197
and lipopolysaccharide, 189-197
Virus-induced immunodeficiency 511-523
and AIDS, 511
see Immunosuppression

Weissbach's reaction-positive substance of **Vibrio** sp. 191
Wheat germ agglutinin, 32

Xenopus frog skin,antimicrobial, 270
Xanthomonas sp., 86

Yersinia enterocolitica, 50
Y. pseudotuberculosis, 185-187
Y. sp., 46

Zymosan 361-363

GPSR Compliance
The European Union's (EU) General Product Safety Regulation (GPSR) is a set of rules that requires consumer products to be safe and our obligations to ensure this.

If you have any concerns about our products, you can contact us on

ProductSafety@springernature.com

In case Publisher is established outside the EU, the EU authorized representative is:

Springer Nature Customer Service Center GmbH
Europaplatz 3
69115 Heidelberg, Germany

www.ingramcontent.com/pod-product-compliance
Ingram Content Group UK Ltd.
Pitfield, Milton Keynes, MK11 3LW, UK
UKHW051132260726
13967UKWH00010B/2995

* 9 7 8 1 4 7 5 7 5 1 4 1 3 *